Molecular Targeted Therapy for Alzheimer's Disease

Edited by

Swarupananda Mukherjee
Department of Pharmaceutical Technology
NSHM Knowledge Campus – Kolkata Group of Institutions
Kolkata, West Bengal
India

Souvik Roy
Department of Pharmaceutical Technology
NSHM Knowledge Campus – Kolkata Group of Institutions
Kolkata, West Bengal
India

&

Dipanjan Karati
Department of Pharmaceutical Technology
School of Pharmacy
Techno India University
West Bengal, Kolkata
India

Molecular Targeted Therapy for Alzheimer's Disease

Editors: Swarupananda Mukherjee, Souvik Roy & Dipanjan Karati

ISBN (Online): 979-8-89881-564-6

ISBN (Print): 979-8-89881-565-3

ISBN (Paperback): 979-8-89881-566-0

First published in 2026.

need for a court order if at any point you breach any terms of this License Agreement. In no event will any delay or failure by Bentham Science Publishers in enforcing your compliance with this License Agreement constitute a waiver of any of its rights.

3. You acknowledge that you have read this License Agreement, and agree to be bound by its terms and conditions. To the extent that any other terms and conditions presented on any website of Bentham Science Publishers conflict with, or are inconsistent with, the terms and conditions set out in this License Agreement, you acknowledge that the terms and conditions set out in this License Agreement shall prevail.

Bentham Science Publishers Pte. Ltd.
No. 9 Raffles Place
Office No. 26-01
Singapore 048619
Singapore
Email: subscriptions@benthamscience.net

BENTHAM SCIENCE

CONTENTS

FOREWORD

Alzheimer's disease continues to challenge scientists, clinicians, and caregivers alike as one of the most complex and devastating neurodegenerative disorders of our time. Despite decades of research, effective long-term treatments remain elusive. However, recent advances in molecular biology, pharmacology, and neuroimmunology have begun to reshape our understanding of the disease's underlying mechanisms, offering hope for new and more effective therapeutic strategies.

This timely and compelling book, "Molecular Targeted Therapy for Alzheimer's Disease," provides a comprehensive and forward-looking exploration into the evolving landscape of Alzheimer's research. It brings together emerging perspectives on the pathophysiology of the disease, highlighting innovative molecular targets, cutting-edge drug development, and integrative therapeutic approaches that extend beyond the traditional amyloid- and tau-focused paradigms.

The chapters, authored by experts in the field, offer readers a deep dive into critical areas such as neuroinflammation, mitochondrial dysfunction, axl kinase disregulation, tau protein hyperphosphorylation, miRNA, and biopolymer-based therapeutic approaches. This book not only elucidates the science behind these developments but also discusses the translational challenges and future directions necessary to bridge laboratory findings with clinical practice.

Whether you are a researcher, clinician, student, or stakeholder in neurodegenerative disease care and policy, this book serves as an invaluable resource. It encourages a multidisciplinary approach and fosters a renewed sense of urgency and innovation in tackling one of the most pressing public health concerns of the 21st century.

In a field that is rapidly evolving, "Molecular Targeted Therapy for Alzheimer's Disease" stands as a testament to the resilience and ingenuity of the scientific community. It is with great admiration and hope that I commend this work to all readers who are committed to making a difference in the battle against Alzheimer's disease.

Debasis Bagchi
Department of Pharmaceutical Sciences
Texas Southern University
Houston, Texas, USA

PREFACE

Due to the loss of mental faculties, millions of individuals worldwide are deprived of their right to cognitive freedom by Alzheimer's disease (AD), a neurodegenerative illness of exceptional magnitude. Despite significant advances in understanding and devising therapeutic management, existing medications give only limited symptom relief and fail to arrest or reverse the process of the disease. The glaring treatment barriers prompted scientists to focus on the molecular basis of Alzheimer's, leading to the development of more accurate and possibly revolutionary approaches to treatment.

Its central goal of Molecular Targeted Therapy for Alzheimer's Disease is to provide a thorough analysis of innovative methods of research in order to analyse and intervene into key molecular pathways of AD. The book covers a great number of key areas such as the role of amyloid-beta and tau proteins, neuroinflammation, oxidative stress, and synaptic dysfunction.

This book aims to assist researchers, clinicians, graduate students, and healthcare specialists who participate in the study of Alzheimer's disease, which is characterized by numerous complex mechanisms. Suggesting a comprehensive review of molecular targets and associated possibilities for therapy, we enable new directions for further research and interdisciplinary collaboration in the treatment of this difficult disorder.

To all those who contributed detailed knowledge and devoted their labor to this volume, we offer our heartfelt thanks. We hope that this compilation will become an indispensable guide, an inspiration for future improvement and development in new therapeutics aiming at a molecular-level treatment for Alzheimer's disease.

Sincerely,

Swarupananda Mukherjee
Department of Pharmaceutical Technology
NSHM Knowledge Campus – Kolkata Group of Institutions
Kolkata, West Bengal
India

Souvik Roy
Department of Pharmaceutical Technology
NSHM Knowledge Campus – Kolkata Group of Institutions
Kolkata, West Bengal
India

&

Dipanjan Karati
Department of Pharmaceutical Technology
School of Pharmacy
Techno India University
West Bengal, Kolkata
India

List of Contributors

Abhishek Jana	Department of Pharmaceutical Technology, JIS Institute of Pharmacy, Kalyani, West Bengal, India
Amima Arshad	Department of Pharmacy, NSHM Knowledge Campus Kolkata – Group of Institutions, Kolkata, West Bengal, India
Ankita Parui	Department of Pharmacy, NSHM Knowledge Campus Kolkata – Group of Institutions, Kolkata, West Bengal, India
Asmita Nag Sarkar	Department of Pharmacy, NSHM Knowledge Campus Kolkata – Group of Institutions, Kolkata, West Bengal, India
Arvind Kumar	Department of Pharmaceutical Technology, NSHM Knowledge Campus Kolkata – Group of Institutions, Kolkata, West Bengal, India
Biplab Debnath	Department of Pharmaceutical Technology, Bharat Technology, Uluberia, West Bengal, India
Biswajit Basu	Department of Pharmaceutical Technology, Adamas University, Kolkata, West Bengal, India
Bramhajit Chatterjee	Department of Pharmaceutical Technology, Brainware University, Kolkata, West Bengal, India
Chowdhury Mobaswar Hossain	Department of Pharmaceutical Technology, Maulana Abul Kalam Azad University of Technology, Haringhata, West Bengal, India
Debankini Dasgupta	Department of Pharmaceutical Technology, MGM College of Pharmacy, Patna, Bihar, India
Dipanjan Karati	Department of Pharmaceutical Technology, School of Pharmacy, Techno India University, Kolkata, West Bengal, India
Dishani Sukul	Department of Pharmaceutical Technology, Maulana Abul Kalam Azad University of Technology, Haringhata, West Bengal, India
Maitreyee Mukherjee	Department of Pharmaceutical Technology, NSHM Knowledge Campus Kolkata – Group of Institutions, Kolkata, West Bengal, India
Md Alfaj Uddin	Department of Pharmaceutical Technology, Maulana Abul Kalam Azad University of Technology, Haringhata, West Bengal, India
Monosiz Rahaman	Department of Pharmaceutical Technology, Adamas University, Kolkata, West Bengal, India
Moumita Kundu	Department of Pharmaceutical Technology, JIS University, Kolkata, West Bengal, India Department of Pharmacology, Anand College of Pharmacy, Midnapore, West Bengal, India
Nipa Roy	Department of Pharmacy, NSHM Knowledge Campus Kolkata – Group of Institutions, Kolkata, West Bengal, India
Nilanjan Sarkar	Department of Pharmaceutical Technology, NSHM Knowledge Campus Kolkata – Group of Institutions, Kolkata, West Bengal, India

Nilanjan Pahari	Department of Pharmaceutical Technology, Calcutta Institute of Pharmaceutical Technology and Allied Health Sciences, Uluberia, West Bengal, India
Piyali Khamkat	Department of Pharmaceutical Technology, Brainware University, Kolkata, West Bengal, India
Poulomi Sen	Department of Pharmaceutical Technology, NSHM Knowledge Campus Kolkata – Group of Institutions, Kolkata, West Bengal, India
Priyanka Banerjee	Department of Pharmaceutical Technology, Adamas University, Kolkata, West Bengal, India
Puneet Samaiya	Department of Pharmacy, Shri G.S. Institute of Technology and Science, Indore, Madhya Pradesh, India
Rajdip Goswami	Department of Pharmaceutical Technology, Adamas University, Kolkata, West Bengal, India
Rudradeep Hazra	Department of Pharmacy, NSHM Knowledge Campus Kolkata – Group of Institutions, Kolkata, West Bengal, India
Saheli Naskar	Department of Pharmaceutical Technology, NSHM Knowledge Campus Kolkata – Group of Institutions, Kolkata, West Bengal, India
Sajal Kumar Jha	Department of Pharmaceutical Technology, Adamas University, Kolkata, West Bengal, India
Sairam Krishnamurthy	Department of Pharmaceutical Engineering and Technology, Indian Institute of Technology (Banaras Hindu University), Varanasi, Uttar Pradesh, India
Sakuntala Gayen	Department of Pharmacy, NSHM Knowledge Campus Kolkata – Group of Institutions, Kolkata, West Bengal, India
Saptarshi Sanyal	Department of Pharmaceutical Technology, Adamas University, Kolkata, West Bengal, India
Santosh Kumar Prajapati	Department of Pharmaceutical Engineering and Technology, Indian Institute of Technology (Banaras Hindu University), Varanasi, Uttar Pradesh, India Department of Neurosurgery and Brain Repair, University of South Florida, Tampa, Florida, USA
Shreyasi Meur	Department of Pharmaceutical Technology, NSHM Knowledge Campus Kolkata – Group of Institutions, Kolkata, West Bengal, India
Shreyasi Majumdar	Department of Pharmaceutical Engineering and Technology, Indian Institute of Technology (Banaras Hindu University), Varanasi, Uttar Pradesh, India Department of Pharmaceutical Technology, Adamas University, Kolkata, West Bengal, India
Sinjini Sarkar	Department of Pharmaceutical Technology, SVKM's Narsee Monjee Institute of Management Studies, Mumbai, Maharashtra, India
Siuli Sen	Department of Pharmaceutical Technology, School of Pharmacy, Techno India University, Kolkata, West Bengal, India
Soumen Dhara	Department of Pharmaceutical Technology, NSHM Knowledge Campus Kolkata – Group of Institutions, Kolkata, West Bengal, India
Soumyadeep Chatterjee	Department of Pharmacy, NSHM Knowledge Campus Kolkata – Group of Institutions, Kolkata, West Bengal, India

Souvik Roy	Department of Pharmacy, NSHM Knowledge Campus Kolkata – Group of Institutions, Kolkata, West Bengal, India
Swagata Bhattacharya	Department of Pharmaceutical Engineering and Technology, Indian Institute of Technology (Banaras Hindu University), Varanasi, Uttar Pradesh, India
Swarupananda Mukherjee	Department of Pharmaceutical Technology, NSHM Knowledge Campus Kolkata – Group of Institutions, Kolkata, West Bengal, India
Suman Sahu	Department of Pharmacognosy, Bharat Technology, Uluberia, West Bengal, India
Tanwi Garai	Department of Pharmaceutical Technology, School of Pharmacy, Techno India University, Kolkata, West Bengal, India
Tathagata Roy	Department of Pharmaceutical Technology, NSHM Knowledge Campus Kolkata – Group of Institutions, Kolkata, West Bengal, India
Tiyas Pal	Department of Pharmaceutical Technology, NSHM Knowledge Campus Kolkata – Group of Institutions, Kolkata, West Bengal, India
Vishal Singh	Department of Pharmaceutical Technology, Exemed Pharmaceuticals, Vadodara, Gujarat, India
Vivek Barik	Department of Pharmaceutical Technology, Brainware University, Kolkata, West Bengal, India

CHAPTER 1

Unveiling the Role of Glutamate and NMDA Receptors in Alzheimer's Disease

Dipanjan Karati[1,*], **Shreyasi Meur**[2], **Poulomi Sen**[2], **Swarupananda Mukherjee**[2] and **Priya Ghosh**[2]

[1] *Department of Pharmaceutical Technology, School of Pharmacy, Techno India University, Kolkata, West Bengal, India*

[2] *Department of Pharmaceutical Technology, NSHM Knowledge Campus, Kolkata - Group of Institutions, Kolkata, West Bengal, India*

Abstract: Alzheimer's disease (AD) is a neurological condition that affects people as they age. Clinically, this illness is typified by changes in behavior, personality, and overall cognitive impairment, including memory loss. The hippocampus and neocortex, two delicate brain regions involved in memory and cognition, have been linked to a progressive decline in form and function as AD progresses. N-methyl-D-aspartate receptor (NMDAR)-mediated excitatory glutamatergic neurotransmission is essential for neuron survival and synaptic plasticity. However, increased NMDAR activity leads to cell death and excitotoxicity, which may be the mechanism behind the neurodegeneration that occurs in AD. Research suggests that regionalized receptor activity, followed by diverse downstream signaling pathways, is responsible for the various NMDAR-mediated responses. Synaptic NMDAR activation promotes cell survival and initiates plasticity. On the other hand, memantine, an AD medication that specifically inhibits the activity of extrasynaptic NMDARs, can prevent the activation of extrasynaptic NMDARs, which causes cell death and hence contributes to the etiology of AD. This chapter aims to outline the role of glutamate and NMDA receptors in AD.

Keywords: Alzheimer's disease, Glutamate, Memantine, N-methyl-D-aspartate receptor (NMDAR), Neurodegeneration.

INTRODUCTION

Named after the German psychiatrist Alois Alzheimer, Alzheimer's disease (AD) is the most prevalent form of dementia. Neuritic plaques and neurofibrillary tangles are the hallmarks of this condition, which is brought on by the build-up of

* **Corresponding author Dipanjan Karati:** Department of Pharmaceutical Technology, School of Pharmacy, Techno India University, Kolkata, West Bengal, India; E-mail: karatibabai@gmail.com

amyloid-beta peptide (Aβ) in the brain's most affected regions, the medial temporal lobe and neocortical structures [1]. As AD progresses, these brain areas undergo significant degeneration, leading to the cognitive and functional impairments associated with the disease. AD shows results in abnormalities in the pulmonary and circulatory systems, low oxygen levels in the blood, vitamin B12 insufficiency, nutritional deficits, and others, which lead to a progressive loss of cognitive functions [2, 3]. The AD is predicted to impact 131.5 million people by 2050 if no new treatments are found [4].

The development of AD has been attributed to cholinergic deficiency [5], tau protein hyperphosphorylation [6], amyloid beta (Aβ) toxicity [7], synaptic dysfunction [8], oxidative stress [9, 10], and neuroinflammation [11]. Synapse loss was found to have a substantial correlation with cognitive impairment in AD when compared to other biochemical measures, such as senile plaques and neurofibrillary tangles (NFTs) [12]. By 2050, there will be 12.7 million people in the US living with AD dementia, up from the present 6.2 million. Apart from persons with AD in the advanced stages of dementia, around 10 million Americans suffer from moderate cognitive impairment (MCI), with 5 million of them having MCI as a result of AD. There are 11.2 million people in the US who have MCI from AD and AD dementia, which are symptomatic manifestations of the disease [13]. $355 billion was projected to be spent on Alzheimer's disease and related dementias (ADRD) care in 2021. By 2050, the number of people affected by AD dementia worldwide will triple from 50 to 150 million, with the majority residing in low- and middle-income nations [14]. AD is categorized as: (i) late-onset AD (LOAD) or sporadic, and (ii) early-onset AD (EOAD) or familial [15]. Their pathophysiologies are remarkably similar [16, 17]. Approximately 5–6% of AD patients have an early-onset disease (EOAD) before the age of 65 [18], and a significant proportion of these patients show severe language or visuospatial deficits. Significant non-cognitive neuropsychiatric symptoms (NPS) (apathy, sadness, anxiety, agitation, violence, and psychosis) are also brought on by AD, regardless of the age at which symptoms first appear [19, 20].

Neurotransmission is the process by which a signal is sent from one neuron to another using endogenous signalling chemicals called neurotransmitters [21]. After being released from the axon terminal of a neuron, neurotransmitters cross the synaptic cleft and bind to receptors on the dendrites of another neuron, then convert those receptors into electrical impulses. The tripartite structure of the synapse, or neuronal junction, is composed of presynaptic and postsynaptic nerve terminals as well as the intimate association of glial cells [22]. Through a feedback mechanism, glial cells—particularly astrocytes—play a significant role in controlling neurotransmission [22]. Signals are transmitted between neurons by neurotransmitters binding to certain postsynaptic receptors [21]. Postsynaptic receptors are characterized as ionotropic receptors, which function as ligand-gated channels, and metabotropic receptors, which act by signal transduction [23]. There are various types of neurotransmitters, such as cholinergic and monoaminergic neurotransmitters. Critical cholinergic neurotransmitters in AD pathogenesis include acetylcholine (ACh) and gamma-aminobutyric acid (GABA), while critical monoaminergic neurotransmitters include histamine, dopamine (DA), and serotonin (5-HT) [24, 25]. Neurotransmitter inhibitors, including acetylcholinesterase inhibitors (AChEI) donepezil, rivastigmine, memantine, and galantamine, have a well-established treatment promise in AD [23]. As AD progresses, pathological alterations include reduced GABA levels, monoaminergic neuron loss, glutamatergic neuron dysfunction, and cholinergic neuron loss. Dopaminergic and 5-hydroxytryptaminergic monoaminergic neurons are subtypes of monoaminergic neurons. Neurotransmitters send messages to the following neuron by binding to postsynaptic membrane receptors [26]. Neuronal dysfunction can be brought on by modifications to the synthesis, storage, transport, and breakdown of neurotransmitters, which can lead to AD-related dementia (Fig. **1**).

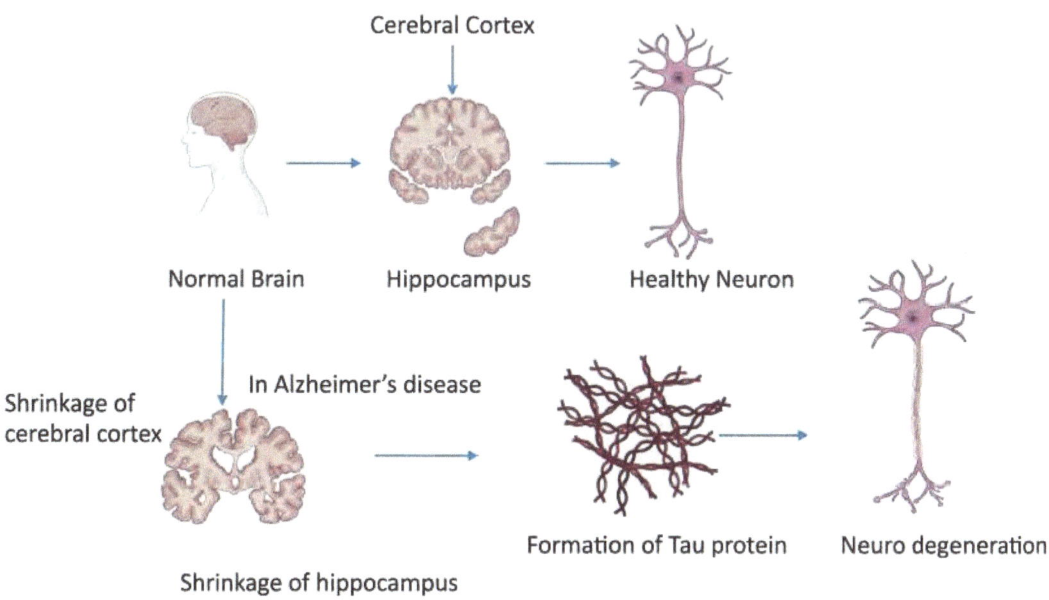

Fig. (1). Neuronal physiology in healthy brains versus brains with AD.

GLUTAMATE NEUROTRANSMISSION

The Fundamentals of Glutamate as a Neurotransmitter

Glutamate, an excitatory neurotransmitter that does not pass through the blood-brain barrier, is dispersed throughout the central nervous system (CNS) and plays a vital role in brain activities. Neurons and glial cells synthesize glutamate by using glucose and α-ketoglutarate as precursors [27]. In the resting condition of the synaptic cleft, the concentration of glutamate is approximately 0.6 μM [28], and during presynaptic neuronal depolarization, it rises to above 10 μM [29]. Glutamate is released into synapses by presynaptic neurons, where it is absorbed and causes glutamatergic receptors to become active. Following receptor activation, astrocytes utilize their excitatory amino acid transporters (EAAT) 1 and 2 to absorb the excess glutamate. Glutamate is transformed into glutamine in glial cells in the presence of the glutamine synthase enzyme [30]. Through the activity of phosphate-activated glutaminase (PAG), presynaptic neurons transform glutamine into glutamate [31]. In the presence of vesicular glutamate transporters (VGLUT1/2), glutamate is transferred into synaptic vesicles. This entire glutamate/glutamine cycle is depicted in the figure below and was discovered in the 1970s [32, 33].

The development of learning, memory, spine maturation, circuit development, and synaptic plasticity are just a few of the cognitive and neurological processes wherein glutamate receptors are involved [34]. Although glutamate plays a vital role in a healthy central nervous system (CNS), high glutamate levels or hyperactivity of glutamatergic nerve terminals can cause neuronal injury and may even play a role in neurodegenerative diseases [35, 36]. Metabotropic glutamate receptors (mGluRs) and ionotropic glutamate receptors (iGluRs) are the two subtypes of these receptors. Synaptic transmissions throughout the central nervous system are guided by the non-selective ion channels known as iGluRs, which are activated by glutamate [37]. Based on their ability to bind ligands, these channels are classified as delta receptors, kainate, N-methyl-D-aspartate (NMDA), 2-amino-3(3-hydroxy-5-methylisoxazol-4-yl) propionate (AMPA), or kainate [38]. On the other hand, ion channel proteins are modified by the mGluRs through the action of a second messenger and metabolic cascades [39]. Based on their structure and function, the eight different types of mGluRs (mGluR1–mGluR8) are divided into three groups.

Glutamate's Function in the Brain and Nervous System

Alzheimer's disease occurrence and progression are strongly correlated with glutamate's excitatory neurotoxicity. Nevertheless, mounting data indicate that glutamate has a dual role in the onset of Alzheimer's disease, contributing to its excitotoxicity as a neurotransmitter and its disruption of metabolic homeostasis. The balance of glutamate metabolism in the brain, which is primarily governed by glutamate intake, glutamate circulation, intracellular mitochondrial transport, and mitochondrial metabolism, is one of the major factors affecting the health of the central nervous system [40]. The postsynaptic neurons' membrane potential is raised by glutamate released into the synaptic cleft, increasing the likelihood that they will produce an action potential. It is also essential for long-term potentiation [41], synaptic plasticity [42], learning and memory [43], and a number of other cognitive processes [44]. In addition to serving as an energy substrate for oxidative metabolism and contributing to glutathione's antioxidant qualities, glutamate regulates the formation and maturation of synapses. Glutamate is a precursor to the production of GABA, which is an inhibitory neurotransmitter and a building block for the synthesis of non-ribosomal peptides [45]. Moreover, glutamate regulates brain progenitor cell migration, proliferation, differentiation, and survival [46].

REGULATION OF GLUTAMATE RELEASE AND UPTAKE

Glutamate Uptake

An essential component of CNS activity is the uptake and recycling of astrocyte glutamate. Excitatory amino acid transporters 1 and 2 (EAAT1 and EAAT2), two astrocytic glutamate transporters that account for the majority of glutamate absorption, are essential components of this apparatus. The solute carrier 1A family of transporters (SLC1A) includes the astrocytic glutamate transporters EAAT1 and EAAT2, as well as the two alanine serine cysteine transporters, ACST1 and ACST2, and the five excitatory amino acid transporters, EAAT1–5 [47]. Using ion concentration gradients of its co- and counter-transported ions (Na+, H+, and K+), the electrogenic secondary-active transporters, or EAATs, accelerate glutamate transport against its concentration gradient into the cell [48]. Astrocytes are able to manage any fluxes caused by this transport process because of their highly expressed membrane K+ channels (especially KIR4.1), Na+/H+ exchangers, and Na+/NCO3− cotransporters. They can also adjust pH and membrane potential [49]. It is very true that numerous brain disorders or neurodegenerative diseases have been linked to decreases in the expression and functionality of the astrocytic glutamate transporters. In order to facilitate efficient synaptic transmission, low extracellular glutamate levels must be maintained by glutamate transporter-1, or GLT-1. It accounts for around 90% of glutamate uptake in the adult dorsal forebrain [50]. Unlike prokaryotes, all eukaryotic transporters have glutamate uptake mediated by the electrochemical gradient for Na+ and H+ ions; the counter-transport of one K+ ion across the membrane is the rate-limiting step [51].

Glutamate Release

When an action potential arrives, glutamate is ready to be released from its storage in the synaptic region and packaged into synaptic vesicles. This release causes voltage-dependent calcium channels to activate, which raises the concentration of intracellular calcium (Ca^{2+}) (Fig. **2**). Neurotransmitters are released into the synaptic cleft when vesicles attach to the plasma membrane, facilitated by the (Ca^{2+}) influx [52]. The family of proteins known as the soluble N-ethylmaleimide-sensitive factor attachment protein receptor (SNARE) is crucial to this process. These proteins are divided into two groups: the vesicular v-SNARE, which is particularly abundant in the vesicles, and the target t-SNARE, which is abundantly expressed in the target zone of the cellular membrane [53]. A trans-SNARE complex, or interaction between v- and t-SNAREs, is required to release the neurotransmitter; the main v-SNAREs are synaptobrevin, synaptotagmin, and syntaxin, while the predominant t-SNARE is SNAP-25. Not only do neurons express SNAREs, but astrocytes also produce gliotransmitters with the help of SNAREs [54]. The production of synaptobrevin II and glutamate by cultured astrocytes, which is blocked by the neuronal exocytosis inhibitors botulinum toxin-A and botulinum toxin-C, suggests the expression of SNAP-25 and syntaxin in astrocytes [55]. Action potential initiation at synapses results in membrane depolarization and an influx of (Ca^{2+}) through transmembrane channels implicated in the action potential response. This, in turn, sets off a series of signalling events that culminate in vesicular release [56]. According to recent research, astrocytes release glutamate through interactions between the metabotropic receptor PAR-1 and either the (Ca^{2+})-activated Bestrophin-1 (Best-1) chloride channel or the two-pore domain potassium channel (TREK-1). Fast glutamate transient currents are enabled by the interface between the TREK-1 intracellular domain and PAR-1, in contrast to the slow transient currents that arise from the contact between Best-1 and PAR-1. Glutamate is released from the intracellular compartment as a result of this action. When taken as a whole, the data support the theory that neurons and astrocytes work together to affect glutamatergic signalling [57, 58].

NMDA RECEPTORS

Structure and Function of NMDA Receptors

The brain contains a substantial number of NMDA receptors, and extensive research has explored their roles in both physiological and pathological processes [59]. N-methyl-D-aspartate receptors (NMDARs) are glutamate-gated ion channels abundantly expressed throughout the central nervous system, playing crucial roles in brain development and synaptic plasticity. Both hyperactivity and hypo-function of NMDARs are detrimental to neuronal health and have been implicated in several neuropsychiatric disorders, including schizophrenia, epilepsy, autism spectrum disorders, and intellectual disability.

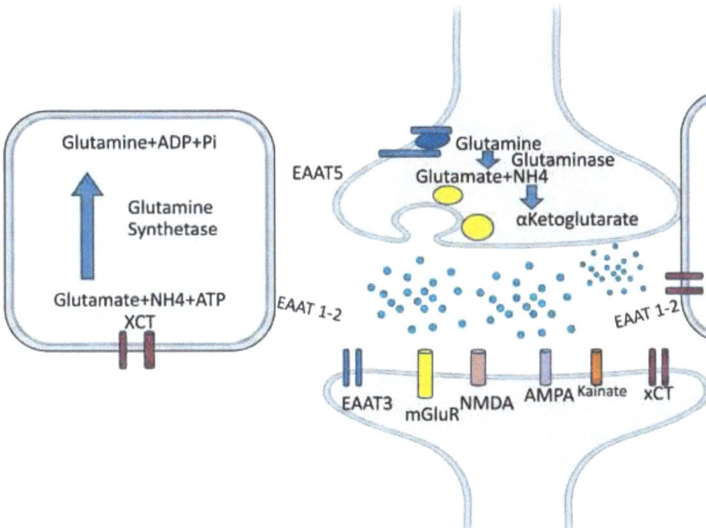

Fig. (2). Glutamate release and uptake, the Xc-antiporter, and the glutamate/glutamine cycle. In glial cells, reuptake of glutamate is converted to glutamine by glutamine synthetase.

A complex regulatory network finely tunes NMDAR signaling, thereby preventing excessive receptor-mediated transmission. This regulation involves numerous endogenous molecules that directly bind to NMDARs and modulate their activity in a subunit-specific manner [60]. Structurally, these receptors are composed of GluN1, GluN2 (A–D), and GluN3 (A, B) subunits. Each functional receptor requires two GluN1 subunits, while the remaining two can be either two GluN2 subunits or one GluN2 and one GluN3 subunit [37, 61 - 64].

Full activation of NMDARs in neurons requires simultaneous binding of glutamate and the co-agonist glycine, along with the displacement of Mg^{2+} ions that block the channel at resting membrane potential. Upon activation, the receptor allows Na^+ and (Ca^{2+}) influx, triggering downstream signaling events. In addition to glycine, astrocytes release D-serine, another potent co-agonist for NMDARs [65].

NMDARs possess multiple ligand-binding sites, including the allosteric site on the amino-terminal domain (ATD), the glutamate and glycine binding sites, and the ion channel pore—each modulating receptor activity in a subtype-specific manner [66, 67]. Interestingly, NMDARs in astrocytes are not inhibited by Mg^{2+} blockade and can even be activated at negative resting potentials [68]. Moreover, the expression patterns of NMDAR subunits in astrocytes vary across brain regions, leading to distinct receptor activation properties and diverse contributions to neuronal and glial signaling [69].

While NMDAR hypo-function has long been associated with neurological and psychiatric disorders such as schizophrenia, intellectual disability, and age-related cognitive decline, overactivation of these receptors—as observed during stroke or traumatic brain injury—can lead to excitotoxic neuronal death [60]. Additionally, different glutamate transporters can directly interact with arachidonic acid, which is generated upon activation of metabotropic glutamate receptors in astrocytes and NMDARs in neurons, producing varied effects. For instance, arachidonic acid modestly enhances glutamate uptake *via* EAAT3, inhibits uptake *via* EAAT1, and increases uptake *via* EAAT2 [70 - 72].

Subtypes of NMDA Receptors

The N-methyl-D-aspartate receptor (NMDAR), a subtype of ionotropic glutamate receptors, plays a pivotal role in regulating synaptic transmission and plasticity within the nervous system [73]. NMDARs are heterotetrameric complexes composed of GluN1, GluN2, and GluN3 subunits. The GluN1 subunit exists in eight splice isoforms, while the GluN2 family comprises four subtypes (GluN2A–D) and the GluN3 family includes two members (GluN3A and GluN3B) [74]. Structurally, each receptor consists of an intracellular C-terminal domain (CTD), transmembrane domains (TMDs), and a large extracellular region that includes an amino-terminal domain (ATD) and a ligand-binding domain (LBD).

Glutamate, the primary agonist, binds to the GluN2 subunits, while the co-agonists glycine or D-serine bind to GluN1 subunits. The GluN2 subunits confer specific biophysical and pharmacological properties to the receptor. Beyond these properties, NMDAR subtypes exhibit distinctive trafficking behaviors that have been extensively characterized [74 - 77]. Structural studies have revealed that NMDAR subunits assemble as dimers of GluN1–GluN2 heterodimers through ATD–LBD interfaces, forming the functional receptor complex [78 - 80].

A defining feature of the NMDAR family is its remarkable subunit diversity, which allows for functional specialization across different brain regions. Various combinations of GluN1–3 subunits give rise to a range of di- and tri-heteromeric NMDAR subtypes with distinct electrophysiological and pharmacological profiles. The selective targeting of NMDAR subtypes offers promising therapeutic opportunities, as numerous studies have demonstrated the spatiotemporal diversity of these receptors throughout brain development and function [81 - 84].

Developing highly subtype-specific modulators would not only deepen our understanding of the biological roles of NMDARs in neurodevelopment and synaptic function but could also lead to novel therapies for neurological disorders. For instance, GluN2B-containing NMDARs are emerging as therapeutic targets for neuropathic pain, schizophrenia, neurodegenerative diseases, and ischemic stroke [85 - 88]. Moreover, GluN2C/2D-containing NMDARs are selectively expressed in specific brain regions relevant to certain pathologies, while GluN2A/2B-containing receptors are predominant in the adult brain. Notably, GluN2D subunits are highly expressed in cortical GABAergic neurons, where NMDAR hypo-function has been implicated in the pathophysiology of schizophrenia [89 - 92].

Mechanism of NMDA Receptor Activation and Signalling Pathways

As NMDARs play a crucial role in neural development, their dysregulation has been implicated in the onset and progression of numerous neurodegenerative disorders [93, 94]. The phosphorylation of the C-terminal domain (CTD) serves as a key mechanism for regulating NMDAR activity and synaptic plasticity [95, 96]. Protein kinase C (PKC), a family of serine/threonine kinases, functions as an essential signal transducer involved in modulating NMDAR activity under both physiological and pathological conditions [97, 98].

NMDAR channels are activated by the simultaneous binding of glutamate to the GluN2 subunits and glycine to the GluN1 subunits [99]. Upon agonist binding, conformational changes occur within the bilobed clamshell-like agonist-binding domains (ABDs), which are transmitted to the transmembrane domains (TMDs) through linker regions connecting these domains. This process triggers the movement of the M3 transmembrane helix, resulting in the rearrangement of the channel gate's crossing helical bundle. Consequently, a cation-selective pore opens, allowing Na^+ and (Ca^{2+}) ions to enter the cell along their electrochemical gradients [100, 101].

The amino-terminal domains (ATDs) act as subunit-specific regulatory regions, capable of mediating intra-subunit allosteric effects on agonist binding and channel gating, as well as interacting with various extracellular allosteric modulators [102]. Meanwhile, the C-terminal domains (CTDs) anchor NMDARs to the postsynaptic cytoskeletal network, provide docking sites for post-translational modifications, and serve as scaffolding regions for the association of signaling molecules such as (Ca^{2+})/calmodulin-dependent protein kinase II (CaMKII) [102].

Overall, NMDAR activation leads to membrane depolarization and a sustained increase in intracellular (Ca^{2+}) concentration—key processes that contribute to the slow component of excitatory synaptic transmission [37, 102].

Role of NMDA Receptors in Alzheimer's Disease

Alzheimer's disease, a progressive neurodegenerative disorder, is characterized by the deterioration of cognitive functions and memory, driven by the pathological accumulation of amyloid-beta plaques and tau neurofibrillary tangles [103]. These deposits induce synaptotoxicity, severely disrupting synaptic integrity and neuronal communication [104]. A critical factor in this process is the dysregulation of NMDA receptors, which, when excessively activated, lead to excitotoxicity and neuronal apoptosis. The primary determinants of NMDAR signaling in AD are glutamate availability and NMDAR channel function regulation [105].

Impact of Amyloid-beta on NMDA Receptoractivity

The hallmarks of AD include excitotoxic quantities of extracellular glutamate, soluble amyloid-beta (Aβ) buildup, and hyperphosphorylated tau protein, which ultimately results in the death of neuronal cells [106, 107]. Research indicates that soluble Aβ buildup causes synaptic failure, possibly by altering the glutamatergic system [106 - 113]. Early stages of the disease, as seen in rat models of AD and mild cognitive impairment (MCI), exhibit a surge in glutamatergicpresynaptic boutons [114, 115] and an enhanced excitability of pyramidal neurons [116 - 118]. Aβ inhibits glutamatergic synaptic transmission at synapses [119], resulting in a decrease in surface glutamate receptors as well as othersynaptic components in cultivated hippocampal neurons [120, 121]. Aβ, similar to NMDA, causes an instantaneousincrease in (Ca^{2+}) by activating NMDARs in cultured cortical neurons that contain GluN2B [122]. Aβ oligomer buildup appears to bemostly located in excitatory synapses bearing the GluN2B subunit of NMDARs in the AD brain as well as human cortical neurons [123]. Aβ oligomers have been shown to disrupt LTP at dentate gyrus and hippocampal CA1 synapses, which is dependent on NMDARs [124]. Furthermore, according to someresearch, Aβ oligomers could attach to a surface tyrosine kinase, EphB2, which binds NMDARs to preserve their integrity. The degradation of EphB2 leads to a reduction in LTP, loss of NMDAR activity [125], and a decrease in the surface distribution of NMDA receptor subunits such as GluN2B [123]. Additionally, at low concentrations, a GluN2B-selective antagonist can stop the suppression of LTP caused by Aβ [126]. Furthermore, itis possible to mitigate the impairment of LTP caused by Aβ in AD by reducing the amounts of extracellular glutamate and inhibiting p38MAPK or calpain, which are triggered specifically by extrasynaptic NMDARs [127].

Certain findings indicate a pathway whereby Aβ promotes the activation of NMDARs, which then regulate the synthesis of Aβ. In primary cultures of cortical neurons, NMDAR activation [128]—more specifically, extrasynaptic activation [129]—increased Aβ production and secretion. This was preceded by a change in APP processing from α-secretase to β-secretase, which was followed by a transition from APP695 towards Kunitz protease inhibitory domain (KPI) comprising amyloid-β precursor protein (KPIAPP), the isoforms displaying an essential high amyloidogenic potential [130]. According to an *in vivo* study, the influence on Aβ generation may be regulated by the degree of NMNDAR activation: Aβ generation is increased by low levels of NMDA receptor activation, whereas Aβ production is decreased by higher levels [131]. In primary neuronal cultures and rat and mouse hippocampus slices, Aβ-induced early neuronal dysfunctionis mediated by activation of GluN2B-containing NMDAR [132]. Furthermore, administering Aβ oligomers to rat organotypic slices harboring pyramidal neurons reduces the density of dendritic spines and the amount of calcium influx mediated by NMDAR into active spines [133]. In addition to having considerably lower GluN1 mRNA levels, postmortem human AD brain regions, including the cortex and hippocampus, which are vulnerable to the disease, also had lower GluN2A as well as GluN2B levels [134]. While GluN2B subunits seem to increase neuronal susceptibility, GluN2A subunits are linked to protective mechanisms. Reduction in GluN2B subunit and activation of GluN2A may be an effort to alleviate Aβ-induced neuronal dysfunction [135]. By controlling the quantity of NMDARs, Aβ decreases glutamatergic transmission and prevents synaptic plasticity. Applying Aβ to cortical neurons *in vitro* increases NMDAR endocytosis and reduces NMDAR expression [120]. Likewise, Aβ reduces glutamatergic synaptic currents in rat hippocampus neurons. Hence, Aβ seems to control synaptic NMDARs, upsetting the equilibrium of extrasynaptic and synaptic NMDAR signaling.

Tau Pathology and NMDA Receptor Dysfunction

Tau is an integral component of the NFT, which is a pathological feature of AD [136]. Similar to Aβ, tau has been associated with synaptic dysfunction and glutamate excitotoxicity. Tau phosphorylation causes synaptic impairment by tau mislocalization from axon to dendritic spines, as well as reduced AMPA receptor expression, and LTP impairments [137]. Acute tau phosphorylation upregulation promotes NMDAR transmission, which in turn helps to facilitate LTD [138] and BDNF-dependent morphological plasticity [139]. Both the activation of the NMDA receptor and incubation with Aβ can cause tau to become phosphorylated.

Although tau phosphorylation after five days of exposure to Aβ is irreversible, tau phosphorylation caused by the NMDA receptor is not [138]. The tyrosine kinase Fyn initiates the phosphorylation of GluN2B receptor subunits at Tyr1472 in dendritic spines, strengthening its connection with PSD95 in PSD. Fyn is bound to dendritic spines by Tau, which also facilitates its transit. Tau reductions fail to shuttle Fyn kinase to dendritic spines, cease Aβ-induced excitability and memory deficits [140]. Endogenous tau appears in postsynaptic regions, where it binds the PSD95-NMDAR complex in addition to Fyn. Tau phosphorylation at specific locations is induced by NMDAR activation, and this regulates tau's interaction with the PSD95-NMDAR complex and Fyn. Additionally, tau phosphorylation promotes LTD facilitation and NMDA receptor transmission [138].

A GluN2B selective antagonist called Ifenprodil can inhibit the cell death caused by overexpression of human tau within primary neuronal cultures, indicating that tau-induced neurotoxicity is mediated through the stimulation of extrasynaptic NMDARs bearing the GluN2B component. Calpain breaks down tau protein into poisonous N-terminal peptides that cause cell death when (Ca^{2+}) influx is stimulated through NMDAR [141]. Memantine treatment reduces tau phosphorylation, excitotoxicity, and preferentially blocks E-NMDARs [142]. In rat hippocampal slices, tau phosphorylation is regulated by NMDA receptors that contain GluN2A. Tau phosphorylation is reduced by the GluN2A-containing NMDA receptor through the PKC/GSK-3 pathway [143]. Tau plays a role in triggering Aβ-induced deaths of neurons and can independently generate synaptic dysfunction, despite the fact that research into its contribution to glutamate excitotoxicity is still in its early stages [144].

ALTERED NMDA RECEPTOR SIGNALLING IN AD

Glial NMDA Receptor

Recent data indicate that astrocytic NMDARs exhibit unique structural and functional characteristics, such as reduced (Ca^{2+}) permeability and limited susceptibility to Mg^{2+} blockage [145]. Astrocytic NMDARs can be activated by glutamate or QUIN, which then increases (Ca^{2+}) influx and triggers a signaling cascade [146]. It has been demonstrated that astrocytic functional NMDA receptors can react to glutamatergic input from neurons. This response is accompanied by a dynamic increase in intracellular (Ca^{2+}), which in turn triggers gliotransmitter-mediated modulation of synaptic activity [145, 147, 148]. Notably, because astrocytic NMDARs facilitate glutamate excitotoxicity, it is possible that they contribute to AD [146, 149].

Studies have revealed that antagonistic treatment of astrocytic GluN2A and GluN2B can worsen Aβ-induced early synaptotoxicity, and nerve growth factor (β-NGF) may operate as a mediator during the synaptoprotection of astrocytic GluN2 stimulation [121]. ERK1/2 phosphorylation is significantly increased in microglia upon NMDAR activation. In neurons, ERK phosphorylation—or the interaction between NMDAR and mitogen-activated protein kinase (MAPK) signaling—is dependent on both CaM and NCS1, whereas in microglia, NMDAR signaling is only dependent on CaM. Microglia obtained from APPSw, Ind transgenic mice showed potentiated NMDAR function, suggesting that the NCS1–NMDAR connection is important for receptor function within the AD animal model's microglia [150].

Presynaptic NMDA Receptor

Presynaptic NMDARs, also known as preNMDARs, can control presynaptic glutamate release and modify the shape and transmission of synapses [74, 151 - 153]. PreNMDARs can regulate evoked release through a frequency-dependent approach by depending on the more traditional Mg^{2+}-dependent route, but they can also govern spontaneous release, independent of Mg^{2+} and (Ca^{2+}) [74, 154 - 156]. According to Abrahamsson *et al.*, preNMDARs within L5 pyramidal cells control both spontaneous and evoked release through pathways that are dependent on JNK2 and RIM1αβ, respectively [155]. PreNMDARs are necessary not just for LTD induction but also for LTP induction [157]. According to Park *et al.*, preNMDARs are essential for LTP induction across corticostriatal synapses in mice. PreNMDAR activation enhances (Ca^{2+}) signals within axonal terminals, which causes BDNF production, suggesting that preNMDARs are just as important for LTP induction as postsynaptic NMDARs [158]. Bell *et al.*, observed that the glutamatergic presynaptic bouton density among individuals with mild cognitive impairment (MCI) showed a counterintuitive rise, which subsequently depletes and lowers with the advancement of the condition. These findings demonstrated that, in the latter stages of AD, dystrophic neurite production and decreased presynaptic bouton densities had a deleterious effect on neurotransmission and cognitive performance [115].

Metabotropic NMDAR

Contemporary, intriguing research suggests that NMDAR may function as a metabotropic receptor that sends out metabotropic signals without requiring (Ca^{2+}) influx into the channel [159 - 163]. According to recent findings, glutamate binding on its own is sufficient to cause NMDAR conformational changes, which in turn set off p38 MAPK signaling cascades and induce LTD [160, 162, 164]. It is interesting to note that an increase in (Ca^{2+}) can cause LTP, yet maintaining intracellular (Ca^{2+}) at the baseline level is essential for the activation of metabotropic NMDAR, resulting in synaptic depression [165]. According to this metabotropic signaling, preNMDARs have the ability to regulate spontaneous release without the need for Mg^{2+} or (Ca^{2+}), whereas evoked release was Mg^{2+}-sensitive [154, 155].

Furthermore, certain research findings indicate that astrocytic NMDARs could potentially function *via* metabotropic signaling pathways [65, 166]. These routes could entail phospholipase C-induced elevation of (Ca^{2+}) in the endoplasmic reticulum as well as activation of protein kinase Cδ [65]. However, further investigation is necessary to elucidate the intricate mechanism [146]. Elevated Aβ oligomer levels are linked to early synaptic dysfunction in AD, resulting in rapid spine loss and NMDAR-dependent synaptic depression [74, 133]. However, additional studies revealed that AP-5, but not MK-801, was able to prevent Aβ-induced NMDA receptor-dependent synaptic depression without the need for ion flux through the receptor, indicating that NMDARs' metabotropic action plays a role in Aβ-induced synaptic dysfunction [159, 167, 168]. There might be a similar mechanism behind both Aβ-induced synaptic depression and metabotropic NMDAR-dependent LTD [162, 169].

SYNAPTIC DYSFUNCTION AND COGNITIVE IMPAIRMENT IN AD

Aβ-induced NMDAR DYs function and Synapticplasticity Disruption

Aβ can impair synaptic plasticity in the early stages of AD by interfering with synaptic glutamatergic receptor function in addition to causing damage to synaptic function by means of internalization and intracellular accumulation [170]. According to studies, Aβ oligomers have the ability to act on NMDARs either directly or indirectly, dysregulate their activity, and interfere with calcium influx, which causes LTD to increase and LTP to be suppressed [133, 171, 172]. The impairment of synaptic plasticity is more pronounced when Aβ-induced NMDAR dysregulation occurs [173]. Aβ oligomers have the ability to suppress LTP by activating extrasynaptic NMDARs in addition to downregulating synaptic NMDAR activity *via* enhancing NMDAR endocytosis [174]. Aβ causes α7 nAChR-mediated astrocytic glutamate release at extrasynaptic regions to activate GluN2B-containing NMDA receptors, which in turn causes the abnormal activation of p38 mitogen-activated kinase (MAPK), suppression of cAMP response element-binding (CREB) signaling, along with disruption of LTP [127, 175]. Extrasynaptic NMDA receptor activation also causes a decrease in synaptic plasticity as well as cognitive function by promoting proteasome-dependent disintegration of BRCA1, a DNA repair factor [176].

A study revealed that the toxic peptide soluble Aβ1-42 significantly raised the extrasynaptic NMDA responses and (Ca^{2+}) flow *via* extrasynaptic NMDARs containing GluN2B [177, 178], which in turn hampered spatial cognition and inhibited LTP [177]. Aβ1-42 has the ability to expedite the phosphorylation process of GluN2B subunit tyrosine and initiate a temporary activation of Akt that is sensitive to Ifenprodil [179]. Due to the activation of Akt, GSK-3β is phosphorylated, which obviously hinders synaptic plasticity, including LTP, from being induced [180, 181]. Nonetheless, the primary cause of LTP suppression controlled by soluble Aβ1-42 was the hyperactivation of extrasynaptic NMDA receptors, including GluN2B, which further harmed synaptic plasticity and impaired calcium homeostasis. Moreover, it is possible that the overactivation of NMDARs and the suppression of LTP caused by Aβ form a vicious cycle that exacerbates the damage to synaptic plasticity [127].

High levels of Aβ can exacerbate NMDAR activation in pathological conditions [182], leading to delayed cognitive impairment triggered by NMDAR agonists [183]. Lower levels of Aβ can specifically hinder glutamatergic synaptic transmission, LTD expression, and LTP by triggering the activation of p38 MAPK and JNK [184 - 186]. As a result, it is evident that greater Aβ production raises NMDAR activation, which in turn raises Aβ production within limits. Cognitive impairment in AD is ultimately caused by overactivation of NMDAR or Aβ deposition, which can both affect synaptic plasticity once the homeostatic equilibrium between NMDA activation and Aβ generation is disrupted [187]. Additionally, some synaptotoxic Aβ assemblies affect cellular prion protein (PrPC), a protein involved in the Aβ-mediated production of LTD [188, 189]. At the postsynaptic density, Aβ, PrPC, and mGlu5R can combine to generate the Aβ-PrPC-mGlu5R triad complex. In addition to increasing mGlu5R-dependent LTD, the Aβ-PrPC-mGlu5R triad also suppresses NMDAR-dependent LTP, exacerbating the impairment of synaptic plasticity [190].

Implications for Learning and Memory Deficits in AD

Phenotypic effects of glutamatergic dysfunction stemming from dysregulation of synaptic components include impaired memory and learning capacities. In AD patients, there exists a presynaptic correlation between a decrease in cognitive state and the duration of the disease, as well as decreases in VGluT1 and VGluT2 [191]. In APP/PS1 mice, increased hippocampal glutamate release also exhibited a negative correlation with cognitive function preceding cognitive damage [118]. S-NMDARs, which are necessary for LTP conduction, are inhibited by soluble Aβ [93, 192]. Treatment with the selective NMDA antagonist (2R)-amino-5-phosphonovaleric acid (D-AP5) reduces LTP *in vivo*, indicating that NMDARs are involved in LTP [193]. D-AP5 treatment, however, was able to reverse the LTP impairment seen in GLT-1 mutant animals, indicating that NMDAR blockage and overactivation can both affect LTP [194]. This effect could be explained by the role of E-NMDARs, since Aβ-mediated LTP impairments are prevented by inhibiting E-NMDARs [127, 195]. The noncompetitive GluN2 receptor antagonist memantine, which has FDA approval for treating AD [196], has demonstrated effectiveness in enhancing Morris water maze test performance [197 - 199] and blocking Aβ suppression of LTP in 3xTg-AD hippocampus slices [200, 201]. Consequently, it may be concluded that non-competitive inhibition of the GluN2B subunit of NMDARs acts as a counterbalance to the inhibition of S-NMDARs and the overactivation of E-NMDARs.

Aβ-induced reduction of LTP as well as potentiation of LTD are both mediated by mGluRs [70, 195, 202]. Impeding mGluR5 can prevent Aβ-mediated LTP deficits [195, 202]. By virtue of their mechanistic coupling, NMDARs and mGluRs can cause persistent activation, which in AD can result in synaptic failure [195, 203]. Since both mGluR5 and E-NMDARs increase intracellular (Ca^{2+}), it is possible that (Ca^{2+}) dysregulation and CREB dephosphorylation are the causes of this failure [204 - 209]. Furthermore, it has been demonstrated that mGluR1 contributes to LTP in the CA1 and synaptic plasticity [210, 211]. Notably, agonism of mGluR1 as well as mGluR5 with 3-hydroxyphenylglycine exacerbated the neurotoxicity induced by NMDAR, which contrasted with the neuroprotective effects of agonism of mGluR2 [212, 213] and further indicated a negative correlation between NMDAR and mGluRs regarding LTP and excitotoxicity. Moreover, soluble Aβ-mediated LTD augmentation requires mGluRs [70, 89, 214]. Reduced surface expression of AMPARs during LTD is the result of treatment with 3,5-dihydroxyphenylglycine, a Group I mGluR agonist [89], revealing another mechanism whereby soluble Aβ affects memory signal conduction and learning.

THERAPEUTIC APPROACHES TARGETING GLUTAMATE AND NMDA RECEPTORS

Current Pharmacological Treatments

Currently available treatments for AD consist of two classes of drugs: the non-competitive NMDA receptor antagonist memantine (authorized for use in moderate to severe AD) and cholinesterase inhibitors (ChEIs), which include galantamine, rivastigmine, and donepezil (authorized for use in mild to moderate AD) [215, 216]. However, the benefits of these drugs in AD are merely symptomatic [217]. Current research indicates that these drugs, which target the NMDA receptors' downstream signaling pathways and function, can effectively treat AD by reestablishing the neural network [218].

As non-competitive antagonists targeting NMDA receptors, phencyclidine (PCP), memantine, ketamine, and MK-801 are used to treat AD (Table **1**). However, MK-801 (dizocilpine), phencyclidine, and ketamine have serious side effects that impede their therapeutic utilization, including high affinity and long dwell times on the receptor [219]. Memantine, on the other hand, has been utilized to treat mild to severe AD because of its reduced affinity and good tolerance [220 - 222]. It has been demonstrated that combination therapy involving memantine and the cholinesterase inhibitor donepezil is more effective than memantine used alone [223]. Patients with AD who consumed memantine and donepezil at daily concentrations of 10 mg and 28 mg, respectively, reported positive effects in the treatment of symptoms including behavior, language, and cognition [216, 224]. Yet, patients with mild-to-moderate AD have not responded satisfactorily to this combination medication [225].

Remarkably, Riluzole, a novel inhibitor of postsynaptic glutamate receptor signaling and glutamate release, is currently being examined in a phase II clinical trial in individuals with mild AD [226].

Table 1. List of Non-competitive NMDA receptor antagonists or blockers.

Antagonist/ Blocker Drug	Mechanism of Action	IC_{50}	Drawback	Outcome	Indication	Clinical/Pre-clinical status	Refs.
Memantine	Inhibitory action on NMDAR-mediated excitotoxicity, rapid unblocking kinetic features, significant voltage dependency, it inhibits the NMDAR and does not release it in the event of a pathological tonic over-activation of the receptor, but itpermits the transmission of brief physiologicalsignals essential for learning and memory processes	1.04 ± 0.26 μM	Provides only symptomatic relief	Enhances cognition, decelerates the progression of disease, decreases the phosphorylation of tau.	Moderate to severe AD	USFDA and EMEA Approved	[192, 227-231]

(Table 1) cont.....

Antagonist/ Blocker Drug	Mechanism of Action	IC_{50}	Drawback	Outcome	Indication	Clinical/Pre-clinical status	Refs.
Phencyclidine (PCP)	Prevents the channel in the NMDA receptor complex from opening.	1.51 μM	Exhibit a high degree of affinity. and sustained cohesion on the receptor, associated with serious adverse effects such as developmental defects, hallucinations, and coma	Psychotomimetic.	-	No clinical applications.	[219]
MK801 (Dizocilpine)	NMDA receptor antagonist that inhibits excitatory aminoacid transmitters.	2.23 ± 0.3 μM		Increase dopamine turnover in the nucleus accumbens.	-	No clinical applications	[219, 232]
Ketamine	Blocks the channel in the NMDA receptor complex from opening.	0.43 ± 0.10 μM		Psychotomimetic	Depression and agitation associated with dementia	No clinical applications	[219, 227, 233]

NOVEL THERAPEUTIC COMPOUNDS UNDER INVESTIGATION

The development, research, and discovery of drugs for AD are arduous and challenging. Currently, 187 trials assessing 141 unique treatments are being studied in clinical trials to treat AD, after hundreds of treatments have been shown to fail. Only two drugs—aducanumab and lecanemab—have been approved for market since 2021, following a 17-year hiatus in the approvals of disease-modifying treatments (DMTs) for AD [234]. Ongoing research focusing on the glutamate and NMDA receptors poses a novel avenue to offer a breakthrough and facilitate the availability of diverse AD treatments. A few of such research findings are discussed in the following Table **2**, which lists some of the novel therapeutic drugs that act on the glutamatergic system.

Table 2. List of novel compounds or drugs that modulate glutamatergic receptors.

Receptor	Antagonist/ Agonist	Mechanism of Action	IC_{50}	Outcome	Pre-clinical Studies	Refs.
NMDA	Nitro Memantine	Selectively inhibits extrasynaptic NMDAR.	2.4 μM	Ameliorates synaptic loss induced by Aβ.	*In vivo* studies in 3×Tg AD α7nAChR-knockout, and hAPP-J20 Tg mice	[192, 234, 235]
GluN2B (Non-competitive)	Ifenprodil	Functions as a non-competitive antagonistin a use-dependent and voltage-independent manner by binding to the N-terminal lysine/isoleucine/valine-binding protein (LIVBP) like domain of GluN2B.	0.34 μM	Ameliorates persistent deficits in sensorimotor and spatial learning.	*In vivo* studies in rat SAH model	[236, 237]
GluN2B (Non-competitive)	Traxoprodil	Inhibits the tyrosine phosphorylation of GluN2B and its interactions with Fyn.	10 nM	Rescued memory deficits of Aβ-injectedmice	*In vivo* studies in Wistar rat embryos	[238, 239]

(Table 2) cont.....

Receptor	Antagonist/ Agonist	Mechanism of Action	IC_{50}	Outcome	Pre-clinical Studies	Refs.
GluN2D (Non-competitive)	NAB-14	Inhibits GluN2D-mediated synapticcurrents in mouse hippocampal interneurons and rat subthalamic neurons.	580 nM	Shows highersystemicexposure, brain penetrance, and is rapidly metabolized *in vivo*.	*In vitro* studies in *Xenopus* oocytes, hippocampal slices of mice C57BL/6 and Sprague Dawley rats. *In vivo* studies in C57BL/6 mice and Wistar rats.	[240]
GluN2B	Rhynchophylline (oxindole alkaloid)	Prevents over-activation of $A\beta_{1-42}$- generated postsynaptic extrasynaptic NMDARs.	43.2 μM	Restored LTP impairment and spatial dysfunctioncaused by $A\beta_{1-42}$. Limited use because of poorbioavailability, low concentration in brain tissue, and low water solubility.	*In vivo* studies in adult Sprague Dawley rats and C57BL/6 mice	[177, 241, 242]
GluN2B	Xanthoceraside (triterpenoid saponin)	Reversed the expression levels of pY1472-GluN2B and GluN2B in synaptic and extrasynaptic pools by significantly reducing STEP61 and pY531-Fyn.	-	Alleviated learning-memory deficits and increased the LTP.	*In vivo* studies in APP/PS1 transgenic mice.	[243]
AMPA (GluA1 subunit) and NMDA	Anemoside A3 (triterpenoid saponin)	Increased GluA1 phosphorylation at Ser831 and Ser845. It is also a low-affinity, non-competitive NMDAR modulator having slow on-rate inhibition and voltage independence that inhibits NMDAR activity.	18.48 and 20.19 μM at − 50 and +50 mV NMDA evoked current	Improvedsynapticstrength and memory, facilitateshippocampal LTP	*In vivo* studies in C57BL/6(C57) mice and *in vitro* studies in mouse hippocampal slices.	[244]
AMPA	PAM-AMPA	Positive allosteric modulation of AMPA receptors.	-	Restored synaptic integrity and cognitive performance. Reverted stress/Aβ-drivensynapticmissorting of Tau and tau accumulation.	*In vivo* studies in male Wistar rats.	[245]
mGluR5-selective	CTEP	As a negative allosteric modulator, it blocks mGluR5 signaling and provides neuroprotection.	11.4 nM	Rescued memory deficits, reduced Aβ oligomer concentrations, and plaque formation.	*In vivo* studies in APPswe/ PS1ΔE9 and 3xTg-AD mouse models of AD and CTEP are analogous to the clinical trial phase II moleculeBasimglurant (RO4917523)	[246, 247]
mGluR5-selective	MTEP	Weakens the interaction between PrP^C and Myc-mGluR5.	5 nM	Alleviated synapticdysfunction and improved memory and learning	*In vivo* studies in APPswe/ PS1ΔE9 and APP/PS1 transgenic mouse models of AD	[248-250]
mGluR1/5	DHPG	Potent agonist of group I mGluR.	-	Prevented Aβ-induced LTD	*In vivo* studies in male Wistar rats	[251]
mGluR5	BMS-984923	Significantly decreases the interaction between mGluR5 and the cellular prion protein (PrP^C) anchored to Aβo *via* silent allosteric modulation of mGluR5.	10 nM (for Aβo)	Inhibited Aβ induced signal transduction, restored memory deficits, and rescued from synaptic depletion.	*In vitro* studies in HEK293T cells *In vivo* studies in APPswe/ PS1DE9 (APP/PS1) transgenic model mice.	[252]
mGluR5	CDPPB	Positive allosteric modulation of mGluR5 offers neuroprotection.	27 nM (EC_{50})	Improved neuronal survival and prevented memory deficits, increased neuronal viability, and reduced gliosis.	*In vivo* studies in T41 and C57BL/6 mice.	[253, 254]
mGluR1/5 (non-selective)	LY341495	Non-selectively inhibits Group I/II mGluR.	7.8 μM (for mGluR1a), 8.2 μM (for mGluR5a)	Completely blocked Aβ-induced LTD.	*In vivo* studies in male Wistar rats.	[251, 255]

(Table 2) cont.....

Receptor	Antagonist/ Agonist	Mechanism of Action	IC_{50}	Outcome	Pre-clinical Studies	Refs.
mGluR2/3 (non-selective)	LY341495	Non-selectively antagonises mGluR2/3.	21 nM (for mGluR2), 14 nM (mGluR3)	Blocked the release of $A\beta_{42}$.	*In vitro* studies in cultured astrocytes and cultured neurons lacking mGlu2 receptors. *In vivo* studies in TgCRND8 mice overexpressing a mutant human APP 695.	[255-257]
mGluR2/3	LY379268	Provides neuroprotection through orthosteric agonism of mGluR2/3.	2.69 nM (for mGlu2), 4.48 nM (for mGlu3); EC_{50}	Protect neurons by producing TGF-β and GDNF.	*In vitro* studies in mixed cultures of mouse cortical cells. *In vivo* studies in mGlu2 and mGlu3 receptor knockout mice.	[256, 258-260]

CONCLUSION

Glutamate plays a central role in the development of Alzheimer's disease (AD) due to its involvement in excitatory signaling within the central nervous system (CNS). The delicate balance of glutamate levels is crucial, as both excessive and insufficient glutamate can be harmful, leading to disruptions in neurotransmission that may trigger or exacerbate AD. The overactivation of glutamate receptors, particularly the NMDA receptors, results in excitotoxicity, which is a major contributor to neuronal damage and cognitive decline in AD. Although current treatments like memantine, an NMDA receptor antagonist, aim to reduce glutamate-induced excitotoxicity, they offer only partial protection and do not fully halt disease progression. The failure of many drugs in clinical trials underscores the complexity of the glutamatergic system, which includes multiple receptor subtypes with distinct and sometimes opposing roles. As such, a deeper understanding of the glutamatergic pathways is crucial for developing more effective therapies.

Looking forward, the future of AD treatment lies in the development of disease-modifying therapies that can more effectively target the glutamatergic system and its complex interactions. This includes the exploration of novel pharmacological agents that could restore synaptic function and cognitive abilities by modulating different components of the glutamatergic system. Furthermore, the selective inhibition of NMDA receptor subtypes, particularly those that mediate excitotoxicity, offers a promising avenue for reducing synaptic dysfunction and slowing disease progression. The potential of medicinal compounds, like those found in certain herbs, to modulate these pathways further broadens the scope of treatment possibilities. Future therapies may involve multi-drug approaches that not only modulate NMDAR activity but also address other components of the glutamatergic system, such as AMPA receptors and metabotropic glutamate receptors (mGluRs), and this may offer the best hope for slowing down AD progression and improving cognitive outcomes in patients. Although current therapies have not yet provided a cure or significantly improved life expectancy in AD patients, ongoing research into these pathways holds the potential for more effective interventions that could delay the onset and progression of this devastating disease.

LIST OF ABBREVIATIONS

AD	Alzheimer's Disease
Akt	Protein kinase B
AMPA	A-amino-3-hydroxy-5-methyl-4isoxasolepropionic Acid
APP	Amyloid Precursor Protein
Aβ	Amyloid-β
BDNF	Brain-derived Neurotrophic Factor
BRCA1	Breast Cancer Type 1 Susceptibilityprotein
CA1	Cornuammonis 1
CaM	Calmodulin
CNS	Central Nervous System
CREB	Cyclic Adenosine Monophosphate Response Element Binding Protein
CTEP	2-chloro-4-[2-[2,5-dimethyl-1-[4-(trifluoromethoxy)phe-nyl]imidazol-4-yl]ethynyl]pyridine
D-AP5	(2R)-Amino-5-phosphonovaleric Acid
DHPG	3,5-dihydroxyphenylglycone
DMTs	Disease Modifying Treatments
E-NMDARs	Extrasynaptic N-Methyl-D-Aspartate Receptors
EphB2	Ephrin Type-B Receptor 2
ERK	Extracellular Signal-related Kinase
GDNF	Glial Cell Line-derived Neurotrophic Factors
GSK3β	Glycogen Synthase Kinase 3-β
JNK	c-Jun N-terminal Kinase
KPIAPP	Kunitzprotease Inhibitory Domain (KPI) Comprisingamyloid-β Precursorprotein
LTD	Long-Term Depression
LTP	Long-Term Potentiation
MAPK	Mitogen-Activated Protein Kinase
MCI	Mild Cognitive Impairment
mRNA	Messenger Ribonucleicacid
MTEP	3-((2-Methyl-1,3-thiazol-4-yl)ethynyl)pyridine

NCS1	Neuronal (Ca^{2+}) Sensorprotein 1
NFTs	Neurofibrillary Tangles
NMDA	N-methyl-D-Aspartate
p38MAPK	p38 Mitogen-activatedprotein Kinase
PAM	Positive Allosteric Modulator
PKC	Protein Kinase C
PrP^c	Cellular Prion Protein
PSD	Postsynaptic Density
PSD95	Postsynaptic density protein 95
QUIN	Quinolinic Acid
STEP61	Striatal-Enriched Protein Tyrosine Phosphatase 61
TGF-β	Transforming growth factor β
VGLUT1/2	Vesicular Glutamate Transporters 1 and 2
β-NGF	Nerve Growth Factor

REFERENCES

[1] De-Paula VJ, Radanovic M, Diniz BS, Forlenza OV. Alzheimer's Disease. In: James Harris, editor. Protein Aggregation and Fibrillogenesis in Cerebral and Systemic Amyloid Disease. Subcellular Biochemistry. Vol. 65. Dordrecht: Springer; 2012. p. 329–352.
[http://dx.doi.org/10.1007/978-94-007-5416-4_14] [PMID: 23225010]

[2] Terry RD, Davies P. Dementia of the Alzheimer type. Annu Rev Neurosci 1980; 3(1): 77-95.
[http://dx.doi.org/10.1146/annurev.ne.03.030180.000453] [PMID: 6251745]

[3] Rathmann KL, Conner CS. Alzheimer's disease: clinical features, pathogenesis, and treatment. Drug Intell Clin Pharm 1984; 18(9): 684-91.
[http://dx.doi.org/10.1177/106002808401800902] [PMID: 6383752]

[4] Cummings J, Aisen PS, DuBois B, *et al.* Drug development in Alzheimer's disease: the path to 2025. Alzheimers Res Ther 2016; 8(1): 39.
[http://dx.doi.org/10.1186/s13195-016-0207-9] [PMID: 27646601]

[5] Ferreira-Vieira TH, Guimaraes IM, Silva FR, Ribeiro FM. Alzheimer's disease: Targeting the Cholinergic System. Curr Neuropharmacol 2016; 14(1): 101-15.
[http://dx.doi.org/10.2174/1570159X13666150716165726] [PMID: 26813123]

[6] Lewis J, Dickson DW. Propagation of tau pathology: hypotheses, discoveries, and yet unresolved questions from experimental and human brain studies. Acta Neuropathol 2016; 131(1): 27-48.
[http://dx.doi.org/10.1007/s00401-015-1507-z] [PMID: 26576562]

[7] Selkoe DJ, Hardy J. The amyloid hypothesis of Alzheimer's disease at 25 years. EMBO Mol Med 2016; 8(6): 595-608.
[http://dx.doi.org/10.15252/emmm.201606210] [PMID: 27025652]

[8] Briggs CA, Chakroborty S, Stutzmann GE. Emerging pathways driving early synaptic pathology in Alzheimer's disease. Biochem Biophys Res Commun 2017; 483(4): 988-97.
[http://dx.doi.org/10.1016/j.bbrc.2016.09.088] [PMID: 27659710]

[9] Kumar A, Singh A. A review on mitochondrial restorative mechanism of antioxidants in Alzheimer's disease and other neurological conditions. Front Pharmacol 2015; 6: 206.

[http://dx.doi.org/10.3389/fphar.2015.00206] [PMID: 26441662]

[10] Kumar A, Singh A, Ekavali . A review on Alzheimer's disease pathophysiology and its management: an update. Pharmacol Rep 2015; 67(2): 195-203. [http://dx.doi.org/10.1016/j.pharep.2014.09.004] [PMID: 25712639]

[11] Calsolaro V, Edison P. Neuroinflammation in Alzheimer's disease: Current evidence and future directions. Alzheimers Dement 2016; 12(6): 719-32. [http://dx.doi.org/10.1016/j.jalz.2016.02.010] [PMID: 27179961]

[12] Terry RD, Masliah E, Salmon DP, *et al.* Physical basis of cognitive alterations in alzheimer's disease: Synapse loss is the major correlate of cognitive impairment. Ann Neurol 1991; 30(4): 572-80. [http://dx.doi.org/10.1002/ana.410300410] [PMID: 1789684]

[13] Alzheimer's Association. 2021 Alzheimer's disease facts and figures. Alzheimers Dement 2021; 17(3): 327-406. [http://dx.doi.org/10.1002/alz.12328] [PMID: 33756057]

[14] Scheltens P, De Strooper B, Kivipelto M, *et al.* Alzheimer's disease. Lancet 2021; 397(10284): 1577-90. [http://dx.doi.org/10.1016/S0140-6736(20)32205-4] [PMID: 33667416]

[15] Reitz C, Rogaeva E, Beecham GW. Late-onset *vs* nonmendelian early-onset Alzheimer disease. Neurol Genet 2020; 6(5): e512. [http://dx.doi.org/10.1212/NXG.0000000000000512] [PMID: 33225065]

[16] Reitz C, Mayeux R. Alzheimer disease: Epidemiology, diagnostic criteria, risk factors and biomarkers. Biochem Pharmacol 2014; 88(4): 640-51. [http://dx.doi.org/10.1016/j.bcp.2013.12.024] [PMID: 24398425]

[17] Cruchaga C, Del-Aguila JL, Saef B, *et al.* Polygenic risk score of sporadic late-onset Alzheimer's disease reveals a shared architecture with the familial and early-onset forms. Alzheimers Dement 2018; 14(2): 205-14. [http://dx.doi.org/10.1016/j.jalz.2017.08.013] [PMID: 28943286]

[18] Mendez MF. Early-onset alzheimer disease and its variants. Continuum (Minneap Minn) 2019; 25(1): 34-51. [http://dx.doi.org/10.1212/CON.0000000000000687] [PMID: 30707186]

[19] Fernández M, Gobartt AL, Balañá M. Behavioural symptoms in patients with Alzheimer's disease and their association with cognitive impairment. BMC Neurol 2010; 10(1): 87. [http://dx.doi.org/10.1186/1471-2377-10-87] [PMID: 20920205]

[20] Lyketsos CG, Carrillo MC, Ryan JM, *et al.* Neuropsychiatric symptoms in Alzheimer's disease. Alzheimers Dement 2011; 7(5): 532-9. [http://dx.doi.org/10.1016/j.jalz.2011.05.2410] [PMID: 21889116]

[21] McEnery MW, Siegel RE. Neurotransmitter receptors. 2nd ed. Oxford: Elsevier Inc. 2014; pp. 552-64.

[22] Araque A, Parpura V, Sanzgiri RP, Haydon PG. Tripartite synapses: glia, the unacknowledged partner. Trends Neurosci 1999; 22(5): 208-15. [http://dx.doi.org/10.1016/S0166-2236(98)01349-6] [PMID: 10322493]

[23] Kandimalla R, Reddy PH. Therapeutics of neurotransmitters in alzheimer's disease. J Alzheimers Dis 2017; 57(4): 1049-69. [http://dx.doi.org/10.3233/JAD-161118] [PMID: 28211810]

[24] Reddy PH. A critical assessment of research on neurotransmitters in alzheimer's disease. J Alzheimers Dis 2017; 57(4): 969-74. [http://dx.doi.org/10.3233/JAD-170256] [PMID: 28409748]

[25] Wong KY, Roy J, Fung ML, Heng BC, Zhang C, Lim LW. Relationships between mitochondrial dysfunction and neurotransmission failure in alzheimer's disease. Aging Dis 2020; 11(5): 1291-316.

[http://dx.doi.org/10.14336/AD.2019.1125] [PMID: 33014538]

[26] Heine M, Heck J, Ciuraszkiewicz A, Bikbaev A. Dynamic compartmentalization of calcium channel signalling in neurons. Neuropharmacology 2020; 169: 107556. [http://dx.doi.org/10.1016/j.neuropharm.2019.02.038] [PMID: 30851307]

[27] Frisardi V, Panza F, Farooqui AA. Late-life depression and Alzheimer's disease: The glutamatergic system inside of this mirror relationship. Brain Res Brain Res Rev 2011; 67(1-2): 344-55. [http://dx.doi.org/10.1016/j.brainresrev.2011.04.003] [PMID: 21570126]

[28] Bouvier M, Szatkowski M, Amato A, Attwell D. The glial cell glutamate uptake carrier countertransports pH-changing anions. Nature 1992; 360(6403): 471-4. [http://dx.doi.org/10.1038/360471a0] [PMID: 1448171]

[29] Clements JD, Lester RAJ, Tong G, Jahr CE, Westbrook GL. The time course of glutamate in the synaptic cleft. Science 1992; 258(5087): 1498-501. [http://dx.doi.org/10.1126/science.1359647] [PMID: 1359647]

[30] Conway ME. Alzheimer's disease: targeting the glutamatergic system. Biogerontology 2020; 21(3): 257-74. [http://dx.doi.org/10.1007/s10522-020-09860-4] [PMID: 32048098]

[31] Walton H, Dodd P. Glutamate–glutamine cycling in Alzheimer's disease. Neurochem Int 2007; 50(7-8): 1052-66. [http://dx.doi.org/10.1016/j.neuint.2006.10.007] [PMID: 17141374]

[32] Hertz L. Functional interactions between neurons and astrocytes I. Turnover and metabolism of putative amino acid transmitters. Prog Neurobiol 1979; 13(3): 277-323. [http://dx.doi.org/10.1016/0301-0082(79)90018-2] [PMID: 42117]

[33] Van Den Berg CJ, Garfinkel D. A simulation study of brain compartments. Metabolism of glutamate and related substances in mouse brain. Biochem J 1971; 123(2): 211-8. [http://dx.doi.org/10.1042/bj1230211] [PMID: 5164952]

[34] Mahan VL. Neurointegrity and europhysiology: astrocyte, glutamate, and carbon monoxide interactions. Med Gas Res 2019; 9(1): 24-45. [http://dx.doi.org/10.4103/2045-9912.254639] [PMID: 30950417]

[35] Meldrum BS. Glutamate as a neurotransmitter in the brain: review of physiology and pathology. J Nutr. 2000; 130(4S Suppl): 1007S-15S.

[36] Miladinovic T, Nashed M, Singh G. Overview of glutamatergic dysregulation in central pathologies. Biomolecules 2015; 5(4): 3112-41. [http://dx.doi.org/10.3390/biom5043112] [PMID: 26569330]

[37] Traynelis SF, Wollmuth LP, McBain CJ, *et al.* Glutamate receptor ion channels: structure, regulation, and function. Pharmacol Rev 2010; 62(3): 405-96. [http://dx.doi.org/10.1124/pr.109.002451] [PMID: 20716669]

[38] Tao W, Ma C, Bemben MA, *et al.* Mechanisms underlying the synaptic trafficking of the glutamate delta receptor GluD1. Mol Psychiatry 2019; 24(10): 1451-60. [http://dx.doi.org/10.1038/s41380-019-0378-4] [PMID: 30824864]

[39] Gabriel L, Lvov A, Orthodoxou D, Rittenhouse AR, Kobertz WR, Melikian HE. The acid-sensitive, anesthetic-activated potassium leak channel, KCNK3, is regulated by 14-3-3β-dependent, protein kinase C (PKC)-mediated endocytic trafficking. J Biol Chem 2012; 287(39): 32354-66. [http://dx.doi.org/10.1074/jbc.M112.391458] [PMID: 22846993]

[40] Song J, Yang X, Zhang M, Wang C, Chen L. Glutamate metabolism in mitochondria is closely related to alzheimer's disease. J Alzheimers Dis 2021; 84(2): 557-78. [http://dx.doi.org/10.3233/JAD-210595] [PMID: 34602474]

[41] Miyamoto E. Molecular mechanism of neuronal plasticity: induction and maintenance of long-term

potentiation in the hippocampus. J Pharmacol Sci 2006; 100(5): 433-42. [http://dx.doi.org/10.1254/jphs.CPJ06007X] [PMID: 16799259]

[42] Barnes JR, Mukherjee B, Rogers BC, Nafar F, Gosse M, Parsons MP. The relationship between glutamate dynamics and activity-dependent synaptic plasticity. J Neurosci 2020; 40(14): 2793-807. [http://dx.doi.org/10.1523/JNEUROSCI.1655-19.2020] [PMID: 32102922]

[43] Balschun D, Wetzel W. Inhibition of mGluR5 blocks hippocampal LTP *in vivo* and spatial learning in rats. Pharmacol Biochem Behav 2002; 73(2): 375-80. [http://dx.doi.org/10.1016/S0091-3057(02)00847-X] [PMID: 12117592]

[44] Peng S, Zhang Y, Zhang J, Wang H, Ren B. Glutamate receptors and signal transduction in learning and memory. Mol Biol Rep 2011; 38(1): 453-60. [http://dx.doi.org/10.1007/s11033-010-0128-9] [PMID: 20364330]

[45] Sieber SA, Marahiel MA. Molecular mechanisms underlying nonribosomal peptide synthesis: approaches to new antibiotics. Chem Rev 2005; 105(2): 715-38. [http://dx.doi.org/10.1021/cr0301191] [PMID: 15700962]

[46] Jansson LC, Louhivuori L, Wigren HK, *et al.* Effect of glutamate receptor antagonists on migrating neural progenitor cells. Eur J Neurosci 2013; 37(9): 1369-82. [http://dx.doi.org/10.1111/ejn.12152] [PMID: 23383979]

[47] Freidman N, Chen I, Wu Q, *et al.* Amino acid transporters and exchangers from the SLC1A family: Structure, mechanism and roles in physiology and cancer. Neurochem Res 2020; 45(6): 1268-86. [http://dx.doi.org/10.1007/s11064-019-02934-x] [PMID: 31981058]

[48] Grewer C, Gameiro A, Rauen T. SLC1 glutamate transporters. Pflugers Arch 2014; 466(1): 3-24. [http://dx.doi.org/10.1007/s00424-013-1397-7] [PMID: 24240778]

[49] Verkhratsky A, Parpura V, Vardjan N, Zorec R. Physiology of Astroglia. Adv Exp Med Biol 2019; 1175: 45-91. [http://dx.doi.org/10.1007/978-981-13-9913-8_3] [PMID: 31583584]

[50] Danbolt NC. Glutamate uptake. Prog Neurobiol 2001; 65(1): 1-105. [http://dx.doi.org/10.1016/S0301-0082(00)00067-8] [PMID: 11369436]

[51] Zerangue N, Kavanaugh MP. Flux coupling in a neuronal glutamate transporter. Nature 1996; 383(6601): 634-7. [http://dx.doi.org/10.1038/383634a0] [PMID: 8857541]

[52] de Wit H, Walter AM, Milosevic I, *et al.* Synaptotagmin-1 docks secretory vesicles to syntaxin-1/SNAP-25 acceptor complexes. Cell 2009; 138(5): 935-46. [http://dx.doi.org/10.1016/j.cell.2009.07.027] [PMID: 19716167]

[53] Han J, Pluhackova K, Böckmann RA. The multifaceted role of SNARE proteins in membrane fusion. Front Physiol 2017; 8: 5. [http://dx.doi.org/10.3389/fphys.2017.00005] [PMID: 28163686]

[54] Crippa D, Schenk U, Francolini M, *et al.* Synaptobrevin2-expressing vesicles in rat astrocytes: insights into molecular characterization, dynamics and exocytosis. J Physiol 2006; 570(3): 567-82. [http://dx.doi.org/10.1113/jphysiol.2005.094052] [PMID: 16322057]

[55] Jeftinija SD, Jeftinija KV, Stefanovic G. Cultured astrocytes express proteins involved in vesicular glutamate release. Brain Res 1997; 750(1-2): 41-7. [http://dx.doi.org/10.1016/S0006-8993(96)00610-5] [PMID: 9098527]

[56] Guerra-Gomes S, Sousa N, Pinto L, Oliveira JF. Functional roles of astrocyte calcium elevations: From synapses to behavior. Front Cell Neurosci 2018; 11: 427. [http://dx.doi.org/10.3389/fncel.2017.00427] [PMID: 29386997]

[57] Lalo U, Rasooli-Nejad S, Bogdanov A, More L, Koh W, Muller J, *et al.* Synergy between vesicular and non-vesicular gliotransmission regulates synaptic plasticity and working memory. bioRxiv 2021.

[58] Woo DH, Han KS, Shim JW, *et al.* TREK-1 and Best1 channels mediate fast and slow glutamate release in astrocytes upon GPCR activation. Cell 2012; 151(1): 25-40. [http://dx.doi.org/10.1016/j.cell.2012.09.005] [PMID: 23021213]

[59] Lakhan SE, Caro M, Hadzimichalis N. NMDA receptor activity in neuropsychiatric disorders. Front Psychiatry 2013; 4: 52. [http://dx.doi.org/10.3389/fpsyt.2013.00052] [PMID: 23772215]

[60] Mony L, Paoletti P. Mechanisms of NMDA receptor regulation. Curr Opin Neurobiol 2023; 83: 102815. [http://dx.doi.org/10.1016/j.conb.2023.102815] [PMID: 37988826]

[61] Schorge S, Elenes S, Colquhoun D. Maximum likelihood fitting of single channel NMDA activity with a mechanism composed of independent dimers of subunits. J Physiol 2005; 569(2): 395-418. [http://dx.doi.org/10.1113/jphysiol.2005.095349] [PMID: 16223763]

[62] Ulbrich MH, Isacoff EY. Rules of engagement for NMDA receptor subunits. Proc Natl Acad Sci USA 2008; 105(37): 14163-8. [http://dx.doi.org/10.1073/pnas.0802075105] [PMID: 18779583]

[63] Salussolia CL, Prodromou ML, Borker P, Wollmuth LP. Arrangement of subunits in functional NMDA receptors. J Neurosci. 2011 Aug 3; 31(31): 11295-304.

[64] Henneberger C, Papouin T, Oliet SHR, Rusakov DA. Long-term potentiation depends on release of d-serine from astrocytes. Nature 2010; 463(7278): 232-6. [http://dx.doi.org/10.1038/nature08673] [PMID: 20075918]

[65] Jimenez-Blasco D, Santofimia-Castaño P, Gonzalez A, Almeida A, Bolaños JP. Astrocyte NMDA receptors' activity sustains neuronal survival through a Cdk5–Nrf2 pathway. Cell Death Differ 2015; 22(11): 1877-89. [http://dx.doi.org/10.1038/cdd.2015.49] [PMID: 25909891]

[66] Hardy J. A hundred years of Alzheimer's disease research. Neuron 2006; 52(1): 3-13. [http://dx.doi.org/10.1016/j.neuron.2006.09.016] [PMID: 17015223]

[67] Higgins GA, Silenieks LB, MacMillan C, Sevo J, Zeeb FD, Thevarkunnel S. Enhanced attention and impulsive action following NMDA receptor GluN2B-selective antagonist pretreatment. Behav Brain Res 2016; 311: 1-14. [http://dx.doi.org/10.1016/j.bbr.2016.05.025] [PMID: 27180168]

[68] Conti F, DeBiasi S, Minelli A, Melone M. Expression of NR1 and NR2A/B subunits of the NMDA receptor in cortical astrocytes. Glia 1996; 17(3): 254-8. [http://dx.doi.org/10.1002/(SICI)1098-1136(199607)17:3<254::AID-GLIA7>3.0.CO;2-0] [PMID: 8840166]

[69] Luque JM, Richards JG. Expression of NMDA 2B receptor subunit mRNA in bergmann glia. Glia 1995; 13(3): 228-32. [http://dx.doi.org/10.1002/glia.440130309] [PMID: 7782108]

[70] Alsaad HA, DeKorver NW, Mao Z, Dravid SM, Arikkath J, Monaghan DT. In the telencephalon, GluN2C NMDA receptor subunit mRNA is predominately expressed in glial cells and GluN2D mRNA in interneurons. Neurochem Res 2019; 44(1): 61-77. [http://dx.doi.org/10.1007/s11064-018-2526-7] [PMID: 29651654]

[71] Palygin O, Lalo U, Pankratov Y. Distinct pharmacological and functional properties of NMDA receptors in mouse cortical astrocytes. Br J Pharmacol 2011; 163(8): 1755-66. [http://dx.doi.org/10.1111/j.1476-5381.2011.01374.x] [PMID: 21449975]

[72] Chan PH, Kerlan R, Fishman RA. Reductions of gamma-aminobutyric acid and glutamate uptake and (Na+ + K+)-ATPase activity in brain slices and synaptosomes by arachidonic acid. J Neurochem 1983; 40(2): 309-16. [http://dx.doi.org/10.1111/j.1471-4159.1983.tb11284.x] [PMID: 6130123]

[73] Bourinet E, Altier C, Hildebrand ME, Trang T, Salter MW, Zamponi GW. Calcium-permeable ion channels in pain signaling. Physiol Rev 2014; 94(1): 81-140. [http://dx.doi.org/10.1152/physrev.00023.2013] [PMID: 24382884]

[74] Paoletti P, Bellone C, Zhou Q. NMDA receptor subunit diversity: impact on receptor properties, synaptic plasticity and disease. Nat Rev Neurosci 2013; 14(6): 383-400. [http://dx.doi.org/10.1038/nrn3504] [PMID: 23686171]

[75] Horak M, Petralia RS, Kaniakova M, Sans N. ER to synapse trafficking of NMDA receptors. Front Cell Neurosci 2014; 8: 394. [http://dx.doi.org/10.3389/fncel.2014.00394] [PMID: 25505872]

[76] Lussier MP, Sanz-Clemente A, Roche KW. Dynamic regulation of n-methyl-d-aspartate (NMDA) and α-amino-3-hydroxy-5-methyl-4-isoxazolepropionic acid (AMPA) receptors by posttranslational modifications. J Biol Chem 2015; 290(48): 28596-603. [http://dx.doi.org/10.1074/jbc.R115.652750] [PMID: 26453298]

[77] Lau CG, Zukin RS. NMDA receptor trafficking in synaptic plasticity and neuropsychiatric disorders. Nat Rev Neurosci 2007; 8(6): 413-26. [http://dx.doi.org/10.1038/nrn2153] [PMID: 17514195]

[78] Furukawa H, Gouaux E. Mechanisms of activation, inhibition and specificity: crystal structures of the NMDA receptor NR1 ligand-binding core. EMBO J 2003; 22(12): 2873-85. [http://dx.doi.org/10.1093/emboj/cdg303] [PMID: 12805203]

[79] Furukawa H, Singh SK, Mancusso R, Gouaux E. Subunit arrangement and function in NMDA receptors. Nature 2005; 438(7065): 185-92. [http://dx.doi.org/10.1038/nature04089] [PMID: 16281028]

[80] Karakas E, Simorowski N, Furukawa H. Subunit arrangement and phenylethanolamine binding in GluN1/GluN2B NMDA receptors. Nature 2011; 475(7355): 249-53. [http://dx.doi.org/10.1038/nature10180] [PMID: 21677647]

[81] Monyer H, Burnashev N, Laurie DJ, Sakmann B, Seeburg PH. Developmental and regional expression in the rat brain and functional properties of four NMDA receptors. Neuron 1994; 12(3): 529-40. [http://dx.doi.org/10.1016/0896-6273(94)90210-0] [PMID: 7512349]

[82] Akazawa C, Shigemoto R, Bessho Y, Nakanishi S, Mizuno N. Differential expression of five N-methyl-D-aspartate receptor subunit mRNAs in the cerebellum of developing and adult rats. J Comp Neurol 1994; 347(1): 150-60. [http://dx.doi.org/10.1002/cne.903470112] [PMID: 7798379]

[83] Laurie DJ, Seeburg PH. Regional and developmental heterogeneity in splicing of the rat brain NMDAR1 mRNA. J Neurosci 1994; 14(5): 3180-94. [http://dx.doi.org/10.1523/JNEUROSCI.14-05-03180.1994] [PMID: 8182465]

[84] Sheng M, Cummings J, Roldan LA, Jan YN, Jan LY. Changing subunit composition of heteromeric NMDA receptors during development of rat cortex. Nature 1994; 368(6467): 144-7. [http://dx.doi.org/10.1038/368144a0] [PMID: 8139656]

[85] Baron R, Binder A, Wasner G. Neuropathic pain: diagnosis, pathophysiological mechanisms, and treatment. Lancet Neurol 2010; 9(8): 807-19. [http://dx.doi.org/10.1016/S1474-4422(10)70143-5] [PMID: 20650402]

[86] Nickel FT, Seifert F, Lanz S, Maihöfner C. Mechanisms of neuropathic pain. Eur Neuropsychopharmacol 2012; 22(2): 81-91. [http://dx.doi.org/10.1016/j.euroneuro.2011.05.005] [PMID: 21672666]

[87] Latremoliere A, Woolf CJ. Central sensitization: a generator of pain hypersensitivity by central neural plasticity. J Pain 2009; 10(9): 895-926. [http://dx.doi.org/10.1016/j.jpain.2009.06.012] [PMID: 19712899]

[88] Dickson DW. Neuropathology of Parkinson disease. Parkinsonism RelatDisord. 2018 Jan; 46 Suppl 1(Suppl 1):S30-S33.
[http://dx.doi.org/10.1016/j.parkreldis.2017.07.033]

[89] Cohen SM, Tsien RW, Goff DC, Halassa MM. The impact of NMDA receptor hypofunction on GABAergic neurons in the pathophysiology of schizophrenia. Schizophr Res 2015; 167(1-3): 98-107.
[http://dx.doi.org/10.1016/j.schres.2014.12.026] [PMID: 25583246]

[90] Nakazawa K, Jeevakumar V, Nakao K. Spatial and temporal boundaries of NMDA receptor hypofunction leading to schizophrenia. NPJ Schizophr 2017; 3(1): 7.
[http://dx.doi.org/10.1038/s41537-016-0003-3] [PMID: 28560253]

[91] von Engelhardt J, Bocklisch C, Tönges L, Herb A, Mishina M, Monyer H. GluN2D-containing NMDA receptors-mediate synaptic currents in hippocampal interneurons and pyramidal cells in juvenile mice. Front Cell Neurosci 2015; 9: 95.
[http://dx.doi.org/10.3389/fncel.2015.00095] [PMID: 25859181]

[92] Standaert DG, Bernhard Landwehrmeyer G, Kerner JA, Penney JB Jr, Young AB. Expression of NMDAR2D glutamate receptor subunit mRNA in neurochemically identified interneurons in the rat neostriatum, neocortex and hippocampus. Brain Res Mol Brain Res 1996; 42(1): 89-102.
[http://dx.doi.org/10.1016/S0169-328X(96)00117-9] [PMID: 8915584]

[93] Collingridge GL, Bliss TVP. Memories of NMDA receptors and LTP. Trends Neurosci 1995; 18(2): 54-6.
[http://dx.doi.org/10.1016/0166-2236(95)80016-U] [PMID: 7537406]

[94] Butler AK, Uryu K, Chesselet MF. A role for N-methyl-D-aspartate receptors in the regulation of synaptogenesis and expression of the polysialylated form of the neural cell adhesion molecule in the developing striatum. Dev Neurosci 1998; 20(2-3): 253-62.
[http://dx.doi.org/10.1159/000017319] [PMID: 9691199]

[95] Chen BS, Roche KW. Regulation of NMDA receptors by phosphorylation. Neuropharmacology 2007; 53(3): 362-8.
[http://dx.doi.org/10.1016/j.neuropharm.2007.05.018] [PMID: 17644144]

[96] Rebola N, Srikumar BN, Mulle C. Activity-dependent synaptic plasticity of NMDA receptors. J Physiol 2010; 588(1): 93-9.
[http://dx.doi.org/10.1113/jphysiol.2009.179382] [PMID: 19822542]

[97] Mao J, Price DD, Mayer DJ. Thermal hyperalgesia in association with the development of morphine tolerance in rats: roles of excitatory amino acid receptors and protein kinase C. J Neurosci 1994; 14(4): 2301-12.
[http://dx.doi.org/10.1523/JNEUROSCI.14-04-02301.1994] [PMID: 7908958]

[98] Lan J, Skeberdis VA, Jover T, *et al.* Protein kinase C modulates NMDA receptor trafficking and gating. Nat Neurosci 2001; 4(4): 382-90.
[http://dx.doi.org/10.1038/86028] [PMID: 11276228]

[99] Hansen KB, Ogden KK, Yuan H, Traynelis SF. Distinct functional and pharmacological properties of triheteromeric GluN1/GluN2A/GluN2B NMDA receptors. Neuron 2014; 81(5): 1084-96.
[http://dx.doi.org/10.1016/j.neuron.2014.01.035] [PMID: 24607230]

[100] Tajima N, Karakas E, Grant T, *et al.* Activation of NMDA receptors and the mechanism of inhibition by ifenprodil. Nature 2016; 534(7605): 63-8.
[http://dx.doi.org/10.1038/nature17679] [PMID: 27135925]

[101] Twomey EC, Sobolevsky AI. Structural mechanisms of gating in ionotropic glutamate receptors. Biochemistry 2018; 57(3): 267-76.
[http://dx.doi.org/10.1021/acs.biochem.7b00891] [PMID: 29037031]

[102] Hansen KB, Wollmuth LP, Bowie D, *et al.* Structure, function, and pharmacology of glutamate receptor ion channels. Pharmacol Rev 2021; 73(4): 1469-658.

[http://dx.doi.org/10.1124/pharmrev.120.000131] [PMID: 34753794]

[103] Gutierrez BA, Limon A. Synaptic disruption by soluble oligomers in patients with Alzheimer's and Parkinson's disease. Biomedicines 2022; 10(7): 1743. [http://dx.doi.org/10.3390/biomedicines10071743] [PMID: 35885050]

[104] Wang R, Reddy PH. Role of glutamate and NMDA receptors in Alzheimer's disease. J Alzheimers Dis 2017; 57(4): 1041-8. [http://dx.doi.org/10.3233/JAD-160763] [PMID: 27662322]

[105] Hiruma H, Katakura T, Takahashi S, Ichikawa T, Kawakami T. Glutamate and amyloid β-protein rapidly inhibit fast axonal transport in cultured rat hippocampal neurons by different mechanisms. J Neurosci 2003; 23(26): 8967-77. [http://dx.doi.org/10.1523/JNEUROSCI.23-26-08967.2003] [PMID: 14523099]

[106] Kopeikina K, Hyman B, Spires-Jones T. Soluble forms of tau are toxic in Alzheimer's disease. Transl Neurosci 2012; 3(3): 223-33. [http://dx.doi.org/10.2478/s13380-012-0032-y] [PMID: 23029602]

[107] Walsh DM, Klyubin I, Fadeeva JV, *et al.* Naturally secreted oligomers of amyloid β protein potently inhibit hippocampal long-term potentiation *in vivo*. Nature 2002; 416(6880): 535-9. [http://dx.doi.org/10.1038/416535a] [PMID: 11932745]

[108] Wang HW, Pasternak JF, Kuo H, *et al.* Soluble oligomers of β amyloid (1-42) inhibit long-term potentiation but not long-term depression in rat dentate gyrus. Brain Res 2002; 924(2): 133-40. [http://dx.doi.org/10.1016/S0006-8993(01)03058-X] [PMID: 11750898]

[109] Barghorn S, Nimmrich V, Striebinger A, *et al.* Globular amyloid β-peptide $_{1-42}$ oligomer – a homogenous and stable neuropathological protein in Alzheimer's disease. J Neurochem 2005; 95(3): 834-47. [http://dx.doi.org/10.1111/j.1471-4159.2005.03407.x] [PMID: 16135089]

[110] Cleary JP, Walsh DM, Hofmeister JJ, *et al.* Natural oligomers of the amyloid-β protein specifically disrupt cognitive function. Nat Neurosci 2005; 8(1): 79-84. [http://dx.doi.org/10.1038/nn1372] [PMID: 15608634]

[111] Selkoe DJ. Soluble oligomers of the amyloid β-protein impair synaptic plasticity and behavior. Behav Brain Res 2008; 192(1): 106-13. [http://dx.doi.org/10.1016/j.bbr.2008.02.016] [PMID: 18359102]

[112] Ferreira ST, Klein WL. The Aβ oligomer hypothesis for synapse failure and memory loss in Alzheimer's disease. Neurobiol Learn Mem 2011; 96(4): 529-43. [http://dx.doi.org/10.1016/j.nlm.2011.08.003] [PMID: 21914486]

[113] Hascup ER, Broderick SO, Russell MK, *et al.* Diet-induced insulin resistance elevates hippocampal glutamate as well as VGLUT 1 and GFAP expression in Aβ PP / PS 1 mice. J Neurochem 2019; 148(2): 219-37. [http://dx.doi.org/10.1111/jnc.14634] [PMID: 30472734]

[114] Bell KFS, Bennett DA, Cuello AC. Paradoxical upregulation of glutamatergic presynaptic boutons during mild cognitive impairment. J Neurosci 2007; 27(40): 10810-7. [http://dx.doi.org/10.1523/JNEUROSCI.3269-07.2007] [PMID: 17913914]

[115] Grutzendler J, Helmin K, Tsai J, Gan WB. Various dendritic abnormalities are associated with fibrillar amyloid deposits in Alzheimer's disease. Ann N Y Acad Sci 2007; 1097(1): 30-9. [http://dx.doi.org/10.1196/annals.1379.003] [PMID: 17413007]

[116] Šišková Z, Justus D, Kaneko H, *et al.* Dendritic structural degeneration is functionally linked to cellular hyperexcitability in a mouse model of Alzheimer's disease. Neuron 2014; 84(5): 1023-33. [http://dx.doi.org/10.1016/j.neuron.2014.10.024] [PMID: 25456500]

[117] Hascup KN, Hascup ER. Altered neurotransmission prior to cognitive decline in AβPP/PS1 mice, a model of Alzheimer's disease. J Alzheimers Dis 2015; 44(3): 771-6.

[http://dx.doi.org/10.3233/JAD-142160] [PMID: 25374106]

[118] Kamenetz F, Tomita T, Hsieh H, *et al.* APP processing and synaptic function. Neuron 2003; 37(6): 925-37.
[http://dx.doi.org/10.1016/S0896-6273(03)00124-7] [PMID: 12670422]

[119] Snyder EM, Nong Y, Almeida CG, *et al.* Regulation of NMDA receptor trafficking by amyloid-β. Nat Neurosci 2005; 8(8): 1051-8.
[http://dx.doi.org/10.1038/nn1503] [PMID: 16025111]

[120] Li Y, Chang L, Song Y, *et al.* Astrocytic GluN2A and GluN2B oppose the synaptotoxic effects of amyloid-β 1-40 in hippocampal cells. J Alzheimers Dis 2016; 54(1): 135-48.
[http://dx.doi.org/10.3233/JAD-160297] [PMID: 27497478]

[121] Ferreira IL, Bajouco LM, Mota SI, Auberson YP, Oliveira CR, Rego AC. Amyloid beta peptide 1–42 disturbs intracellular calcium homeostasis through activation of GluN2B-containing N-methyl-d-aspartate receptors in cortical cultures. Cell Calcium 2012; 51(2): 95-106.
[http://dx.doi.org/10.1016/j.ceca.2011.11.008] [PMID: 22177709]

[122] Shi XD, Sun K, Hu R, *et al.* Blocking the interaction between EphB2 and ADDLs by a small peptide rescues impaired synaptic plasticity and memory deficits in a mouse model of Alzheimer's disease. J Neurosci 2016; 36(47): 11959-73.
[http://dx.doi.org/10.1523/JNEUROSCI.1327-16.2016] [PMID: 27881781]

[123] Danysz W, Parsons CG. Alzheimer's disease, β-amyloid, glutamate, NMDA receptors and memantine – searching for the connections. Br J Pharmacol 2012; 167(2): 324-52.
[http://dx.doi.org/10.1111/j.1476-5381.2012.02057.x] [PMID: 22646481]

[124] Dalva MB, Takasu MA, Lin MZ, *et al.* EphB receptors interact with NMDA receptors and regulate excitatory synapse formation. Cell 2000; 103(6): 945-56.
[http://dx.doi.org/10.1016/S0092-8674(00)00197-5] [PMID: 11136979]

[125] Hu NW, Klyubin I, Anwyl R, Rowan MJ. GluN2B subunit-containing NMDA receptor antagonists prevent Aβ-mediated synaptic plasticity disruption *in vivo*. Proc Natl Acad Sci USA 2009; 106(48): 20504-9.
[http://dx.doi.org/10.1073/pnas.0908083106] [PMID: 19918059]

[126] Li S, Jin M, Koeglsperger T, Shepardson NE, Shankar GM, Selkoe DJ. Soluble Aβ oligomers inhibit long-term potentiation through a mechanism involving excessive activation of extrasynaptic NR2B-containing NMDA receptors. J Neurosci 2011; 31(18): 6627-38.
[http://dx.doi.org/10.1523/JNEUROSCI.0203-11.2011] [PMID: 21543591]

[127] Lesné S, Ali C, Gabriel C, *et al.* NMDA receptor activation inhibits α-secretase and promotes neuronal amyloid-β production. J Neurosci 2005; 25(41): 9367-77.
[http://dx.doi.org/10.1523/JNEUROSCI.0849-05.2005] [PMID: 16221845]

[128] Bordji K, Becerril-Ortega J, Nicole O, Buisson A. Activation of extrasynaptic, but not synaptic, NMDA receptors modifies amyloid precursor protein expression pattern and increases amyloid-ß production. J Neurosci 2010; 30(47): 15927-42.
[http://dx.doi.org/10.1523/JNEUROSCI.3021-10.2010] [PMID: 21106831]

[129] Hoey SE, Williams RJ, Perkinton MS. Synaptic NMDA receptor activation stimulates α-secretase amyloid precursor protein processing and inhibits amyloid-β production. J Neurosci 2009; 29(14): 4442-60.
[http://dx.doi.org/10.1523/JNEUROSCI.6017-08.2009] [PMID: 19357271]

[130] Verges DK, Restivo JL, Goebel WD, Holtzman DM, Cirrito JR. Opposing synaptic regulation of amyloid-β metabolism by NMDA receptors *in vivo*. J Neurosci 2011; 31(31): 11328-37.
[http://dx.doi.org/10.1523/JNEUROSCI.0607-11.2011] [PMID: 21813692]

[131] Rönicke R, Mikhaylova M, Rönicke S, *et al.* Early neuronal dysfunction by amyloid β oligomers depends on activation of NR2B-containing NMDA receptors. Neurobiol Aging 2011; 32(12): 2219-28.

[http://dx.doi.org/10.1016/j.neurobiolaging.2010.01.011] [PMID: 20133015]

[132] Shankar GM, Bloodgood BL, Townsend M, Walsh DM, Selkoe DJ, Sabatini BL. Natural oligomers of the Alzheimer amyloid-β protein induce reversible synapse loss by modulating an NMDA-type glutamate receptor-dependent signaling pathway. J Neurosci 2007; 27(11): 2866-75. [http://dx.doi.org/10.1523/JNEUROSCI.4970-06.2007] [PMID: 17360908]

[133] Mishizen-Eberz AJ, Rissman RA, Carter TL, Ikonomovic MD, Wolfe BB, Armstrong DM. Biochemical and molecular studies of NMDA receptor subunits NR1/2A/2B in hippocampal subregions throughout progression of Alzheimer's disease pathology. Neurobiol Dis 2004; 15(1): 80-92. [http://dx.doi.org/10.1016/j.nbd.2003.09.016] [PMID: 14751773]

[134] Liu Y, Wong TP, Aarts M, *et al.* NMDA receptor subunits have differential roles in mediating excitotoxic neuronal death both *in vitro* and *in vivo*. J Neurosci 2007; 27(11): 2846-57. [http://dx.doi.org/10.1523/JNEUROSCI.0116-07.2007] [PMID: 17360906]

[135] Meur S, Karati D. Fyn kinase in alzheimer's disease: unraveling molecular mechanisms and therapeutic implications. Mol Neurobiol 2024; 62(1): 643-60. [PMID: 38890236]

[136] Hoover BR, Reed MN, Su J, *et al.* Tau mislocalization to dendritic spines mediates synaptic dysfunction independently of neurodegeneration. Neuron 2010; 68(6): 1067-81. [http://dx.doi.org/10.1016/j.neuron.2010.11.030] [PMID: 21172610]

[137] Mondragón-Rodríguez S, Trillaud-Doppia E, Dudilot A, *et al.* Interaction of endogenous tau protein with synaptic proteins is regulated by N-methyl-D-aspartate receptor-dependent tau phosphorylation. J Biol Chem 2012; 287(38): 32040-53. [http://dx.doi.org/10.1074/jbc.M112.401240] [PMID: 22833681]

[138] Chen Q, Zhou Z, Zhang L, *et al.* Tau protein is involved in morphological plasticity in hippocampal neurons in response to BDNF. Neurochem Int 2012; 60(3): 233-42. [http://dx.doi.org/10.1016/j.neuint.2011.12.013] [PMID: 22226842]

[139] Ittner LM, Ke YD, Delerue F, *et al.* Dendritic function of tau mediates amyloid-β toxicity in Alzheimer's disease mouse models. Cell 2010; 142(3): 387-97. [http://dx.doi.org/10.1016/j.cell.2010.06.036] [PMID: 20655099]

[140] Amadoro G, Ciotti MT, Costanzi M, Cestari V, Calissano P, Canu N. NMDA receptor mediates tau-induced neurotoxicity by calpain and ERK/MAPK activation. Proc Natl Acad Sci USA 2006; 103(8): 2892-7. [http://dx.doi.org/10.1073/pnas.0511065103] [PMID: 16477009]

[141] Song MS, Rauw G, Baker GB, Kar S. Memantine protects rat cortical cultured neurons against β-amyloid-induced toxicity by attenuating tau phosphorylation. Eur J Neurosci 2008; 28(10): 1989-2002. [http://dx.doi.org/10.1111/j.1460-9568.2008.06498.x] [PMID: 19046381]

[142] De Montigny A, Elhiri I, Allyson J, Cyr M, Massicotte G. NMDA reduces Tau phosphorylation in rat hippocampal slices by targeting NR2A receptors, GSK3β, and PKC activities. Neural Plast 2013; 2013(1): 261593. [http://dx.doi.org/10.1155/2013/261593] [PMID: 24349798]

[143] Reifert J, Hartung-Cranston D, Feinstein SC. Amyloid β-mediated cell death of cultured hippocampal neurons reveals extensive Tau fragmentation without increased full-length tau phosphorylation. J Biol Chem 2011; 286(23): 20797-811. [http://dx.doi.org/10.1074/jbc.M111.234674] [PMID: 21482827]

[144] Hogan-Cann AD, Anderson CM. Physiological roles of non-neuronal NMDA receptors. Trends Pharmacol Sci 2016; 37(9): 750-67. [http://dx.doi.org/10.1016/j.tips.2016.05.012] [PMID: 27338838]

[145] Lee MC, Ting KK, Adams S, Brew BJ, Chung R, Guillemin GJ. Characterisation of the expression of

NMDA receptors in human astrocytes. PLoS One 2010; 5(11): e14123.
[http://dx.doi.org/10.1371/journal.pone.0014123] [PMID: 21152063]

[146] Kato H, Narita M, Miyatake M, Yajima Y, Suzuki T. Role of neuronal NR2B subunit-containing NMDA receptor-mediated (Ca^{2+}) influx and astrocytic activation in cultured mouse cortical neurons and astrocytes. Synapse 2006; 59(1): 10-7.
[http://dx.doi.org/10.1002/syn.20213] [PMID: 16235228]

[147] Lalo U, Pankratov Y, Kirchhoff F, North RA, Verkhratsky A. NMDA receptors mediate neuron-t--glia signaling in mouse cortical astrocytes. J Neurosci 2006; 26(10): 2673-83.
[http://dx.doi.org/10.1523/JNEUROSCI.4689-05.2006] [PMID: 16525046]

[148] Mota SI, Ferreira IL, Rego AC. Dysfunctional synapse in Alzheimer's disease – A focus on NMDA receptors. Neuropharmacology 2014; 76(Pt A): 16-26.
[http://dx.doi.org/10.1016/j.neuropharm.2013.08.013] [PMID: 23973316]

[149] Franco R, Aguinaga D, Reyes I, *et al.* N-methyl-D-aspartate receptor link to the MAP kinase pathway in cortical and hippocampal neurons and microglia is dependent on calcium sensors and is blocked by α-Synuclein, Tau, and Phospho-Tau in non-transgenic and transgenic APPSw, Ind mice. Front Mol Neurosci 2018; 11: 273.
[http://dx.doi.org/10.3389/fnmol.2018.00273] [PMID: 30233307]

[150] Corlew R, Wang Y, Ghermazien H, Erisir A, Philpot BD. Developmental switch in the contribution of presynaptic and postsynaptic NMDA receptors to long-term depression. J Neurosci 2007; 27(37): 9835-45.
[http://dx.doi.org/10.1523/JNEUROSCI.5494-06.2007] [PMID: 17855598]

[151] Banerjee A, Larsen RS, Philpot BD, Paulsen O. Roles of presynaptic NMDA receptors in neurotransmission and plasticity. Trends Neurosci 2016; 39(1): 26-39.
[http://dx.doi.org/10.1016/j.tins.2015.11.001] [PMID: 26726120]

[152] Dore K, Stein IS, Brock JA, Castillo PE, Zito K, Sjöström PJ. Unconventional NMDA receptor signaling. J Neurosci 2017; 37(45): 10800-7.
[http://dx.doi.org/10.1523/JNEUROSCI.1825-17.2017] [PMID: 29118208]

[153] Kunz PA, Roberts AC, Philpot BD. Presynaptic NMDA receptor mechanisms for enhancing spontaneous neurotransmitter release. J Neurosci 2013; 33(18): 7762-9.
[http://dx.doi.org/10.1523/JNEUROSCI.2482-12.2013] [PMID: 23637168]

[154] Abrahamsson T, Chou CYC, Li SY, *et al.* Differential regulation of evoked and spontaneous release by presynaptic NMDA receptors. Neuron 2017; 96(4): 839-855.e5.
[http://dx.doi.org/10.1016/j.neuron.2017.09.030] [PMID: 29033205]

[155] Bouvier G, Larsen RS, Rodríguez-Moreno A, Paulsen O, Sjöström PJ. Towards resolving the presynaptic NMDA receptor debate. Curr Opin Neurobiol 2018; 51: 1-7.
[http://dx.doi.org/10.1016/j.conb.2017.12.020] [PMID: 29454833]

[156] McGuinness L, Taylor C, Taylor RDT, *et al.* Presynaptic NMDARs in the hippocampus facilitate transmitter release at theta frequency. Neuron 2010; 68(6): 1109-27.
[http://dx.doi.org/10.1016/j.neuron.2010.11.023] [PMID: 21172613]

[157] Park H, Popescu A, Poo M. Essential role of presynaptic NMDA receptors in activity-dependent BDNF secretion and corticostriatal LTP. Neuron 2014; 84(5): 1009-22.
[http://dx.doi.org/10.1016/j.neuron.2014.10.045] [PMID: 25467984]

[158] Kessels HW, Nabavi S, Malinow R. Metabotropic NMDA receptor function is required for β-amyloid–induced synaptic depression. Proc Natl Acad Sci USA 2013; 110(10): 4033-8.
[http://dx.doi.org/10.1073/pnas.1219605110] [PMID: 23431156]

[159] Nabavi S, Kessels HW, Alfonso S, Aow J, Fox R, Malinow R. Metabotropic NMDA receptor function is required for NMDA receptor-dependent long-term depression. Proc Natl Acad Sci USA 2013; 110(10): 4027-32.

[http://dx.doi.org/10.1073/pnas.1219454110] [PMID: 23431133]

[160] Stein IS, Gray JA, Zito K. Non-ionotropic NMDA receptor signaling drives activity-induced dendritic spine shrinkage. J Neurosci 2015; 35(35): 12303-8.
[http://dx.doi.org/10.1523/JNEUROSCI.4289-14.2015] [PMID: 26338340]

[161] Gray JA, Zito K, Hell JW. Non-ionotropic signaling by the NMDA receptor: controversy and opportunity. F1000 Res 2016; 5: 1010.
[http://dx.doi.org/10.12688/f1000research.8366.1] [PMID: 27303637]

[162] Sanders EM, Nyarko-Odoom AO, Zhao K, *et al.* Separate functional properties of NMDARs regulate distinct aspects of spatial cognition. Learn Mem 2018; 25(6): 264-72.
[http://dx.doi.org/10.1101/lm.047290.118] [PMID: 29764972]

[163] Carter BC, Jahr CE. Postsynaptic, not presynaptic NMDA receptors are required for spike-timin--dependent LTD induction. Nat Neurosci 2016; 19(9): 1218-24.
[http://dx.doi.org/10.1038/nn.4343] [PMID: 27399842]

[164] Chung C. NMDA receptor as a newly identified member of the metabotropic glutamate receptor family: clinical implications for neurodegenerative diseases. Mol Cells 2013; 36(2): 99-104.
[http://dx.doi.org/10.1007/s10059-013-0113-y] [PMID: 23740429]

[165] Montes de Oca Balderas P, Aguilera P. A metabotropic-like flux-independent NMDA receptor regulates (Ca^{2+}) exit from endoplasmic reticulum and mitochondrial membrane potential in cultured astrocytes. PLoS One 2015; 10(5): e0126314.
[http://dx.doi.org/10.1371/journal.pone.0126314] [PMID: 25954808]

[166] Tamburri A, Dudilot A, Licea S, Bourgeois C, Boehm J. NMDA-receptor activation but not ion flux is required for amyloid-beta induced synaptic depression. PLoS One 2013; 8(6): e65350.
[http://dx.doi.org/10.1371/journal.pone.0065350] [PMID: 23750255]

[167] Birnbaum JH, Bali J, Rajendran L, Nitsch RM, Tackenberg C. Calcium flux-independent NMDA receptor activity is required for Aβ oligomer-induced synaptic loss. Cell Death Dis 2015; 6(6): e1791.
[http://dx.doi.org/10.1038/cddis.2015.160] [PMID: 26086964]

[168] Foster TC, Kyritsopoulos C, Kumar A. Central role for NMDA receptors in redox mediated impairment of synaptic function during aging and Alzheimer's disease. Behav Brain Res 2017; 322(Pt B): 223-32.
[http://dx.doi.org/10.1016/j.bbr.2016.05.012] [PMID: 27180169]

[169] Ripoli C, Cocco S, Li Puma DD, *et al.* Intracellular accumulation of amyloid-β (Aβ) protein plays a major role in Aβ-induced alterations of glutamatergic synaptic transmission and plasticity. J Neurosci 2014; 34(38): 12893-903.
[http://dx.doi.org/10.1523/JNEUROSCI.1201-14.2014] [PMID: 25232124]

[170] Shankar GM, Li S, Mehta TH, *et al.* Amyloid-β protein dimers isolated directly from Alzheimer's brains impair synaptic plasticity and memory. Nat Med 2008; 14(8): 837-42.
[http://dx.doi.org/10.1038/nm1782] [PMID: 18568035]

[171] Tu S, Okamoto S, Lipton SA, Xu H. Oligomeric Aβ induced synaptic dysfunction in Alzheimer's disease. Mol Neurodegener 2014; 9(1): 48.
[http://dx.doi.org/10.1186/1750-1326-9-48] [PMID: 25394486]

[172] Coan EJ, Irving AJ, Collingridge GL. Low-frequency activation of the NMDA receptor system can prevent the induction of LTP. Neurosci Lett 1989; 105(1-2): 205-10.
[http://dx.doi.org/10.1016/0304-3940(89)90038-4] [PMID: 2577224]

[173] Hu R, Wei P, Jin L, *et al.* Overexpression of EphB2 in hippocampus rescues impaired NMDA receptors trafficking and cognitive dysfunction in Alzheimer model. Cell Death Dis 2017; 8(3): e2717.
[http://dx.doi.org/10.1038/cddis.2017.140] [PMID: 28358367]

[174] Talantova M, Sanz-Blasco S, Zhang X, *et al.* Aβ induces astrocytic glutamate release, extrasynaptic NMDA receptor activation, and synaptic loss. Proc Natl Acad Sci USA 2013; 110(27): E2518-27.

[http://dx.doi.org/10.1073/pnas.1306832110] [PMID: 23776240]

[175] Suberbielle E, Djukic B, Evans M, *et al.* DNA repair factor BRCA1 depletion occurs in Alzheimer brains and impairs cognitive function in mice. Nat Commun 2015; 6(1): 8897. [http://dx.doi.org/10.1038/ncomms9897] [PMID: 26615780]

[176] Zhou JY, Mo ZX, Zhou SW. Rhynchophylline down-regulates NR2B expression in cortex and hippocampal CA1 area of amphetamine-induced conditioned place preference rat. Arch Pharm Res 2010; 33(4): 557-65. [http://dx.doi.org/10.1007/s12272-010-0410-3] [PMID: 20422365]

[177] Yang Y, Ji W, Zhu Z, Wu Y, Zhang Z, Qu S. Rhynchophylline suppresses soluble $A\beta_{1-42}$-induced impairment of spatial cognition function *via* inhibiting excessive activation of extrasynaptic NR2B-containing NMDA receptors. Neuropharmacology 2018; 135: 100-12. [http://dx.doi.org/10.1016/j.neuropharm.2018.03.007] [PMID: 29510187]

[178] Abbott JJ, Howlett DR, Francis PT, Williams RJ. Aβ1–42 modulation of Akt phosphorylation *via* α7 nAChR and NMDA receptors. Neurobiol Aging 2008; 29(7): 992-1001. [http://dx.doi.org/10.1016/j.neurobiolaging.2007.01.003] [PMID: 17292512]

[179] Hooper C, Markevich V, Plattner F, *et al.* Glycogen synthase kinase-3 inhibition is integral to long-term potentiation. Eur J Neurosci 2007; 25(1): 81-6. [http://dx.doi.org/10.1111/j.1460-9568.2006.05245.x] [PMID: 17241269]

[180] Peineau S, Taghibiglou C, Bradley C, *et al.* LTP inhibits LTD in the hippocampus *via* regulation of GSK3β. Neuron 2007; 53(5): 703-17. [http://dx.doi.org/10.1016/j.neuron.2007.01.029] [PMID: 17329210]

[181] Kawamoto EM, Lepsch LB, Boaventura MFC, *et al.* Amyloid β-peptide activates nuclear factor-κB through an N-methyl-D-aspartate signaling pathway in cultured cerebellar cells. J Neurosci Res 2008; 86(4): 845-60. [http://dx.doi.org/10.1002/jnr.21548] [PMID: 17969100]

[182] Nakamura S, Murayama N, Noshita T, Katsuragi R, Ohno T. Cognitive dysfunction induced by sequential injection of amyloid-β and ibotenate into the bilateral hippocampus; protection by memantine and MK-801. Eur J Pharmacol 2006; 548(1-3): 115-22. [http://dx.doi.org/10.1016/j.ejphar.2006.07.049] [PMID: 16952349]

[183] Origlia N, Righi M, Capsoni S, *et al.* Receptor for advanced glycation end product-dependent activation of p38 mitogen-activated protein kinase contributes to amyloid-β-mediated cortical synaptic dysfunction. J Neurosci 2008; 28(13): 3521-30. [http://dx.doi.org/10.1523/JNEUROSCI.0204-08.2008] [PMID: 18367618]

[184] Origlia N, Bonadonna C, Rosellini A, *et al.* Microglial receptor for advanced glycation end product-dependent signal pathway drives β-amyloid-induced synaptic depression and long-term depression impairment in entorhinal cortex. J Neurosci 2010; 30(34): 11414-25. [http://dx.doi.org/10.1523/JNEUROSCI.2127-10.2010] [PMID: 20739563]

[185] Falcicchia C, Tozzi F, Arancio O, Watterson DM, Origlia N. Involvement of p38 MAPK in synaptic function and dysfunction. Int J Mol Sci 2020; 21(16): 5624. [http://dx.doi.org/10.3390/ijms21165624] [PMID: 32781522]

[186] Parihar MS, Brewer GJ. Amyloid-β as a modulator of synaptic plasticity. J Alzheimers Dis 2010; 22(3): 741-63. [http://dx.doi.org/10.3233/JAD-2010-101020] [PMID: 20847424]

[187] Laurén J, Gimbel DA, Nygaard HB, Gilbert JW, Strittmatter SM. Cellular prion protein mediates impairment of synaptic plasticity by amyloid-β oligomers. Nature 2009; 457(7233): 1128-32. [http://dx.doi.org/10.1038/nature07761] [PMID: 19242475]

[188] Nicoll AJ, Panico S, Freir DB, *et al.* Amyloid-β nanotubes are associated with prion protein-dependent synaptotoxicity. Nat Commun 2013; 4(1): 2416.

[http://dx.doi.org/10.1038/ncomms3416] [PMID: 24022506]

[189] Um JW, Kaufman AC, Kostylev M, *et al.* Metabotropic glutamate receptor 5 is a coreceptor for Alzheimer aβ oligomer bound to cellular prion protein. Neuron 2013; 79(5): 887-902. [http://dx.doi.org/10.1016/j.neuron.2013.06.036] [PMID: 24012003]

[190] Kashani A, Lepicard È, Poirel O, *et al.* Loss of VGLUT1 and VGLUT2 in the prefrontal cortex is correlated with cognitive decline in Alzheimer disease. Neurobiol Aging 2008; 29(11): 1619-30. [http://dx.doi.org/10.1016/j.neurobiolaging.2007.04.010] [PMID: 17531353]

[191] Parsons CG, Stöffler A, Danysz W. Memantine: a NMDA receptor antagonist that improves memory by restoration of homeostasis in the glutamatergic system - too little activation is bad, too much is even worse. Neuropharmacology 2007; 53(6): 699-723. [http://dx.doi.org/10.1016/j.neuropharm.2007.07.013] [PMID: 17904591]

[192] Davis S, Butcher SP, Morris RG. The NMDA receptor antagonist D-2-amino-5-phosphonopentanoate (D-AP5) impairs spatial learning and LTP *in vivo* at intracerebral concentrations comparable to those that block LTP *in vitro*. J Neurosci 1992; 12(1): 21-34. [http://dx.doi.org/10.1523/JNEUROSCI.12-01-00021.1992] [PMID: 1345945]

[193] Katagiri H, Tanaka K, Manabe T. Requirement of appropriate glutamate concentrations in the synaptic cleft for hippocampal LTP induction. Eur J Neurosci 2001; 14(3): 547-53. [http://dx.doi.org/10.1046/j.0953-816x.2001.01664.x] [PMID: 11553304]

[194] Rammes G, Hasenjäger A, Sroka-Saidi K, Deussing JM, Parsons CG. Therapeutic significance of NR2B-containing NMDA receptors and mGluR5 metabotropic glutamate receptors in mediating the synaptotoxic effects of β-amyloid oligomers on long-term potentiation (LTP) in murine hippocampal slices. Neuropharmacology 2011; 60(6): 982-90. [http://dx.doi.org/10.1016/j.neuropharm.2011.01.051] [PMID: 21310164]

[195] Parsons CG, Danysz W, Quack G. Glutamate in CNS disorders as a target for drug development: an update. Drug News Perspect 1998; 11(9): 523-69. [http://dx.doi.org/10.1358/dnp.1998.11.9.863689] [PMID: 15616669]

[196] Barnes CA, Danysz W, Parsons CG. Effects of the uncompetitive NMDA receptor antagonist memantine on hippocampal long-term potentiation, short-term exploratory modulation and spatial memory in awake, freely moving rats. Eur J Neurosci 1996; 8(3): 565-71. [http://dx.doi.org/10.1111/j.1460-9568.1996.tb01241.x] [PMID: 8963448]

[197] Van Dam D, Abramowski D, Staufenbiel M, De Deyn PP. Symptomatic effect of donepezil, rivastigmine, galantamine and memantine on cognitive deficits in the APP23 model. Psychopharmacology (Berl) 2005; 180(1): 177-90. [http://dx.doi.org/10.1007/s00213-004-2132-z] [PMID: 15654502]

[198] Banerjee PK, Billings Luhrs L, LeFerla FM. P1–001: Memantine reverses cognitive deficits in transgenic mice with both plaques and tangles. Alzheimers Dement 2006; 2(3S_Part_4): S94. [http://dx.doi.org/10.1016/j.jalz.2006.05.376]

[199] Parsons CG, Albrecht M, Rammes G. P1-017: Memantine reverses ß-amyloid oligomers-induced deficits in long term potentiation (LTP) in murine hippocampal slices. Alzheimer's & Dementia. 2009 Jul;5(4S_Part_6):P176-.

[200] Martinez-Coria H, Green KN, Billings LM, *et al.* Memantine improves cognition and reduces Alzheimer's-like neuropathology in transgenic mice. Am J Pathol 2010; 176(2): 870-80. [http://dx.doi.org/10.2353/ajpath.2010.090452] [PMID: 20042680]

[201] Wang Q, Walsh DM, Rowan MJ, Selkoe DJ, Anwyl R. Block of long-term potentiation by naturally secreted and synthetic amyloid β-peptide in hippocampal slices is mediated *via* activation of the kinases c-Jun N-terminal kinase, cyclin-dependent kinase 5, and p38 mitogen-activated protein kinase as well as metabotropic glutamate receptor type 5. J Neurosci 2004; 24(13): 3370-8. [http://dx.doi.org/10.1523/JNEUROSCI.1633-03.2004] [PMID: 15056716]

[202] Kervern M, Angeli A, Nicole O, *et al.* Selective impairment of some forms of synaptic plasticity by oligomeric amyloid-β peptide in the mouse hippocampus: implication of extrasynaptic NMDA receptors. J Alzheimers Dis 2012; 32(1): 183-96. [http://dx.doi.org/10.3233/JAD-2012-120394] [PMID: 22785392]

[203] Chen QS, Wei WZ, Shimahara T, Xie CW. Alzheimer amyloid β-peptide inhibits the late phase of long-term potentiation through calcineurin-dependent mechanisms in the hippocampal dentate gyrus. Neurobiol Learn Mem 2002; 77(3): 354-71. [http://dx.doi.org/10.1006/nlme.2001.4034] [PMID: 11991763]

[204] Hardingham GE, Fukunaga Y, Bading H. Extrasynaptic NMDARs oppose synaptic NMDARs by triggering CREB shut-off and cell death pathways. Nat Neurosci 2002; 5(5): 405-14. [http://dx.doi.org/10.1038/nn835] [PMID: 11953750]

[205] Hardingham GE, Bading H. The Yin and Yang of NMDA receptor signalling. Trends Neurosci 2003; 26(2): 81-9. [http://dx.doi.org/10.1016/S0166-2236(02)00040-1] [PMID: 12536131]

[206] Verkhratsky A, Kirchhoff F. Glutamate-mediated neuronal–glial transmission. J Anat 2007; 210(6): 651-60. [http://dx.doi.org/10.1111/j.1469-7580.2007.00734.x] [PMID: 17504269]

[207] Yamin G. NMDA receptor–dependent signaling pathways that underlie amyloid β-protein disruption of LTP in the hippocampus. J Neurosci Res 2009; 87(8): 1729-36. [http://dx.doi.org/10.1002/jnr.21998] [PMID: 19170166]

[208] Zhang Y, Li P, Feng J, Wu M. Dysfunction of NMDA receptors in Alzheimer's disease. Neurol Sci 2016; 37(7): 1039-47. [http://dx.doi.org/10.1007/s10072-016-2546-5] [PMID: 26971324]

[209] Neyman S, Manahan-Vaughan D. Metabotropic glutamate receptor 1 (mGluR1) and 5 (mGluR5) regulate late phases of LTP and LTD in the hippocampal CA1 region *in vitro*. Eur J Neurosci 2008; 27(6): 1345-52. [http://dx.doi.org/10.1111/j.1460-9568.2008.06109.x] [PMID: 18364018]

[210] Rudy CC, Hunsberger HC, Weitzner DS, Reed MN. The role of the tripartite glutamatergic synapse in the pathophysiology of Alzheimer's disease. Aging Dis 2015; 6(2): 131-48. [http://dx.doi.org/10.14336/AD.2014.0423] [PMID: 25821641]

[211] Buisson A, Choi DW. The inhibitory mGluR agonist, s-4-carboxy-3-hydroxy-phenylglycine selectively attenuates NMDA neurotoxicity and oxygen-glucose deprivation-induced neuronal death. Neuropharmacology 1995; 34(8): 1081-7. [http://dx.doi.org/10.1016/0028-3908(95)00073-F] [PMID: 8532157]

[212] Tyszkiewicz JP, Yan Z. β-Amyloid peptides impair PKC-dependent functions of metabotropic glutamate receptors in prefrontal cortical neurons. J Neurophysiol 2005; 93(6): 3102-11. [http://dx.doi.org/10.1152/jn.00939.2004] [PMID: 15659527]

[213] Palop JJ, Mucke L. Amyloid-β–induced neuronal dysfunction in Alzheimer's disease: from synapses toward neural networks. Nat Neurosci 2010; 13(7): 812-8. [http://dx.doi.org/10.1038/nn.2583] [PMID: 20581818]

[214] Patel L, Grossberg GT. Combination therapy for Alzheimer's disease. Drugs Aging 2011; 28(7): 539-46. [http://dx.doi.org/10.2165/11591860-000000000-00000] [PMID: 21721598]

[215] Deardorff WJ, Grossberg GT. Pharmacotherapeutic strategies in the treatment of severe Alzheimer's disease. Expert Opin Pharmacother 2016; 17(13): 1789-800. [http://dx.doi.org/10.1080/14656566.2016.1215431] [PMID: 27450461]

[216] Salomone S, Caraci F, Leggio GM, Fedotova J, Drago F. New pharmacological strategies for treatment of Alzheimer's disease: focus on disease modifying drugs. Br J Clin Pharmacol 2012; 73(4):

504-17.
[http://dx.doi.org/10.1111/j.1365-2125.2011.04134.x] [PMID: 22035455]

[217] Zong N, Li F, Deng Y, Shi J, Jin F, Gong Q. Icariin, a major constituent from Epimedium brevicornum, attenuates ibotenic acid-induced excitotoxicity in rat hippocampus. Behav Brain Res 2016; 313: 111-9.
[http://dx.doi.org/10.1016/j.bbr.2016.06.055] [PMID: 27368415]

[218] Ellison G. The N-methyl-d-aspartate antagonists phencyclidine, ketamine and dizocilpine as both behavioral and anatomical models of the dementias. Brain Res Brain Res Rev 1995; 20(2): 250-67.
[http://dx.doi.org/10.1016/0165-0173(94)00014-G] [PMID: 7795658]

[219] Reisberg B, Doody R, Stöffler A, Schmitt F, Ferris S, Möbius HJ. Memantine in moderate-to-severe Alzheimer's disease. N Engl J Med 2003; 348(14): 1333-41.
[http://dx.doi.org/10.1056/NEJMoa013128] [PMID: 12672860]

[220] Pierson TM, Yuan H, Marsh ED, *et al.* *GRIN2A* mutation and early-onset epileptic encephalopathy: personalized therapy with memantine. Ann Clin Transl Neurol 2014; 1(3): 190-8.
[http://dx.doi.org/10.1002/acn3.39] [PMID: 24839611]

[221] Song X, Jensen MØ, Jogini V, *et al.* Mechanism of NMDA receptor channel block by MK-801 and memantine. Nature 2018; 556(7702): 515-9.
[http://dx.doi.org/10.1038/s41586-018-0039-9] [PMID: 29670280]

[222] Howard R, McShane R, Lindesay J, *et al.* Donepezil and memantine for moderate-to-severe Alzheimer's disease. N Engl J Med 2012; 366(10): 893-903.
[http://dx.doi.org/10.1056/NEJMoa1106668] [PMID: 22397651]

[223] Kabir MT, Uddin MS, Mamun AA, *et al.* Combination drug therapy for the management of Alzheimer's disease. Int J Mol Sci 2020; 21(9): 3272.
[http://dx.doi.org/10.3390/ijms21093272] [PMID: 32380758]

[224] Farlow M, Anand R, Messina J Jr, Hartman R, Veach J. A 52-week study of the efficacy of rivastigmine in patients with mild to moderately severe Alzheimer's disease. Eur Neurol 2000; 44(4): 236-41.
[http://dx.doi.org/10.1159/000008243] [PMID: 11096224]

[225] Graham WV, Bonito-Oliva A, Sakmar TP. Update on Alzheimer's disease therapy and prevention strategies. Annu Rev Med 2017; 68(1): 413-30.
[http://dx.doi.org/10.1146/annurev-med-042915-103753] [PMID: 28099083]

[226] Parsons CG, Panchenko VA, Pinchenko VO, Tsyndrenko AY, Krishtal OA. Comparative patch clamp studies with freshly dissociated rat hippocampal and striatal neurons on the NMDA receptor antagonistic effects of amantadine and memantine. Eur J Neurosci 1996; 8(3): 446-54.
[http://dx.doi.org/10.1111/j.1460-9568.1996.tb01228.x] [PMID: 8963435]

[227] Lipton SA. Paradigm shift in neuroprotection by NMDA receptor blockade: Memantine and beyond. Nat Rev Drug Discov 2006; 5(2): 160-70.
[http://dx.doi.org/10.1038/nrd1958] [PMID: 16424917]

[228] Li L, Sengupta A, Haque N, Grundke-Iqbal I, Iqbal K. Memantine inhibits and reverses the Alzheimer type abnormal hyperphosphorylation of tau and associated neurodegeneration. FEBS Lett 2004; 566(1-3): 261-9.
[http://dx.doi.org/10.1016/j.febslet.2004.04.047] [PMID: 15147906]

[229] Möbius HJ, Stöffler A, Graham SM. Memantine hydrochloride: pharmacological and clinical profile. Drugs of Today (Barcelona, Spain: 1998). 2004 Aug 1; 40(8): 685-95.

[230] Marum R. Update on the use of memantine in Alzheimer's disease. Neuropsychiatr Dis Treat 2009; 5: 237-47.
[http://dx.doi.org/10.2147/NDT.S4048] [PMID: 19557118]

[231] Vandame D, Desmadryl G, Becerril Ortega J, *et al.* Comparison of the pharmacological properties of

GK11 and MK801, two NMDA receptor antagonists: towards an explanation for the lack of intrinsic neurotoxicity of GK11. J Neurochem 2007; 103(4): 1682-96.
[http://dx.doi.org/10.1111/j.1471-4159.2007.04925.x] [PMID: 17908242]

[232] Kapoor A, Peguero Estevez T, Chan C, Yamagata N, Doumlele K, Tampi R. Is there evidence for using ketamine among individuals with dementia? J Int Med Res 2024; 52(6): 03000605241258473.
[http://dx.doi.org/10.1177/03000605241258473] [PMID: 38907362]

[233] Cummings J, Zhou Y, Lee G, Zhong K, Fonseca J, Cheng F. Alzheimer's disease drug development pipeline: 2023. Alzheimers Dement (N Y) 2023; 9(2): e12385.
[http://dx.doi.org/10.1002/trc2.12385] [PMID: 37251912]

[234] Takahashi H, Xia P, Cui J, *et al.* Pharmacologically targeted NMDA receptor antagonism by NitroMemantine for cerebrovascular disease. Sci Rep 2015; 5(1): 14781.
[http://dx.doi.org/10.1038/srep14781] [PMID: 26477507]

[235] Sun J, Zhao S, Wang H, *et al.* Ifenprodil improves long-term neurologic deficits through antagonizing glutamate-induced excitotoxicity after experimental subarachnoid hemorrhage. Transl Stroke Res 2021; 12(6): 1067-80.
[http://dx.doi.org/10.1007/s12975-021-00906-4] [PMID: 33713028]

[236] Williams K. Ifenprodil discriminates subtypes of the N-methyl-D-aspartate receptor: selectivity and mechanisms at recombinant heteromeric receptors. Mol Pharmacol 1993; 44(4): 851-9.
[http://dx.doi.org/10.1016/S0026-895X(25)13275-6] [PMID: 7901753]

[237] Gomes GM, Dalmolin GD, Bär J, *et al.* Inhibition of the polyamine system counteracts β-amyloid peptide-induced memory impairment in mice: involvement of extrasynaptic NMDA receptors. PLoS One 2014; 9(6): e99184.
[http://dx.doi.org/10.1371/journal.pone.0099184] [PMID: 24921942]

[238] Chenard BL, Bordner J, Butler TW, *et al.* (1S,2S)-1-(4-hydroxyphenyl)-2-(4-hyroxy-4-phenylpiperidino)-1-propanol: a potent new neuroprotectant which blocks N-methyl-D-aspartate responses. J Med Chem 1995; 38(16): 3138-45.
[http://dx.doi.org/10.1021/jm00016a017] [PMID: 7636876]

[239] Swanger SA, Vance KM, Acker TM, *et al.* A novel negative allosteric modulator selective for GluN2C/2D-containing NMDA receptors inhibits synaptic transmission in hippocampal interneurons. ACS Chem Neurosci 2018; 9(2): 306-19.
[http://dx.doi.org/10.1021/acschemneuro.7b00329] [PMID: 29043770]

[240] Kang TH, Murakami Y, Matsumoto K, *et al.* Rhynchophylline and isorhynchophylline inhibit NMDA receptors expressed in Xenopus oocytes. Eur J Pharmacol 2002; 455(1): 27-34.
[http://dx.doi.org/10.1016/S0014-2999(02)02581-5] [PMID: 12433591]

[241] Xu R, Wang J, Xu J, *et al.* Rhynchophylline loaded-mPEG-PLGA nanoparticles coated with tween-80 for preliminary study in Alzheimer's disease. Int J Nanomedicine 2020; 15: 1149-60.
[http://dx.doi.org/10.2147/IJN.S236922] [PMID: 32110013]

[242] Zhu L, Yang L, Zhao X, *et al.* Xanthoceraside modulates NR2B-containing NMDA receptors at synapses and rescues learning-memory deficits in APP/PS1 transgenic mice. Psychopharmacology (Berl) 2018; 235(1): 337-49.
[http://dx.doi.org/10.1007/s00213-017-4775-6] [PMID: 29124300]

[243] Ip FCF, Fu WY, Cheng EYL, *et al.* Anemoside A3 enhances cognition through the regulation of synaptic function and neuroprotection. Neuropsychopharmacology 2015; 40(8): 1877-87.
[http://dx.doi.org/10.1038/npp.2015.37] [PMID: 25649278]

[244] Monteiro-Fernandes D, Silva JM, Soares-Cunha C, *et al.* Allosteric modulation of AMPA receptors counteracts Tau-related excitotoxic synaptic signaling and memory deficits in stress- and Aβ-evoked hippocampal pathology. Mol Psychiatry 2021; 26(10): 5899-911.
[http://dx.doi.org/10.1038/s41380-020-0794-5] [PMID: 32467647]

[245] Hamilton A, Vasefi M, Vander Tuin C, McQuaid RJ, Anisman H, Ferguson SSG. Chronic pharmacological mGluR5 inhibition prevents cognitive impairment and reduces pathogenesis in an Alzheimer disease mouse model. Cell Rep 2016; 15(9): 1859-65. [http://dx.doi.org/10.1016/j.celrep.2016.04.077] [PMID: 27210751]

[246] Lindemann L, Jaeschke G, Michalon A, *et al.* CTEP: a novel, potent, long-acting, and orally bioavailable metabotropic glutamate receptor 5 inhibitor. J Pharmacol Exp Ther 2011; 339(2): 474-86. [http://dx.doi.org/10.1124/jpet.111.185660] [PMID: 21849627]

[247] Haas LT, Kostylev MA, Strittmatter SM. Therapeutic molecules and endogenous ligands regulate the interaction between brain cellular prion protein (PrPC) and metabotropic glutamate receptor 5 (mGluR5). J Biol Chem 2014; 289(41): 28460-77. [http://dx.doi.org/10.1074/jbc.M114.584342] [PMID: 25148681]

[248] Hamilton A, Esseltine JL, DeVries RA, Cregan SP, Ferguson SSG. Metabotropic glutamate receptor 5 knockout reduces cognitive impairment and pathogenesis in a mouse model of Alzheimer's disease. Mol Brain 2014; 7(1): 40. [http://dx.doi.org/10.1186/1756-6606-7-40] [PMID: 24886239]

[249] Lea PM IV, Faden AI. Metabotropic glutamate receptor subtype 5 antagonists MPEP and MTEP. CNS Drug Rev 2006; 12(2): 149-66. [http://dx.doi.org/10.1111/j.1527-3458.2006.00149.x] [PMID: 16958988]

[250] Chen X, Lin R, Chang L, *et al.* Enhancement of long-term depression by soluble amyloid β protein in rat hippocampus is mediated by metabotropic glutamate receptor and involves activation of p38MAPK, STEP and caspase-3. Neuroscience 2013; 253: 435-43. [http://dx.doi.org/10.1016/j.neuroscience.2013.08.054] [PMID: 24012839]

[251] Haas LT, Salazar SV, Smith LM, *et al.* Silent allosteric modulation of mGluR5 maintains glutamate signaling while rescuing Alzheimer's mouse phenotypes. Cell Rep 2017; 20(1): 76-88. [http://dx.doi.org/10.1016/j.celrep.2017.06.023] [PMID: 28683325]

[252] Kinney GG, O'Brien JA, Lemaire W, *et al.* A novel selective positive allosteric modulator of metabotropic glutamate receptor subtype 5 has *in vivo* activity and antipsychotic-like effects in rat behavioral models. J Pharmacol Exp Ther 2005; 313(1): 199-206. [http://dx.doi.org/10.1124/jpet.104.079244] [PMID: 15608073]

[253] Bellozi PMQ, Gomes GF, da Silva MCM, *et al.* A positive allosteric modulator of mGluR5 promotes neuroprotective effects in mouse models of Alzheimer's disease. Neuropharmacology 2019; 160: 107785. [http://dx.doi.org/10.1016/j.neuropharm.2019.107785] [PMID: 31541651]

[254] Kingston AE, Ornstein PL, Wright RA, *et al.* LY341495 is a nanomolar potent and selective antagonist of group II metabotropic glutamate receptors. Neuropharmacology 1998; 37(1): 1-12. [http://dx.doi.org/10.1016/S0028-3908(97)00191-3] [PMID: 9680254]

[255] Caraci F, Molinaro G, Battaglia G, *et al.* Targeting group II metabotropic glutamate (mGlu) receptors for the treatment of psychosis associated with Alzheimer's disease: selective activation of mGlu2 receptors amplifies β-amyloid toxicity in cultured neurons, whereas dual activation of mGlu2 and mGlu3 receptors is neuroprotective. Mol Pharmacol 2011; 79(3): 618-26. [http://dx.doi.org/10.1124/mol.110.067488] [PMID: 21159998]

[256] Kim SH, Fraser PE, Westaway D, St George-Hyslop PH, Ehrlich ME, Gandy S. Group II metabotropic glutamate receptor stimulation triggers production and release of Alzheimer's amyloid(β)42 from isolated intact nerve terminals. J Neurosci 2010; 30(11): 3870-5. [http://dx.doi.org/10.1523/JNEUROSCI.4717-09.2010] [PMID: 20237257]

[257] Battaglia G, Molinaro G, Riozzi B, *et al.* Activation of mGlu3 receptors stimulates the production of GDNF in striatal neurons. PLoS One 2009; 4(8): e6591. [http://dx.doi.org/10.1371/journal.pone.0006591] [PMID: 19672295]

[258] Monn JA, Valli MJ, Massey SM, *et al.* Synthesis, pharmacological characterization, and molecular modeling of heterobicyclic amino acids related to (+)-2-aminobicyclo[3.1.0] hexane-2,6-dicarboxylic acid (LY354740): identification of two new potent, selective, and systemically active agonists for group II metabotropic glutamate receptors. J Med Chem 1999; 42(6): 1027-40. [http://dx.doi.org/10.1021/jm980616n] [PMID: 10090786]

[259] Battaglia G, Riozzi B, Bucci D, *et al.* Activation of mGlu3 metabotropic glutamate receptors enhances GDNF and GLT-1 formation in the spinal cord and rescues motor neurons in the SOD-1 mouse model of amyotrophic lateral sclerosis. Neurobiol Dis 2015; 74: 126-36. [http://dx.doi.org/10.1016/j.nbd.2014.11.012] [PMID: 25434487]

[260] Corti C, Battaglia G, Molinaro G, *et al.* The use of knock-out mice unravels distinct roles for mGlu2 and mGlu3 metabotropic glutamate receptors in mechanisms of neurodegeneration/neuroprotection. J Neurosci 2007; 27(31): 8297-308. [http://dx.doi.org/10.1523/JNEUROSCI.1889-07.2007] [PMID: 17670976]

CHAPTER 2

Tau Protein in Alzheimer's Disease

Maitreyee Mukherjee[1], **Soumen Dhara**[1], **Abhishek Jana**[2] and **Tathagata Roy**[1,*]

[1] *Department of Pharmaceutical Technology, NSHM Knowledge Campus, Kolkata - Group of Institutions, Kolkata, West Bengal, India*

[2] *Department of Pharmaceutical Technology, JIS Institute of Pharmacy, Kalyani, West Bengal, India*

Abstract: In Alzheimer's disease (AD) and other tauopathies, tau, a protein linked to microtubules, creates insoluble filaments that form as neurofibrillary tangles. Compared to the healthy human brain, tau is around three to four times more hyperphosphorylated in the brain of an AD patient. In this hyperphosphorylated condition, tau polymerizes into paired helical filaments mixed with straight filaments to create neurofibrillary tangles. During development, anesthesia, and hypothermia, tau is hyperphosphorylated; however, not to the same extent as in the brain of an AD patient. The potency of the abnormally hyperphosphorylated tau in AD brain to sequester healthy tau, microtubule-associated protein 1 (MAP1), and microtubule-associated protein 2 (MAP2), break microtubules, and self-assemble into PHF/SF, differentiates it from hyperphosphorylated tau. Due to oligomerization, the cytosolically hyperphosphorylated tau is sedimentable and loses its capacity to sequester normal MAPs during self-assembly into PHF/SF. For AD and associated tauopathies, inhibition of dysfunctional tau hyperphosphorylation will serve as a possible therapeutic target in the near future.

Keywords: Alzheimer's disease, Microtubule-associated protein 1, Neurofibrillary tangles, Neurodegenerative disorder, Tau protein.

INTRODUCTION

Alzheimer's disease (AD) is a neurodegenerative disorder associated with age progression and affects the thoughts, memory, and behavioural pattern of a person [1, 2]. Approximately 40-44 million people suffer from dementia, among them 60-80% of cases are due to AD [3, 4]. Considering the present-day demographic condition, 10% individuals in the age range above 65 years suffer from AD, and that increases to 32% over the age bar of 85 years. Gender based study indicates two-thirds of AD patients are women, this may be due to the higher life expectancy of women in comparison to men [5]. Predictive data suggests that

* **Corresponding author Tathagata Roy:** Department of Pharmaceutical Technology, NSHM Knowledge Campus, Kolkata - Group of Institutions, Kolkata, West Bengal, India; E-mail: tathagata.roy@nshm.com

Swarupananda Mukherjee, Souvik Roy & Dipanjan Karati (Eds.)

approximately 65.7 million people may suffer from dementia in 2023, and projections are high in the case of 2050, which is around 115.4 million [4].

A complex relationship exists between proteins and AD. AD is characterised by two hallmarks. Firstly, amyloid plaque formation by accumulation of Amyloid-beta (Aβ) peptide, and secondly, from intraneuronal neurofibrillary tangles (NFTs) due to hyperphosphorylation of Tau protein [1, 6, 7]. Tau is a key microtubule-associated protein (MAP) found in ocular neurons and the central nervous system (CNS), and it stabilizes neuronal microtubules [2]. Microtubules (MTs) play a crucial role in the functioning of intracellular signal transduction and the structural maintenance of neurons.

In normal physiologic conditions, the tau protein is moderately phosphorylated, whereas in abnormal conditions, the tau protein is hyperphosphorylated [8]. In this hyper phosphorylated tau first tends to detach from MTs, followed by aggregation in the form of Paired Helical Filaments (PHFs), leading to NFTs formation [8, 9]. This abnormal aggregation of tau protein subsequently causes breakdown of MTs and neuroinflammation, ultimately leading to neuronal degradation [10]. This suggests that the presence of tau does not cause AD; rather, in atypical conditions, it helps in the formation of plaques and tangles in the brain to spawn AD.

After identifying the pivotal role of the Tau protein in AD, researchers are finding various ways to control AD by utilizing the Tau protein. From a diagnostic reference point, tau imaging is now used for early diagnosis of AD [11, 12]. In AD treatment, tau targeting is also gaining significant focus as a potential therapy, with methods like Tau aggregation inhibitors [13], phosphorylation modulators [14, 15], and immunotherapy [16, 17], showing promising future applications.

STRUCTURE AND ACTIVATION OF TAU

Structural Elucidation of the Tau Protein

Tau is an abundant neuronal protein that is linked to microtubules. Tau is a protein that aids in maintaining the internal framework of neurons, which are nerve cells. Nutrients and other necessary materials pass through this tube-like structure to reach different areas of the neuron.

The microtubule-associated protein tau (MAPT) gene mutation, which is responsible for frontotemporal dementia with Parkinsonism associated with chromosome 17 (FTLD-17), was a groundbreaking discovery. It came up with genetic proof that demonstrated tau dysfunction was sufficient to initiate neurodegeneration, even in the absence of ß-amyloid peptide (Aß) [18]. The tau proteins with a molecular weight of 50,000-68,000 are found in the adult brain, while the fetal brain only contains one band with an apparent molecular weight of 48,000 [19]. Tau is mostly in axons. It is a highly soluble protein, generally an unfolded protein that interacts with tubulin to promote microtubule assembly and helps in the stabilization of microtubule structure under proper physiological conditions. The latest research suggests that tau has other functions, for example, by sustaining ß-catenin, phosphorylation of tau allows neurons to avoid apoptotic death [20]. Additionally, tau regulates the anterograde transport by kinesin and the retrograde transport by dynein, which is crucial for maintaining the equilibrium of microtubule-dependent axonal transport of organelles and biomolecules [21].

Six isoforms of tau are expressed in the adult human brain. These isoforms are formed by alternative splicing of the MAPT gene, which is found on chromosome 17q21 [22]. The splicing of exons 2 and 3 can be altered to produce variants with zero (0N), one (1N), or two (2N) embeds at the N-terminus. Furthermore, tau proteins with three (3R) or four (4R) C-terminal microtubule-binding domains are generated based on the presence or absence of exon 10, where 3R tau isoforms bind microtubules less firmly than 4R tau. A total of six tau isoforms are reported, and these are 3R0N, 3R1N, 3R2N, 4R0N, 4R1N, and 4R2N. The ratio of 3R to 4R tau expression levels is 1:1 in the human brain. The alterations in the 3R:4R tau ratio are a hallmark of many tauopathies. For example, a higher proportion of 4R tau is located in some mutated exon 10 with FTDP-17 families, which elevates the ability of tau to interact with microtubules [18, 22].

Tau is modulated by a number of posttranslational changes, such as nitration, glycosylation, ubiquitination, glycation, and oxidation, during both normal homeostasis and stress-induced reactions. Phosphorylation is the posttranslational change that has been studied the most. About 2–3 residues of tau are phosphorylated in a healthy human brain. The level of phosphorylation of tau is higher, with around nine phosphates per molecule in AD and other types of tauopathies. Tau may become hyperphosphorylated at serine, threonine, and tyrosine when the activity of tau kinases and tau phosphatases is interrupted. Although the exact effects of this event are still being studied, it decreases the affinity of tau for microtubules. It increases tau's susceptibility to neutral proteases activated by calcium and the ubiquitin-proteosome pathway, which degrades tau [22]. The fibrillization and aggregation into neurofibrillary tangles are controlled by tau hyperpolarisation. Glycogen-synthase kinase-3ß (GSK3ß), cAMP-dependent protein kinase (PKA), mitogen-activated protein kinases (MAPK), cyclin-dependent protein kinase 5 (CDK5), calcium-calmoduli--dependent kinase-II (CaMK II), and microtubule affinity-regulating kinase (MARK) are a few significant tau kinases. According to research on transgenic mice models of AD, inflammation, poor brain glucose metabolism, and Aß with overlapping pathways that lead to aberrant hyperphosphorylation of tau. Determining the cellular processes responsible for tau's posttranslational alterations is important for identifying potential treatment targets [22, 23].

MECHANISM OF SECRETION AND CIRCULATION OF TAU

An infectious misfolded protein, prions, which has the ability to migrate from one cell to another and transfer their misfolded conformation, or "a prion template," to its native, "healthy," forms in the cells that were not already affected. This enables the pathology to spread in a way that is determined by the template. At the same time, not prions per se, many proteins involved in neurodevelopmental diseases do have characteristics similar to prions, such as tau and alpha-synuclein (α-syn). This indicates that misfolded structures of some of these proteins may spread across an affected cell to a healthy neuron, where they could trigger additional misfolding and aggregation of the protein's original forms.

The following processes are involved in the prion-like spread of tauopathies: (1) formation of tau to spread the tauopathies; (2) secretion of tau proteins that can transmit, (3) intake of tau that is capable of spreading by an undamaged cell; and (4) templated misfolding that produces new tau seeds in the recipient cell. Aggregation of tau can be triggered by a single misfolded protein in a particular form [24]. According to study reports from Sharma *et al.*, in 2018, tau monomers that are seed-competent can generate morphologically distinct "strains" in various tauopathies. This implies that the distinctive kind of inclusions, rate of spread, and pattern of the neuropathological lesion in each illness are determined by the tau conformation in a specific seed [25]. In the procedure of cell-to-cell transmission *in vitro* and *in vivo*, all of these characteristics can be mimicked. A number of studies have shown that tau strains obtained from different tauopathies can be injected intracranially into healthy animals, and this can lead to the development of tau pathology characteristics that are comparable to the original tauopathy [26, 27]. To spread, pathogenic seeds must leave donor cells and enter the tau disorder. Through possible secretion routes, they can come to the extracellular space. The three methods are translocation across the plasma membrane, membrane-based organelle-based secretion (MOBS), and ectosomal secretion that could be involved in tau secretion [28, 29].

Tau does not diffuse randomly but instead follows a disease-specific spatiotemporal arrangement, with tau being released by a presynaptic neuron and taken up by a postsynaptic neuron. It is probable that neural activity is essential for trans-synaptic transmission.

According to the experiment, there are other pathways for tau to be sent from cell to cell than the activity-stimulated trans-synaptic transfer, since the process can also go backward through a network of neurons. Therefore, the propagation process is also probably aided by microglia-assisted or interstitial diffusion processes [30, 31]. Tau that has been secreted either arrives on a recipient neuron's surface unencumbered or enclosed in extracellular vesicles. According to current research, monomeric tau can undergo slower actin-dependent macropinocytosis, while aggregated and free tau can be ingested quickly *via* dynamin-dependent endocytosis without the need for clathrin [32]. Based on the report highlighted by Morozova *et al.*, in 2019 and Rauch *et al.*, in 2020, tau endocytosis may be triggered by the M1/M3 muscarinic receptor and low-density lipoprotein receptor-related protein 1 (LRP1) [33, 34]. It is probable that tau, a cytosolic leaderless protein that is typically bound to microtubules, will follow unique secretory pathways. Lots of studies have demonstrated that tau is released through a variety of non-conventional secretory pathways instead of the ER-Golgi pathway.

TAU TRANSLOCATION THROUGH THE PLASMA MEMBRANE

Certain proteins found in the cytosol pass straight through the plasma membrane and into the extracellular space, where they exist as free proteins. The bulk of tau in human CSF or extracellular medium is a vesicle-free protein. Fibroblast growth factor 2, or FGF2, is a secreted growth factor that does not have a signal peptide. It is the most explored protein that adheres to this secretory pathway. Recent research has shown that tau is another protein that uses the same secretory pathway as FGF2. The major steps in tau secretion are as follows: (1) tau is attracted to the plasma membrane through interaction with immobilized PIP2; (2) tau is phosphorylated by Tec-kinase at tyrosine 82 [35]; (3) tau is oligomerized and membrane pores form in a phosphatidylinositol 4,5-bisphosphate (PI(4,5)P2)-dependent manner and (4) tau molecules are translocated to the extracellular side through binding to heparan-sulfate chains of cell surface heparin sulfate proteoglycans (HSPGs) (Fig. **1**). Free tau can also derive from autophagy-based secretion and lysosomal secretion, two subtypes of membranous organelle-based secretion (MOBS), along with translocation across the plasma membrane. However, it has been found that tau secretion is independent of both ATP and Ca2+, strongly indicating that membrane fusion events are not involved in this process among the cells, eliminating MOBS. The secretion pathways based on exosomes, autophagy, and lysosomes are the three known MOBS sub-pathways [36, 37].

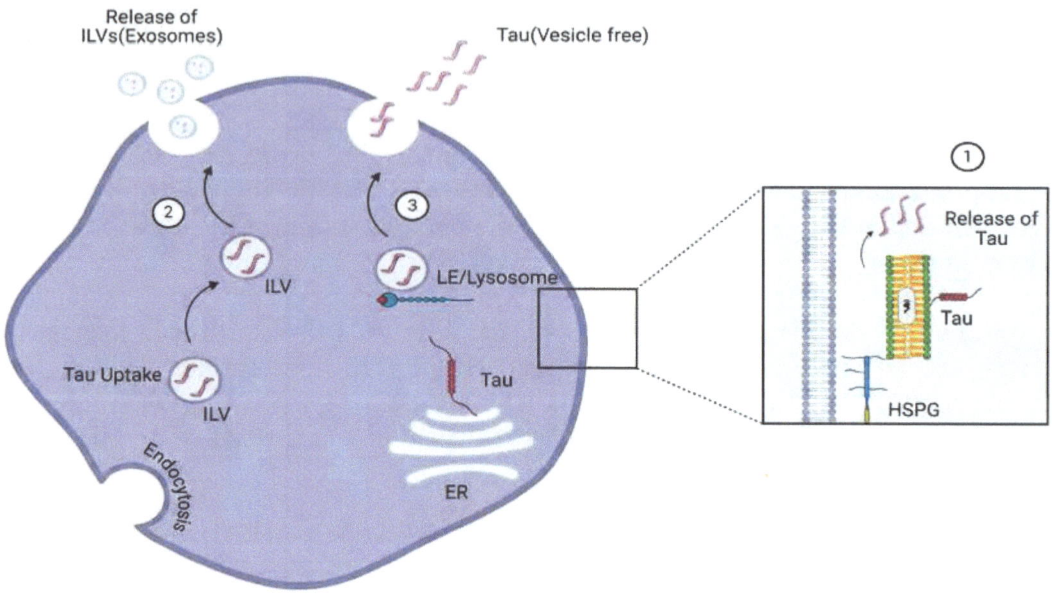

Fig. (1). Pathways of tau translocation. (1) Translocation of tau through the plasma membrane, (2) Exosome-mediated tau release, (3) Endosome/ Lysosome-mediated tau secretion.

Exosome-mediated Tau Release

Exosome-dependent release is the first and most extensively studied theory for tau secretion. Intraluminal vesicles (ILVs) contain cytosolic proteins that are taken up by the inward budding of the endosomal membrane (Fig. **1**). ILV development can sequester a random section of the cytosol and accumulate material unselectively, or it can function very precisely to detect certain molecules. The consequent multivesicular bodies (MVBs) would either come together with a lysosome to destroy their contents or interact with the plasma membrane to release the ILVs into the extracellular space. The mechanism that regulates the "fusion fate" of MVBs is unknown. There is a possibility of the presence of multiple MVB populations capable of fusing with the plasma membrane. These populations could emerge from various sorting processes, leading to unique cargo within ILVs and specific results for MVBs. To sort proteins for degradation, for example, lipid microdomain-dependent ILVs may be necessary, which leads to a population of MVBs that fuse with lysosomes; however, endosomal sorting complexes required for transport-dependent ILVs may sort proteins for secretion, leading to a population of MVBs that fuse with the plasma membrane. In addition, MVBs' fusion with the plasma membrane may be regulated by the lipid microdomains on their membrane. MVBs driven toward secretion translocate along microtubules, dock at the plasma membrane, and undergo Ca2+-regulated fusion to provide abundant extra levels of regulation of exosomal secretion. This mechanism is based on soluble N-ethylmaleimide-sensitive factor attachment protein receptors (SNAREs). Exosomes from immortal cell lines, rodent neuronal cultures, human iPSC neurons, mouse brain, human iPSC neurons, and CSF of AD patients have all been found to have endogenous and overexpressed tau [36, 38]. Based on other research, the CSF of AD patients or controls had more oligomerized tau in their exosomes than in drug action on the nervous system [39]. The neuronally derived extracellular vesicles (NDEVs) from AD and AD model systems, as well as from patients with mild cognitive impairment (MCI), were able to propagate tau pathology over long distances, seed tau aggregation in cell culture, and move pathological tau to unaffected cells [40].

Endosome/Lysosome Influenced Tau Secretion

Cytosolic proteins come into the LE/lysosomes with the help of chaperone-mediated autophagy (CMA) [36]. Heat shock cognate protein with molecular weight 71 kDa (Hsc70) and its co-chaperones distinguish cytosolic proteins with a KFERQ-like motif regularly in CMA. This is trailed by unfolding-coupled translocation to the lumen of LE/lysosome, which is mediated by LAMP2A protein on this organelle's membrane [41]. Misfolding-associated protein secretion pathway (MAPS) is the identical organelle entrance mechanism utilized for LE/lysosomal secretion of misfolded proteins. MAPS acts to translocate misfolded cytosolic proteins, like tau and other neurodegenerative disease-associated proteins, to LEs/lysosomes for secretion to the extracellular space during cellular stress and overloading of the ubiquitin-proteasome system. In this mechanism, a misfolded cytosolic protein at the extracellular surface of the ER is captured by ubiquitin carboxyl-terminal hydrolase 19 (USP19) utilizing its chaperone activity. The cargo protein is translocated into the lumen of the LE/lysosome that connects with the ER following Hsc70 and its co-chaperone DnaJ heat shock protein family member C5 (DNAJC5); during this process, DNAJC5 translocates into the lumen of the LE/lysosome and undergoes secretion in conjunction with a cargo protein. The MAPS pathway is for misfolded proteins and can translocate them to the LE/lysosome without the need for unfolding, whereas the CMA pathway binds to proteins with the KFERQ-like motif and requires unfolding during translocation. The LE/lysosomal secretion needs three more processes in addition to cargo loading. First, LEs and lysosomes are moved from perinuclear and cytosolic regions to the cell periphery along microtubules in response to stimulation; this translocation modifies the characteristics of these organelles (Fig. **1**). Compared to perinuclear LEs/lysosomes, peripheral LEs/lysosomes are slightly different in composition, less acidic, and show less proteolytic activity. The SNARE complex, which is made up of the plasma membrane's SNAP23 along with syntaxin-4, LE/lysosomal VAMP7 or VAMP8, and the plasma membrane, firmly binds LEs/lysosomes to the membrane. A limited rise in intracellular Ca2+ levels enables LE/lysosomes to fuse with the plasma membrane during the last step of the process. A tau secretion mechanism that depends on the DNAJC5-Hsc70 complex was identified by Fontaine and his colleagues in 2016 [42]. The mechanism necessitates the packing of cargo into an unknown membranous compartment that merges with the plasma membrane. However, Xu Y. *et al.*, in 2018 presented their data two years later, and it became clearer that tau is one of the MAPS cargos and that the mechanism Fontaine highlighted is MAPS [40, 43].

PATHOPHYSIOLOGY OF ALZHEIMER'S DISEASE

Alzheimer's Disease

AD is a neurodegenerative disorder that is characterised by severe dementia, *i.e.*, loss of cognitive function of the brain. It is a progressive disease; it slowly destroys the brain's ability to recall simple things [44]. The deposition of β-amyloid (Aβ) peptides in the extracellular surface of neurons and the formation of neurofibrillary tangles arising from the accumulation of hyperphosphorylated Tau protein inside the cell are the hallmarks of AD [3]. The lack of the neurotransmitter acetylcholine (ACh) and oxidative stress caused by glutamatergic transmission are also related to AD [45]. In AD, the atrophy of the hippocampus and cerebral cortex appears due to age [46]. Amyloid plaques or senile plaques formation is possible to observe microscopically [47].

Amyloid Hypothesis and Protein Tau

The existence of neurofibrillary tangles and amyloid beta (Aβ) fragments, which are important markers for AD, is what defines the amyloid hypothesis [48]. Amyloid precursor protein (APP) is changed into amyloid beta (Aβ) peptide by the enzymes β- and γ-secretase [49]. Tau protein provides microtubule stability by promoting a certain type of tubulin assembly. The last phase of the pathophysiology of AD is represented by tau protein aggregation and Aβ accumulation [2]. Another harmful feature of AD is the formation of senile plaques (SP), which are caused by the deposition of Aβ [50]. An imbalance between the synthesis and clearance of Aβ can lead to many types of dangerous oligomers, including fibrils, plaques, and protofibrils, depending on the degree of oligomerization. The genesis of AD is linked to several mechanisms, such as mitochondrial failure, oxidative stress, amyloid/tau toxicity, and cholinergic dysfunction [51].

More than 20 phosphorylation sites that are absent from healthy brains are present in tau that has been isolated from AD brains [52]. A number of protein kinases have been investigated as possible therapeutic targets for treating tau neuropathology. These include GSK3, cdk5, Erk2, JNK, MARK, and PKA. These kinases have the ability to phosphorylate tau at several locations [53].

Inflammatory Mechanism and Mitochondrial Dysfunction

Aβ fragment deposits and abnormal Tau protein are thought to have an impact on mitochondrial dysfunction in brain cells, particularly on the reduction of mitochondrial oxidative metabolism [54]. Benevento's research on the existence of Aβ peptides allowed him to more precisely determine that these peptides may be directly harmful to neuronal mitochondria [55].

Genetic Mechanism of AD

Most AD instances are sporadic in nature. AD is inherited. Three genes are altered in AD: the AAP gene, Presenilin 1 (PSEN1), and Presenilin 2 (PSEN2). Mutations in the APP may increase the generation and accumulation of Aβ. Similar to this, mutations in PSEN1 and PSEN2 stop γ-secretase from processing, which results in Aβ accumulation in the brain [56]. Apolipoprotein E (APOE) is a lipid metabolism regulator with a preference for the Aβ protein. There are three alleles of the Apolipoprotein E gene: ε2, ε3, and ε4. The ε4 allele of the APOE gene is one of the main genetic risk factors for AD [57].

Oxidative Stress

Oxidative stress brought on by Aβ is essential to the onset and course of AD [58]. The brain is a highly dynamic organ. The brain gets its energy from a process called mitochondrial oxidative phosphorylation, which also generates a lot of reactive oxygen species (ROS). Oxidative stress is caused by the overproduction of ROS [59]. Neurons are more susceptible to excitotoxic injury when ROS begin to collect. However, this process depends on the build-up of Aβ fragments and promotes the reduction of iron and copper in the brain, two important elements that initiate oxidative stress. Elevated levels of iron (Fe), copper (Cu), and other trace metals are linked to AD [60].

Cholinergic Hypothesis

Early in the disease, cholinergic neurons in the entorhinal cortex and basal nucleus are lost; however, by the time the disease reaches an advanced stage, over 90% of the cholinergic neurons in the basal nucleus have been eliminated [61]. Due to the loss of central cholinergic transmission and the death of cholinergic neurons in the basal forebrain, patients with AD have both cognitive and non-cognitive symptoms [62]. The cholinergic theory also includes the removal of cholinergic neurons in the Meynert basal nucleus and a significant decrease in the concentration of acetyltransferase, which is required for the generation of acetylcholine in the cortex and hippocampus [63].

How people with AD are affected by the APOE genotype in terms of the therapeutic effectiveness of acetylcholinesterase inhibitors (AChEIs) [64]. Neuropsychiatric symptoms are associated with a decrease in cholinergic receptor binding in certain brain regions in mild to severe AD [65].

TAU IN AD

Tau protein seems to be the primary microtubule-associated protein (MAP) of a grown-up neuron, along with MAP1 and MAP2. The microtubule-associated protein tau (MAPT) gene, with 16 exons and located on chromosome 17, is primarily responsible for encoding tau. In physiological conditions, tau is a highly soluble, naturally unfolded protein [66]. It works with tubulin to promote microtubule assembly, which helps to stabilize the structure of the microtubules, and its action is regulated by tau phosphorylation. Microtubule development is facilitated through the 2-3 moles of phosphate per mole found in normal brain tau [67 - 69].

The most typical cause of dementia in elderly people is Alzheimer's disease (AD). Amyloid-β (Aβ) plaques and tau neurofibrillary tangles in the brain, together with the subsequent loss of synapses and neurons, are pathological features of AD that inevitably lead to dementia [70].

Research has shown that unusual forms of hyperphosphorylated Tau, which polymerize into paired helical filament structures mixed with straight filaments to form neurofibrillary tangles, are present in all tauopathies, including AD.

Phosphorylation, acetylation, glycosylation, nitration, glycation, methylation, ubiquitination, sumoylation, truncation, and prolyl-isomerization are a few examples of the post-translational modifications (PTMs) that can take place on tau. Abundant lines of evidence suggest that PTMs influence both the pathology of tauopathies like AD and tau function [66].

Phosphorylation of the Tau Protein

The longest tau isoform (2N4R) detected in the human brain has 85 putative phosphorylation sites (45 Ser, 35 Thr, and 5 Tyr); of these, over 47 phosphorylation sites have been learned. Numerous protein kinases and phosphatases control tau phosphorylation. The classification of tau kinases is like: (1) Protein kinases that are Ser/Thr, like CDK5, glycogen synthase kinase 3β (GSK3β), mitogen-activated protein kinase, Ca2+/calmodulin-dependent protein kinase II, microtubule-affinity regulating kinase, protein kinase A (PKA), protein kinase C, Akt, TTBK1/2, CK1, DYRK1A, and (2) tyrosine kinases, such as Fyn, Src, Syk, and c-Abl [71].

Several protein phosphatases, like protein phosphatase 1 (PP1), PP2A, PP2B, and PP5, can dephosphorylate Tau. PHFs (paired helical filaments) are present in abundance in hyperphosphorylated tau observed in the brains of AD patients or AD mouse models. Since elevated levels of phosphorylated tau are found in the CSF of prospective AD patients at an early stage of the disease and correspond with cognitive impairment, tau hyperphosphorylation may represent an early event during AD pathogenesis. As a result, it is suggested that phosphorylated tau species in human CSF act as a biomarker for AD diagnosis. Both pathological and healthy tau function can be altered by tau phosphorylation and hyperphosphorylation. Although synchronous hyperphosphorylation of tau at numerous sites causes tau to dissociate from microtubules and increases tau aggregation, phosphorylation has an impact on tau's ability to connect to microtubules. In order to further modify synaptic function, tau phosphorylation also modulates its distribution to dendritic spines. Although the induction and maintenance of hippocampal LTD primarily depend on phosphorylation at S396, the distribution of mutant tau hyperphosphomimetic Ser/Thr isoforms to dendritic spines is promoted, which adversely affects synaptic function.

The histone acetyltransferases P300 and CREB-binding protein can acetylate tau. Catalytic Cys291 and Cys322 residues in the microtubule binding domain can autoacetylate tau. SIRT1 and HDAC6 can deacetylate tau [72]. Due to its correlation with AD, tau acetylation at Lys174, Lys274, Lys280, and Lys281 has been studied. Particularly, acetylation of tau at Lys280 is specific to AD and 4R tauopathies, including PSP and corticobasal degeneration. In addition, in the brains of AD patients at different stages of the disease, elevated amounts of acetylated tau at Lys174, Lys274, and Lys281 have been detected [73]. Acetylation may provide tau with its unsafe characteristics and impair its normal activity. Tau binding to microtubules is hindered by acetylation of tau at Lys274, Lys280, and Lys281 residues within the microtubule binding domain. While acetylation of Lys274 and Lys281 increases tau distribution to the soma and dendrites, which leads to synaptic and cognitive impairment, acetylation of Lys280 improves fibrillization [74, 75]. Tau acetylation at Lys174 results in cognitive impairments and decreases tau turnover. Since both ubiquitination and acetylation are changes on Lys residues, acetylation may reduce tau ubiquitination by competitive attenuation, hence reducing proteasome-mediated tau breakdown. Acetylation may also influence other PTMs in tau [76].

Acetylation at specific Lys residues is necessary for the effect of tau acetylation on tau phosphorylation. Lys residues inside the KXGS motif that are acetylated decrease tau phosphorylation; Lys274 and Lys281 acetylation generally have no effect on tau phosphorylation; and Lys280 acetylation modifies certain tau phosphoresidues [77]. Thus, for AD and kindred tauopathies, suppression of acetylation at some but not all of tau's Lys residues may be helpful. Because tau in paired helical filaments (PHFs) is predominantly monoubiquitinated rather than polyubiquitinated, tau monoubiquitination may prevent tau from being destroyed by UPS, which typically promotes the destruction of polyubiquitinated protein. Furthermore, abnormal PHF binding to proteasomes impairs proteasomal activity, which in turn promotes the accumulation of ubiquitinated tau in the AD brain [66, 78].

Glycosylation in Tau

Tau has been shown to have both N- and O-linked glycosylation [79, 80]. In PHF-tau isolated from AD brains, N-glycosylation has been found, but not in healthy brains [79]. It is unclear how N-glycosylation affects tau pathobiology. N-glycosylated tau appears to exhibit less aggregation but is susceptible to phosphorylation, according to a number of studies [81, 82]. It has been possible to pinpoint six O-linked Ser and ThrGlcNAcylated sites in tau [83]. Due to some overlap between the Ser and Thr targets for O-GlcNAcylation and phosphorylation, O-GlcNAcylation adversely affects tau phosphorylation. While O-GlcNAcase inhibition lowers tau phosphorylation, downregulation of O-GlcNAc transferase causes decreased O-GlcNAcylation and increased tau phosphorylation [84, 85].

Reduced amounts of O-GlcNAcylated tau have been seen in the brains of AD patients; these levels are inversely correlated with tau phosphorylation at several sites, which may be an indicator of abnormality in glucose metabolism among AD patients [84]. These study data indicate that reduced tau O-GlcNAcylation plays a role in the pathophysiology of AD.

Truncation of the Tau Protein

Proteolytic processing generates truncated tau species. Only the cleaved tau, which are the products of caspase-2, 3, and 6, have been associated with AD [86 - 88].

Tau can be cleaved by caspase-1, 2, 3, 6, and 7 *in vitro*. Increased levels of truncated tau-314 have been seen in the brains of AD patients, where caspase-2 cleaves tau at Asp314. To cause synaptic and cognitive impairment, tau-314 dissociates from microtubules and encourages the distribution of both full-length tau and tau-314 to dendritic spines. Indeed, in rTg4510 tau transgenic mice, downregulation of caspase-2 partially restores memory deficits [86]. Tau is mainly cleaved at Asp421, generating a tau-421 species by Caspase-3 [87]. In AD, as well as PSP, elevated levels of tau-421 and caspase-3 have been reported [89, 90].

In the human AD brain, tau-421 co-localizes with NFTs and is correlated with both NFT development and cognitive decline in old mice [87]. Tau detaches from microtubules and increases tau aggregation because of caspase-3 cleavage [87, 91]. Also, tau-421 has been detected in PSD fractions from primary neuronal cultures, suggesting that it plays a function in synaptic development. In fact, a tau-421 transgenic mouse model showed memory problems [92]. Our team has recently discovered that appoptosin is a positive regulator of tau cleavage mediated by caspase-3. Elevated levels of appoptosinare linked to the SNP rs1768208(C/T), which is related to AD, PSP, and FTD-T.

In JNPL3 tau transgenic mice, the overexpression of appoptosin stimulates caspase-3-dependent tau destruction and activates caspase-3, which exacerbates motor impairment. Appoptosin is an upstream regulator of caspase-3, and since caspase-3 activation occurs before NFT formation [93], appoptosin probably has a role in the early stages of tau pathogenesis in AD and other tauopathies. Asp13 (tau-13) and Asp402 (tau-402) are the sites where caspase-6 can cleave tau [94]. In the brains of AD patients, neuritic plaques and NFTs contained active caspase-6 and tau-402. Furthermore, tau-402 levels in CSF are correlated with older people's or AD patients' cognitive ability [94]. These results suggest that tau-402 could be an effective biomarker for AD and a pathogenic indicator. It is yet undetermined, nevertheless, if tau-402 has an impact on tau conformation and function. Consequently, it is uncertain whether tau breakage by caspase-6 contributes to the pathophysiology of AD. It is evident that the pathogenic event of tau damage in AD is triggered by caspase. Numerous truncated tau isoforms, such as the 17 kDa tau45–230 and 24 kDa tau243–441 products, are generated by the cleavage of tau by caspase, which are calcium-dependent cysteine proteases [95, 96]. Brain samples from AD and many other tauopathies have been found to exhibit increased calpain activity and tau45–230 levels, whereas the tau transgenic Tg601 mouse model shows raised tau243–441 levels [96, 97]. While tau45-230's effects on neuronal cell death are contradicted by *in vitro* research, a recent study using tau45-230 transgenic mice shows that tau45-230 is neurotoxic and may lead to synaptic and cognitive impairment [95, 98, 99]. Tau 243–441 isoforms may be damaging because they can encourage tau aggregation and propagation, even though they do not appear to have any effects on microtubule assembly [96]. The phosphorylation of tau by PKA decreases calpain-mediated tau proteolysis, and NFTs are resistant to calpain cleavage, indicating that phosphorylation negatively affects calpain-mediated tau cleavage [100]. As a result, tau cleavage by calpain could take place early in the course of AD. AEP (δ-secretase), is a cysteine protease that is specific to asparagine. At Asn167, Asn255, and Asn368, tau can be cleaved by AEP [101]. The tau-368 isoform, which is shortened as a consequence of AEP cleavage, has a greater tendency to form PHFs *in vitro* and less augmentation in microtubule assembly. Tau-368 was demonstrated to rise with aging and in the AD brain, and raised AEP activity was first observed in old mouse and human brains [101]. Only minimal traces of tau-368 were identified in insoluble tau aggregates in the AD brain, and a subsequent investigation found no change in soluble tau-368 in the brains of AD patients [101, 102]. Microglia are the primary cells in which AEP is expressed [103]. AEP cleaves tau without causing tau to accumulate in microglia. Therefore, rather than increasing tau aggregation, it is more plausible that AEP modulates tau breakdown [103]. More research is needed to determine the specific function that AEP and AEP-cleaved tau serve in the etiology of AD [78].

CONCLUSION

AD is a polygenetic and multifactorial neurodegenerative disorder mainly affecting cognitive behaviour. Abnormal phosphorylation of tau protein and intraneuronal neurofibrillary tangles play a pivotal role in the development and pathogenesis of AD. The multifaceted character of AD is reflected in the ongoing uncovering of new signalling pathways. It is important to address this complexity in patient management for improved treatment outcomes. Targeting the pathological characteristics of AD, like hyperphosphorylated tau and neurofibrillary tangles, is an important approach for the pharmacotherapy of AD. An urgent need to develop a potent drug is required to treat AD patients as well as those having a chance of developing AD.

REFERENCES

[1] Stefanoska K, Gajwani M, Tan ARP, *et al.* Alzheimer's disease: Ablating single master site abolishes tau hyperphosphorylation. Sci Adv 2022; 8(27): eabl8809. [http://dx.doi.org/10.1126/sciadv.abl8809] [PMID: 35857446]

[2] Muralidar S, Ambi SV, Sekaran S, Thirumalai D, Palaniappan B. Role of tau protein in Alzheimer's disease: The prime pathological player. Int J Biol Macromol 2020; Vol. 163: 1599-617.

[3] Ashrafian H, Zadeh EH, Khan RH. Review on Alzheimer's disease: Inhibition of amyloid beta and tau tangle formation. Int J Biol Macromol 2021; Vol. 167: 382-94.

[4] Gao Y, Tan L, Yu JT, Tan L. Tau in alzheimer's disease: mechanisms and therapeutic strategies. Curr Alzheimer Res 2018; 15(3): 283-300. [http://dx.doi.org/10.2174/1567205014666170417111859] [PMID: 28413986]

[5] Rosende-Roca M, Abdelnour C, Esteban E, *et al.* The role of sex and gender in the selection of Alzheimer patients for clinical trial pre-screening. Alzheimers Res Ther 2021; 13(1): 95. [http://dx.doi.org/10.1186/s13195-021-00833-4] [PMID: 33952308]

[6] Laurent C, Buée L, Blum D. Tau and neuroinflammation: What impact for Alzheimer's Disease and Tauopathies? Biomed J 2018; 41(1): 21-33.
[http://dx.doi.org/10.1016/j.bj.2018.01.003] [PMID: 29673549]

[7] Choi H, Kim HJ, Yang J, *et al.* Acetylation changes tau interactome to degrade tau in Alzheimer's disease animal and organoid models. Aging Cell 2020; 19(1): e13081.
[http://dx.doi.org/10.1111/acel.13081] [PMID: 31763743]

[8] Drummond E, Pires G, MacMurray C, *et al.* Phosphorylated tau interactome in the human Alzheimer's disease brain. Brain 2020; 143(9): 2803-17.
[http://dx.doi.org/10.1093/brain/awaa223] [PMID: 32812023]

[9] Breijyeh Z, Karaman R. Comprehensive review on Alzheimer's disease: causes and treatment. Molecules. 2020; 25(24): 5789.
[http://dx.doi.org/10.3390/molecules25245789]

[10] Amir Mishan M, Rezaei Kanavi M, Shahpasand K, Ahmadieh H. Pathogenic tau protein species: Promising therapeutic targets for ocular neurodegenerative diseases. J Ophthalmic Vis Res 2019; 14(4): 491-505.
[http://dx.doi.org/10.18502/jovr.v14i4.5459]

[11] Betthauser TJ, Koscik RL, Jonaitis EM, *et al.* Amyloid and tau imaging biomarkers explain cognitive decline from late middle-age. Brain 2020; 143(1): 320-35.
[http://dx.doi.org/10.1093/brain/awz378] [PMID: 31886494]

[12] Villemagne VL, Leuzy A, Bohorquez SS, *et al.* CenTauR: Toward a universal scale and masks for standardizing tau imaging studies. Alzheimers Dement (Amst) 2023; 15(3): e12454.
[http://dx.doi.org/10.1002/dad2.12454] [PMID: 37424964]

[13] Liu X, She W, Sung HHY, Williams ID, Qian P. Tau-aggregation inhibitors derived from Streptomyces tendae MCCC 1A01534 protect HT22 cells against okadaic acid-induced damage. Int J Biol Macromol 2023; 231: 123170.
[http://dx.doi.org/10.1016/j.ijbiomac.2023.123170] [PMID: 36621732]

[14] Su J, Xiao Y, Wei L, *et al.* Generation of tau dephosphorylation-targeting chimeras for the treatment of Alzheimer's disease and related tauopathies. Sci Bull (Beijing) 2024; 69(8): 1137-52.
[http://dx.doi.org/10.1016/j.scib.2024.01.019] [PMID: 38341350]

[15] Oliveira AC, Santos M, Pinho M, Lopes CS. String/Cdc25 phosphatase is a suppressor of Tau-associated neurodegeneration. Dis Model Mech 2023; 16(1): dmm049693.
[http://dx.doi.org/10.1242/dmm.049693] [PMID: 36601903]

[16] Bittar A, Bhatt N, Kayed R. Advances and considerations in AD tau-targeted immunotherapy. Neurobiol Dis 2020; 134: 104707.
[http://dx.doi.org/10.1016/j.nbd.2019.104707] [PMID: 31841678]

[17] Shahpasand K, Sepehri Shamloo A, Nabavi SM, Ping Lu K, Zhen Zhou X. "Tau immunotherapy: Hopes and hindrances". Hum Vaccin Immunother 2018; 14(2): 277-84.
[http://dx.doi.org/10.1080/21645515.2017.1393594]

[18] Hutton M, Lendon CL, Rizzu P, *et al.* Association of missense and 5′-splice-site mutations in tau with the inherited dementia FTDP-17. Nature 1998; 393(6686): 702-5.
[http://dx.doi.org/10.1038/31508] [PMID: 9641683]

[19] Goedert M, Spillantini MG, Jakes R, Rutherford D, Crowther RA. Multiple isoforms of human microtubule-associated protein tau: sequences and localization in neurofibrillary tangles of Alzheimer's disease. Neuron 1989; 3(4): 519-26.
[http://dx.doi.org/10.1016/0896-6273(89)90210-9] [PMID: 2484340]

[20] Li HL, Wang HH, Liu SJ, *et al.* Phosphorylation of tau antagonizes apoptosis by stabilizing β-catenin, a mechanism involved in Alzheimer's neurodegeneration. Proc Natl Acad Sci USA 2007; 104(9): 3591-6.

[http://dx.doi.org/10.1073/pnas.0609303104] [PMID: 17360687]

[21] Stokin GB, Lillo C, Falzone TL, *et al.* Axonopathy and transport deficits early in the pathogenesis of Alzheimer's disease. Science 2005; 307(5713): 1282-8. [http://dx.doi.org/10.1126/science.1105681] [PMID: 15731448]

[22] Medeiros R, Baglietto-Vargas D, LaFerla FM. The role of tau in Alzheimer's disease and related disorders. CNS Neurosci Ther 2011; 17(5): 514-24. [http://dx.doi.org/10.1111/j.1755-5949.2010.00177.x] [PMID: 20553310]

[23] Wei X, Du P, Zhao Z. Impacts of DNA methylation on Tau protein related genes in the brains of patients with Alzheimer's disease. Neurosci Lett 2021; 763: 136196. [http://dx.doi.org/10.1016/j.neulet.2021.136196] [PMID: 34437990]

[24] Mirbaha H, Chen D, Morazova OA, *et al.* Inert and seed-competent tau monomers suggest structural origins of aggregation. eLife 2018; 7: e36584. [http://dx.doi.org/10.7554/eLife.36584] [PMID: 29988016]

[25] Sharma AM, Thomas TL, Woodard DR, Kashmer OM, Diamond MI. Tau monomer encodes strains. eLife 2018; 7: e37813. [http://dx.doi.org/10.7554/eLife.37813] [PMID: 30526844]

[26] Kaufman SK, Sanders DW, Thomas TL, *et al.* Tau prion strains dictate patterns of cell pathology, progression rate, and regional vulnerability *In vivo.* Neuron 2016; 92(4): 796-812. [http://dx.doi.org/10.1016/j.neuron.2016.09.055] [PMID: 27974162]

[27] Narasimhan S, Guo JL, Changolkar L, *et al.* Pathological tau strains from human brains recapitulate the diversity of tauopathies in nontransgenic mouse brain. J Neurosci 2017; 37(47): 11406-23. [http://dx.doi.org/10.1523/JNEUROSCI.1230-17.2017] [PMID: 29054878]

[28] Kang S, Son SM, Baik SH, Yang J, Mook-Jung I. Autophagy-mediated secretory pathway is responsible for both normal and pathological tau in neurons. J Alzheimers Dis 2019; 70(3): 667-80. [http://dx.doi.org/10.3233/JAD-190180] [PMID: 31256134]

[29] Pernègre C, Duquette A, Leclerc N. Tau secretion: Good and bad for neurons. Front Neurosci 2019; 13: 649. [http://dx.doi.org/10.3389/fnins.2019.00649] [PMID: 31293374]

[30] Ahmed Z, Cooper J, Murray TK, *et al.* A novel *in vivo* model of tau propagation with rapid and progressive neurofibrillary tangle pathology: the pattern of spread is determined by connectivity, not proximity. Acta Neuropathol 2014; 127(5): 667-83. [http://dx.doi.org/10.1007/s00401-014-1254-6] [PMID: 24531916]

[31] Asai H, Ikezu S, Tsunoda S, *et al.* Depletion of microglia and inhibition of exosome synthesis halt tau propagation. Nat Neurosci 2015; 18(11): 1584-93. [http://dx.doi.org/10.1038/nn.4132] [PMID: 26436904]

[32] Brunello CA, Merezhko M, Uronen RL, Huttunen HJ. Mechanisms of secretion and spreading of pathological tau protein. Cellular and Molecular Life Sciences. 2020 May; 77(9): 1721-44.

[33] Evans LD, Wassmer T, Fraser G, *et al.* Extracellular monomeric and aggregated tau efficiently enter human neurons through overlapping but distinct pathways. Cell Rep 2018; 22(13): 3612-24. [http://dx.doi.org/10.1016/j.celrep.2018.03.021] [PMID: 29590627]

[34] Morozova V, Cohen LS, Makki AEH, *et al.* Normal and pathological tau uptake mediated by M1/M3 muscarinic receptors promotes opposite neuronal changes. Front Cell Neurosci 2019; 13: 403. [http://dx.doi.org/10.3389/fncel.2019.00403] [PMID: 31555098]

[35] Rauch JN, Luna G, Guzman E, *et al.* LRP1 is a master regulator of tau uptake and spread. Nature 2020; 580(7803): 381-5. [http://dx.doi.org/10.1038/s41586-020-2156-5] [PMID: 32296178]

[36] Ebert AD, Laußmann M, Wegehingel S, *et al.* Tec-kinase-mediated phosphorylation of fibroblast

growth factor 2 is essential for unconventional secretion. Traffic 2010; 11(6): 813-26. [http://dx.doi.org/10.1111/j.1600-0854.2010.01059.x] [PMID: 20230531]

[37] Rabouille C. Pathways of unconventional protein secretion. Trends Cell Biol 2017; 27(3): 230-40. [http://dx.doi.org/10.1016/j.tcb.2016.11.007] [PMID: 27989656]

[38] Saman S, Kim W, Raya M, *et al.* Exosome-associated tau is secreted in tauopathy models and is selectively phosphorylated in cerebrospinal fluid in early Alzheimer disease. J Biol Chem 2012; 287(6): 3842-9. [http://dx.doi.org/10.1074/jbc.M111.277061] [PMID: 22057275]

[39] Dujardin S, Bégard S, Caillierez R, *et al.* Ectosomes: a new mechanism for non-exosomal secretion of tau protein. PLoS One 2014; 9(6): e100760. [http://dx.doi.org/10.1371/journal.pone.0100760] [PMID: 24971751]

[40] Merezhko M, Uronen RL, Huttunen HJ. The cell biology of tau secretion. Front Mol Neurosci 2020; 13: 569818. [http://dx.doi.org/10.3389/fnmol.2020.569818] [PMID: 33071756]

[41] Kaushik S, Bandyopadhyay U, Sridhar S, *et al.* Chaperone-mediated autophagy at a glance. J Cell Sci 2011; 124(4): 495-9. [http://dx.doi.org/10.1242/jcs.073874] [PMID: 21282471]

[42] Fontaine SN, Zheng D, Sabbagh JJ, *et al.* DnaJ/Hsc70 chaperone complexes control the extracellular release of neurodegenerative-associated proteins. EMBO J 2016; 35(14): 1537-49. [http://dx.doi.org/10.15252/embj.201593489] [PMID: 27261198]

[43] Xu Y, Du S, Marsh JA, *et al.* TFEB regulates lysosomal exocytosis of tau and its loss of function exacerbates tau pathology and spreading. Mol Psychiatry 2021; 26(10): 5925-39. [http://dx.doi.org/10.1038/s41380-020-0738-0] [PMID: 32366951]

[44] Matej R, Tesar A, Rusina R. Alzheimer's disease and other neurodegenerative dementias in comorbidity: A clinical and neuropathological overview. Clin Biochem 2019; 73: 26-31. [http://dx.doi.org/10.1016/j.clinbiochem.2019.08.005] [PMID: 31400306]

[45] Yang Z, Zou Y, Wang L. Neurotransmitters in Prevention and Treatment of Alzheimer's Disease. Vol. 24. Int J Mol Sci 2023.

[46] Pardo-Moreno T, González-Acedo A, Rivas-Domínguez A, *et al.* Therapeutic Approach to Alzheimer's Disease: Current Treatments and New Perspectives. Pharmaceutics 2022; 14(6): 1117. [http://dx.doi.org/10.3390/pharmaceutics14061117] [PMID: 35745693]

[47] Forestier A, Douki T, De Rosa V, Béal D, Rachidi W. Combination of Aβ secretion and oxidative stress in an Alzheimer-like cell line leads to the over-expression of the nucleotide excision repair proteins DDB2 and XPC. Int J Mol Sci 2015; 16(8): 17422-44. [http://dx.doi.org/10.3390/ijms160817422] [PMID: 26263968]

[48] Kamble SM, Patil KR, Upaganlawar AB. Etiology, pathogenesis of Alzheimer's disease and amyloid beta hypothesis. In: Alzheimer's disease and advanced drug delivery strategies. 2024. p. 1–11. [http://dx.doi.org/10.1016/B978-0-443-13205-6.00022-4]

[49] Funamoto S, Tagami S, Okochi M, Morishima-Kawashima M. Successive cleavage of β-amyloid precursor protein by γ-secretase. Semin Cell Dev Biol 2020; 105: 64-74. [http://dx.doi.org/10.1016/j.semcdb.2020.04.002] [PMID: 32354467]

[50] Armstrong RA. The molecular biology of senile plaques and neurofibrillary tangles in Alzheimer's disease. Folia Neuropathol 2009; 47(4): 289-99. [PMID: 20054780]

[51] Fišar Z. Linking the amyloid, tau, and mitochondrial hypotheses of alzheimer's disease and identifying promising drug targets. Biomolecules 2022; 12(11): 1676. [http://dx.doi.org/10.3390/biom12111676] [PMID: 36421690]

[52] Duka V, Lee JH, Credle J, *et al.* Identification of the sites of tau hyperphosphorylation and activation of tau kinases in synucleinopathies and Alzheimer's diseases. PLoS One 2013; 8(9): e75025. [http://dx.doi.org/10.1371/journal.pone.0075025] [PMID: 24073234]

[53] Martin L, Latypova X, Wilson CM, *et al.* Tau protein kinases: Involvement in Alzheimer's disease. Ageing Res Rev 2013; 12(1): 289-309. [http://dx.doi.org/10.1016/j.arr.2012.06.003]

[54] Tobore TO. On the central role of mitochondria dysfunction and oxidative stress in Alzheimer's disease. Neurol Sci 2019; 40(8): 1527-40. [http://dx.doi.org/10.1007/s10072-019-03863-x] [PMID: 30982132]

[55] dos Santos Picanco LC, Ozela PF, de Fatima de Brito Brito M, *et al.* Alzheimer's disease: A review from the pathophysiology to diagnosis, new perspectives for pharmacological treatment. Curr Med Chem 2018; 25(26): 3141-59. [http://dx.doi.org/10.2174/0929867323666161213101126] [PMID: 30191777]

[56] Tsering W, Prokop S. Neuritic plaques — gateways to understanding alzheimer's disease. Mol Neurobiol 2024; 61(5): 2808-21. [http://dx.doi.org/10.1007/s12035-023-03736-7] [PMID: 37940777]

[57] Yamazaki Y, Zhao N, Caulfield TR, Liu CC, Bu G. Apolipoprotein E and Alzheimer disease: pathobiology and targeting strategies. Nat Rev Neurol 2019; 15(9): 501-18. [http://dx.doi.org/10.1038/s41582-019-0228-7] [PMID: 31367008]

[58] Caruso G, Spampinato SF, Cardaci V, Caraci F, Sortino MA, Merlo S. β-amyloid and oxidative stress: Perspectives in drug development. Curr Pharm Des 2020; 25(45): 4771-81. [http://dx.doi.org/10.2174/1381612825666191209115431] [PMID: 31814548]

[59] Singh A, Kukreti R, Saso L, Kukreti S. Oxidative stress: A key modulator in neurodegenerative diseases. Vol. 24. Molecules 2019; 24(8): 1583. [http://dx.doi.org/10.3390/molecules24081583]

[60] Cilliers K. Trace element alterations in Alzheimer's disease: A review. Clin Anat 2021; 34(5): 766-73. [http://dx.doi.org/10.1002/ca.23727] [PMID: 33580904]

[61] Chen ZR, Huang JB, Yang SL, Hong FF. Role of cholinergic signaling in Alzheimer's disease. Molecules. 2022; 27(6): 1816. [http://dx.doi.org/10.3390/molecules27061816]

[62] Giacobini E, Cuello AC, Fisher A. Reimagining cholinergic therapy for Alzheimer's disease. Brain 2022; 145(7): 2250-75. [http://dx.doi.org/10.1093/brain/awac096]

[63] Ferreira-Vieira TH, Guimarães IM, Silva FR, Ribeiro FM. Alzheimer's disease: targeting the cholinergic system. Curr Neuropharmacol. 2016; 14(1): 101–115. [http://dx.doi.org/10.2174/1570159x13666150716165726]

[64] Cheng YC, Huang YC, Liu HC. Effect of apolipoprotein e ε4 carrier status on cognitive response to acetylcholinesterase inhibitors in patients with alzheimer's disease: A systematic review and meta-analysis. Dement Geriatr Cogn Disord 2018; 45(5-6): 335-52. [http://dx.doi.org/10.1159/000490175] [PMID: 30041236]

[65] Stanciu GD, Luca A, Rusu RN, *et al.* Alzheimer's disease pharmacotherapy in relation to cholinergic system involvement. Biomolecules. 2020;10(1):40.

[66] Liu F, Zaidi T, Iqbal K, Grundke-Iqbal I, Merkle RK, Gong CX. Role of glycosylation in hyperphosphorylation of tau in Alzheimer's disease. FEBS Lett 2002; 512(1-3): 101-6. [http://dx.doi.org/10.1016/S0014-5793(02)02228-7] [PMID: 11852060]

[67] Nichols E, Steinmetz JD, Vollset SE, *et al.* Estimation of the global prevalence of dementia in 2019 and forecasted prevalence in 2050: an analysis for the Global Burden of Disease Study 2019. Lancet

Public Health 2022; 7(2): e105-25.
[http://dx.doi.org/10.1016/S2468-2667(21)00249-8] [PMID: 34998485]

[68] Panza F, Lozupone M, Logroscino G, Imbimbo BP. A critical appraisal of amyloid-β-targeting therapies for Alzheimer disease. Nat Rev Neurol 2019; 15(2): 73-88.
[http://dx.doi.org/10.1038/s41582-018-0116-6] [PMID: 30610216]

[69] Jeremic D, Jiménez-Díaz L, Navarro-López JD. Past, present and future of therapeutic strategies against amyloid-β peptides in Alzheimer's disease: a systematic review. Ageing Res Rev 2021; 72: 101496.
[http://dx.doi.org/10.1016/j.arr.2021.101496] [PMID: 34687956]

[70] Congdon EE, Ji C, Tetlow AM, Jiang Y, Sigurdsson EM. Tau-targeting therapies for Alzheimer disease: current status and future directions. Nat Rev Neurol 2023; 19(12): 715-36.
[http://dx.doi.org/10.1038/s41582-023-00883-2] [PMID: 37875627]

[71] Min SW, Cho SH, Zhou Y, *et al.* Acetylation of tau inhibits its degradation and contributes to tauopathy. Neuron 2010; 67(6): 953-66.
[http://dx.doi.org/10.1016/j.neuron.2010.08.044] [PMID: 20869593]

[72] Min SW, Chen X, Tracy TE, *et al.* Critical role of acetylation in tau-mediated neurodegeneration and cognitive deficits. Nat Med 2015; 21(10): 1154-62.
[http://dx.doi.org/10.1038/nm.3951] [PMID: 26390242]

[73] Irwin DJ, Cohen TJ, Grossman M, *et al.* Acetylated tau, a novel pathological signature in Alzheimer's disease and other tauopathies. Brain 2012; 135(3): 807-18.
[http://dx.doi.org/10.1093/brain/aws013] [PMID: 22366796]

[74] Tracy TE, Sohn PD, Minami SS, *et al.* Acetylated tau obstructs KIBRA-mediated signaling in synaptic plasticity and promotes tauopathy-related memory loss. Neuron 2016; 90(2): 245-60.
[http://dx.doi.org/10.1016/j.neuron.2016.03.005] [PMID: 27041503]

[75] Morris M, Knudsen GM, Maeda S, *et al.* Tau post-translational modifications in wild-type and human amyloid precursor protein transgenic mice. Nat Neurosci 2015; 18(8): 1183-9.
[http://dx.doi.org/10.1038/nn.4067] [PMID: 26192747]

[76] Vogelsberg-Ragaglia V, Schuck T, Trojanowski JQ, Lee VMY. PP2A mRNA expression is quantitatively decreased in Alzheimer's disease hippocampus. Exp Neurol 2001; 168(2): 402-12.
[http://dx.doi.org/10.1006/exnr.2001.7630] [PMID: 11259128]

[77] Guo T, Zhang D, Zeng Y, Huang TY, Xu H, Zhao Y. Molecular and cellular mechanisms underlying the pathogenesis of Alzheimer's disease. Mol Neurodegener 2020; 15(1): 40.
[http://dx.doi.org/10.1186/s13024-020-00391-7] [PMID: 32677986]

[78] Wang JZ, Grundke-Iqbal I, Iqbal K. Glycosylation of microtubule–associated protein tau: An abnormal posttranslational modification in Alzheimer's disease. Nat Med 1996; 2(8): 871-5.
[http://dx.doi.org/10.1038/nm0896-871] [PMID: 8705855]

[79] Arnold CS, Johnson GW, Cole RN, Dong DLY, Lee M, Hart GW. The microtubule-associated protein tau is extensively modified with O linked N acetylglucosamine. J Biol Chem 1996; 271(46): 28741-4.
[http://dx.doi.org/10.1074/jbc.271.46.28741] [PMID: 8910513]

[80] Liu F, Shi J, Tanimukai H, *et al.* Reduced O-GlcNAcylation links lower brain glucose metabolism and tau pathology in Alzheimer's disease. Brain 2009; 132(7): 1820-32.
[http://dx.doi.org/10.1093/brain/awp099] [PMID: 19451179]

[81] Losev Y, Paul A, Frenkel-Pinter M, *et al.* Novel model of secreted human tau protein reveals the impact of the abnormal N-glycosylation of tau on its aggregation propensity. Sci Rep 2019; 9(1): 2254.
[http://dx.doi.org/10.1038/s41598-019-39218-x] [PMID: 30783169]

[82] Yuzwa SA, Yadav AK, Skorobogatko Y, Clark T, Vosseller K, Vocadlo DJ. Mapping O-GlcNAc modification sites on tau and generation of a site-specific O-GlcNAc tau antibody. Amino Acids 2011;

40(3): 857-68.
[http://dx.doi.org/10.1007/s00726-010-0705-1] [PMID: 20706749]

[83] Wang Y, Balaji V, Kaniyappan S, *et al.* The release and trans-synaptic transmission of Tau *via* exosomes. Mol Neurodegener 2017; 12(1): 5.
[http://dx.doi.org/10.1186/s13024-016-0143-y] [PMID: 28086931]

[84] Yuzwa SA, Macauley MS, Heinonen JE, *et al.* A potent mechanism-inspired O-GlcNAcase inhibitor that blocks phosphorylation of tau *in vivo.* Nat Chem Biol 2008; 4(8): 483-90.
[http://dx.doi.org/10.1038/nchembio.96] [PMID: 18587388]

[85] Jouanne M, Rault S, Voisin-Chiret AS. Tau protein aggregation in Alzheimer's disease: An attractive target for the development of novel therapeutic agents. European Journal of Medicinal Chemistry. Elsevier Masson SAS 2017; Vol. 139: pp. 153-67.

[86] Zhao X, Kotilinek LA, Smith B, *et al.* Caspase-2 cleavage of tau reversibly impairs memory. Nat Med 2016; 22(11): 1268-76.
[http://dx.doi.org/10.1038/nm.4199] [PMID: 27723722]

[87] Gamblin TC, Chen F, Zambrano A, *et al.* Caspase cleavage of tau: Linking amyloid and neurofibrillary tangles in Alzheimer's disease. Proc Natl Acad Sci USA 2003; 100(17): 10032-7.
[http://dx.doi.org/10.1073/pnas.1630428100] [PMID: 12888622]

[88] Rissman RA, Poon WW, Blurton-Jones M, *et al.* Caspase-cleavage of tau is an early event in Alzheimer disease tangle pathology. J Clin Invest 2004; 114(1): 121-30.
[http://dx.doi.org/10.1172/JCI200420640] [PMID: 15232619]

[89] Jicha GA, Berenfeld B, Davies P. Sequence requirements for formation of conformational variants of tau similar to those found in Alzheimer's disease. J Neurosci Res 1999; 55(6): 713-23.
[http://dx.doi.org/10.1002/(SICI)1097-4547(19990315)55:6<713::AID-JNR6>3.0.CO;2-G] [PMID: 10220112]

[90] Zhao Y, Tseng IC, Heyser CJ, *et al.* Appoptosin-mediated caspase cleavage of tau contributes to progressive supranuclear palsy pathogenesis. Neuron 2015; 87(5): 963-75.
[http://dx.doi.org/10.1016/j.neuron.2015.08.020] [PMID: 26335643]

[91] Barini E, Antico O, Zhao Y, *et al.* Metformin promotes tau aggregation and exacerbates abnormal behavior in a mouse model of tauopathy. Mol Neurodegener 2016; 11(1): 16.
[http://dx.doi.org/10.1186/s13024-016-0082-7] [PMID: 26858121]

[92] Kim Y, Choi H, Lee W, *et al.* Caspase-cleaved tau exhibits rapid memory impairment associated with tau oligomers in a transgenic mouse model. Neurobiol Dis 2016; 87: 19-28.
[http://dx.doi.org/10.1016/j.nbd.2015.12.006] [PMID: 26704708]

[93] de Calignon A, Fox LM, Pitstick R, *et al.* Caspase activation precedes and leads to tangles. Nature 2010; 464(7292): 1201-4.
[http://dx.doi.org/10.1038/nature08890] [PMID: 20357768]

[94] Horowitz PM, Patterson KR, Guillozet-Bongaarts AL, *et al.* Early N-terminal changes and caspase-6 cleavage of tau in Alzheimer's disease. J Neurosci 2004; 24(36): 7895-902.
[http://dx.doi.org/10.1523/JNEUROSCI.1988-04.2004] [PMID: 15356202]

[95] Park SY, Ferreira A. The generation of a 17 kDa neurotoxic fragment: an alternative mechanism by which tau mediates β-amyloid-induced neurodegeneration. J Neurosci 2005; 25(22): 5365-75.
[http://dx.doi.org/10.1523/JNEUROSCI.1125-05.2005] [PMID: 15930385]

[96] Matsumoto SE, Motoi Y, Ishiguro K, *et al.* The twenty-four KDa C-terminal tau fragment increases with aging in tauopathy mice: implications of prion-like properties. Hum Mol Genet 2015; 24(22): 6403-16.
[http://dx.doi.org/10.1093/hmg/ddv351] [PMID: 26374846]

[97] Ferreira A, Bigio EH. Calpain-mediated tau cleavage: a mechanism leading to neurodegeneration shared by multiple tauopathies. Mol Med 2011; 17(7-8): 676-85.

[http://dx.doi.org/10.2119/molmed.2010.00220] [PMID: 21442128]

[98] Garg S, Timm T, Mandelkow EM, Mandelkow E, Wang Y. Cleavage of Tau by calpain in Alzheimer's disease: the quest for the toxic 17 kD fragment. Neurobiol Aging 2011; 32(1): 1-14. [http://dx.doi.org/10.1016/j.neurobiolaging.2010.09.008] [PMID: 20961659]

[99] Lang AE, Riherd Methner DN, Ferreira A. Neuronal degeneration, synaptic defects, and behavioral abnormalities in tau45-230 transgenic mice. Neuroscience 2014; 275: 322-39. [http://dx.doi.org/10.1016/j.neuroscience.2014.06.017] [PMID: 24952329]

[100] Liu MC, Kobeissy F, Zheng W, Zhang Z, Hayes RL, Wang KKW. Dual vulnerability of tau to calpains and caspase-3 proteolysis under neurotoxic and neurodegenerative conditions. ASN Neuro 2011; 3(1): AN20100012. [http://dx.doi.org/10.1042/AN20100012] [PMID: 21359008]

[101] Zhang Z, Song M, Liu X, *et al.* Cleavage of tau by asparagine endopeptidase mediates the neurofibrillary pathology in Alzheimer's disease. Nat Med 2014; 20(11): 1254-62. [http://dx.doi.org/10.1038/nm.3700] [PMID: 25326800]

[102] Schlegel K, Awwad K, Heym RG, *et al.* N368-Tau fragments generated by legumain are detected only in trace amount in the insoluble Tau aggregates isolated from AD brain. Acta Neuropathol Commun 2019; 7(1): 177. [http://dx.doi.org/10.1186/s40478-019-0831-2] [PMID: 31722749]

[103] Zhang Z, Obianyo O, Dall E, *et al.* Inhibition of delta-secretase improves cognitive functions in mouse models of Alzheimer's disease. Nat Commun 2017; 8(1): 14740. [http://dx.doi.org/10.1038/ncomms14740] [PMID: 28345579]

CHAPTER 3

Axl Kinase in Alzheimer's Disease

Dipanjan Karati[1,*] and **Shreyasi Meur**[2]

[1] *Department of Pharmaceutical Technology, School of Pharmacy, Techno India University, Kolkata, West Bengal, India*

[2] *Department of Pharmaceutical Technology, NSHM Knowledge Campus- Group of Institution, Kolkata, West Bengal, India*

Abstract: Alzheimer's disease (AD) is a debilitating neurodegenerative disorder characterized by progressive cognitive decline, neuroinflammation, and the accumulation of amyloid-beta plaques and neurofibrillary tangles. These pathological features result in significant neuronal loss and impaired brain function, underscoring the urgent need for effective therapeutic interventions. Axl kinase, a member of the TAM receptor family, has emerged as a promising target due to its neuroprotective properties. Activation of Axl by its ligand, growth arrest-specific protein 6 (Gas6), modulates several critical signaling pathways that are integral to reducing neuroinflammation, promoting neuronal survival, and enhancing the clearance of amyloid-beta and hyperphosphorylated tau. Additionally, Axl influences ApoE metabolism, further impacting amyloid-beta clearance. The strategic modulation of Axl-mediated pathways supports an anti-inflammatory environment and bolsters microglial phagocytic activity, thereby mitigating the progression of AD. Current therapeutic strategies range from plant-based small molecule inhibitors to recombinant Gas6, focusing on the selective activation of Axl kinase to ensure optimal blood-brain barrier penetration and minimal off-target effects. Critical information regarding the structural aspects of Axl kinase, along with its protective role in the central nervous system (CNS), its capability to modulate hallmarks of AD as well as neuroinflammation, and finally, the therapeutic regulation of Axl and Gas6 has been discussed here. As our understanding of the molecular mechanisms underlying Axl signaling in the CNS deepens, the development of Axl-targeted therapies promises a hopeful trajectory towards effective and sustainable treatments for Alzheimer's disease, ultimately improving patient outcomes and quality of life.

Keywords: Alzheimer's disease, Axl kinase, Gene expression, Microglia, Neurodegeneration.

* **Corresponding author Dipanjan Karati:** Department of Pharmaceutical Technology, School of Pharmacy, Techno India University, Kolkata, West Bengal, India; E-mail: karatibabai@gmail.com

Swarupananda Mukherjee, Souvik Roy & Dipanjan Karati (Eds.)

INTRODUCTION

Alzheimer's disease (AD), a progressive neurodegenerative disorder, has emerged as a critical global health concern, particularly in the context of an aging population [1]. AD accounts for 60-80% of dementia cases worldwide, currently affecting approximately 50 million people, with projections suggesting this figure could triple by 2050 [2] (World Health Organization, 2020). The pathogenesis of AD involves the accumulation of amyloid-beta plaques and neurofibrillary tangles composed of hyperphosphorylated tau proteins, which disrupt neuronal communication and function, ultimately leading to neuronal death [3]. In the quest for effective treatments, kinase-targeted therapies have garnered significant attention due to their role in modulating various signaling pathways implicated in Alzheimer's disease.

Among the kinases, the TAM (Tyro3, Axl, and MerTK) receptor tyrosine kinase family plays a pivotal role in the regulation of immune responses and cellular debris clearance in the central nervous system (CNS) [4]. Analysis of TAM gene mutations in mice led to the discovery of the function of TAM receptors within the mouse immune system. Chronic inflammation was also observed in mice deficient in all three of the TAM receptors [5]. Numerous published studies have demonstrated that TAMs control a variety of microglial processes, such as phagocytosis, the removal of apoptotic cells, and the clearance of cellular debris [6, 7]. It was recently found that neurodegenerative disorders are associated with a subtype of disease-associated microglia (DAM) [8]. In this subtype, they found evidence of brain injury in the guise of neurodegeneration-associated molecular patterns or NAMPs, which they linked to the activation of a defense mechanism through pattern recognition receptors (PRRs) [9]. In contrast to the control population, Axl was significantly elevated inside the DAM of the AD model, indicating that TAM receptors may be involved in degenerative disorders [9].

Axl kinase, structurally characterized by its extracellular domains that facilitate ligand binding and its intracellular kinase domain, is instrumental in the phagocytosis of apoptotic cells and the suppression of inflammatory responses [10]. Studies have shown that Axl is upregulated in response to amyloid-beta, suggesting a compensatory mechanism aimed at mitigating amyloid burden and inflammation [11]. The activation of Axl is primarily mediated by its ligand growth-arrest-specific gene 6 (Gas6), which binds to the extracellular domain of Axl, leading to receptor dimerization and autophosphorylation of the intracellular tyrosine kinase domain. This activation triggers a cascade of intracellular signaling pathways, including the PI3K/Akt, MAPK/ERK, and NF-κBpathways, which are crucial for cell survival, autophagy, and inflammatory response modulation. Axl activation enhances the phagocytic activity of microglia, the brain's resident immune cells, facilitating the clearance of Aβ and apoptotic neurons [12].

A connection has been found between microglial function and innate immune responses in up to 50% of AD gene variations [12]. Positron emission tomography (PET) has directly demonstrated increased microglial activity in the brains of AD patients [13]. Thus, the microglial-expressed Axl kinase may be at the nexus of neuroinflammation as well as neurodegenerative illnesses. The purpose of our study is to delve into the molecular pathways involving Axl, evaluate the therapeutic potential of targeting Axl, and assess the outcomes of preclinical and clinical studies. By including a comprehensive analysis of activation and regulation of Axl kinase, protective role, real-world studies, therapeutic potential, and future directions, this chapter aims to provide a thorough understanding of Axl kinase's role in AD and its potential as a therapeutic target. Our study emphasizes the importance of continuing research to develop targeted therapies that can effectively mitigate the progression of Alzheimer's disease.

AXL RECEPTOR TYROSINE KINASE: AN OVERVIEW

Structure and Biological Function

Axl kinase is a receptor tyrosine kinase that belongs to the TAM family, which also includes Tyro3 and Mer (Mertk). This family is named after the first three letters of its members: Tyro3, Axl, and Mer [4]. Axl was initially identified in chronic myelogenous leukemia cells, and its gene is located on chromosome 19q13.2 [14]. The name "AXL" means "uncontrolled," and it originates from the Greek term "anexelekto". The Axl receptor consists of an extracellular domain, a single-pass transmembrane domain, and an intracellular tyrosine kinase domain [15]. The extracellular region is composed of two immunoglobulin-like (Ig-like) domains and two fibronectin type III (FroIII) domains, which facilitate ligand binding and receptor dimerization and bear a resemblance to neural cell adhesion molecules (NCAMs) [16]. Upon ligand binding, typically by growth arrest-specific 6 (Gas6), a protein of 75kDa, Axl undergoes dimerization and autophosphorylation of its tyrosine residues within the intracellular domain [17]. This phosphorylation initiates a cascade of downstream signaling pathways, including the PI3K/Akt, MAPK/ERK, and NF-κB pathways, which regulate diverse cellular processes such as survival, proliferation, migration, and immune responses [18]. The intracellular domain of Axl kinase contains the TAM family-specific KW(I/L)A(I/L)ES sequence, which is involved in tyrosine kinase activity and shares considerable homology with Axl-relatedreceptor tyrosine kinases (RTKs) like Rearranged during transfection (RET) [19]. It controls a variety of processes, including platelet aggregation, natural killer cell differentiation, cell survival, and the non-inflammatory phagocytic cell clearance of apoptotic cells [17, 20 - 22].

Axl Gene Expression Regulation

Axl gene expression is intricately regulated at multiple levels, including transcriptional, post-transcriptional, and epigenetic mechanisms. The Axl geneis predominantly regulated by the SP1/SP3 transcription factors, which bind to the GC-rich promoter region of the Axl gene to initiate transcription [23]. There are four other transcription factors that interact with the Axl promoter: hypoxia inducible factor 1α (HIF1α), YAP/TAZ/TEAD [24], myeloid zinc finger 1 (MZF-1) protein [25] and activator protein 1 (AP1) [26]. In addition to transcriptional regulation, Axl expression is also modulated by microRNAs (miRNAs), small non-coding RNAs that bind to the 3' untranslated region (UTR) of mRNA, leading to mRNA degradation or translational repression. Notably, miR-34a and miR-199a/b have been identified as negative regulators of Axl expression, with their downregulation leading to increased Axl levels in various pathological conditions, including cancer and neuroinflammation [27, 28]. Axl mRNA is upregulated in dendritic cells as well as macrophages upon Toll-like receptor (TLR) signaling activation [29, 30]. Epigenetic modifications further influence Axl gene expression. DNA methylation and histone modifications at the Axl promoter region play critical roles in the transcriptional regulation of Axl [23, 31]. Hypomethylation of CpG islands within the Axl promoter is associated with increased Axl expression, whereas hypermethylation leads to transcriptional silencing [32]. Additionally, histone acetylation and methylation marks, such as H3K27ac and H3K4me3, are correlated with active transcription of the Axl gene [33]. The actual measured molecular weight of Axl kinase fluctuates from 100 to 140 kDa because of post-transcriptional modulation of the activated Axl receptor through glycosylation, phosphorylation, and numerous sites of monoubiquitination, despite the fact that full-length Axl has 894 amino acids that encode a preset protein of 98 kDa [34 - 38].

Receptor Activation

Axl activation is primarily mediated by its high-affinity ligand, namely, growth arrest-specific 6 or Gas6, although other ligands like TULP-1 have also been reported [39]. Upon binding of Gas6 onto Axl's extracellular domain, receptor dimerization occurs, prompting autophosphorylation of key tyrosine residues within the intracellular kinase domain, including Tyr779, Tyr821, and Tyr866 [40]. These phosphorylated tyrosines serve as binding sites for SH2 domain-containing proteins, such as Growth Factor Receptor Bound Protein 2 (Grb2) and phosphoinositide 3-kinase (PI3K), which propagate the signal downstream [40,

41]. This process is tightly regulated to ensure appropriate cellular responses. For instance, in the context of neuroinflammation and ischemic injury, Gas6-Axl signaling has been shown to inhibit the TLR and TRAF/NF-κB pathways, therefore encouraging anti-inflammatory responses and decreasing the generation of pro-inflammatory cytokines [12]. This anti-inflammatory effect is particularly relevant in neurodegenerative diseases like AD, where chronic inflammation is a key pathological feature. Furthermore, through Vav regulation, Axl activation causes actin mobilization and phagocytosis. Lastly, Axl reduces the expression of proinflammatory cytokines that are triggered by TLR [11].

Expression and Regulation in the Brain

Expression of Axl occurs in the Schwann cells in the PNS (Peripheral nervous system) and oligodendrocytes, astrocytes, and microglia within the cerebellum as well as hippocampus [17]. Its expression is tightly regulated and can be influenced by several factors, including inflammatory cytokines, oxidative stress, and cellular damage. Microglia, the resident immune cells of the brain, exhibit high levels of Axl expression, which can be further upregulated in response to brain injury or disease [42]. The regulation of Axl expression involves both transcriptional and post-transcriptional mechanisms. For instance, inflammatory signals such as lipopolysaccharide (LPS) and interleukin-1β (IL-1β) can induce Axl expression through the activation of transcription factors like Nuclear factor kappa-light-chain-enhancer of activated B cells (NF-κB) and Signal transducer and activator of transcription 1 (STAT1) [43]. Additionally, miRNAs have been shown to modulate Axl expression post-transcriptionally, providing another layer of regulation [44]. The upregulation of Axl in microglia during neuroinflammatory conditions suggests a critical role for Axl in modulating the brain's immune response [45].

Role in Normal Neural Processes

Axl kinase plays a multifaceted role in the normal functioning of the neural environment. One of its primary functions is the regulation of microglial activity [45]. Microglia are essential for maintaining homeostasis in the CNS, performing tasks such as clearing apoptotic cells and debris, and modulating inflammatory responses [46]. Axl, upon activation by Gas6, enhances the phagocytic activity of microglia, facilitating the removal of apoptotic cells and reducing the liberation of pro-inflammatory cytokines. This process is crucial for preventing chronic inflammation and promoting tissue repair [47]. Furthermore, TAM signaling (which includes Axl signaling) is involved in the maintenance of the blood-brain barrier (BBB) integrity, neuronal survival, and synaptic plasticity [17]. Additionally, Axl has been implicated in the differentiation and maturation of oligodendrocytes, which are responsible for myelination in the CNS [48]. Moreover, Axl's role extends to synaptic regulation and plasticity, which are critical for learning and memory. The MAPK/ERK pathway, another downstream signaling route of Axl [49], is known to influence synaptic strength and plasticity. Through this pathway, Axl can modulate the expression of synaptic proteins and receptors, thereby impacting synaptic transmission and plasticity [50]. Additionally, Axl's interaction with its ligand, Gas6, has trophic effects, promoting the survival and growth of neurons and glial cells under stress conditions. In the hippocampus, Axl activation has been shown to protect neurons from excitotoxic injury and promote synaptic remodeling, underscoring its significance in cognitive functions [11].

PROTECTIVE ROLE OF AXL KINASE IN THE CNS

Conventionally, the Ig domain of Axl receptor is bound by the SHBG-like domain located at the C-terminal region of Gas-6 ligand (Fig. **1**) [51, 52]. This TAM receptor subsequently utilizes auto-phosphorylation of tyrosine residues to dimerize and activate its RTK domain within the cytoplasmic region [53]. Following that, signaling pathways that are downstream and linked to cell proliferation, survival, and migration, as well as phagocytosis, attenuation of inflammation, and the removal of cellular debris and apoptotic cells (ACs), will be triggered. There are two approaches to modulating the activation of receptor kinase. The first is the typical pathway, which was previously discussed. The other, known as atypical activation, is distinguished by receptor dimerization among all three TAMs or heterotypic cross-talk between Axl and various other receptors (for instance, IFNAR or EGFR) [29, 54, 55]. For instance, by receptor heterodimerization, ProS1/Tyro3 or ProS1/Mertk might indirectly activate Axl [56].

ENHANCEMENT OF CELL PROLIFERATION, SURVIVAL, AND MIGRATION

Axl kinase, when activated by its ligand Growth Arrest Specific 6 (Gas6), initiates a series of complex signaling cascades that are vital for cellular proliferation, survival, and migration. Specifically, the engagement of Axl leads to the activation and phosphorylation of the PI3K/Akt and MAPK/ERK pathways [41, 57]. These pathways are instrumental in ensuring cell survival and promoting proliferation. By attaching to the proline-rich area of PI3K's regulatory subunit (p85) and the SH3 domain of Grb2, Axl activated Protein kinase-B(Akt) and improved the proliferation and survival of cells [58]. Axl engaged in a PI3K/Akt signaling pathway interaction with Gas6 to enhance oligodendrocyte survival [48]. Gas6-induced viability of NIH3T3 cells that were serum-starved was shown to need PI3K, Rac, and Rho [59]. The activation of PI3K/Akt signaling by Axl has been shown to enhance cell survival by inhibiting apoptotic processes and promoting cellular growth and repair [41]. Similarly, the MAPK/ERK pathway contributes to the regulation of gene expression and cellular responses that support neuronal resilience and plasticity. Axl's interaction with Gas6 also activated the PI3K/Ras pathway along with its downstream protein kinases Rac as well as p38 MAPK, which in turn helped Gonadotropin-releasing hormone (GnRH) neurons migrate into the hypothalamus, which promoted reproduction [60].

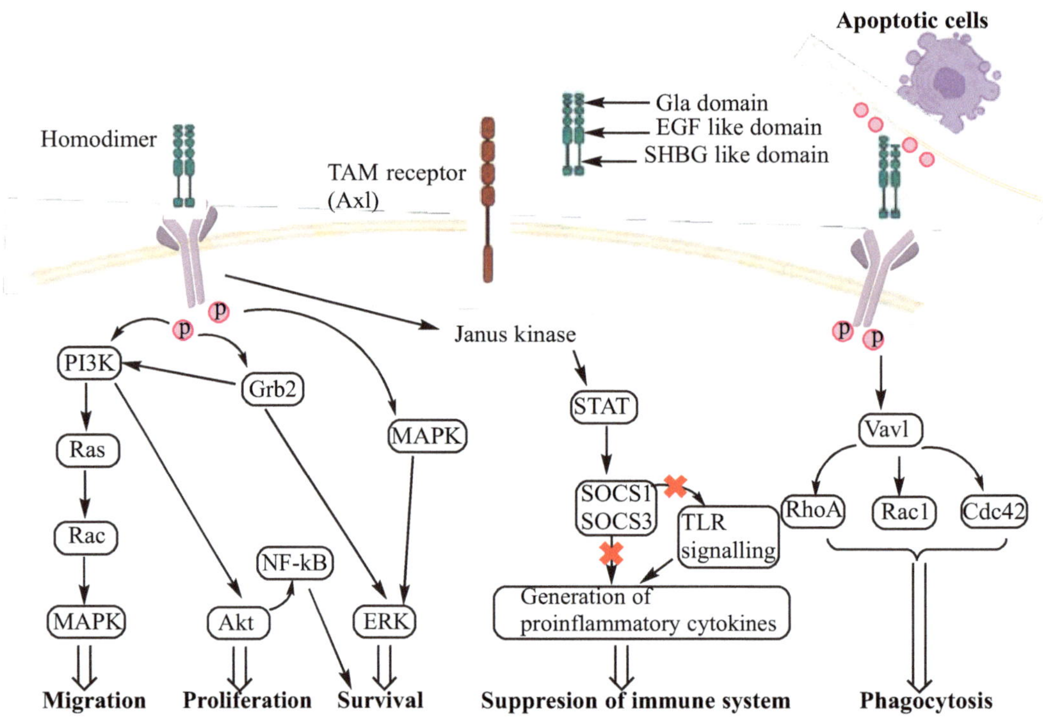

Fig. (1). CNS protection by Axl kinase.

Additionally, proliferating neural progenitors express TAM receptors, which work in concert with neurotrophins to provide intrinsic functional contributions to proliferation as well as differentiation [61 - 63]. Neurogenesis decreased while astrogenesis and hippocampus neural stem cells (NSCs)proliferation increased in neural progenitors when ProS1 was genetically ablated. Additionally, the researchers revealed that the ProS1 effect over NSC quiescence was partially caused by the Notch-1 signaling pathway [64]. Moreover, ProS1's inhibitory function in the Bmi-1-dependent self-renewal of adult and embryonic hippocampus NSCs was emphasized in their subsequent study [65]. Thus, ProS1 may serve as a novel regulator of the brain's homeostasis by controlling quiescence, proliferation, and cell fate determination. It is still unclear, nevertheless, if Axl receptors are involved in these processes.

REGULATION OF PHAGOCYTOSIS

Axl, together with Mertk, plays a pivotal role in the phagocytic function of microglia, the brain's resident immune cells. These receptors are essential for the recognition and engulfment of apoptotic cells and amyloid-beta (Aβ) plaques, processes critical for maintaining brain homeostasis. Ligands mediate an efferocytosis pathway by functioning as "bridging molecules" between the TAM receptors and apoptotic cells (ACs) [66, 67]. On their surface, ACs present "eat-me" signals (also known as apoptotic cell-associated molecular patterns [68]) that phagocytes can identify. PtdSer is the signal with the greatest characterization. It is a typical phospholipid occurring mostly on the inside of the membrane bilayers of every eukaryotic cell [69]. It becomes a signal between cells when it translocates to the external leaflet of the cellular membrane [70]. Aided by Vitamin K, ligands can attach to PtdSer by γ-carboxylation of Gla domains in the presence of Ca^{2+} ions, perhaps guaranteeing structural stability [71]. Following PtdSer recognition, Axl receptors bind to the particular ligand in a 2:1 stoichiometric ratio, which phosphorylates Vav1 and activates the downstream members of Rho, such as Rac1, RhoA, and Cdc42 [72]. When cytoskeleton dynamics eventually change, the ACs are absorbed in a "silent" non-inflammatory manner without the release of pro-inflammatory cytokines [73]. TAM-dependent phagocytic processes are routinely observed in certain normal, healthy cells. For instance, Axl kinase aids Sertoli cells in eliminating germ cells that cause apoptosis in the testes. The accumulation of dead apoptotic germ cells within seminiferous tubules may eventually cause progressive germ cell death and sterility [74, 75].

Efferocytosis has a critical role in controlling inflammatory reactions as well. Inadequate efferocytosis can cause auto-antigen release and secondary necrosis, which can result in long-term autoimmune diseases [76, 77]. In macrophages, tolerance-inducing stimuli like dexamethasone decrease Axl expression while promoting Mertk expression. On the other hand, inflammatory mediators, including poly (I:C) and LPS, increase the expression of Axl while inhibiting the expression of Mertk. Scientists refer to this pattern of expression as "yin and yang" for these two receptors [30]. Microglia also followed the same pattern [45]. Thus, Axl exhibits burst increase expression in response to various inflammatory stimuli and usually plays a role in the cessation of inflammation [73]. Neurogenesis has also been shown to benefit from TAM receptors' phagocytic function. Neurogenesis is primarily initiated by neural stem cells (NSCs), which occur within the subventricular zone (SVZ) proximal to the lateral ventricle as well as the subgranular zone (SGZ) located within the hippocampus's dentate gyrus. To preserve the volume of neurogenesis in a steady-state, "resting stage," microglia phagocytize all these apoptotic cells [70, 78]. In mice models of microglial Mertk and Axl deficiency, ACs gathered and became trapped in the SVZ. Here, the microglia underwent a transformation into active "amoeboid" morphologies. Mertk and Axl work in concert as the primary executors of the eradication of ACs, where ProS1 and Gas6 operate as mediators of the engulfment [79].

SUPPRESSION OF THE IMMUNE SYSTEM

For innate immune responses, the TAM system's anti-inflammatory mechanism has been thoroughly investigated using dendritic cells (DCs) [29]. Axl starts SOCS1 and SOCS3's downstream transcription, which prevents TLR activation as well as IFNAR signaling. In human macrophages, chronic TLR4 stimulation resulted in a substantial increase in TAM expression. Consequently, the secretion of proinflammatory cytokines was downregulated, and SOCS3 was increased in an Axl-dependent manner [80]. When combined, the activation of Axl will obstruct and hijack the preceding route, causing the IFNAR signaling to switch from proinflammatory signaling to immunosuppressive signaling. Lately, it was verified that Gas6 and Axl suppress TLR-induced inflammatory reactions in mouse microglia, in addition to decreased TNF-α production as well as an altered amoeboid microglial shape [45]. The link between the TAM and TLR signaling pathways is further supported by this discovery. Furthermore, following the type I IFN-mediated suppression of TNF-α production in collaboration with Axl, the Twist transcriptional repressor was activated, which then bound to the TNF-α promoter and finally impeded the transcription of downstream genes [81]. These discoveries offer fresh perspectives on the control of inflammation while also expanding the anti-inflammatory functions performed by Axl receptors. The polarization ofM1/M2 phenotypes of microglia, which in itself is crucial in neurodegeneration, can be regulated by the Axl receptors [82]. Furthermore, the TAM signaling pathway has been shown to be able to suppress the transcription of some pro-inflammatory cytokines [83]. By curbing the production of inflammatory mediators, Axl helps maintain a balanced immune response, thus protecting neurons from the deleterious effects of prolonged inflammation and contributing to a more favorable environment for neuronal survival and function.

AXL IN ALZHEIMER'S DISEASE PATHOPHYSIOLOGY

Axl and Amyloid-beta Pathology

Axl kinase is significantly implicated in the modulation of amyloid-beta (Aβ) accumulation, a significant hallmark of AD. Aβ peptides, derived from the amyloid precursor protein (APP), aggregate to form plaques that contribute to neurotoxicity and neuroinflammation [84]. Studies have shown that Axl activation influences the phagocytic activity of microglia, which is crucial for clearing Aβ. Plaques surrounded by microglia displayed heightened immunological responses and increased the expression of phagocytic genes, such as Axl [85]. In the presence of Aβ, Gas6 binding to Axl enhances microglial phagocytosis and reduces Aβ burden, thereby exerting a neuroprotective effect. This is particularly important in the early stages of AD, where efficient clearance of Aβ can mitigate the formation of plaques and slow disease progression [86]. The interaction between Gas6 and Axl may have numerous other effects, such as lowering the amount of toxic Aβ that causes neuronal death, influencing the removal of apoptotic nerve cells in AD, reducing the amount of plaque by removing apoptotic neurons before the cells can produce further pathological Aβ, and possibly even having an impact on neurogenesis [9]. For instance, Gas6 shields cortical neurons against harmful Aβ species *in vitro*, preventing their death [87]. Axl in AD has been described in Fig. (**2**).

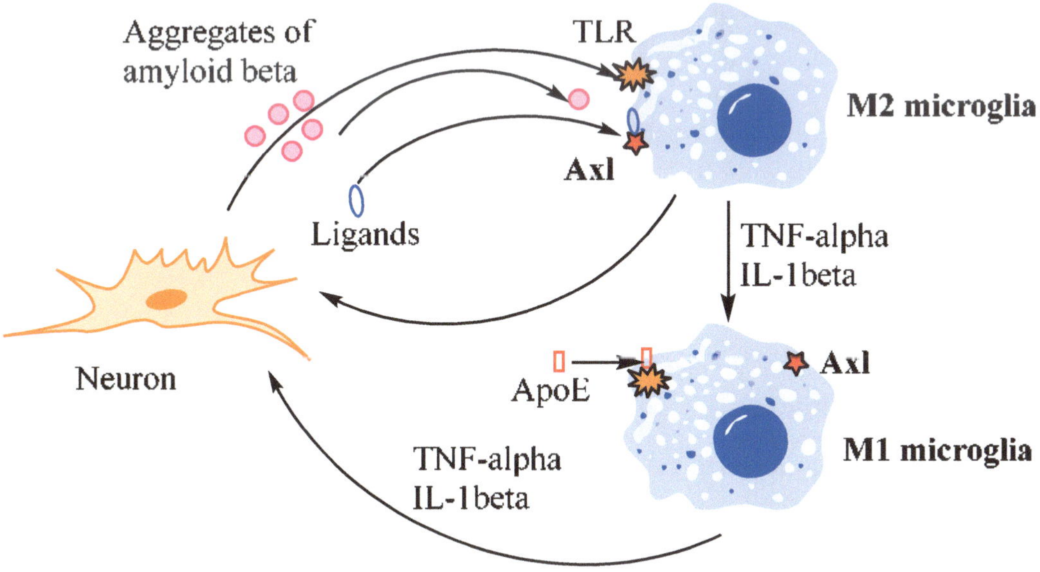

Fig. (2). Axl receptors in AD.

Additionally, Axl influences the metabolism of Apolipoprotein E (ApoE), which is crucial for Aβ clearance. ApoE isoforms, particularly ApoE4, have been shown to differentially affect Aβ aggregation and clearance [88]. In apoE-TR mice, ApoE haploinsufficiency reduced amyloid accumulation in all APOE genotypes [89, 90]. Intraperitoneal injection of anti-apoE antibody into AD mice has resulted in decreased brain Aβ burden and enhanced cognitive performance [91]. Axl signaling negatively influences the production and secretion of ApoE in glial cells, particularly astrocytes, which are the prime sources of ApoE inside the brain. Upon Axl activation, there is suppression in the expression of ATP-binding cassette transporter A1 (ABCA1), a protein involved in the lipidation and secretion of ApoE. Proper lipidation of ApoE is crucial for its role in lipid transport and Aβ clearance. Dysregulation of Axl signaling can lead to impaired lipidation of ApoE, affecting its ability to forge high-density lipoprotein (HDL)-like particles and consequently its efficiency in Aβ clearance. An Axl kinase inhibitor, namely AZ7235, was initially found to increase ApoE in astrocytes as well as microglia [92].

Axl kinase modulates the expression and activity of enzymes involved in Aβ production. Through the downregulation of the NF-κB cascade, Gas6 can downregulate the expression of beta-secretase 1 (BACE1), an enzyme critical for the cleavage of APP into Aβ peptides [93, 94]. This regulatory mechanism suggests that Axl activation can decrease the production of Aβ, further reducing plaque formation. The neurotoxicity of Aβ is caused by an imbalance in intracellular Ca^{2+} concentration, which was dramatically reduced by the inclusion of Gas6 into the primary cell cultures of cortical nerve cells [87]. Moreover, it prevented Aβ-induced demise *in vitro* in cortical neurons [87]. Vitamin K is necessary for the proper functioning of γ-carboxylation in the Gla domain of ligands. Researchers have demonstrated that vitamin K2—whose metabolism was impaired in AD—is essential for healthy brain growth and function. According to a recent study, Gas6/Axl may use the PI3K/Akt/Bad signaling pathway to partially shield cells from the cytotoxicity of Aβ when vitamin K2 is applied [95]. These findings point to a potential protective function of the Gas6/Axl receptor signaling cascade in the survival of brain cells in AD.

Axl and Tau Pathology

Tau pathology, characterized by the generation of neurofibrillary tangles (NFTs) comprising hyperphosphorylated tau protein, is another critical aspect of AD [96]. Growth arrest-specific 6 (Gas6)-mediated activation of Axl initiates the PI3K/Akt pathway, which subsequently inhibits glycogen synthase kinase-3β (GSK-3β), an enzyme directly involved in tau phosphorylation [41, 97]. By inhibiting GSK-3β [98], Axl activation can reduce the hyperphosphorylation of tau, thereby decreasing the formation of NFTs and protecting neuronal structure and function. Axl's interaction with ApoE isoforms plays a significant role in tau pathology [99]. Regarding tauopathy, tau transgenic mice exhibiting human ApoE knock-in had notable atrophy of the brain along with neuroinflammation, while ApoE knockout tau mice were mainly shielded from these alterations [100]. ApoE4, which is the most detrimental isoform of ApoE in the case of AD, is inhibited by Axl signaling, thereby influencing tau hyperphosphorylation and aggregation [99, 100]. In a particular investigation, melatonin-treated male 3xTg mice showed decreased tau phosphorylation along with lower serum levels of Gas6 [101], thereby underscoring a link between Gas6, which is the ligand of Axl kinase, and tau pathology.

IMPACT ON NEUROINFLAMMATION AND GLIAL CELL FUNCTION

Neuroinflammation is a central feature of Alzheimer's disease, and Axl kinase is a crucial regulator of inflammatory responses in the central nervous system (CNS). Axl's neuroprotective functions are largely mediated through its ability to modulate microglial activity and inflammatory responses in the central nervous system (CNS) [47]. Activation of Axl by its ligand, growth arrest-specific protein 6 (Gas6), initiates a cascade of anti-inflammatory signaling pathways that help dampen the immune response. One crucial mechanism involves the suppression of the TLR/TRAF/NF-κB pathway, which is known to drive the production of pro-inflammatory cytokines such as TNF-α, IL-1β, and IL-6. By inhibiting NF-κB, Axl activation reduces the secretion of these cytokines, thereby mitigating the chronic inflammatory state characteristic of AD [11]. In experimental neuroinflammatory conditions, it has been found that Axl deficiency leads to impaired clearance of myelin debris and increased axonal damage. Studies have shown that $Axl^{-/-}$ mice exhibit larger inflammatory lesions and reduced numbers of activated microglia and macrophages at the lesion sites compared to wild-type mice [102]. This indicates that Axl is crucial for the recruitment and activation of phagocytic microglia, which are essential for clearing debris and reducing inflammation.

Axl kinase significantly impacts glial cell function, particularly in microglia and astrocytes, which are vital for maintaining CNS homeostasis and responding to injury [103]. In the context of AD, effective microglial function is critical for clearing amyloid-beta (Aβ) plaques and limiting neuroinflammation [104]. Axl activation supports microglial migration to sites of injury and promotes the phagocytosis of apoptotic neurons and debris, processes that are impaired in Axl-deficient models. The absence of Axl leads to an accumulation of myelin debris and a hyper-inflammatory state, as seen in EAE models, underscoring the importance of Axl in maintaining glial cell function and reducing neuroinflammation [102].

The interaction between Axl and ApoE in glial cells is particularly relevant to understanding the mechanisms of neuroinflammation in AD. Researchers have discovered that plasma from ApoE4 carriers had higher concentrations of inflammatory biomarkers than from non-carriers [105]. When lipopolysaccharide (LPS) was administered to ApoE-TR mice in experiments, ApoE4-TR mice displayed a greater inflammatory response than ApoE3-TR mice, as seen by raised levels of pro-inflammatory cytokines in the brain [106, 107]. Thus, the suppression of ApoE expression through Axl activation can be considered as a therapeutic avenue.

Axl's role in maintaining endothelial BBB integrity is linked to its maintenance of co-localization of Tight junction (TJ) proteins. Studies using a broad-spectrum TAM signaling inhibitor revealed that mice treated with West Nile Virus (WNV)were more susceptible to death and had greater blood-brain barrier permeability. During infection, the $Axl^{-/-}$ phenotype was linked to noticeably impaired BBB integrity, suggesting that Axl possesses the ability to sustain BBB during viral infection [108]. Disruption of Axl signaling can lead to BBB breakdown, allowing peripheral immune cells to infiltrate the brain and exacerbate neuroinflammation. Furthermore, a gene that mediates the damage to the BBB, MMP-9, was downregulated by Gas6 [74]. Gas6 may therefore aid in preserving the integrity of the BBB and preventing immune cells from penetrating the central nervous system.

Evidence from Human Studies

Researchers studying the gene expression of plaque-associated microglia in postmortem brain tissues from individuals with early-onset AD (EOAD) discovered an upregulation of Axl inside the brain's plaque regions [109]. It is postulated that in the early stages of the illness, Axl may be activated to serve a protective function in immunological reconstitution. Clinical investigations provide more hints about the relationship between Axl and AD. In this case, the changes in TAMs/ligands present within cerebrospinal fluid (CSF) or in serum could possibly be useful indicators for diagnosis and prognosis. In human AD, increased levels of sAxl complex in conjunction with Gas6 within CSF are predictive of the onset and course of the illness [7, 86]. Scientists who recently obtained access to several enhanced CSF neuroinflammation indicators discovered a strong correlation between sAxl and larger brain structure, as well as preserved cognition throughout the pre-dementia phases observed in AD. The scientists believed that these spikes in soluble Axl concentrations were markers of

Axl expression as well as activity, suggesting that Axl might serve as a defense mechanism [110]. There is a substantial correlation between the baseline Axl level in the CSF and the decline of Aβ_{42}. It is proposed that this criterion, which is clinically reliable for diagnosing AD, can also be used to anticipate the early stages of AD's development of Aβ pathology [111]. Additionally, by examining plasma samples, it can be confirmed that Axl assists in estimating the brain Aβ burden of AD [112]. In the CSF of AD patients, the protein levels of Gas6 ligand of Axl were markedly raised and exhibited an inverse relationship with cognitive decline [113].

THERAPEUTIC STRATEGIES FOR TARGETING AXL AND GAS6

Targeting Axl kinase within the context of AD holds promise owing to its role in the modulation of inflammatory responses and facilitation of protein clearance through the TAM system. Effective drug discovery strategies for targeting Axl kinase must prioritize achieving substantial penetration across the blood-brain barrier (BBB), a critical factor for treating central nervous system (CNS) disorders. This requirement underscores the necessity for drug candidates with optimal pharmacokinetic properties, ensuring adequate CNS exposure while maintaining efficacy. Moreover, the complexity of neurodegenerative diseases necessitates early detection and sustained therapeutic intervention to halt or slow disease progression effectively. Nevertheless, the challenge remains in balancing therapeutic efficacy with safety, as prolonged immune suppression could potentially create a milieu conducive to other pathological conditions, including malignancies and infections. Therefore, a nuanced approach to drug development is essential, one that carefully calibrates the degree of immune modulation to avoid adverse effects while harnessing the beneficial aspects of Axl kinase activation. The therapeutic strategies discovered so far have been discussed below.

Plant-based Small Molecule Regulators of Axl

A number of cutting-edge plant-based drugs that improve AD pathogenesis in an Axl-dependent way have recently been discovered by scientists. Ganoderic acid A (GAA), which is a tetracyclic triterpenoid, has been identified as the main active ingredient in *Ganoderma lucidum*. It possesses many bioactivities, including immunological modulation and anti-tumor properties. Qi *et al.*, conducted a study where it was found that GAA therapy dramatically decreased the amounts of intracellular Aβ_{42} in microglial cells [114]. Furthermore, elevated LC3B-II levels indicated that GAA triggered autophagy, which in turn was triggered by upregulating Axl and Pak1 (p21-activated kinase 1) phosphorylation. R428, an Axl inhibitor, reversed the impact of GAA, removing Aβ by autophagy. In line with the cell-based assay, GAA improved cognitive impairment and decreased Aβ_{42} levels within a mouse model of AD. Moreover, GAA treatment increased the expression of LC3B in the hippocampal regions; however, R428 reversed these GAA-specific effects. Thus, GAA improved cognitive deficit *in vivo* and reduced the Aβ_{42} load in microglia by promoting autophagy *via* Axl/Pak1.

A triterpene saponin called Jujuboside A (JuA) was extracted from *Semen ZiziphiSpinosae*. Numerous biological actions of JuA have been documented, including anti-oxidant, anti-inflammatory, anti-apoptotic, and neuroprotective properties. In an AD animal model, JuA improved learning and memory deficit by promoting Aβ clearance *via* the Axl/ERK pathway, maintaining the activation of peroxisome proliferator-activated receptor γ (PPARγ) inside the microglia of APP/PS1 transgenic mice. This study by Zhang *et al.*, showed that *via* upregulating HSP90β expression, JuA considerably restored the amount and functionality of PPARγ in BV2 cell lines as well as in primary microglia [115]. Nuclear receptors like liver X receptor (LXR), retinoid X receptor (RXR), PPARγ, and PPARδ license Axl's ability to phagocytose [116]. Hence, Aβ clearance is facilitated by positive feedback provided by the Axl as well as the PPARγ signaling pathways. Additionally, their investigation revealed that JuA prevented tau protein phosphorylation produced by Aβ or DL-homocysteine [116].

Immunotherapeutic Agent

In a study by Jun *et al.*, a section derived from an Aβ-targeting monoclonal antibody was substituted for Gas6's Gla domain to create the phagocytosis inducer fusion protein known as αAβ-Gas6 [117]. Through this modification, αAβ-Gas6 is able to identify Aβ in particular and facilitate Aβ elimination. By means of TAM receptor-dependent phagocytosis, the chimeric protein αAβ–Gas6 selectively removes Aβ plaques without triggering reactive gliosis or NF-kB-mediated inflammatory reactions. Additionally, αAβ–Gas6 can cause a synergistic clearance of Aβ by triggering astrocytic and microglial phagocytosis. This leads to improved behavioral outcomes in a mouse model of AD, as well as cerebral amyloid angiopathy, with significantly less microhemorrhage and synapse elimination than when Aβ antibody treatment is used. As a viable immunotherapeutic approach for AD, it could mitigate the pro-inflammatory as well as neuronally-toxic adverse effects of traditional immune treatment aducanumab. Additionally, single-cell RNA sequencing suggested that αAβ-Gas6 therapy might produce a type 1 IFN-responsive microglial population.

ADAM Metalloproteases Inhibitor

The TAM receptors are cleavable in proximity to the region of the cell membrane. It is the ADAM metalloproteases that generate the soluble forms of Axl, sAxl. Compared to total Axl, sAxl has a higher affinity for binding Gas6 [118]. Through the sequestration of Gas6 and blockade of the Gas6/Axl pathway, it acts as an antagonist for Gas6. Also, in a study conducted by Orme *et al.*, it was discovered that the Axl ectodomain is shed from leukocytes through the action of the proteases ADAM10 as well as TACE [119]. The cleavage of surface Axl on certain leukocytes is facilitated by ADAM matrix metalloproteases, namely ADAM10 and TACE (ADAM17). Under normal circumstances, Twist-mediated inhibition of inflammatory cytokines is how Axl transduces an anti-inflammatory signal in macrophages [18]. They showed that Axl-mediated anti-inflammatory action is abolished both *in vitro* and *in vivo* when surface Axl is lost. In response to Gas6, Axl-deficient and lupus-prone mice macrophages are unable to trigger Twist or inhibit the production of IL-6 and TNF-α. Inhibiting ADAM10/17 together can save the anti-inflammatory properties of Axl as well as the resistance of lupus-prone macrophages to Gas6 [119]. Therefore, ADAM10/17 inhibitor-induced Axl function restoration may be beneficial for AD therapeutic intervention.

RECOMBINANT GAS6 ADMINISTRATION

Numerous illness models in animals have demonstrated the neuroprotective effects of recombinant Gas6 (rGas6). For instance, in a stroke model, rGas6 therapy activated Axl to reduce neuroinflammation and alleviate neurological impairments. In addition to improving neurologic impairment scores and reducing brain infarction, rGas6 also lowered TRAF3 and TRAF6 expression. It also lowered the expression of inflammatory mediators, namely TNF-α, IL-1β, and IL-6. RGas6 enhanced long-term neurological functioning and memory, four weeks following MCAO (Middle cerebral artery occlusion). The brain protection provided by rGas6 was abolished by blockage of the Axl/TLR/TRAF/NF-κB pathway [120]. Following the delivery of rGas6, a mouse model of intracerebral hemorrhage showed comparable outcomes. In this instance, there was an increase in Axl phosphorylation alongside cleavage of soluble Axl (sAxl), as well as elevated SOCS1 and SOCS3 were observed [121]. Rgas6 also improved recovery and remyelination in the cuprizone as well as the EAE model of Multiple Sclerosis [122, 123]. In another study conducted on a subarachnoid hemorrhage (SAH) model, rGas6 treatment alleviated inflammation, enhanced microglia efferocytosis, and mitigated neurological impairments and BBB disintegration brought on by SAH. Axl and Rac1 inhibition or knockdown abrogated the positive effects of rGas6. It was found that rGas6 inhibited the onset of early brain damage in mice following SAH, which is partially reliant on Axl activation [47]. While the precise function of rGas6 in the pathogenesis of AD has not yet been investigated, these findings will help devise therapy plans for AD.

CONCLUSION

Throughout this discourse, the multifaceted role of Axl kinase in modulating key signaling pathways pertinent to AD has been elucidated with considerable depth. Axl kinase, a critical component of the TAM receptor family, demonstrates profound neuroprotective properties by influencing several signaling cascades, including MAPK/ERK, TLR/TRAF/NF-κB, PI3K/AKT, and GSK-3β pathways. These pathways are pivotal in regulating neuroinflammation, neuronal survival, and the clearance of pathogenic proteins such as amyloid-beta and hyperphosphorylated tau. Activation of Axl kinase by its ligand, Gas6, fosters an anti-inflammatory environment, enhances microglial phagocytic activity, and supports neuronal resilience against stressors, thereby mitigating the progression of AD. The strategic modulation of Axl-mediated pathways underscores its potential as a therapeutic target, offering a promising avenue to slow or halt the neurodegenerative processes characteristic of AD.

Future therapeutic strategies should focus on the precise activation of Axl kinase to harness its neuroprotective effects while ensuring minimal adverse outcomes. Drug development must prioritize compounds with optimal blood-brain barrier (BBB) penetration and selectivity to avoid off-target effects and maintain safety. Furthermore, exploring combination therapies that integrate Axl activation with other treatments, such as anti-amyloid agents, tau inhibitors, and neuroprotective compounds, may yield synergistic benefits. This multi-pronged approach could address the complex pathology of AD more effectively than monotherapy. Advancing our understanding of the molecular mechanisms underlying Axl signaling in the CNS will be crucial. Comprehensive preclinical as well as clinical studies are essential to evaluate the long-term efficacy and safety of Axl-targeted therapies. Additionally, investigating biomarkers for early detection and monitoring therapeutic responses will enhance the clinical management of AD, ultimately improving patient outcomes and quality of life. The neuroprotective promise of Axl kinase activation in AD offers a hopeful trajectory towards developing effective and sustainable treatments for this debilitating neurodegenerative disorder.

LIST OF ABBREVIATIONS

ABCA1 ATP-Binding Cassette Transporter A1

ACs Apoptotic Cells

AD Alzheimer's Disease

ADAM10	ADAM Metallopeptidase Domain 10
Akt	Protein kinase-B
AP1	Activator Protein 1
ApoE	Apolipoprotein E
BACE1	beta-secretase 1
BBB	Blood Brain Barrier
DAM	Disease-Associated Microglia
EAE	Experimental Autoimmune Encephalomyelitis
EGFR	Epidermal Growth Factor Receptor
EOAD	Early-onset AD
ERK	Extracellular Signal-regulated Kinase
GAA	Ganoderic Acid A
Gas6	Growth Arrest-specific Protein 6
Grb2	Growth Factor Receptor Bound Protein 2
GSK-3β	Glycogen Synthase Kinase-3
HDL	High-Density Lipoprotein
HIF1α	Hypoxia Inducible Factor 1α
IFN	Interferons
IFNAR	type I IFN Receptor
IL-1β	Interleukin-1 Beta
IL-6	Interleukin-6
JuA	Jujuboside A
LC3B II	LC3-phosphatidylethanolamine Conjugate
LPS	Lipopolysaccharide
LXR	Nuclear Receptors like the Liver X Receptor
MAPK	Mitogen-Activated Protein Kinase
MCAO	Middle Cerebral Artery Occlusion
MMP-9	Matrix Metallopeptidase 9
MZF-1	Myeloid Zinc Finger 1 Protein
NAMPs	Neurodegeneration-Associated Molecular Patterns
NF-κB	Nuclear Factor Kappa-light-chain-enhancer Of Activated B Cells
NIH3T3	Mouse Embryonic Fibroblast Cell Line
NSCs	Neural Stem Cells
Pak1	p21-activated Kinase 1
PI3K	phosphoinositide 3-Kinase

PPARγ	Peroxisome Proliferator-activated Receptor γ
ProS1	Protein S1
PRRs	Pattern Recognition Receptors
rGas6	Recombinant Gas6
RTKs	Receptor Tyrosine Kinases
RXR	Retinoid X Receptor
SAH	Subarachnoid Hemorrhage
SHBG	Serum Sex Hormone-binding Globulin
SOCS1	Suppressor of Cytokine Signaling 1
SOCS3	Suppressor of Cytokine Signaling 3
STAT1	Signal Transducer and Activator of Transcription 1
TACE/ADAM17	Metalloprotease TNF-α Converting Enzyme
TLR	Toll-Like Receptor
TNF-α	Tumour Necrosis Factor Alpha
TRAF	Tumor Necrosis Factor Receptor–associated Factor
TRAF3	Tumor Necrosis Factor Receptor-associated Factor 3
TRAF6	Tumor Necrosis Factor Receptor-associated Factor 6
TULP-1	Tubby-Related Protein 1
WNV	West Nile Virus

REFERNCES

[1] Guzman-Martinez L, Calfío C, Farias GA, Vilches C, Prieto R, Maccioni RB. New frontiers in the prevention, diagnosis, and treatment of Alzheimer's disease. J Alzheimers Dis 2021; 82(s1): S51-63. [http://dx.doi.org/10.3233/JAD-201059] [PMID: 33523002]

[2] Kim AY, Al Jerdi S, MacDonald R, Triggle CR. Alzheimer's disease and its treatment–yesterday, today, and tomorrow. Front Pharmacol 2024; 15: 1399121. [http://dx.doi.org/10.3389/fphar.2024.1399121] [PMID: 38868666]

[3] Meur S, Mukherjee S, Roy S, Karati D. Role of PIM kinase inhibitor in the treatment of alzheimer's disease. Mol Neurobiol 2024; 61(12): 10941-55. [http://dx.doi.org/10.1007/s12035-024-04257-7] [PMID: 38816674]

[4] Wang ZY, Wang PG, An J. The multifaceted roles of TAM receptors during viral infection. Virol Sin 2021; 36(1): 1-12. [http://dx.doi.org/10.1007/s12250-020-00264-9] [PMID: 32720213]

[5] Lu Q, Lemke G. Homeostatic regulation of the immune system by receptor tyrosine kinases of the Tyro 3 family. Science 2001; 293(5528): 306-11. [http://dx.doi.org/10.1126/science.1061663] [PMID: 11452127]

[6] Pampuscenko K, Morkuniene R, Sneideris T, *et al.* Extracellular tau induces microglial phagocytosis of living neurons in cell cultures. J Neurochem 2020; 154(3): 316-29. [http://dx.doi.org/10.1111/jnc.14940] [PMID: 31834946]

[7] Huang Y, Happonen KE, Burrola PG, *et al.* Microglia use TAM receptors to detect and engulf amyloid

β plaques. Nat Immunol 2021; 22(5): 586-94.
[http://dx.doi.org/10.1038/s41590-021-00913-5] [PMID: 33859405]

[8] Keren-Shaul H, Spinrad A, Weiner A, *et al.* A unique microglia type associated with restricting development of Alzheimer's disease. Cell 2017; 169(7): 1276-1290.e17.
[http://dx.doi.org/10.1016/j.cell.2017.05.018] [PMID: 28602351]

[9] Deczkowska A, Keren-Shaul H, Weiner A, Colonna M, Schwartz M, Amit I. Disease-associated microglia: a universal immune sensor of neurodegeneration. Cell 2018; 173(5): 1073-81.
[http://dx.doi.org/10.1016/j.cell.2018.05.003] [PMID: 29775591]

[10] Seitz HM. The role of Axl/Mertk/Tyro3 receptor tyrosine kinases in the clearance of apoptotic cells. The University of North Carolina at Chapel Hill 2006.

[11] Owlett LD. Owlett M. Modulation of acute inflammation and Alzheimer's disease pathology by Gas6-Axl interaction [PhD thesis on the Internet]. Rochester (NY): University of Rochester; 2020.

[12] Zhou S, Li Y, Zhang Z, Yuan Y. An insight into the TAM system in Alzheimer's disease. Int Immunopharmacol 2023; 116: 109791.
[http://dx.doi.org/10.1016/j.intimp.2023.109791] [PMID: 36738678]

[13] Shen Z, Bao X, Wang R. Clinical PET imaging of microglial activation: implications for microglial therapeutics in Alzheimer's disease. Front Aging Neurosci 2018; 10: 314.
[http://dx.doi.org/10.3389/fnagi.2018.00314] [PMID: 30349474]

[14] Feneyrolles C, Spenlinhauer A, Guiet L, *et al.* Axl kinase as a key target for oncology: focus on small molecule inhibitors. Mol Cancer Ther 2014; 13(9): 2141-8.
[http://dx.doi.org/10.1158/1535-7163.MCT-13-1083] [PMID: 25139999]

[15] Liu E, Hjelle B, Bishop JM. Transforming genes in chronic myelogenous leukemia. Proc Natl Acad Sci USA 1988; 85(6): 1952-6.
[http://dx.doi.org/10.1073/pnas.85.6.1952] [PMID: 3279421]

[16] Goyette MA, Côté JF. AXL receptor tyrosine kinase as a promising therapeutic target directing multiple aspects of cancer progression and metastasis. Cancers (Basel) 2022; 14(3): 466.
[http://dx.doi.org/10.3390/cancers14030466] [PMID: 35158733]

[17] Yamagata M, Sanes JR, Weiner JA. Synaptic adhesion molecules. Curr Opin Cell Biol 2003; 15(5): 621-32.
[http://dx.doi.org/10.1016/S0955-0674(03)00107-8] [PMID: 14519398]

[18] Burstyn-Cohen T, Hochberg A. TAM signaling in the nervous system. Brain Plast 2021; 7(1): 33-46.
[http://dx.doi.org/10.3233/BPL-210125] [PMID: 34631419]

[19] Kimani SG, Kumar S, Bansal N, *et al.* Small molecule inhibitors block Gas6-inducible TAM activation and tumorigenicity. Sci Rep 2017; 7(1): 43908.
[http://dx.doi.org/10.1038/srep43908] [PMID: 28272423]

[20] Toledo RA, Qin Y, Cheng ZM, *et al.* Recurrent mutations of chromatin-remodeling genes and kinase receptors in pheochromocytomas and paragangliomas. Clin Cancer Res 2016; 22(9): 2301-10.
[http://dx.doi.org/10.1158/1078-0432.CCR-15-1841] [PMID: 26700204]

[21] Scaltriti M, Elkabets M, Baselga J. Molecular pathways: AXL, a membrane receptor mediator of resistance to therapy. Clin Cancer Res 2016; 22(6): 1313-7.
[http://dx.doi.org/10.1158/1078-0432.CCR-15-1458] [PMID: 26763248]

[22] Meertens L, Labeau A, Dejarnac O, *et al.* Axl mediates ZIKA virus entry in human glial cells and modulates innate immune responses. Cell Rep 2017; 18(2): 324-33.
[http://dx.doi.org/10.1016/j.celrep.2016.12.045] [PMID: 28076778]

[23] Fujimori T, Grabiec AM, Kaur M, *et al.* The Axl receptor tyrosine kinase is a discriminator of macrophage function in the inflamed lung. Mucosal Immunol 2015; 8(5): 1021-30.
[http://dx.doi.org/10.1038/mi.2014.129] [PMID: 25603826]

[24] Mudduluru G, Allgayer H. The human receptor tyrosine kinase *Axl* gene – promoter characterization and regulation of constitutive expression by Sp1, Sp3 and CpG methylation. Biosci Rep 2008; 28(3): 161-76.
[http://dx.doi.org/10.1042/BSR20080046] [PMID: 18522535]

[25] Mudduluru G, Leupold JH, Stroebel P, Allgayer H. PMA up-regulates the transcription of Axl by AP-1 transcription factor binding to TRE sequences *via* the MAPK cascade in leukaemia cells. Biol Cell 2011; 103(1): 21-33.
[http://dx.doi.org/10.1042/BC20100094] [PMID: 20977427]

[26] Rankin EB, Fuh KC, Castellini L, *et al.* Direct regulation of GAS6/AXL signaling by HIF promotes renal metastasis through SRC and MET. Proc Natl Acad Sci USA 2014; 111(37): 13373-8.
[http://dx.doi.org/10.1073/pnas.1404848111] [PMID: 25187556]

[27] Mudduluru G, Vajkoczy P, Allgayer H. Myeloid zinc finger 1 induces migration, invasion, and *in vivo* metastasis through Axl gene expression in solid cancer. Mol Cancer Res 2010; 8(2): 159-69.
[http://dx.doi.org/10.1158/1541-7786.MCR-09-0326] [PMID: 20145042]

[28] Mudduluru G, Ceppi P, Kumarswamy R, Scagliotti GV, Papotti M, Allgayer H. Regulation of Axl receptor tyrosine kinase expression by miR-34a and miR-199a/b in solid cancer. Oncogene 2011; 30(25): 2888-99.
[http://dx.doi.org/10.1038/onc.2011.13] [PMID: 21317930]

[29] Mishra S, Sarkar S, Pandey A, *et al.* Crosstalk between miRNA and protein expression profiles in nitrate-exposed brain cells. Mol Neurobiol 2023; 60(7): 3855-72.
[http://dx.doi.org/10.1007/s12035-023-03316-9] [PMID: 36971918]

[30] Rothlin CV, Ghosh S, Zuniga EI, Oldstone MBA, Lemke G. TAM receptors are pleiotropic inhibitors of the innate immune response. Cell 2007; 131(6): 1124-36.
[http://dx.doi.org/10.1016/j.cell.2007.10.034] [PMID: 18083102]

[31] Zagórska A, Través PG, Lew ED, Dransfield I, Lemke G. Diversification of TAM receptor tyrosine kinase function. Nat Immunol 2014; 15(10): 920-8.
[http://dx.doi.org/10.1038/ni.2986] [PMID: 25194421]

[32] Ott M, Litzenburger UM, Sahm F, Rauschenbach KJ, Tudoran R, Hartmann C, Marquez VE, von Deimling A, Wick W, Platten M. Promotion of glioblastoma cell motility by enhancer of zeste homolog 2 (EZH2) is mediated by AXL receptor kinase.

[33] Xu D, Wang G, Li J, *et al.* Tissue-Specific monoallelic expression of bovine AXL is associated with DNA methylation of promoter DMR. Biochem Genet 2019; 57(6): 801-12.
[http://dx.doi.org/10.1007/s10528-019-09925-1] [PMID: 31073794]

[34] McCornack C, Woodiwiss T, Hardi A, Yano H, Kim AH. The function of histone methylation and acetylation regulators in GBM pathophysiology. Front Oncol 2023; 13: 1144184.
[http://dx.doi.org/10.3389/fonc.2023.1144184] [PMID: 37205197]

[35] Valverde P. Effects of Gas6 and hydrogen peroxide in Axl ubiquitination and downregulation. Biochem Biophys Res Commun 2005; 333(1): 180-5.
[http://dx.doi.org/10.1016/j.bbrc.2005.05.086] [PMID: 15958209]

[36] Sather S, Kenyon KD, Lefkowitz JB, *et al.* A soluble form of the Mer receptor tyrosine kinase inhibits macrophage clearance of apoptotic cells and platelet aggregation. Blood 2007; 109(3): 1026-33.
[http://dx.doi.org/10.1182/blood-2006-05-021634] [PMID: 17047157]

[37] O'Bryan JP, Frye RA, Cogswell PC, *et al.* axl, a transforming gene isolated from primary human myeloid leukemia cells, encodes a novel receptor tyrosine kinase. Mol Cell Biol 1991; 11(10): 5016-31.
[http://dx.doi.org/10.1128/mcb.11.10.5016-5031.1991] [PMID: 1656220]

[38] Lu Q, Gore M, Zhang Q, *et al.* Tyro-3 family receptors are essential regulators of mammalian spermatogenesis. Nature 1999; 398(6729): 723-8.

[http://dx.doi.org/10.1038/19554] [PMID: 10227296]

[39] Mosesson Y, Shtiegman K, Katz M, *et al.* Endocytosis of receptor tyrosine kinases is driven by monoubiquitylation, not polyubiquitylation. J Biol Chem 2003; 278(24): 21323-6. [http://dx.doi.org/10.1074/jbc.C300096200] [PMID: 12719435]

[40] Caberoy NB, Zhou Y, Li W. Tubby and tubby-like protein 1 are new MerTK ligands for phagocytosis. EMBO J 2010; 29(23): 3898-910. [http://dx.doi.org/10.1038/emboj.2010.265] [PMID: 20978472]

[41] Graham DK, DeRyckere D, Davies KD, Earp HS. The TAM family: phosphatidylserine-sensing receptor tyrosine kinases gone awry in cancer. Nat Rev Cancer 2014; 14(12): 769-85. [http://dx.doi.org/10.1038/nrc3847] [PMID: 25568918]

[42] Stenhoff J, Dahlbäck B, Hafizi S. Vitamin K-dependent Gas6 activates ERK kinase and stimulates growth of cardiac fibroblasts. Biochem Biophys Res Commun 2004; 319(3): 871-8. [http://dx.doi.org/10.1016/j.bbrc.2004.05.070] [PMID: 15184064]

[43] Zhou H, Hu L, Li J, *et al.* AXL kinase-mediated astrocytic phagocytosis modulates outcomes of traumatic brain injury. J Neuroinflammation 2021; 18(1): 154. [http://dx.doi.org/10.1186/s12974-021-02201-3] [PMID: 34233703]

[44] Duan J, Zhao Q, He Z, Tang S, Duan J, Xing W. Current understanding of macrophages in intracranial aneurysm: relevant etiological manifestations, signaling modulation and therapeutic strategies. Front Immunol 2024; 14: 1320098. [http://dx.doi.org/10.3389/fimmu.2023.1320098] [PMID: 38259443]

[45] Jones TA, Jeyapalan JN, Forshew T, *et al.* Molecular analysis of pediatric brain tumors identifies microRNAs in pilocytic astrocytomas that target the MAPK and NF-κB pathways. Acta Neuropathol Commun 2015; 3(1): 86. [http://dx.doi.org/10.1186/s40478-015-0266-3]

[46] Gilchrist SE, Goudarzi S, Hafizi S. Gas6 inhibits toll-like receptor-mediated inflammatory pathways in mouse microglia *via* Axl and Mer. Front Cell Neurosci 2020; 14: 576650. [http://dx.doi.org/10.3389/fncel.2020.576650] [PMID: 33192322]

[47] Kabba JA, Xu Y, Christian H, *et al.* Microglia: housekeeper of the central nervous system. Cell Mol Neurobiol 2018; 38(1): 53-71. [http://dx.doi.org/10.1007/s10571-017-0504-2] [PMID: 28534246]

[48] Tang J, Jin Y, Jia F, *et al.* Gas6 promotes microglia efferocytosis and suppresses inflammation through activating Axl/Rac1 signaling in subarachnoid hemorrhage mice. Transl Stroke Res 2023; 14(6): 955 69. [http://dx.doi.org/10.1007/s12975-022-01099-0] [PMID: 36324028]

[49] Shankar SL, O'Guin K, Kim M, *et al.* Gas6/Axl signaling activates the phosphatidylinositol 3-kinase/Akt1 survival pathway to protect oligodendrocytes from tumor necrosis factor α-induced apoptosis. J Neurosci 2006; 26(21): 5638-48. [http://dx.doi.org/10.1523/JNEUROSCI.5063-05.2006] [PMID: 16723520]

[50] Wu X, Liu X, Koul S, Lee CY, Zhang Z, Halmos B. AXL kinase as a novel target for cancer therapy. Oncotarget 2014; 5(20): 9546-63. [http://dx.doi.org/10.18632/oncotarget.2542] [PMID: 25337673]

[51] Mazzucchelli C, Brambilla R. Ras-related and MAPK signalling in neuronal plasticity and memory formation. Cell Mol Life Sci 2000; 57(4): 604-11. [http://dx.doi.org/10.1007/PL00000722] [PMID: 11130460]

[52] Tanabe K, Nagata K, Ohashi K, Nakano T, Arita H, Mizuno K. Roles of γ-carboxylation and a sex hormone-binding globulin-like domain in receptor-binding and in biological activities of Gas6. FEBS Lett 1997; 408(3): 306-10. [http://dx.doi.org/10.1016/S0014-5793(97)00448-1] [PMID: 9188782]

[53] Evenäs P, Dahlbäck B, Frutos PG. The first laminin G-type domain in the SHBG-like region of protein S contains residues essential for activation of the receptor tyrosine kinase sky. [http://dx.doi.org/10.1515/BC.2000.027]

[54] Lemmon MA, Schlessinger J. Cell signaling by receptor tyrosine kinases. Cell 2010; 141(7): 1117-34. [http://dx.doi.org/10.1016/j.cell.2010.06.011] [PMID: 20602996]

[55] Vouri M, Croucher DR, Kennedy SP, An Q, Pilkington GJ, Hafizi S. Axl-EGFR receptor tyrosine kinase hetero-interaction provides EGFR with access to pro-invasive signalling in cancer cells. Oncogenesis 2016; 5(10): e266. [http://dx.doi.org/10.1038/oncsis.2016.66] [PMID: 27775700]

[56] Brown JE, Krodel M, Pazos M, Lai C, Prieto AL. Cross-phosphorylation, signaling and proliferative functions of the Tyro3 and Axl receptors in Rat2 cells. PLoS One 2012; 7(5): e36800. [http://dx.doi.org/10.1371/journal.pone.0036800] [PMID: 22606290]

[57] Ray AK, DuBois JC, Gruber RC, *et al.* Loss of G as6 and A xl signaling results in extensive axonal damage, motor deficits, prolonged neuroinflammation, and less remyelination following cuprizone exposure. Glia 2017; 65(12): 2051-69. [http://dx.doi.org/10.1002/glia.23214] [PMID: 28925029]

[58] Li Y, Jia L, Liu C, *et al.* Axl as a downstream effector of TGF-β1 *via* PI3K/Akt-PAK1 signaling pathway promotes tumor invasion and chemoresistance in breast carcinoma. Tumour Biol 2015; 36(2): 1115-27. [http://dx.doi.org/10.1007/s13277-014-2677-3] [PMID: 25327287]

[59] Weinger JG, Gohari P, Yan Y, Backer JM, Varnum B, Shafit-Zagardo B. In brain, Axl recruits Grb2 and the p85 regulatory subunit of PI3 kinase; *in vitro* mutagenesis defines the requisite binding sites for downstream Akt activation. J Neurochem 2008; 106(1): 134-46. [http://dx.doi.org/10.1111/j.1471-4159.2008.05343.x] [PMID: 18346204]

[60] Goruppi S, Ruaro E, Varnum B, Schneider C. Gas6-mediated survival in NIH3T3 cells activates stress signalling cascade and is independent of Ras. Oncogene 1999; 18(29): 4224-36. [http://dx.doi.org/10.1038/sj.onc.1202788] [PMID: 10435635]

[61] Nielsen-Preiss SM, Allen MP, Xu M, *et al.* Adhesion-related kinase induction of migration requires phosphatidylinositol-3-kinase and ras stimulation of rac activity in immortalized gonadotropin-releasing hormone neuronal cells. Endocrinology 2007; 148(6): 2806-14. [http://dx.doi.org/10.1210/en.2007-0039] [PMID: 17332061]

[62] Ji R, Tian S, Lu HJ, *et al.* TAM receptors affect adult brain neurogenesis by negative regulation of microglial cell activation. J Immunol 2013; 191(12): 6165-77. [http://dx.doi.org/10.4049/jimmunol.1302229] [PMID: 24244024]

[63] Ji R, Johnson K. TAM receptors: two pathways to regulate adult neurogenesis. Neural Regen Res 2015; 10(3): 344-5. [http://dx.doi.org/10.4103/1673-5374.153671] [PMID: 25878570]

[64] Ji R, Meng L, Li Q, Lu Q. TAM receptor deficiency affects adult hippocampal neurogenesis. Metab Brain Dis 2015; 30(3): 633-44. [http://dx.doi.org/10.1007/s11011-014-9636-y] [PMID: 25487541]

[65] Zelentsova K, Talmi Z, Abboud-Jarrous G, *et al.* Protein S regulates neural stem cell quiescence and neurogenesis. Stem Cells 2017; 35(3): 679-93. [http://dx.doi.org/10.1002/stem.2522] [PMID: 27753164]

[66] Zelentsova-Levytskyi K, Talmi Z, Abboud-Jarrous G, Capucha T, Sapir T, Burstyn-Cohen T. Protein S negatively regulates neural stem cell self-renewal through Bmi-1 signaling. Front Mol Neurosci 2017; 10: 124. [http://dx.doi.org/10.3389/fnmol.2017.00124] [PMID: 28512399]

[67] Nagata S, Hanayama R, Kawane K. Autoimmunity and the clearance of dead cells. Cell 2010; 140(5):

619-30.
[http://dx.doi.org/10.1016/j.cell.2010.02.014] [PMID: 20211132]

[68] Boada-Romero E, Martinez J, Heckmann BL, Green DR. The clearance of dead cells by efferocytosis. Nat Rev Mol Cell Biol 2020; 21(7): 398-414.
[http://dx.doi.org/10.1038/s41580-020-0232-1] [PMID: 32251387]

[69] Kumar S, Birge RB. Efferocytosis. Curr Biol 2016; 26(13): R558-9.
[http://dx.doi.org/10.1016/j.cub.2016.01.059] [PMID: 27404247]

[70] Leventis PA, Grinstein S. The distribution and function of phosphatidylserine in cellular membranes. Annu Rev Biophys 2010; 39(1): 407-27.
[http://dx.doi.org/10.1146/annurev.biophys.093008.131234] [PMID: 20192774]

[71] Lemke G. Phosphatidylserine is the signal for TAM receptors and their ligands. Trends Biochem Sci 2017; 42(9): 738-48.
[http://dx.doi.org/10.1016/j.tibs.2017.06.004] [PMID: 28734578]

[72] Nakano T, Ishimoto Y, Kishino J, *et al.* Cell adhesion to phosphatidylserine mediated by a product of growth arrest-specific gene 6. J Biol Chem 1997; 272(47): 29411-4.
[http://dx.doi.org/10.1074/jbc.272.47.29411] [PMID: 9367994]

[73] Sasaki T, Knyazev PG, Clout NJ, *et al.* Structural basis for Gas6–Axl signalling. EMBO J 2006; 25(1): 80-7.
[http://dx.doi.org/10.1038/sj.emboj.7600912] [PMID: 16362042]

[74] Lemke G. How macrophages deal with death. Nat Rev Immunol 2019; 19(9): 539-49.
[http://dx.doi.org/10.1038/s41577-019-0167-y] [PMID: 31019284]

[75] Goudarzi S, Rivera A, Butt AM, Hafizi S. Gas6 promotes oligodendrogenesis and myelination in the adult central nervous system and after lysolecithin-induced demyelination. ASN Neuro 2016; 8(5): 1759091416668430.
[http://dx.doi.org/10.1177/1759091416668430] [PMID: 27630207]

[76] Nakagawa A, Shiratsuchi A, Tsuda K, Nakanishi Y. *In vivo* analysis of phagocytosis of apoptotic cells by testicular Sertoli cells. Mol Reprod Dev 2005; 71(2): 166-77.
[http://dx.doi.org/10.1002/mrd.20278] [PMID: 15791597]

[77] Tajbakhsh A, Farahani N, Gheibihayat SM, *et al.* Autoantigen-specific immune tolerance in pathological and physiological cell death: Nanotechnology comes into view. Int Immunopharmacol 2021; 90: 107177.
[http://dx.doi.org/10.1016/j.intimp.2020.107177] [PMID: 33249046]

[78] Elliott MR, Ravichandran KS. Clearance of apoptotic cells: implications in health and disease. J Cell Biol 2010; 189(7): 1059-70.
[http://dx.doi.org/10.1083/jcb.201004096] [PMID: 20584912]

[79] Diaz-Aparicio I, Paris I, Sierra-Torre V, *et al.* Microglia actively remodel adult hippocampal neurogenesis through the phagocytosis secretome. J Neurosci 2020; 40(7): 1453-82.
[http://dx.doi.org/10.1523/JNEUROSCI.0993-19.2019] [PMID: 31896673]

[80] Zheng S, Hedl M, Abraham C. TAM receptor-dependent regulation of SOCS3 and MAPKs contributes to proinflammatory cytokine downregulation following chronic NOD2 stimulation of human macrophages. J Immunol 2015; 194(4): 1928-37.
[http://dx.doi.org/10.4049/jimmunol.1401933] [PMID: 25567680]

[81] Sharif MN, Šošić D, Rothlin CV, *et al.* Twist mediates suppression of inflammation by type I IFNs and Axl. J Exp Med 2006; 203(8): 1891-901.
[http://dx.doi.org/10.1084/jem.20051725] [PMID: 16831897]

[82] Wu H, Zheng J, Xu S, *et al.* Mer regulates microglial/macrophage M1/M2 polarization and alleviates neuroinflammation following traumatic brain injury. J Neuroinflammation 2021; 18(1): 2.
[http://dx.doi.org/10.1186/s12974-020-02041-7] [PMID: 33402181]

[83] Alciato F, Sainaghi PP, Sola D, Castello L, Avanzi GC. TNF-α, IL-6, and IL-1 expression is inhibited by GAS6 in monocytes/macrophages. J Leukoc Biol 2010; 87(5): 869-75. [http://dx.doi.org/10.1189/jlb.0909610] [PMID: 20103767]

[84] Sun X, Chen WD, Wang YD. β-Amyloid: the key peptide in the pathogenesis of Alzheimer's disease. Front Pharmacol 2015; 6: 221. [http://dx.doi.org/10.3389/fphar.2015.00221] [PMID: 26483691]

[85] Yin Z, Raj D, Saiepour N, *et al.* Immune hyperreactivity of Aβ plaque-associated microglia in Alzheimer's disease. Neurobiol Aging 2017; 55: 115-22. [http://dx.doi.org/10.1016/j.neurobiolaging.2017.03.021] [PMID: 28434692]

[86] Herrera-Rivero M, Heneka M. Expression of the TAM system in frontal cortex of Alzheimer's disease in early stages. In: Degeneration and regeneration in musculoskeletal and neurodegenerative diseases; 2016 Apr; Trelleborg, Sweden. [http://dx.doi.org/10.13140/RG.2.1.1826.8561]

[87] Yagami T, Ueda K, Asakura K, *et al.* Gas6 rescues cortical neurons from amyloid β protein-induced apoptosis. Neuropharmacology 2002; 43(8): 1289-96. [http://dx.doi.org/10.1016/S0028-3908(02)00333-7] [PMID: 12527478]

[88] Saunders AM, Strittmatter WJ, Schmechel D, *et al.* Association of apolipoprotein E allele ϵ 4 with late-onset familial and sporadic Alzheimer's disease. Neurology 1993; 43(8): 1467-72. [http://dx.doi.org/10.1212/WNL.43.8.1467] [PMID: 8350998]

[89] Bien-Ly N, Gillespie AK, Walker D, Yoon SY, Huang Y. Reducing human apolipoprotein E levels attenuates age-dependent Aβ accumulation in mutant human amyloid precursor protein transgenic mice. J Neurosci 2012; 32(14): 4803-11. [http://dx.doi.org/10.1523/JNEUROSCI.0033-12.2012] [PMID: 22492035]

[90] Kim J, Jiang H, Park S, *et al.* Haploinsufficiency of human APOE reduces amyloid deposition in a mouse model of amyloid-β amyloidosis. J Neurosci 2011; 31(49): 18007-12. [http://dx.doi.org/10.1523/JNEUROSCI.3773-11.2011] [PMID: 22159114]

[91] Liao F, Hori Y, Hudry E, *et al.* Anti-ApoE antibody given after plaque onset decreases Aβ accumulation and improves brain function in a mouse model of Aβ amyloidosis. J Neurosci 2014; 34(21): 7281-92. [http://dx.doi.org/10.1523/JNEUROSCI.0646-14.2014] [PMID: 24849360]

[92] Zheng Y, Wang Q, Xiao B, Lu Q, Wang Y, Wang X. Involvement of receptor tyrosine kinase Tyro3 in amyloidogenic APP processing and β-amyloid deposition in Alzheimer's disease models. PLoS One 2012; 7(6): e39035. [http://dx.doi.org/10.1371/journal.pone.0039035] [PMID: 22701746]

[93] Li M, Ye J, Zhao G, *et al.* Gas6 attenuates lipopolysaccharide-induced TNF-α expression and apoptosis in H9C2 cells through NF-κB and MAPK inhibition *via* the Axl/PI3K/Akt pathway. Int J Mol Med 2019; 44(3): 982-94. [http://dx.doi.org/10.3892/ijmm.2019.4275] [PMID: 31524235]

[94] Guglielmotto M, Aragno M, Tamagno E, *et al.* AGEs/RAGE complex upregulates BACE1 *via* NF-κB pathway activation. Neurobiol Aging 2012; 33(1): 196.e13-27. [http://dx.doi.org/10.1016/j.neurobiolaging.2010.05.026] [PMID: 20638753]

[95] Huang SH, Fang ST, Chen YC. Molecular mechanism of vitamin K2 protection against amyloid---induced cytotoxicity. Biomolecules 2021; 11(3): 423. [http://dx.doi.org/10.3390/biom11030423] [PMID: 33805625]

[96] Kempf SJ, Metaxas A. Neurofibrillary tangles in Alzheimer's disease: elucidation of the molecular mechanism by immunohistochemistry and tau protein phospho-proteomics. Neural Regen Res 2016; 11(10): 1579-81. [http://dx.doi.org/10.4103/1673-5374.193234] [PMID: 27904486]

[97] Razani E, Pourbagheri-Sigaroodi A, Safaroghli-Azar A, Zoghi A, Shanaki-Bavarsad M, Bashash D. The PI3K/Akt signaling axis in Alzheimer's disease: a valuable target to stimulate or suppress? Cell Stress Chaperones 2021; 26(6): 871-87. [http://dx.doi.org/10.1007/s12192-021-01231-3] [PMID: 34386944]

[98] Paccez JD, Duncan K, Vava A, *et al.* Inactivation of GSK3β and activation of NF-κB pathway *via* Axl represents an important mediator of tumorigenesis in esophageal squamous cell carcinoma. Mol Biol Cell 2015; 26(5): 821-31. [http://dx.doi.org/10.1091/mbc.E14-04-0868] [PMID: 25568334]

[99] Zhao W, Fan J, Kulic I, *et al.* Axl receptor tyrosine kinase is a regulator of apolipoprotein E. Mol Brain 2020; 13(1): 66. [http://dx.doi.org/10.1186/s13041-020-00609-1] [PMID: 32366277]

[100] Shi Y, Yamada K, Liddelow SA, *et al.* ApoE4 markedly exacerbates tau-mediated neurodegeneration in a mouse model of tauopathy. Nature 2017; 549(7673): 523-7. [http://dx.doi.org/10.1038/nature24016] [PMID: 28959956]

[101] Corpas R, Griñán-Ferré C, Palomera-Ávalos V, *et al.* Melatonin induces mechanisms of brain resilience against neurodegeneration. J Pineal Res 2018; 65(4): e12515. [http://dx.doi.org/10.1111/jpi.12515] [PMID: 29907977]

[102] Weinger JG, Brosnan CF, Loudig O, *et al.* Loss of the receptor tyrosine kinase Axl leads to enhanced inflammation in the CNS and delayed removal of myelin debris during Experimental Autoimmune Encephalomyelitis. J Neuroinflammation 2011; 8(1): 49. [http://dx.doi.org/10.1186/1742-2094-8-49] [PMID: 21569627]

[103] Grommes C, Lee CYD, Wilkinson BL, *et al.* Regulation of microglial phagocytosis and inflammatory gene expression by Gas6 acting on the Axl/Mer family of tyrosine kinases. J Neuroimmune Pharmacol 2008; 3(2): 130-40. [http://dx.doi.org/10.1007/s11481-007-9090-2] [PMID: 18247125]

[104] Cai Z, Hussain MD, Yan LJ. Microglia, neuroinflammation, and beta-amyloid protein in Alzheimer's disease. Int J Neurosci 2014; 124(5): 307-21. [http://dx.doi.org/10.3109/00207454.2013.833510] [PMID: 23930978]

[105] Ringman JM, Elashoff D, Geschwind DH, *et al.* Plasma signaling proteins in persons at genetic risk for Alzheimer disease: influence of APOE genotype. Arch Neurol 2012; 69(6): 757-64. [http://dx.doi.org/10.1001/archneurol.2012.277] [PMID: 22689192]

[106] Lynch JR, Tang W, Wang H, *et al.* APOE genotype and an ApoE-mimetic peptide modify the systemic and central nervous system inflammatory response. J Biol Chem 2003; 278(49): 48529-33. [http://dx.doi.org/10.1074/jbc.M306923200] [PMID: 14507923]

[107] Vitek MP, Brown CM, Colton CA. APOE genotype-specific differences in the innate immune response. Neurobiol Aging 2009; 30(9): 1350-60. [http://dx.doi.org/10.1016/j.neurobiolaging.2007.11.014] [PMID: 18155324]

[108] Miner JJ, Daniels BP, Shrestha B, *et al.* The TAM receptor Mertk protects against neuroinvasive viral infection by maintaining blood-brain barrier integrity. Nat Med 2015; 21(12): 1464-72. [http://dx.doi.org/10.1038/nm.3974] [PMID: 26523970]

[109] Wilson EN, Andreasson KI. TAM-ping down amyloid in Alzheimer's disease. Nat Immunol 2021; 22(5): 543-4. [http://dx.doi.org/10.1038/s41590-021-00918-0] [PMID: 33859407]

[110] Brosseron F, Maass A, Kleineidam L, *et al.* Soluble TAM receptors sAXL and sTyro3 predict structural and functional protection in Alzheimer's disease. Neuron 2022; 110(6): 1009-1022.e4. [http://dx.doi.org/10.1016/j.neuron.2021.12.016] [PMID: 34995486]

[111] Mattsson N, Insel P, Nosheny R, *et al.* CSF protein biomarkers predicting longitudinal reduction of CSF β-amyloid42 in cognitively healthy elders. Transl Psychiatry 2013; 3(8): e293.

[http://dx.doi.org/10.1038/tp.2013.69] [PMID: 23962923]

[112] Kiddle SJ, Thambisetty M, Simmons A, et al. Plasma based markers of [11C] PiB-PET brain amyloid burden. PLoS One. 2012; 7(9): e44260.
[http://dx.doi.org/10.1371/journal.pone.0044260]

[113] Sainaghi PP, Bellan M, Lombino F, *et al.* Growth arrest specific 6 concentration is increased in the cerebrospinal fluid of patients with Alzheimer's disease. J Alzheimers Dis 2016; 55(1): 59-65.
[http://dx.doi.org/10.3233/JAD-160599] [PMID: 27636849]

[114] Qi LFR, Liu S, Liu YC, Li P, Xu X. Ganoderic acid a promotes amyloid-β clearance (*in vitro*) and ameliorates cognitive deficiency in Alzheimer's disease (mouse model) through autophagy induced by activating Axl. Int J Mol Sci 2021; 22(11): 5559.
[http://dx.doi.org/10.3390/ijms22115559] [PMID: 34074054]

[115] Zhang M, Qian C, Zheng ZG, *et al.* Jujuboside A promotes Aβ clearance and ameliorates cognitive deficiency in Alzheimer's disease through activating Axl/HSP90/PPARγ pathway. Theranostics 2018; 8(15): 4262-78.
[http://dx.doi.org/10.7150/thno.26164] [PMID: 30128052]

[116] Savage JC, Jay T, Goduni E, *et al.* Nuclear receptors license phagocytosis by trem2+ myeloid cells in mouse models of Alzheimer's disease. J Neurosci 2015; 35(16): 6532-43.
[http://dx.doi.org/10.1523/JNEUROSCI.4586-14.2015] [PMID: 25904803]

[117] Jung H, Lee SY, Lim S, *et al.* Anti-inflammatory clearance of amyloid-β by a chimeric Gas6 fusion protein. Nat Med 2022; 28(9): 1802-12.
[http://dx.doi.org/10.1038/s41591-022-01926-9] [PMID: 35927581]

[118] Miller MA, Oudin MJ, Sullivan RJ, *et al.* Reduced proteolytic shedding of receptor tyrosine kinases is a post-translational mechanism of kinase inhibitor resistance. Cancer Discov 2016; 6(4): 382-99.
[http://dx.doi.org/10.1158/2159-8290.CD-15-0933] [PMID: 26984351]

[119] Orme JJ, Du Y, Vanarsa K, *et al.* Heightened cleavage of Axl receptor tyrosine kinase by ADAM metalloproteases may contribute to disease pathogenesis in SLE. Clin Immunol 2016; 169: 58-68.
[http://dx.doi.org/10.1016/j.clim.2016.05.011] [PMID: 27237127]

[120] Wu G, McBride DW, Zhang JH. Axl activation attenuates neuroinflammation by inhibiting the TLR/TRAF/NF-κB pathway after MCAO in rats. Neurobiol Dis 2018; 110: 59-67.
[http://dx.doi.org/10.1016/j.nbd.2017.11.009] [PMID: 29196212]

[121] Tong L, Shao A, Ou Y, *et al.* Recombinant Gas6 augments Axl and facilitates immune restoration in an intracerebral hemorrhage mouse model. J Cereb Blood Flow Metab 2017; 37(6): 1971-81.
[http://dx.doi.org/10.1177/0271678X16658490] [PMID: 27389179]

[122] Tsiperson V, Li X, Schwartz GJ, Raine CS, Shafit-Zagardo B. GAS6 enhances repair following cuprizone-induced demyelination. PLoS One 2010; 5(12): e15748.
[http://dx.doi.org/10.1371/journal.pone.0015748] [PMID: 21203420]

[123] Gruber RC, Ray AK, Johndrow CT, *et al.* Targeted GAS6 delivery to the CNS protects axons from damage during experimental autoimmune encephalomyelitis. J Neurosci 2014; 34(49): 16320-35.
[http://dx.doi.org/10.1523/JNEUROSCI.2449-14.2014] [PMID: 25471571]

CHAPTER 4

Role of NFAT Dysregulation in the Pathogenesis and Progression of Alzheimer's Disease

Shreyasi Majumdar[1,2,*], **Santosh Kumar Prajapati**[1,3], **Puneet Samaiya**[4], **Swagata Bhattacharya**[1] and **Sairam Krishnamurthy**[1]

[1] *Department of Pharmaceutical Engineering and Technology, Indian Institute of Technology (Banaras Hindu University), Varanasi, Uttar Pradesh, India*

[2] *Department of Pharmaceutical Technology, School of Health and Medical Sciences, Adamas University, Kolkata, West Bengal, India*

[3] *Department of Neurosurgery and Brain Repair, University of South Florida, Tampa, Florida, USA*

[4] *Department of Pharmacy, Shri G.S. Institute of Technology and Science, Indore, Madhya Pradesh, India*

Abstract: Alzheimer's Disease (AD) is a progressive neurodegenerative condition marked by cognitive deterioration, memory deficits, and neuronal degeneration. Its pathogenesis is multifactorial, involving amyloid-beta (Aβ) plaque accumulation, tau hyperphosphorylation, synaptic dysfunction, and neuroinflammation. Among these pathways, calcium dysregulation and its downstream signaling have emerged as critical contributors. Calcineurin (CN), a calcium-dependent serine/threonine phosphatase, and its downstream target, the nuclear factor of activated T-cells (NFAT), play pivotal roles in AD pathophysiology. Dysregulated CN-NFAT signaling has been linked to neuroinflammation, synaptic plasticity deficits, and enhanced Aβ production, exacerbating AD progression. This chapter elaborated on the preclinical studies, highlighting that CN-mediated NFAT activation promotes astrocyte and microglial activation, increasing pro-inflammatory cytokines like IL-6 and TNF-α. Besides, NFAT also influences amyloid precursor protein (APP) processing, augmenting Aβ generation. Moreover, excessive NFAT activation disrupts synaptic protein expression, leading to cognitive deficits. Here, we have also emphasized clinical studies implicating elevated nuclear NFATc4 levels and dysregulated NFAT signaling pathways in post-mortem AD brain tissues, highlighting their relevance in human pathology. Therapeutic strategies targeting NFAT signaling include CN inhibitors, such as FK506, to reduce Aβ deposition, neuroinflammation, and synaptic loss. Emerging selective NFAT inhibitors, including VIVIT, LxVP peptides, and novel small molecules like Q-134R, have demonstrated efficacy with reduced side effects

* **Corresponding author Shreyasi Majumdar:** Department of Pharmaceutical Engineering and Technology, Indian Institute of Technology (Banaras Hindu University), Varanasi, Uttar Pradesh, India and Department of Pharmaceutical Technology, School of Health and Medical Sciences, Adamas University, Kolkata, West Bengal, India; E-mail: shreyasimajumdar.rs.phe18@itbhu.ac.in

Swarupananda Mukherjee, Souvik Roy & Dipanjan Karati (Eds.)

compared to traditional CN inhibitors. Polyphenols, hydrogen sulfide donors, and gene therapy approaches also offer potential avenues for modulating CN-NFAT activity.

Keywords: Alzheimer's disease, Amyloid-beta, Cyclosporin A, Harmine, Hippocampus, Neuroinflammation, Nuclear factor of activated T-cells (NFAT).

INTRODUCTION

Alzheimer's Disease (AD) is a neurodegenerative disorder characterized by progressive cognitive decline, memory impairment, and changes in executive function and disposition [1, 2]. It is considered the predominant reason for dementia and constitutes a substantial public health challenge, impacting approximately 6.9 million adults over the age of 65 in the United States in 2024 [3]. However, this figure is anticipated to increase to 13.8 million by 2060 [3], thus positioning AD as the fifth predominant reason for mortality among the geriatric community [3, 4]. The prevailing clinical treatment for AD generally encompasses symptomatic therapy aimed at decelerating cognitive deterioration with no medications to cure it [5]. The primary reason is its multifaceted pathophysiology involving amyloid-beta (Aβ) plaque accumulation, tau hyperphosphorylation, synaptic dysfunction, neuroinflammation, and neuronal loss [6, 7]. Moreover, among the several other biochemical pathways associated with AD, calcium dysregulation has been documented to hinder cognitive function and elevate susceptibility to the disease [8, 9]. Further, there are numerous reports that exhibited a direct link between the perturbed intracellular calcium homeostasis and calcium-dependent phosphatase, *i.e.*, calcineurin (CN) protein, that subsequently activates various other pathogenic hallmark proteins of AD [10 - 12]. Among these, the CN-activated nuclear factor of activated T-cells (NFAT) transcription factor has gained attention for its role in exacerbating the disease pathology. This chapter will discuss the role of CN and NFAT dysregulation in AD, drawing on preclinical and clinical evidence to highlight its contribution to the disease progression and its potential as a therapeutic target.

CALCINEURIN

Calcineurin is a calcium/calmodulin-dependent serine/threonine phosphatase that is activated upon fluctuation in the intracellular calcium level [13, 14]. The holoenzyme of the calcium-sensing CN consists of two primary subunits, *i.e.*, a 60 kDa catalytic subunit and a 19 kDa regulatory subunit that includes four Ca^{2+}-binding EF-hand motifs [15]. An increase in the intracellular calcium level causes conformation changes in the calmodulin protein (CaM), thus exposing its hydrophobic binding site, which helps in binding to the regulatory subunit of CN [16]. This increases the phosphatase enzyme activity of CN, which dephosphorylates various cellular proteins that mediate crucial cellular and molecular processes, including inflammation, apoptosis, and memory formation [17, 18]. It has been reported that NFAT is dephosphorylated in the presence of CN and CaM complexes, which largely contribute to the advancement of AD [15, 19, 20]. These cascades of events, in turn, cause the localization of NFAT inside the nucleus, resulting in the transcription of inflammation-related genes like interleukins (ILs), tumor necrosis factor (TNF-α), granulocyte-macrophage stimulating factor, and apoptotic factor FasL [21] (Fig. **1**). Furthermore, aberrant activation of CN-mediated NFAT has also been noted in various other cellular processes often associated with AD, such as astrocyte activation, Aβ production, synaptic plasticity, and cognitive inflexibility [22].

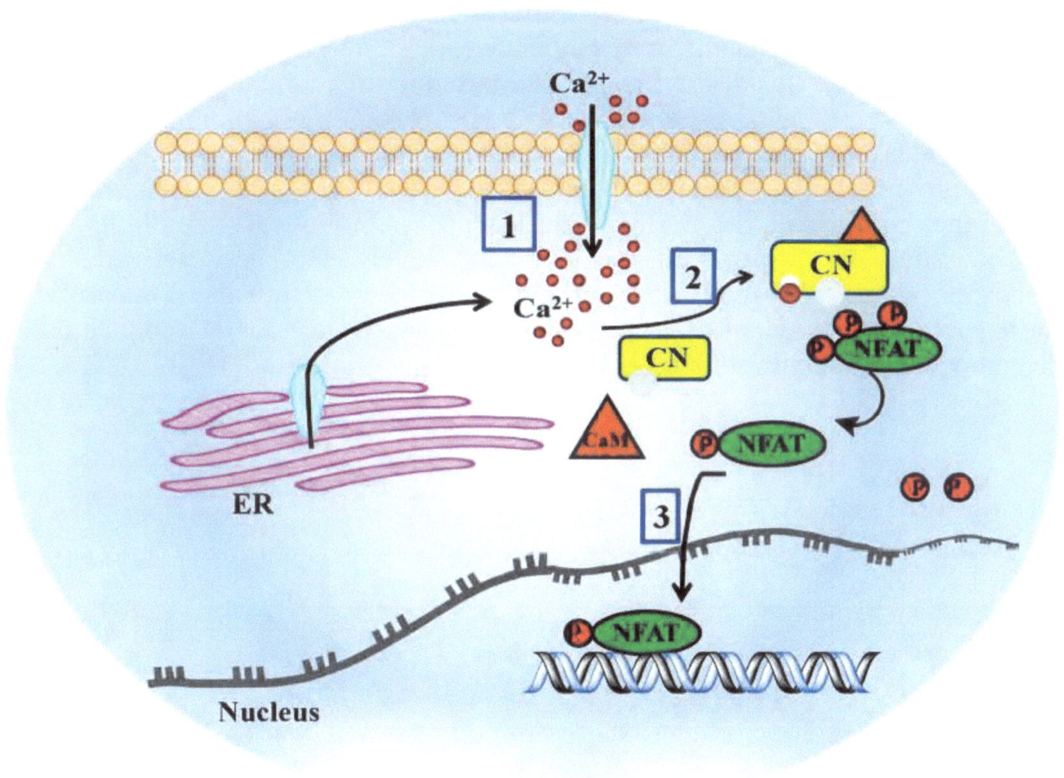

Fig. (1). The mechanism of activation of Nuclear Factor of Activated T-cells (NFAT) post-calcium perturbation *via* the calcium sensor, *i.e.*, calcineurin (CN). This image illustrates the activation pathway of NFAT following an increase in cellular calcium levels (1). Calcium influx triggers the binding to calmodulin (CaM), a calcium-sensingprotein, which in turnactivates CN [2]. CN dephosphorylates NFAT, facilitating its translocation into the nucleus, where it modulates gene expression pertinent to immunological response, neural plasticity, and several cellular functions [3].

NFAT FAMILY PROTEINS

The NFAT (Nuclear Factor of Activated T-cells) family consists of five calcium-regulated proteins: NFAT1 (also known as NFATc2), NFAT2 (also known as NFATc1), NFAT3 (NFATc4), NFAT4 (NFATc3 or NFATx), and NFAT5 (also called tonicity enhancer binding protein (TonEBP)). These proteins are encoded by distinct genes, which are primarily recognized for theiri nvolvement in immune cell activation, including the proliferation of B cells, natural killer (NK) cells, and basophils with simultaneous activation of genes coding various interleukins [23, 24]. The NFAT proteins (NFAT 1-4) comprise the Rel-homologyregion (RHR), the NFAT homology regulatory region (NHR), and a C-terminal domain. However, NFAT 5 is devoid of the NHR unit (25)that normally has been reported to contain the N-terminal transactivation domain (TAD), a CN binding site, a nuclear localization sequence (NLS), and a nuclear export signal (NES) [25] (Fig. **2**). Besides, several serine-based motifs, including SRR1, SRR2, SP1, SP2, and SP3, are present in the NHR regulating domain [19]. In the dormant state, the NHR domain is hyperphosphorylated, maintaining the inactive state of these calcium-regulated proteins, *i.e.*, NFAT, and is primarily situated inside the cytoplasm [26]. However, during pathological conditions with characteristics of elevated intracellular Ca^{2+} levels, CN gets activated and dephosphorylates NFAT, resulting in swift translocation into the nucleus [26]. These cascades of events further activate gene transcription factors connected to the pathogenesis and progression of neurodegenerative diseases [19, 27, 28].

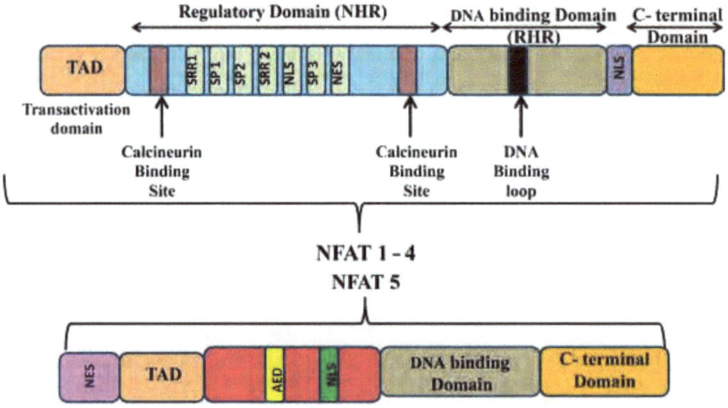

Fig. (2). The general framework of calcineurin and NFAT. The NFAT (NFAT 1-4) proteins are comprised of the Rel-homologyregion (RHR), the NFAT homology regulatory region (NHR), and a C-terminal domain, but NFAT5 lacks the NHR. The NHR comprises an N-terminal transactivation domain (TAD), a calcineurin binding site, a nuclear localization sequence (NLS), and a nuclear export signal (NES). It has many serine-rich motifs, namely SRR1, SRR2, SP1, SP2, and SP3. The RHR consists of the DNA-binding domain and the recognition sites for additionaltranscriptional binding proteins.

NFAT DYSREGULATION IN ALZHEIMER'S DISEASE: PRECLINICAL EVIDENCE

In the neurological system, particularly within neurons, NFATs play crucial roles in regulating synaptic plasticity, neuronal survival, and the expression of genes associated with memory formation [19]. Moreover, prior research has proven that NFAT activation is tightly controlled by intracellular Ca^{2+} level and dephosphorylation of NFAT proteins regulates the transcription of target genes, such as Cox2, which is linked to neuroinflammatory processes associated with the neurodegenerative disorders, including AD [29, 30]. Further, another preclinical study has provided substantial evidence implicating the role of NFAT activation in promoting neuroinflammation, a hallmark of the progression of AD [31]. Besides, in AD, NFAT proteins have been shown to regulate the activation of astrocytes *via* CN along with an elevated expression of pro-inflammatory cytokines such as interleukin-6 (IL-6) and tumor necrosis factor-alpha (TNF-α), both of which are reportedly elevated in various AD animal models [31]. Furthermore, a study conducted using transgenic mice that express human amyloid precursor protein (APP) demonstrated that the activation of NFATc2 increased the IL-6 and TNF-α levels, thereby exacerbating neuroinflammation and promoting synaptic loss [32]. Accumulating pieces of evidence have also highlighted glutamate dysregulation in the pathogenesis of AD and elevated expression of excitatory amino acid transporters 2 (EAAT2) in the hippocampus of rodents [31, 33], further activating the CN-NFAT pathway [31]. On top of that, increased CN-NFAT activity has been observed in post-calcium dysregulation that is linked with the amyloid protein (Aβ) plaque deposition in rodents [34, 35]. Amyloid beta is generated from amyloid precursor protein through the concurrent activity of beta and gamma secretase; it occurs both outside and inside the plasma membrane in the Golgi apparatus and vesicles [36]. Its clearance depends on lysosomal degradation and proteolysis. In the brain samples of AD subjects, the production of Aβ increases beyond physiological value, especially the Aβ1-42 peptide, leading to subsequent neuronal loss and memory impairment. Based on the above-mentioned hypothesis regarding the activity of NFATs in the etiology of AD, several preclinical studies explored the therapeutic potential of inhibiting NFAT signaling in AD models [37]. For instance, calcineurin inhibitors, which block NFAT activation, have exhibited promise in restoring synaptic function and enhancing cognitive performance [38]. In addition, the administration of FK506, a well-known calcineurin inhibitor, to the APP/PS1 transgenic mice resulted in abridged Aβ deposition, reduced neuroinflammation, and improved memory performance in behavioral tests performed in rodents [39]. Additionally, Tideglusib, an inhibitor of glycogen synthase kinase-3 beta (GSK-3β), has also been documented to reduce tau phosphorylation and Aβ production preclinically *via* the downregulation of NFAT activity in various AD models [40, 41].

Therefore, the aforementioned findings underscore the therapeutic potential of targeting NFAT signaling in AD.

NFAT DYSREGULATION IN AD: CLINICAL EVIDENCE

Clinical studies have also provided a multitude of evidence of exacerbated phosphatase protein, *i.e.*, CN and NFAT activity in post-mortem brains [11, 35, 42]. The post-mortem examinations of the brain tissue from AD patients have exhibited elevated levels of nuclear NFATc4 in neurons, particularly in neuroanatomical regions associated with memory formation, such as the hippocampus [43]. Additionally, enhanced expression of NFAT-regulated genes, including those involved in neuroinflammation and synapticplasticity, has also been identified in the AD brains [20]. Similarly, DYRK1A (Dual-specificity tyrosine-phosphorylation-regulated kinase 1A) is a kinase that regulates NFAT signaling along with Aβ aggregation, causing progressive neurodegeneration [44], and DYRK1A inhibitors, such as harmine, have shown promise in preventing tau hyperphosphorylation and reducing cognitive decline [40, 45]. While no clinical trials in AD patients are yet complete, there is growing interest in this approach due to its impact on NFAT signaling. Further, Leucettinib-21, another DYRK1A inhibitor, is in phase 1 clinical trial for its potential anti-AD properties [46]. These outcomes imply that NFAT dysregulation is a characteristic feature of AD pathophysiology in humans, aligning with observations from various animal models.

NFAT INTERACTION WITH AMYLOID PRECURSOR PROTEIN (APP) PROCESSING

Aβ plaques, the preliminary hallmark of the pathophysiology of AD, are generated from the amyloid precursor protein (APP) through the two important enzymes, *i.e.*, β and γ secretase [36]. In AD, the brain production of Aβ increases beyond the physiological limit, which accumulates in the brain and synapses, causing its dysfunction, leading to subsequent neuronal loss and memory impairment. Studies have also reported the transformation of the elevated Aβ into soluble oligomers, fibrils, and senile plaques that cause oxidation and microgliosis, astrocyte activation, and subsequent neuroinflammation leading to progressive cell death [47]. Besides, NFAT also plays a vital role in the processing of APP, the precursor molecule of Aβ [48]. NFAT can interact with transcriptional complexes that regulate APP expression, thereby influencing Aβ production [19, 48]. In an *in vitro* study using cultured cortical neurons, inhibition of NFAT activity resulted in reduced APP expression and a subsequent decrease in Aβ levels [48]. Further, Eloise *et al.*, [48] also reported that genetically coded VIVIT blocked the NFAT accumulation in the nucleus that reversed the loss of synaptic spine connections constitutively triggered by the activated CN-NFAT interactions. This suggests that NFAT dysregulation not only contributes to calcium-mediated neuronal damage and synaptotoxicity but also promotes the accumulation of Aβ, further driving the AD pathology [49].

NFAT IMPACT ON THE SYNAPTIC FUNCTION

NFAT dysregulation plays a crucial role in synaptic function, significantly contributing to the cognitive decline observed in AD. This relationship is underscored by a variety of studies and findings that highlight how alterations in NFAT signaling pathways disrupt synaptic connections, ultimately affecting learning and memory processes [10, 50]. Synaptic plasticity, the capability of synapses to enhance or weaken over time, is essential for learning and memory [51]. A greater synaptic connection enhances memory formation and improves cognitive flexibility. However, during neurodegenerative diseases like AD, preclinical reports have highlighted aberrant NFAT activation linked to the dysregulation of genes involved in synapse formation and maintenance [11]. For instance, NFATc4 was found to be excessively activated in the hippocampus of AD transgenic mice [52], leading to reduced expression of synaptic proteins such as synapsin-1 and PSD-95, and ultimately resulting in synaptic deficits. Further, it has been observed that synaptic plasticity defects in the hippocampus are an early event for AD progression, which is followed by beta-amyloid plaque formation and subsequent tau phosphorylation [53]. Genetically inhibiting calcineurin using a doxycycline-dependent rTA system, reversibly facilitated the long-term potentiation both *in vitro* and *in vivo* [54].

THERAPEUTIC IMPLICATIONS

Given the evidence from various preclinical and clinical studies, NFAT dysregulation represents a promising therapeutic target for AD. Several strategies could be employed to modulate NFAT activity, including:

Calcineurin Inhibitors

While effective in preclinical models, the use of CN inhibitors in humans is limited by their broad effects on immune function. Therefore, more selective approaches are needed.

Selective NFAT Inhibitors

Developing small molecule inhibitors or biologics that selectively target NFAT isoforms implicated in AD could reduce off-target effects. For example, inhibitors that specifically block NFATc4 may provide therapeutic benefits while minimizing adverse effects like immune suppression.

Gene Therapy

Gene therapy approaches to knock down NFAT expression in the brain are being explored using techniques such as RNA interference (RNAi) or CRISPR-Cas9 to silence NFAT genes in the affected neurons.

Combination Therapies

Given the intricate nature of AD, combination therapies targeting multiple pathways, including NFAT signaling, may prove more efficacious than monotherapy. For example, combining NFAT inhibitors with agents that target Aβ or tau pathology may yield synergistic effects (see **Table 1**).

Table 1. The NFAT inhibitors with therapeutic potential for Alzheimer's disease and their mechanism of action.

	NFAT Inhibitors	Mechanism of Action	Refs.
(A) Direct NFAT inhibitors			
1)	VIVIT peptide (16-member linear L-peptide)	Restricts Calcineurin-NFATc interaction	[55]
2)	LxVP peptide	RestrictsCalcineurin-NFATc interaction	[56]
3)	Dipyridamole (Pyramidopyrimidine compound)	DisruptsCalcineurin-NFATc interaction	[57]
4)	Inhibitors of NFAT-Calcineurin Association (INCAs) INCA-6 (Organicmolecule)	Disrupts Calcineurin-NFATc interaction	[58]
5)	A-28522 (Small molecule)	Blocks NFAT activity	[59]
6)	Q-134R (Hydroxyquinoline derivative)	Blocks NFAT activity	[60]
7)	Quercetin (Que) and kaempferol (Kae) (Polyphenols)	Blocks NFATc2 activity	[61]
8)	Hydrogen sulfide (H_2S)	Calcineurin-NFAT Signalling Pathway	[62]
9)	Rubiginosin B	Calcineurin-NFAT Signalling Pathway	[63]
10)	CNI103	Blocks Calcineurin-NFAT Interaction	[64]
(B) Indirect NFAT inhibitors			
1)	**Cyclosporin A** (11 amino acids containing a cyclic peptide)	Inhibits substrate access to the active site of Calcineurin	[65]
2)	FK506 (23-membered polyketide macrolide)	Inhibits substrate access to the active site of Calcineurin	[66]

NFAT INHIBITORS

Direct NFAT Inhibitors

VIVIT

The 16-mer oligopeptide VIVIT demonstrates a significantly enhanced potency, exhibiting a 25-fold greater effectiveness in suppressing NFATc dephosphorylation relative to the original SPRIEIT peptide. Studies have shown that VIVIT effectively inhibits the dephosphorylation of NFATc isoforms, including NFATc1, NFATc2, and NFATc3, while also preventing the nuclear translocation of NFATc2 [19]. Moreover, GFP-tagged VIVIT has been found to suppress the NFAT-mediated transcription of several cytokines and immune-related molecules, including IL-2, IL-3, IL-13, TNF-α, and macrophage inflammatory protein-1α (MIP-1α). Importantly, it does not influence the expression of genes regulated by CsA, such as TNF-β and lymphotoxin-β. Notably, VIVIT has not been associated with any toxicity so far. Therefore, the high specificity of VIVIT in targeting NFAT signaling, without broadly affecting CN activity, positions it as a promising candidate for therapies aimed at reducing toxicity compared to traditional immunosuppressants like CsA and FK506 for AD [55].

LxVP Peptides

LxVP peptides, which are based on the CN-docking sequence found in NFATc, compete for binding with the activated CN. CN demonstrates a high affinity for the LxVP motifs present in NFATc1, NFATc3, and NFATc4, whereas its binding to NFATc2—the primary isoform in activated CD4+ T cells—is comparatively weaker [56].

Dipyridamole (Pyramidopyrimidine Compound)

During screening of the Prestwick Chemical Library, which comprises 880 physiologically active compounds, Mulero and colleagues [57] discovered dipyridamole, a phosphodiesterase 3 inhibitor, as a molecule that competitively binds to the RCAN1 peptide. Functional assessments of the effect of dipyridamole on CN activity exhibited that it does not disrupt the phosphatase function of CN. Instead, its mechanism of action seems to entail a specific interaction with various NFAT proteins. In support of this, dipyridamole was found to inhibit the nuclear translocation of NFAT, hence reducing NFAT activity and suppressing the NFAT-dependent cytokine gene expression. This points to the fact that, beyond its established antiplatelet properties, dipyridamole may potentially have an immunomodulatory effect [57].

INCAs

Inhibitors of NFAT-Calcineurin Association (INCAs) were identified for their ability to compete with the VIVIT peptide for calcineurin binding. Notably, three compounds—INCA-1, INCA-2, and INCA-6 can fully displace VIVIT from CN at low micromolar concentrations by producing an allosteric alteration at the NFAT-binding site. For example, INCA-6 specifically affects NFAT activity, while INCA-2 exerts broader effects by generally inhibiting CN activity. Nevertheless, all INCAs have shown concentration-dependentcytotoxicity, raisingconcerns about theirpotential limitations for use in biologicalsystemsfor AD [58].

A-28522

A-285222, a compound from the bis-trifluoromethyl-pyrazole class, belongs to a group of immunosuppressive compounds that suppresses NFAT activity in both human and non-human primates *via* a mechanism that is not linked to calcineurin [59]. Further, in the intact T cells, A-285222 has been reported to maintain the NFAT proteins in the phosphorylated state and hence is sequestered in the cytoplasm, preventing its nuclear localization without affecting the activation of AP-1 or NF-κB. Consequently, it proficiently inhibits the transcription of NFAT-dependent cytokine genes. Nonetheless, despite its potential as an immunosuppressant, the drug is linked to considerable adverse effects, specifically neurotoxicity [59].

Q-134R

Q134R, a hydroxyquinoline derivative, is known for its capacity to traverse the blood-brain barrier and inhibit the NFAT transcriptional activity as well as caspase-3 activation. Notably, this molecule does not directly affect CN; hence, it circumvents the immunosuppressive side effects commonly associated with other therapeutic agents. Similarly, preclinical investigations have established its safety, stability, and adequate oral bioavailability. Following the successful completion of Phase I/A trials, this drug is now advancing into Phase II clinical trials [60].

Polyphenols

Quercetin (Que) and kaempferol (Kae), two naturally derived flavonoids sourced from plants such as kale, broccoli, and beans [67], and recognized for their antidepressant effects, are attributed to their anti-inflammatory properties and suppression of mastcell activation [68]. In the *in vitro* study, the pretreatment of humanmast cells (HMC-1) with Que or Kae exhibited reduced TNF-α secretion and expression upon stimulation [61]. Both flavonoids also reduced NFAT transcriptional activity and NFATc2 nuclear translocation. Additionally, Que and Kae suppressed the store-operated calcium entry (SOCE), with molecular docking indicating robust binding to the calcium channel ORAI, similar to the ORAI inhibitor YM58483. Further, the oral administration of Que or Kae also reversed the lipopolysaccharide (LPS)-induced depressive behaviors in rodents and diminished mast cell activation in the hippocampus [61].

Hydrogen Sulfide (H_2S)

Hydrogen sulfide (H_2S), a gaseous signaling molecule, is known to be essential for preserving stem cell functionality *via* the regulation of cellular redox homeostasis and inhibition of apoptotic protein, *i.e.*, Caspase activation [69]. In a preclinical study, the effect of H_2S on stem cell ageing was investigated utilizing the bone marrow mesenchymal stem cells (BMMSCs) derived from young (2 months) and old (12 months) mice [62]. Post-H_2S therapy, several senescence markers, ROS production, and cell-cycle-related gene expression were evaluated. It was observed that following the H_2S treatment, osteogenic differentiation and cell senescence in BMMSC were induced, which inhibited bone loss [62]. The aforementioned mechanism by which H_2S delays ageing is purportedly mediated through the calcineurin-NFAT1 pathway [62].

Rubiginosin B

Rubiginosin B (RGB), a chromanemero terpenoid, augments theanti-tumor immune responses by obstructingregulatory T cell (Treg) differentiation *via* the calcineurin-NFAT signaling pathway, suggesting its potential as an adjuvant therapy [63]. Moreover, RGB specifically suppressed the differentiation of TGFβ-induced CD4+Foxp3+ Tregs, overcoming the immunosuppressive tumor microenvironment (TME) and restraining tumor growth in the murine model [70] throughits action on CN, thereby preventing the NFAT dephosphorylation and diminishing Foxp3 expression [63].

CNI103

CNI103 is a potent, easily cell-permeable and metabolically stable peptidyl inhibitor that selectively disrupts the physiological interaction between CN and NFATc3 [64]. The CN inhibitory properties of CNI103 were observed both in the *in vitro* and *in vivo* studies, displaying favorable pharmacokinetic parameters and wide tissue distribution across various administration routes with limited organ toxicity. These findings highlight that CNI103 shows potential as a novel treatment strategy for AD and other inflammatory disease conditions [64].

Indirect NFAT Inhibitors

Cyclosporin A

Cyclophilins, a class of immunophilins, exhibit peptidyl-proline cis-trans isomerase (PPIase) activity, essential for proper protein folding, while cyclosporine A (CsA) inhibits PPIase, which is purportedly unrelated to its immunosuppressive effects [71]. Normally, CsA forms a complex with the proteins, cyclophilin A and CN, thus inhibiting CN's phosphatase activity that prevents the NFAT-mediated inflammatory cascades [72]. Preclinical studies have indicated that the indirect inhibition of NFAT by CsA diminishes the transcription of cytokine genes, including IL-2 and IL-4 [72]. In addition to its effects on the CN/NFAT pathway, CsA also influences the transcription of NF-κB and AP-1, which govern IL-2 production, a peripheral inflammatory factor predominant in post-mortem brains [19, 73]. Furthermore, the neuroprotective effects of CsA in the *in vitro* setup have also been highlighted. Therefore, modulating CN activity pharmacologically can offer neuroprotection, enhance synaptic function, and diminish glial activation in neurodegenerative diseases. Nonetheless, despite its therapeutic potential, CsA's clinical use is constrained by adverse effects including nephrotoxicity, neurotoxicity, and hepatotoxicity [65].

FK506 (Tacrolimus)

FK506 is a macrolide antibiotic with immunosuppressive effects that forms a complex with FKBP12 to inhibit CN-dependent NFAT signaling [74]. Despite structural and mechanistic differences, FK506 and CsA exhibit similar biological effects. On the other hand, unlike CsA, FK506 suppresses IL-2-induced IL-5 production, T-cell proliferation, and decreases IL-7 receptor expression. Additionally, FK506 demonstrates superior efficacy compared to CsA in regulating IL-2 production. Notably, FK506 is also reportedly beneficial in managing steroid-resistant allograft rejection, a condition in which CsA becomes ineffective [66].

CONCLUSION

The dysregulation of NFAT signaling is increasingly being recognized as a pivotal factor in the pathogenesis of AD. Preclinical studies have demonstrated that NFAT activation contributes to neuroinflammation, synaptic dysfunction, and Aβ plaque accumulation, all of which are considered the key features of AD. Besides, clinical evidence also supports the relevance of NFAT dysregulation in the pathogenesis and progression of AD, highlighting its potential as a therapeutic target. Future research should focus on developing selective NFAT inhibitors and exploring their efficacy in clinical trials. Additionally, the identification of

NFAT-related biomarkers could facilitate the early diagnosis and monitoring of AD progression. As our understanding of NFAT's role in AD continues to grow, targeting this pathway may offer new hope for the treatment of a disease that currently lacks effective therapies.

REFERENCES

[1] Prajapati SK, Pathak A, Samaiya PK. Alzheimer's disease: from early pathogenesis to novel therapeutic approaches. Metab Brain Dis 2024; 39(6): 1231-54. [http://dx.doi.org/10.1007/s11011-024-01389-6] [PMID: 39046584]

[2] Manzoor S, Prajapati SK, Majumdar S, Khurana S, Krishnamurthy S, Hoda N. Pharmacological investigations of selected multitarget-direct ligands for the treatment of alzheimer's disease. ChemistrySelect 2022; 7(38): e202200975. [http://dx.doi.org/10.1002/slct.202200975]

[3] Better MA. 2023 Alzheimer's disease facts and figures. Alzheimers Dement 2023; 19(4): 1598-695. [http://dx.doi.org/10.1002/alz.13016] [PMID: 36918389]

[4] Alzheimer's Association. 2022 Alzheimer's disease facts and figures. Alzheimers Dement 2022; 18(4): 700-89. [http://dx.doi.org/10.1002/alz.12638] [PMID: 35289055]

[5] Yiannopoulou KG, Papageorgiou SG. Current and future treatments in Alzheimer disease: an update. J Cent Nerv Syst Dis 2020; 12. [http://dx.doi.org/10.1177/1179573520907397] [PMID: 32165850]

[6] Bellaver B, Povala G, Ferreira PCL, *et al.* Astrocyte reactivity influences amyloid-β effects on tau pathology in preclinical Alzheimer's disease. Nat Med 2023; 29(7): 1775-81. [http://dx.doi.org/10.1038/s41591-023-02380-x] [PMID: 37248300]

[7] Prajapati SK, Shah R, Alford N, *et al.* The triple alliance: microbiome, mitochondria, and metabolites in the context of age-related cognitive decline and Alzheimer's disease. J Gerontol A Biol Sci Med Sci. 2023; 78(12): 2187-202.

[8] Gibson GE, Peterson C. Calcium and the aging nervous system. Neurobiol Aging 1987; 8(4): 329-43. [http://dx.doi.org/10.1016/0197-4580(87)90072-8] [PMID: 3306433]

[9] Thibault O, Gant JC, Landfield PW. Expansion of the calcium hypothesis of brain aging and Alzheimer's disease: minding the store. Aging Cell 2007; 6(3): 307-17. [http://dx.doi.org/10.1111/j.1474-9726.2007.00295.x] [PMID: 17465978]

[10] Abdul HM, Furman JL, Sama MA, Mathis DM, Norris CM. NFATs and Alzheimer's disease. Mol Cell Pharmacol 2010; 2(1): 7-14. [PMID: 20401186]

[11] Abdul HM, Sama MA, Furman JL, *et al.* Cognitive decline in Alzheimer's disease is associated with selective changes in calcineurin/NFAT signaling. J Neurosci 2009, 29(41): 12957-69. [http://dx.doi.org/10.1523/JNEUROSCI.1064-09.2009] [PMID: 19828810]

[12] Asai M, Kinjo A, Kimura S, *et al.* Perturbed calcineurin-NFAT signaling is associated with the development of Alzheimer's disease. Biol Pharm Bull 2016; 39(10): 1646-52. [http://dx.doi.org/10.1248/bpb.b16-00350] [PMID: 27725441]

[13] Rusnak F, Mertz P. Calcineurin: Form and function. Physiol Rev 2000; 80(4): 1483-521. [http://dx.doi.org/10.1152/physrev.2000.80.4.1483] [PMID: 11015619]

[14] Scaramuzzino C, Cuoc EC, Pla P, Humbert S, Saudou F. Calcineurin and huntingtin form a calcium-sensing machinery that directs neurotrophic signals to the nucleus. Sci Adv 2022; 8(1): eabj8812. [http://dx.doi.org/10.1126/sciadv.abj8812] [PMID: 34985962]

[15] Chen L, Song M, Yao C. Calcineurin in development and disease. Genes Dis 2022; 9(4): 915-27. [http://dx.doi.org/10.1016/j.gendis.2021.03.002] [PMID: 35685477]

[16] Kundu P, Nehra A, Gill R, Tuteja N, Gill SS. Unraveling the importance of EF-hand-mediated calcium signaling in plants. S Afr J Bot 2022; 148: 615-33. [http://dx.doi.org/10.1016/j.sajb.2022.04.045]

[17] Zeng J, Hu XF, Sun DS, Hong XY, Ma JZ, Feng Q. Alzheimer-like behavior and synaptic dysfunction in 3 × Tg-AD mice are reversed with calcineurin inhibition. Exp Brain Res 2024; 242(6): 1507-15. [http://dx.doi.org/10.1007/s00221-024-06841-8] [PMID: 38719948]

[18] Rafael-Vidal C, Altabás I, Pérez N, Mourino Rodríguez C, Pego-Reigosa JM, Garcia S. Calcineurin and systemic lupus erythematosus: the rationale for using calcineurin inhibitors in the treatment of lupus nephritis. Int J Mol Sci 2021; 22(3): 1263. [http://dx.doi.org/10.3390/ijms22031263] [PMID: 33514066]

[19] Mackiewicz J, Lisek M, Boczek T. Targeting CaN/NFAT in Alzheimer's brain degeneration. Front Immunol 2023; 14: 1281882. [http://dx.doi.org/10.3389/fimmu.2023.1281882] [PMID: 38077352]

[20] dos Santos JPA, Vizuete AF, Gonçalves CA. Calcineurin-mediated hippocampal inflammatory alterations in streptozotocin-induced model of dementia. Mol Neurobiol 2020; 57(1): 502-12. [http://dx.doi.org/10.1007/s12035-019-01718-2] [PMID: 31388960]

[21] Kiani A, Rao A, Aramburu JJI. Manipulating immune responses with immunosuppressive agents that target NFAT. 2000;12(4):359-72. [http://dx.doi.org/10.1016/S1074-7613(00)80188-0]

[22] Reese LC, Taglialatela G. A role for calcineurin in Alzheimer's disease. Curr Neuropharmacol 2011; 9(4): 685-92. [http://dx.doi.org/10.2174/157015911798376316] [PMID: 22654726]

[23] Vaeth M, Schliesser U, Müller G, *et al.* Dependence on nuclear factor of activated T-cells (NFAT) levels discriminates conventional T cells from Foxp3 $^{+}$ regulatory T cells. Proc Natl Acad Sci USA 2012; 109(40): 16258-63. [http://dx.doi.org/10.1073/pnas.1203870109] [PMID: 22991461]

[24] Shaw JP, Utz PJ, Durand DB, Toole JJ, Emmel EA, Crabtree GR. Identification of a putative regulator of early T cell activation genes. Science 1988; 241(4862): 202-5. [http://dx.doi.org/10.1126/science.3260404] [PMID: 3260404]

[25] Zhang P, Huang C, Liu H, *et al.* The mechanism of the NFAT transcription factor family involved in oxidative stress response. J Cardiol 2024; 83(1): 30-6. [http://dx.doi.org/10.1016/j.jjcc.2023.04.017] [PMID: 37149283]

[26] Vaeth M, Feske S. NFAT control of immune function: New Frontiers for an Abiding Trooper. F1000 Res 2018; 7: 260. [http://dx.doi.org/10.12688/f1000research.13426.1] [PMID: 29568499]

[27] Beals CR, Sheridan CM, Turck CW, Gardner P, Crabtree GR. Nuclear export of NF-ATc enhanced by glycogen synthase kinase-3. Science 1997; 275(5308): 1930-3. [http://dx.doi.org/10.1126/science.275.5308.1930] [PMID: 9072970]

[28] Gwack Y, Sharma S, Nardone J, *et al.* A genome-wide Drosophila RNAi screen identifies DYRK-family kinases as regulators of NFAT. Nature 2006; 441(7093): 646-50. [http://dx.doi.org/10.1038/nature04631] [PMID: 16511445]

[29] Park YJ, Yoo SA, Kim M, Kim WU. The role of calcium–calcineurin–NFAT signaling pathway in health and autoimmune diseases. Front Immunol 2020; 11: 195. [http://dx.doi.org/10.3389/fimmu.2020.00195] [PMID: 32210952]

[30] Ben Haim L, Carrillo-de Sauvage M-A, Ceyzériat K, Escartin C. Elusive roles for reactive astrocytes

in neurodegenerative diseases. Front Cell Neurosci 2015; 9: 278.
[http://dx.doi.org/10.3389/fncel.2015.00278] [PMID: 26283915]

[31] Sompol P, Norris CM. Ca2+, astrocyte activation and calcineurin/NFAT signaling in age-related neurodegenerative diseases. Front Aging Neurosci 2018; 10: 199.
[http://dx.doi.org/10.3389/fnagi.2018.00199] [PMID: 30038565]

[32] Kim C, Beilina A, Smith N, *et al.* LRRK2 mediates microglial neurotoxicity *via* NFATc2 in rodent models of synucleinopathies. Sci Transl Med 2020; 12(565): eaay0399.
[http://dx.doi.org/10.1126/scitranslmed.aay0399] [PMID: 33055242]

[33] Robinson MB, Jackson JG. Astroglial glutamate transporters coordinate excitatory signaling and brain energetics. Neurochem Int 2016; 98: 56-71.
[http://dx.doi.org/10.1016/j.neuint.2016.03.014] [PMID: 27013346]

[34] Hong HS, Hwang JY, Son SM, Kim YH, Moon M, Mook-Jung I. FK506 reduces amyloid plaque burden and induces MMP-9 in AβPP/PS1 double transgenic mice. J Alzheimers Dis 2010; 22(1): 97-105.
[http://dx.doi.org/10.3233/JAD-2010-100261] [PMID: 20847451]

[35] Mohmmad Abdul H, Baig I, LeVine H III, Guttmann RP, Norris CM. Proteolysis of calcineurin is increased in human hippocampus during mild cognitive impairment and is stimulated by oligomeric Abeta in primary cell culture. Aging Cell 2011; 10(1): 103-13.
[http://dx.doi.org/10.1111/j.1474-9726.2010.00645.x] [PMID: 20969723]

[36] Hartmann T, Bieger SC, Brühl B, *et al.* Distinct sites of intracellular production for Alzheimer's disease Aβ40/42 amyloid peptides. 1997;3(9):1016-20.

[37] Rojanathammanee L, Floden AM, Manocha GD, Combs CK. Attenuation of microglial activation in a mouse model of Alzheimer's disease *via* NFAT inhibition. J Neuroinflammation 2015; 12(1): 42.
[http://dx.doi.org/10.1186/s12974-015-0255-2] [PMID: 25889879]

[38] Scaduto P, Marcatti M, Bhatt N, Kayed R, Taglialatela G. Calcineurin inhibition prevents synaptic plasticity deficit induced by brain-derived tau oligomers. Brain Commun 2024; 6(5): fcae277.
[http://dx.doi.org/10.1093/braincomms/fcae277] [PMID: 39239152]

[39] Yan P, Hu X, Song H, *et al.* Matrix metalloproteinase-9 degrades amyloid-β fibrils *in vitro* and compact plaques in situ. J Biol Chem 2006; 281(34): 24566-74.
[http://dx.doi.org/10.1074/jbc.M602440200] [PMID: 16787929]

[40] Demuro S, Di Martino RMC, Ortega JA, Cavalli A. GSK-3β, FYN, and DYRK1A: master regulators in neurodegenerative pathways. Int J Mol Sci 2021; 22(16): 9098.
[http://dx.doi.org/10.3390/ijms22169098] [PMID: 34445804]

[41] Congdon EE, Sigurdsson EM. Tau-targeting therapies for Alzheimer disease. Nat Rev Neurol 2018; 14(7): 399-415.
[http://dx.doi.org/10.1038/s41582-018-0013-z] [PMID: 29895964]

[42] Norris CM, Abdul HM, Kraner SD, Sama MA. P3-367: Alterations in the subcellular localization of calcineurin/NFAT isoforms in Alzheimer's disease: Implications for neuroinflammation. Alzheimer's & Dementia. 2008;4:T629-T.

[43] Hyman BT, Serrano-Pozo A. Systematic review of human post-mortem immunohistochemical studies and bioinformatics analyses unveil the complexity of astrocyte reaction in Alzheimer's. 2021.

[44] Jarhad DB, Mashelkar KK, Kim HR, Noh M, Jeong LS. Dual-specificity tyrosine phosphorylation-regulated kinase 1A (DYRK1A) inhibitors as potential therapeutics. J Med Chem 2018; 61(22): 9791-810.
[http://dx.doi.org/10.1021/acs.jmedchem.8b00185] [PMID: 29985601]

[45] Wu YW, HuangFu WC, Lin TE, *et al.* Identification of selective dual-specificity tyrosine phosphorylation-regulated kinase 1A (DYRK1A) inhibitors and their effects on tau and microtubule. Int J Biol Macromol 2024; 259(Pt 1): 129074.

[http://dx.doi.org/10.1016/j.ijbiomac.2023.129074] [PMID: 38163507]

[46] Meijer L, Chrétien E, Ravel D. Leucettinib-21, a DYRK1A Kinase Inhibitor as Clinical Drug Candidate for Alzheimer's Disease and Down Syndrome. J Alzheimers Dis 2024; 101(s1): S95-S113. [http://dx.doi.org/10.3233/JAD-240078] [PMID: 39422950]

[47] Musiek ES, Holtzman DMJNn. Three dimensions of the amyloid hypothesis: time, space and'wingmen'. 2015;18(6):800-6.

[48] Hudry E, Wu HY, Arbel-Ornath M, *et al.* Inhibition of the NFAT pathway alleviates amyloid β neurotoxicity in a mouse model of Alzheimer's disease. J Neurosci 2012; 32(9): 3176-92. [http://dx.doi.org/10.1523/JNEUROSCI.6439-11.2012] [PMID: 22378890]

[49] Baracaldo-Santamaría D, Avendaño-Lopez SS, Ariza-Salamanca DF, *et al.* Role of calcium modulation in the pathophysiology and treatment of Alzheimer's disease. Int J Mol Sci 2023; 24(10): 9067. [http://dx.doi.org/10.3390/ijms24109067] [PMID: 37240413]

[50] Martinez TP. AKAP-CaN-NFAT Signaling in Alzheimer's Disease: University of Colorado Denver. Anschutz Medical Campus 2024.

[51] Benfenati F. Synaptic plasticity and the neurobiology of learning and memory. Acta Biomed 2007; 78 (Suppl. 1): 58-66. [PMID: 17465325]

[52] Sompol P, Furman JL, Pleiss MM, *et al.* Calcineurin/NFAT signaling in activated astrocytes drives network hyperexcitability in Aβ-bearing mice. J Neurosci 2017; 37(25): 6132-48. [http://dx.doi.org/10.1523/JNEUROSCI.0877-17.2017] [PMID: 28559377]

[53] John A, Reddy PHJArr. Synaptic basis of Alzheimer's disease: Focus on synaptic amyloid beta, P-tau and mitochondria. 2021;65:101208.

[54] Malleret G, Haditsch U, Genoux D, Jones MW, Bliss TV, Vanhoose AM, *et al.* Inducible and reversible enhancement of learning, memory, and long-term potentiation by genetic inhibition of calcineurin. 2001;104(5):675-86. [http://dx.doi.org/10.1016/S0092-8674(01)00264-1]

[55] Aramburu J, Yaffe MB, López-Rodríguez C, Cantley LC, Hogan PG, Rao A. Affinity-driven peptide selection of an NFAT inhibitor more selective than cyclosporin A. Science 1999; 285(5436): 2129-33. [http://dx.doi.org/10.1126/science.285.5436.2129] [PMID: 10497131]

[56] Martínez-Martínez S, Rodríguez A, López-Maderuelo MD, Ortega-Pérez I, Vázquez J, Redondo JM. Blockade of NFAT activation by the second calcineurin binding site. J Biol Chem 2006; 281(10): 6227-35. [http://dx.doi.org/10.1074/jbc.M513885200] [PMID: 16407284]

[57] Mulero MC, Aubareda A, Orzáez M, *et al.* Inhibiting the calcineurin-NFAT (nuclear factor of activated T cells) signaling pathway with a regulator of calcineurin-derived peptide without affecting general calcineurin phosphatase activity. J Biol Chem 2009; 284(14): 9394-401. [http://dx.doi.org/10.1074/jbc.M805889200] [PMID: 19189965]

[58] Kang S, Li H, Rao A, Hogan PG. Inhibition of the calcineurin-NFAT interaction by small organic molecules reflects binding at an allosteric site. J Biol Chem 2005; 280(45): 37698-706. [http://dx.doi.org/10.1074/jbc.M502247200] [PMID: 16148011]

[59] Trevillyan JM, Chiou XG, Chen YW, *et al.* Potent inhibition of NFAT activation and T cell cytokine production by novel low molecular weight pyrazole compounds. J Biol Chem 2001; 276(51): 48118-26. [http://dx.doi.org/10.1074/jbc.M107919200] [PMID: 11592964]

[60] Sompol P, Gollihue JL, Kraner SD, *et al.* Q134R: Small chemical compound with NFAT inhibitory properties improves behavioral performance and synapse function in mouse models of amyloid pathology. Aging Cell 2021; 20(7): e13416.

[http://dx.doi.org/10.1111/acel.13416] [PMID: 34117818]

[61] Su P, Li Z, Yan X, *et al.* Quercetin and Kaempferol inhibit HMC-1 activation *via* SOCE/NFATc2 signaling and suppress hippocampal mast cell activation in lipopolysaccharide-induced depressive mice. Inflamm Res 2024; 73(6): 945-60.
[http://dx.doi.org/10.1007/s00011-024-01876-7] [PMID: 38587532]

[62] Yang S, Su Y, Li X, *et al.* Hydrogen sulfide attenuates mesenchymal stem cell aging progress *via* the calcineurin-NFAT signaling pathway. Stem Cells 2023; 41(10): 916-27.
[http://dx.doi.org/10.1093/stmcls/sxad056] [PMID: 37549235]

[63] Geng CA, Chen FY, Zheng JB, *et al.* Rubiginosin B selectively inhibits Treg cell differentiation and enhances anti-tumor immune responses by targeting calcineurin-NFAT signaling pathway. Phytomedicine 2023; 116: 154898.
[http://dx.doi.org/10.1016/j.phymed.2023.154898] [PMID: 37247590]

[64] Dougherty PG, Karpurapu M, Koley A, *et al.* A peptidyl inhibitor that blocks calcineurin–NFAT interaction and prevents acute lung injury. J Med Chem 2020; 63(21): 12853-72.
[http://dx.doi.org/10.1021/acs.jmedchem.0c01236] [PMID: 33073986]

[65] Handschumacher RE, Harding MW, Rice J, Drugge RJ, Speicher DW. Cyclophilin: a specific cytosolic binding protein for cyclosporin A. Science 1984; 226(4674): 544-7.
[http://dx.doi.org/10.1126/science.6238408] [PMID: 6238408]

[66] Mori A, Suko M, Kaminuma O, *et al.* IL-2-induced IL-5 synthesis, but not proliferation, of human CD4+ T cells is suppressed by FK506. J Immunol. (Baltimore, Md: 1950). 1997; 158(8): 3659-65.

[67] Periferakis A, Periferakis K, Badarau IA, *et al.* Kaempferol: antimicrobial properties, sources, clinical, and traditional applications. Int J Mol Sci 2022; 23(23): 15054.
[http://dx.doi.org/10.3390/ijms232315054] [PMID: 36499380]

[68] Devi KP, Malar DS, Nabavi SF, *et al.* Kaempferol and inflammation: From chemistry to medicine. Pharmacol Res 2015; 99: 1-10.
[http://dx.doi.org/10.1016/j.phrs.2015.05.002] [PMID: 25982933]

[69] Cirino G, Szabo C, Papapetropoulos A. Physiological roles of hydrogen sulfide in mammalian cells, tissues, and organs. Physiol Rev 2023; 103(1): 31-276.
[http://dx.doi.org/10.1152/physrev.00028.2021] [PMID: 35435014]

[70] Deng Y, Lu GH, Xu JY, Luo Q, Du QF. Discovery, biosynthesis, organic synthesis, and bioactivities of meroterpenoids from Rhododendron species. Phytochemistry 2024; 222: 114089.
[http://dx.doi.org/10.1016/j.phytochem.2024.114089] [PMID: 38626831]

[71] Biswas G, Banerjee R. Role of peptidyl-prolyl cis-trans isomerases in infectious diseases and host-pathogen interactions. Curr Sci. 2021; 121(6): 742-752.
[http://dx.doi.org/10.18520/cs/v121/i6/758-768]

[72] Gui Q, Jiang Z, Zhang L. Insights into the modulatory role of cyclosporine A and its research advances in acute inflammation. Int Immunopharmacol 2021; 93: 107420.
[http://dx.doi.org/10.1016/j.intimp.2021.107420] [PMID: 33540245]

[73] Lai KSP, Liu CS, Rau A, *et al.* Peripheral inflammatory markers in Alzheimer's disease: a systematic review and meta-analysis of 175 studies. J Neurol Neurosurg Psychiatry 2017; 88(10): 876-82.
[http://dx.doi.org/10.1136/jnnp-2017-316201] [PMID: 28794151]

[74] Jie J, Li W, Wang G, Xu X. FK506 ameliorates osteoporosis caused by osteoblast apoptosis *via* suppressing the activated CaN/NFAT pathway during oxidative stress. Inflamm Res 2021; 70(7): 789-97.
[http://dx.doi.org/10.1007/s00011-021-01452-3] [PMID: 34165588]

CHAPTER 5

Pathophysiological Insights and Therapeutic Approaches of Oxidative Stress in Alzheimer's Disease

Dipanjan Karati[1,*], **Tanwi Garai**[1], **Siuli Sen**[1], **Swarupananda Mukherjee**[2], **Sajal Kumar Jha**[3] and **Biplab Debnath**[4]

[1] *Department of Pharmaceutical Technology, School of Pharmacy, Techno India University, Kolkata, West Bengal, India*

[2] *Department of Pharmaceutical Technology, NSHM Knowledge Campus, Kolkata - Group of Institutions, Kolkata, West Bengal, India*

[3] *Department of Pharmaceutical Technology, School of Health and Medical Sciences, Adamas University, Kolkata, West Bengal, India*

[4] *Department of Pharmaceutical Technology, Bharat Technology, Uluberia, West Bengal, India*

Abstract: Alzheimer's disease (AD) is the leading neurodegenerative disorder responsible for dementia. Globally, AD is the leading cause of disability among those over 65. The primary pathological features of AD brains include the formation of senile plaques, loss of neurons, and neurofibrillary tangles. Amyloid beta plaque formation, aggregation, and accumulation, disturbedmetal (copper, iron, and zinc) homeostasis, metal-induced abnormal acetylcholinesterase (AChE) activity, neuroinflammation, oxidative stress, and other pathologies are all manifestations of AD, a multifactorial neurodegenerative illness. Therefore, developing treatment methods aimed at preventing AD pathogenesis requires a knowledge of the oxidative stress mechanism and degenerating synapses. The hypothesis of free radicals suggests that the buildup of certain oxidative lesions is at least primarily responsible for the slow and unavoidable process of physiological aging. Environmental risk factors are recognized as a major contributor to the development and progression of AD. Antioxidant combinations may provide an even higher potential benefit for AD, particularly if the medicines show complementary action or operate in distinct cellular compartments. Furthermore, it has been proposed that exposure to heavy metals, pesticides, and particulate matter increases the risk of Alzheimer's disease and, *via* epigenetic pathways, contributes to phenotypic variation. Therefore, gaining a deeper understanding of the mechanisms of antioxidants and biomarkers behind oxidative stress and synaptic degeneration is essential for developing therapeutic approaches aimed at preventing the progression of AD.

* **Corresponding author Dipanjan Karati:** Department of Pharmaceutical Technology, School of Pharmacy, Techno India University, Kolkata, West Bengal, India; E-mail: karatibabai@gmail.com

Keywords: Alzheimer's disease, Biomarker, Intracellular neurofibrillary tangles (NFTs), Oxidative stress.

INTRODUCTION

A progressive neurodegenerative illness, Alzheimer's disease (AD) is defined by memory and learning impairment that causes disruptions in language, perception, and planning. In 1906, German psychiatrist Alois Alzheimer made the initial discovery of AD. It is now thought that AD may impact 10% of the world's population. Millions of individuals throughout the world have been affected by this pandemicillness. By 2050, it is anticipated that the global prevalence will have quadrupled to 106.8 million [1]. Oxidative stress arises when there is an imbalance between pro-oxidants, including reactive oxygen species (ROS), and the body's antioxidant defenses. Oxidative stress is the result of an imbalance between the body's antioxidant defences and pro-oxidants, such as reactive oxygen species (ROS), with the balance shifting in favour of the pro-oxidants [2]. Memory impairment and dementia are caused by AD, which is typified by the accumulation of extracellular senile plaques, neurofibrillary tangles (NFTs), and neurodegeneration. Comprehensive efforts to study the pathophysiology of AD have not yet revealed the precise processes underlying the disease [3]. According to clinical research, persons with AD and those with moderate cognitive impairment had higher plasma cortisol levels (Fig. **1**). Because the hypothalamic-pituitary-adrenal (HPA) axis is frequently activated in physiological reactions to different stresses, causing the release of corticosteroids into the blood [4]. At the cytochrome oxidase complex, over 98% of the molecular oxygen is used by the mitochondrial electron transport chain, with the remainder being converted into superoxide and hydrogenperoxide radicals. The oxygen radical superoxide ($O_2•^-$), the non-radical oxidant hydrogenperoxide (H_2O_2), and hypochlorousacid are formed during regular metabolism and other processes [5]. AD is characterized by the loss of synapses, build-up of extracellular amyloid beta-peptide (Aβ), and formation of senile plaques (SPs) due to amyloid precursor protein (APP) undergoing amyloidogenic transformation. Moreover, there is an increase in intracellular neurofibrillary tangles (NFTs) made up of hyperphosphorylated tau protein that stabilizes microtubules and is associated with this region [6]. Over the past ten or fifteen years, conclusive evidence has been proposed connecting AD to a rise in oxidative stress, partly due to both the enhanced production of reactive oxygen and nitrogen species (ROS and RNS, respectively) and loss of function of numerous antioxidant defence enzymes [7, 8]. Oxidative stress is recognized as a key factor in the development of AD; however, the precise mechanisms leading to redox imbalance and the origins of free radicals remain unclear. This chapter explores how the abnormal deposits of amyloid-beta (Aβ) and tau proteins contribute to oxidative imbalance and the production of free radicals. It highlights processes such as mitochondrial dysfunction and disruptions in transition metal homeostasis as potential sources of oxidative stress. Additionally, it examines how oxidative damage enhances Aβ- and tau-driven neurotoxicity, further accelerating neuronal degeneration in AD [9].

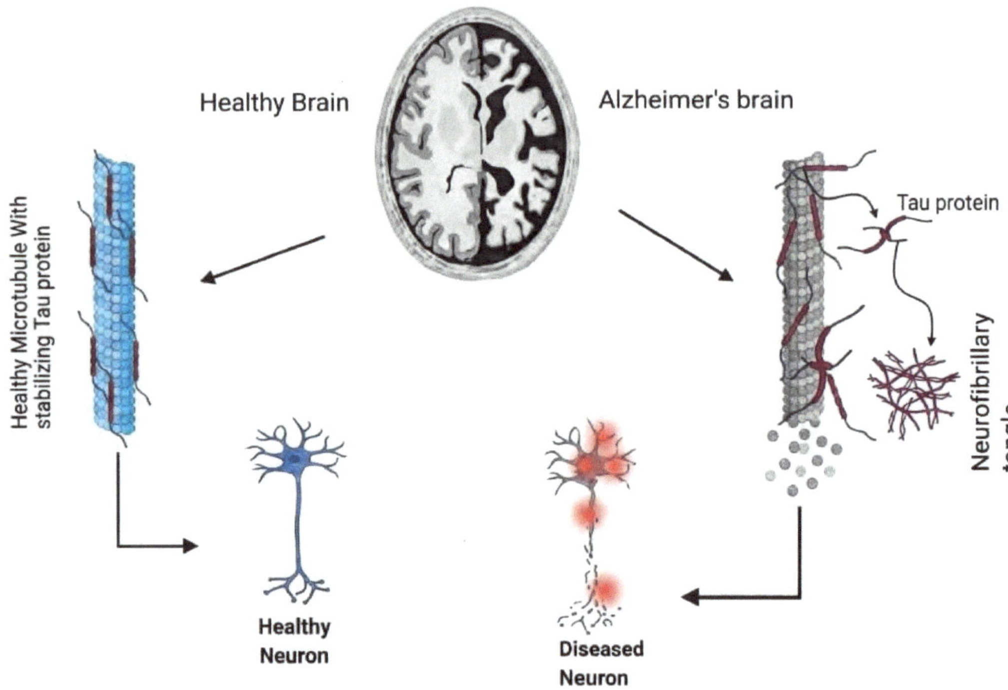

Fig. (1). Comparison between a normal brain and an AD-affected brain.

PATHOPHYSIOLOGY OF ALZHEIMER'S DISEASE

The study of AD pathophysiology is traced back to 1907 when Alzheimer found crucial neuropathological characteristics of the disease, such as amyloid plaques and hyperphosphorylated neurofibrillary tangles (NFTs).

Several theories have been advocated for explaining the complicated disorder on the basis of various causative elements. Some of these hypotheses are the tau hypothesis, cholinergic hypothesis, inflammation hypothesis, and amyloid-beta (Aβ) hypothesis (Fig. **2**) [10].

AMYLOID PLAQUES AND TAU TANGLES

Beta-amyloid plaques are insoluble peptide deposits that arise as a consequence of the pathological cleavage of amyloid precursor protein (APP), whose functionis not exactly known. APP is normally processed by three enzymes: α-secretase, γ-secretase, and β-secretase. On cleavage by β-secretase and then by γ-secretase, a 40-amino acid soluble peptide is generated. But in AD, one of the forms of γ-secretase cleaves APP aberrantly, producing a 42-amino acid peptide called Aβ42 or Aβ. This is not soluble and causes beta-amyloid plaques to be formed. α-secretase acts as a protector by cutting APP at a location that avoids Aβ.

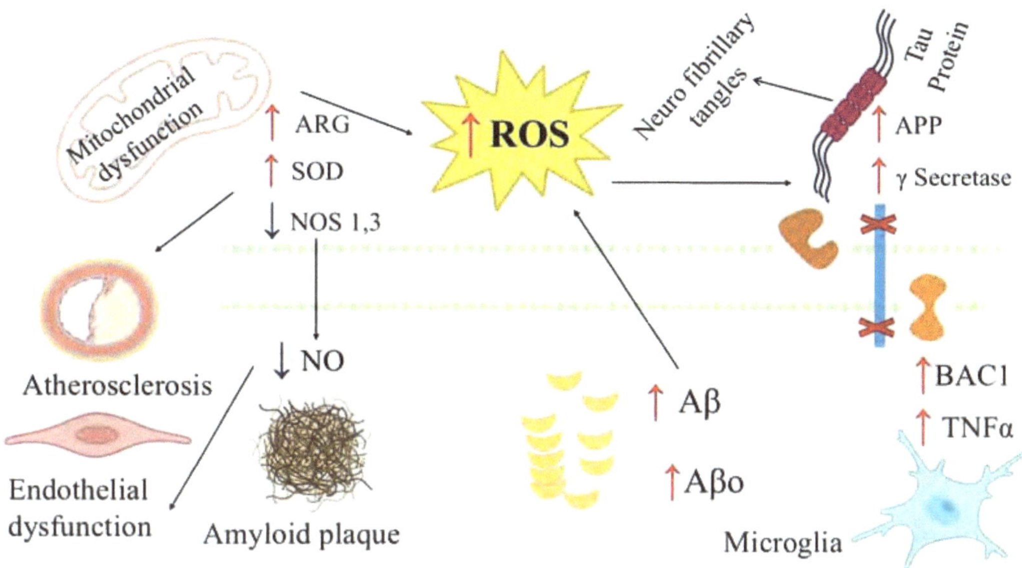

Fig. (2). Pathogenesis of AD.

Neurofibrillary tangles (NFTs) are seen as damaged or deadneurons on histological staining. The tangles result from the degeneration of neuronal microtubules, which happens when their stabilizing protein tau is altered. Microtubules are important in holding the structure of neurons intact, maintaining nutrient transport, and aiding in signal conduction within axons. In Alzheimer's, tau proteins are hyperphosphorylated, leading to the release of the proteinsfrom microtubules. This results in microtubule breakdown, disrupting the transport and communication system of the neuron, leading eventually to cell death. Although the precise causal relationshipis not yetknown, hyperphosphorylation of tau isthought to occur after plaque formation (Fig. **2**) [11].

NEUROINFLAMMATION AND BLOOD-BRAIN BARRIER DISRUPTION

The blood-brain barrier is made up of astrocytes, pericytes, innate immune cells, non-fenestrated special endothelial cells, and the basement membrane [12]. Transport of nucleotides, fatty acids, carbohydrates, hormones, amino acids, vitamins, monocarboxylic acids, organic anions, and cations across the blood-brain barrieris facilitated by solute carricr-mediated transport (CMT). Both from the blood to the brain and from the brain to the blood, transendothelial transport of proteins and peptides is made possible *via* receptor-mediated transcytosis (RMT). Essential ω3 fatty acids are transported into the brain *via* sodium-dependent transport so phosphatidyl choline symporter 1, an important transporter that is also necessary for the establishment of the blood-brain barrier. While RMT removesamyloid-β (Aβ), some types of which are linked to AD, CMT helps the brain to remove excitatory amino acids (such as aspartate and glutamate) from the blood [13].

MITOCHONDRIAL DYSFUNCTION AND CELLULAR METABOLISM

Since they are metabolically active cell organelles, mitochondria are the main producers of biological energy generated in the cell through oxidative phosphorylation (OXPHOS), which yields adenosine triphosphate (ATP). The major source of energy for cells, ATP, is required by both signalling pathways and regular cell functions. Because of their high energy needs and limited glycolytic capacity, which makes them very dependent on OXPHOS, the importance of mitochondria in neuronal cells increases even more. Reactive oxygen species, such as hydrogenperoxide (H_2O_2), hydroxyl (HO•), and superoxide (O_2−•), are also mostly located in mitochondria. They are byproducts of OXPHOS. Electrons are transferred from electron donors to electronacceptors (such as oxygen) in redox reactions in oxidative phosphorylation [1].

UNDERSTANDING OXIDATIVE STRESS

Over the last few decades, the amyloid cascade theory that dominated AD research has been contested in an effort to uncover the underlying causes of the disease [14]. Oxidative stress occurs when there is either an increase in the production of ROS within the cell or when the body's defences against the potentially harmful effects of ROS are not strong enough. This definition naturally states that increased generation of reactive oxygen species (ROS) or reactive nitrogen species (RNS) typically does not give enough leverage to cause pathology as long as the antioxidant defence system is good enough at scavenging the created reactive species [15]. The primary origin of reactive oxygen species (ROS) is the electron transport chain (ETC) located in the inner mitochondrial membrane, where ATP is produced as an energy source [16]. Synapses serve as the connections between neurons, enabling the transmission of signals from one cell to another. In many neurodegenerative diseases, these connections often become impaired or deteriorate. Growing research indicates that synaptic dysfunction and loss may play a key role in the early stages of AD. The degeneration of synapses in AD is closely linked to cognitive decline, reduced synaptic density, and neuronal cell death [17]. A well-functioning brain is safeguarded against oxidative damage by antioxidant defence mechanisms. These defences consist of antioxidant enzymes and molecules that neutralize free radicals, including ascorbate, vitamin E, and protein sulfhydryls. Growing experimental research suggests that a decline in total antioxidant capacity (TAC) is a key factor in the development of AD. In individuals with AD, the activity levels of antioxidant enzymes such as Cu/Zn catalase (CAT) and superoxide dismutase (SOD) are notably diminished in the frontal and temporal cortex [18].

ANTIOXIDANT DEFENCE MECHANISMS

The two self-protection mechanisms using antioxidants present in the human body are the enzymatic (endogenous) and non-enzymatic (exogenous) mechanisms. The non-enzymatic system consists of families of materials such as plant material, minerals, and vitamins, which may be obtained by taking food. Antioxidants function to combat free radicals in a two-fold way: either by preventing them from forming or repairing any damage that has been established. The first of these is associated with the inhibition of chain reactions with their formation, and the second one is the elimination of damaged cells with subsequent reconstitution of cell membranes [19]. As a lipid-soluble antioxidant, vitamin E may counteract the effects of peroxide and protect cell membranes from lipid peroxidation. Water-soluble antioxidant vitamin C serves as a co-factor for antioxidant enzymes and aids in the electron transfer that eliminates free radicals [20]. Moreover, cells can create antioxidants that chelate and/or bind to redox metals to indirectly shield cells from oxidative stress. The first natural scavenger, melatonin, is known to neutralize hypochlorous acid and detoxify a variety of chemical and environmental agents, such as H_2O_2, hydroxylradicals (OH•), peroxyl radicals (ROO•), singlet oxygen ($^1O2$), and reactive nitrogen species (RNS), including nitric oxide radicals (NO•) and peroxynitrite (ONOO−) [21].

OXIDATIVE STRESS AND AD

AD patients' brains exhibit a high degree of oxidative damage linked to aberrantly high Aβ accumulation and neurofibrillary tangle formation [5]. AD is associated with the accumulation of misfolded tau and amyloid-β proteins. It has been hypothesized that oxidative stress and these protein aggregates have a cause-an--effect connection. According to some research, oxidative stress-driven ROS increases with age and may have a role in the development of neural plaque [22].

EFFECTS OF OXIDATIVE STRESS ON AMYLOID-BETA AND TAU PATHOLOGY

Phosphorylated tau accumulates in synapses after Aβ is collected. Early-stage illness is indicated by the buildup of Aβ, whereas late-stage disease is indicated by phosphorylated tau, according to researchers. Through the use of transgenic rat models and human parietal cortex synaptosomes, researchers have been able to comprehend the course of AD. Endosomes, mitochondria, and other components are found in presynaptic structures called synaptosomes. They found that when the amyloid beta percentage rose, so did phosphorylated tau. Because of this, they speculate that tau phosphorylation may be related to Aβ [23].

By promoting tau phosphorylation and the development of neurofibrillary tangles, oxidative stress is thought to be a key early event in the pathophysiology of AD. However, it is still unclear how oxidative stress and tau hyperphosphorylation are related, as well as the underlying processes. A clear connection between the processes by which oxidative stress causes the development of NFTs in AD is offered by fatty acid oxidative products [24].

MITOCHONDRIAL DYSFUNCTION AND OXIDATIVE INJURY

The pathophysiology of AD involves a vicious cycle of oxidative stress and mitochondrial (mt) dysfunction. OS can result in mitochondria that are structurally and functionally flawed, but damaged mitochondria are more likely to produce a lot of ROS, which raises the brain's total oxidative load. Early-stage AD is characterized by mitochondrial dysfunction. In comparison to healthycontrols, it has been noted that the Aβ peptide actively obtains access to the mt-matrix in the brains of transgenic APP mice and AD mice. After interacting with Aβ, the mt-enzyme Aβ-binding alcohol dehydrogenase is inhibited, which causes ROS to be released and impacts important metabolic pathways [25].

There is evidence from a number of studies that AD is associated with increased oxidative damage to DNA and RNA. DNA double-strand breakage, DNA/DNA or DNA/protein crosslinking, and base modification can all result from oxidative DNA damage [26]. mtDNA is especially vulnerable to oxidative damage because it is found close to the ETC, a significant source of ROS, and is not compacted around histones. Moreover, mtDNA contains few or no noncoding regions, which raises the possibility that coding areas will be mutagenic [27].

NEUROINFLAMMATION AND THE ROLE OF MICROGLIA

In relation to disorders of the brain, microglial cells play an essential role in controlling neuroinflammatory reactions. This phagocytic glia contributes to a diverse network that manages development, maintains homeostasis, surveys the parenchyma, and responds to injury and pathogen-associated stimuli. The "amyloid cascade–inflammatory hypothesis of AD" states that misfolded Aβ buildup in microglial innate immune receptors, including G protein-coupled receptors (GPCRs), triggers an inflammatory cascade that causes neuroinflammation. Inflammation and systemic infections cause microglia to age, undergo cell priming, and ultimately lead to neurodegeneration. The emergence of AD is caused by microglial dysfunction and associated neuroinflammation [28, 29].

BIOMARKERS OF OXIDATIVE STRESS IN ALZHEIMER'S DISEASE

The pathophysiology of Alzheimer's disease (AD) relies heavily on oxidative stress, as it accumulates reactive oxygen species (ROS), which induce neurodegeneration. Proteins, lipids, and DNA are among the biological macromolecules affected. Reliable oxidative stress biomarkers can aid in early diagnosis, disease monitoring, and treatment assessment [30].

Several potential biomarkers used for the diagnosis of AD include sensitive cognitive tests, metabolic abnormalities (measured by PET or SPECT), and structural changes (MRI volumetry) [31]. These biomarkers differ in their sensitivity, specificity, cost-effectiveness, level of invasiveness, logistical requirements, and/or technical requirements [32]. For example, Pittsburgh compound B (PIB), which is not commonly available, can scan amyloid *in vivo*. Additionally, 50–60% of patients with moderate cognitive impairment (MCI) and 20–30% of healthy elderly people have PIB-positive results, suggesting the need for other diagnostic techniques [33]. Oxidative stress biomarkers can be divided into the following categories to enhance AD diagnosis and disease monitoring:

Oxidative Damage to Lipids

Lipid peroxidation constitutes one of the most serious consequences of oxidative imbalance–induced brain injury. It affects the permeability and fluidity of cell membranes and decreases the activity of membrane-bound enzymes [34]. Additionally, conjugated diene hydroperoxides and unstable compounds that break down into different aldehydes, including malondialdehyde, 4-hydroxynonenal, and Thiobarbituric Acid Reactive Substances (TBARS), are produced as a result of lipid peroxidation. Plasma or serum TBARS levels in AD patients are substantially greater than in controls, according to some research. In contrast, other investigations found no difference between AD participants and controls (Table **1**) [3].

Table 1. Research investigating the ability of lipidperoxidation indicators in AD to predict outcomes.

Subjects' Characteristics	Specimen	Methodology	Key Findings	Results	References
There were 62 people suffering from AD (average age = 73.3, MMSE 7-20, ADAS-Cog 10-35, GDS >1 or ≤3). 56 subjects (average age of 70.8)	Serum	Mann-Whitney U test	TBARS levels analyzed in AD and control groups	Substantial higher in AD patients and the reference group ($p < 0.0001$).	[41]
50 patients with Alzheimer's disease (22 aged 65-74, 23 aged 75-84, and five aged>85). Exclusion criteria include diabetes, mental impairment, myeloproliferative diseases, uncontrolled hypertension, andmalnutrition. 50 controls (24 subjects aged 65-74, 21 aged 75-84, and five aged over 85).	Erythrocytes (HPLC)	High-Performance Liquid Chromatography (HPLC)	TBARS levels measured in different age groups	AD rates were significantly higher in the 65-74 ($p < 0.001$), 75-84 ($p < 0.001$), and 85-94 ($p < 0.05$) age groups.	[39]
18 patients with Alzheimer's Disease (average age = 76.3). 14 controls (average age: 75.2).	Erythrocytes (HPLC)	HPLC-based TBARS analysis	TBARS concentration comparison between AD and controls	Notably higher in AD ($p < 0.01$).	[43]
40 patients with Alzheimer's disease (median age = 84.2). Criteria for rejection include having a life expectancy of less than four months, using steroids, and being blind or deaf. 34 controls (mean age: 79.1).	Plasma	Spectrophotometric analysis	Oxidative stress marker levels assessed	There is no substantial difference between AD and controls.	[44]

(Table 1) cont.....

Subjects' Characteristics	Specimen	Methodology	Key Findings	Results	References
25 patients with AD (an average of age = 78.2). Among those who are excluded criteria are Vascular injury, diabetes, chronic infection, malignant disease, severerenal, hepatic, cardiorespiratory, or hematological disease, and the use of vitamin supplements. 66 controls (mean age: 70.4).	Serum	ELISA-based detection	TBARS levels compared across groups	AD and controls did not differ significantly.	[45]
29 AD patients (MMSE of 7 to 24; mean age = 74). Additional serious health issues are a criterion for exclusion. 46 controls, whose average age is 73.	Serum	Spectrophotometric method	Oxidative stress markers evaluated	AD and controls did not differ significantly.	[46]
The mean age of 27 AD patients is 72.3. Life expectancy shorter than three months, steroid use, blindness and deafness, iron deficiency, and illness esotherthandementia are also grounds for exclusion. 25 controls, with an average age of 64.4.	Serum	TBARS spectrophotometric assay	Comparison of oxidative stress markers	Notably higher in AD ($p < 0.001$).	[47]
112 AD patients (average age of 78.2). Exclusion criteria include chronic infections, vascular disease, diabetes, cancer, severe cardiac, renal, hepatic, or haematologic illnesses, and the use of vitamin supplements. 85 controls (average age: 74.6).	Serum	Enzymatic analysis	Lipid per oxidation levels in AD patients *vs.* controls	Significantly greater in AD patients ($p < 0.01$).	[36]

There is considerable debate over findings related to erythrocyte TBARS levels in AD. Some research shows no distinction between AD and controls [36 - 38], while others report greater erythrocyte TBARS levels in AD [39]. A meta-analysis of blood TBARS levels among people with AD and moderate cognitive decline found that Alzheimer's disease plasma/serum had significantly higher TBARS levels [40]. However, findings may differ depending on patient selection criteria. For example, some researchers found that AD subjects with MMSE scores between 7 and 24 lacked significantly greater serum TBARS compared to controls. In contrast, others found that AD subjects with scores between 7 and 20 and ADAS-cog scores between 10 and 35 had significantly higher serum TBARS than controls [41].

These results indicate that MMSE alone is unable to distinguish between individuals with higher and lower TBARS. Another study likewise found no correlation between MMSE and TBARS, indicating that MMSE and TBARS are unrelated [42], but that the degree of cognitive dysfunction in AD may raise plasma TBARS levels.

Oxidative Damage to Proteins

Protein oxidation, which produces protein carbonyls, and protein peroxidation, which produces nitrated protein, are two separate indications of free-radical damage to proteins that are being proposed [42 - 49]. (Table **2**). Despite differing patient selection criteria, numerous studies have found that AD is associated with elevated serum/plasma protein carbonyl levels, a peripheral indication of oxidative damage in the brain. According to studies, serum/plasma protein carbonyl levels in AD and controls are not significantly different.

Table 2. Protein Carbonyls in Alzheimer's disease (AD).

Subject Characteristics	Specimen	Methodology	Key Findings	Result	Refs.
110 Alzheimer's disease patients (average age 74.7;). 134 controls (average age of 77.8).	Plasma, erythrocytes, leukocytes	Spectrophotometric assay for proteincarbonyl content	Higher levels in AD *vs.* controls across all samples. Increased severity correlates with higher protein carbonyl levels. Inversely correlated with MMSE.	Significant	[42]
45 Alzheimer's patients, 28 controls.	Serum	ELISA for oxidative stress biomarkers	Protein carbonyl levels are significantly higher in AD.	Proteincarbonyl levels are substantially greater in AD ($P < 0.05$).	[43]

(Table 2) cont.....

Subject Characteristics	Specimen	Methodology	Key Findings	Result	Refs.
25 AD patients (average age: 78) and 14 controls (mean age: 84).	Serum	High-performance liquid chromatography (HPLC) analysis	Notably elevated amounts of protein carbonyl in AD.	Proteincarbonyl level is significantly greater in AD (P< 0.05).	[50]
72 patients with Alzheimer'sdisease (mean age 80). 72 controls (mean age of 75).	Serum	Spectrophotometry	There is no notable difference between the AD and control groups.	Not significant	[51]
15 Alzheimer's patients and 15 controls.	Serum	Oxidative stress biomarker analysis.	The MMSE had an inverse correlation with ox-LDL.	Proteincarbonyl levels are considerably greater in AD. P<0.05	[52]
20 AD men (average age: 70.6,) and 26 AD women (average age: 73.9,). 16 control males (average age: 73.3), and 30 control females (average age: 73.8).	Plasma	Enzyme-linked immunosorbent assay (ELISA)	Compared to controls, AD men and females had greater amounts of protein carbonyl.	P<0.05	[53]
There were 6 Alzheimer's patients (median age at death: 84.5) and 6 controls (median age at death: 85.8).	Brain (hippocampus)	Western blot and 2D-gel electrophoresis.	Identified proteins with considerably increased carbonylation in AD.	P≤0.05P	[54]
5 Alzheimer's patients (median age at death: 85.5), and 5 controls (median age at death: 83).	Brain (neocortex, hippocampus, entorhinal cortex, cerebellum, amygdala, brainstem,)	Mass spectrometry-based proteomics.	Protein carbonyls are significantly elevated in AD.	(□≤0.05).	[55]

(Table 2) cont.....

Subject Characteristics	Specimen	Methodology	Key Findings	Result	Refs.
22 AD patients (mean age: 72, MMSE: 21.3 ± 0.9, illness duration: 2.3 ± 0.3, 12 AD patients APOE4 positive). 18 controls (mean age: 68), 10 of whom were APOE4-positive.	CSF, plasma, serum	Immuno assay-based detection	CSF protein carbonyls were higher in APOE4-negative AD patients compared to APOE4-negative controls. Serum levels were higher in controls compared to AD. There is no substantial change in plasma.	P=0.03, P=0.016, P=0.005	[56]
9 Alzheimer's disease patients (ages 70-89) and 9 controls (ages 74-89).	Plasma	Spectrophotometry	Protein carbonyls are significantly higher in AD.	P<0.05	[57]
11 AD patients (median age: 73.5, mild AD, MMSE: 14-26) and 8 controls (median age: 64.6).	CSF	Western blot analysis	Higher carbonylation of λ chain precursor in AD.	P=0.03	[58]

Oxidative Damage to Antioxidants

According to Table **3**, antioxidants may serve as indirect indicators of how oxidative stress is processed in AD patients' brains. It has been hypothesized that oxidative stress leads to antioxidant consumption, resulting in a drop in levels of antioxidants [59]. Uric acid, vitamins C and E, and vitamin A/carotenoids are some of the nonenzymatic compounds with antioxidant properties. However, since oxidative stress can activate the production of antioxidant enzymes such as glutathione peroxidase (GPx) and superoxide dismutase (SOD) (to raise their level or activity), the behavior of antioxidant enzymes—whether they differ based on the extent of oxidative stress in AD or become consumed (lowering their activity or level) remains unresolved [40].

Table 3. Research investigating the ability of antioxidants to predict AD.

Subjects' Characteristics	Specimen	Methodology	Key Findings	Results	Refs.
35 AD patients (median age of 85.9). 40 controls (median age: 85.5).	Plasma	Case-control study	Investigated plasma uric acid levels in AD and controls.	There is no substantial difference between AD and controls.	[59]

(Table 3) cont.....

Subjects' Characteristics	Specimen	Methodology	Key Findings	Results	Refs.
24 AD patients (mean age of 83). Exclusion criteria included diabetes and the use of any medication that affects blood glucose or lipidlevels. 66 controls (mean age: 85).	Plasma	Case-control study	Examined the effect of metabolic diseases on uric acid levels.	There is no substantial difference between AD and controls.	[60]
101 patients with Alzheimer's disease (median age 73.5). Among the exclusion criteria are diabetes, hypertension, and hyperlipidemia. AD MMSE: 17 ± 5.8. 101 controls (median age = 73.2).	Plasma	Cross-sectional study	Analysis of uric acid levels and cognitive performance in Alzheimer's disease	Significantly decreased in AD (P< 0.0001).	[61]
18 Alzheimer's patients. 11 controls.	Serum	Case-control study	Investigated serum uric acid concentration in AD	Significantlydecreased in AD patients (P<0.02).	[62]
63 AD patients (mean age of 76.8). Exclusion factors include smoking, alcoholism, dyslipidemia, significant organ failure, and malnutrition. 56 controls (mean age: 75.8).	Plasma	Case-control study	Assessed metabolic and oxidative stress markers in AD.	Significantly lower in AD (P< 0.001).	[63]
20 patients with Alzheimer's disease (median age = 80.1). Over six months of follow-up at a memory center with no indication of dietary behavior; median AD duration = 3.9 years; 19 patients on cholinergic medication. 23 controls (median age: 76.0).	Plasma/erythrocytes	Longitudinal study	Evaluated vitamin E levels in plasma and erythrocytes.	Notably, plasma levels in AD (P = 0.002). There is no difference in erythrocyte levels.	[37]
110 AD patients (median age = 74.7; GDS 3 = moderate, GDS 4-5 = intermediate, and GDS 6-7 = severe). No otherexcludingcriteriaexist 134 controls (mean age: 77.8).	Plasma	Case-control study	Examined vitamin E levels at different AD severity stages.	Notably lower in mild AD compared to control, intermediate AD compared to mild AD, and severe AD compared to intermediate AD.	[42]
35 AD patients (mean age of 85.9). 40 controls (median age: 85.5).	Plasma	Case-control study	Investigated vitamin E deficiency in AD patients	AD plasma levels were significantly lower (P< 0.001).	[59]

(Table 3) cont.....

Subjects' Characteristics	Specimen	Methodology	Key Findings	Results	Refs.
44 Alzheimer's sufferers. 37 controls.	Serum/CSF/serum-CSF ratio	Case-control study	Compared vitamin E levels in serum and CSF.	In Alzheimer's disease, serum and CSF levels are significantly lower, but the serum-CSF ratio remains unchanged.	[64]
44 AD patients (MMSE < 24, mean age = 78.5). 20 controls, with an average age of 79.3.	Plasma	Case-control study	Investigated the plasma levels of vitamin E in AD.	There is no substantial difference between AD and controls.	[65]
37 AD patients (cholesterol-adjustedvitamin E levels). 24 controls.	Plasma	Case-control study	Evaluated cholesterol-corrected vitamin E levels.	Decreased (P< 0.05) in AD patients.	[66]
The mean age of 26 AD patients is 73.9. 14 controls, with an average age of 70.3.	CSF/plasma	Case-control study	Compared vitamin E levels in CSF and plasma.	The difference between plasma and CSF is negligible.	[67]
20 Alzheimer's sufferers. 18 controls.	Serum	Case-control study	Investigated serum vitamin E levels in AD	Decrease in AD (P< 0.05).	[68]
25 AD patients (median MMSE: 19, mean age: 74.3). 41 controls (73.4 years old on average).	Plasma	Case-control study	Assessed vitamin E levels and cognitive decline.	AD is much reduced (P = 0.035).	[69]
79 AD individuals with an MMSE range of 10 to 25 and a median age of 79. 58 controls, with an average age of 74.	Plasma	Case-control study	Evaluated plasma vitamin E in AD progression.	Notably reduced in AD (P< 0.01).	[70]
74 Alzheimer's patients. 158 controls.	Serum	Case-control study	Investigated vitamin E levels in mildde mentia	The control group and those with mild dementia are identical.	[71]
40 patients with AD (mean MMSE: 17.3, mean age: 75.9). 39 controls (74.8 years old on average).	Plasma	Case-control study	Examined vitamin E and other indicators of oxidative damage.	Notablyreduced in AD (P< 0.001).	[72]

GENETIC AND ENVIRONMENTAL FACTORS INFLUENCING OXIDATIVE STRESS

Genetic Mutations Linked to Increased Oxidative Stress

Gene mutations have a substantial effect on how well the body regulates oxidative stress, which in turn affects the risk of developing AD. Mutations in genes related to mitochondrial activity, antioxidant enzymes, and amyloid metabolism cause the cell to produce more reactive oxygen species (ROS) while decreasing its defensive capacities. For example, mutations in the SOD2 gene, which lead to the production of manganese superoxide dismutase, have been associated with poor removal of ROS, leading to neuronal oxidative damage [73]. Moreover, mutations in the GPX4 gene, which encodes glutathione peroxidase, result in decreased antioxidant activity, leading to greater levels of lipid peroxidation and more neuronal degeneration [74]. Additionally, mtDNA deletions and point mutations compromise the electron transport chain, which consequently increases oxidative stress in AD neurons [75].

The Role of ApoE in Oxidative Stress and Alzheimer's Disease

Apolipoprotein E (ApoE), which has three main isoforms, is now among the most significant hereditary risk indicators for late-onset Alzheimer's disease (AD): ApoE2, ApoE3, and ApoE4 [76]. ApoE is a protein that is vital for the metabolism of cholesterol and lipid repair in neurons. Because of its effects on mitochondria, lipid peroxidation, and antioxidant function, ApoE can alter oxidative stress. Since ApoE4 has the least amount of antioxidant activity, neurons are severely damaged. ApoE4 is also linked to a higher Aβ burden, inefficient clearance, persistent inflammation, and a breakdown of the blood-brain barrier in AD, all of which exacerbate the illness [77]. The primary goals of translational techniques are to address oxidative stress, modify ApoE function, which is responsible for lipophagy, halt the course of the disease, and directly target neurotoxicity. Recognising the relationship between ApoE, oxidative damage, and AD pathogenesis is essential for therapies to be successful [78].

Factors Related to the Environment and Lifestyle Choices

Lifestyle habits and environmental conditions synergistically influence oxidative stress levels that lead to AD.

Diet and Nutrition

A Mediterranean diet rich in polyphenols, omega-3s, and flavonoids can lower the risk of AD compared to Western diets filled with saturated fats and processed food, which increase oxidative stress and neuroinflammation [79].

Air Pollution

The relentless emission of PM2.5 pollutants and lead- and mercury-containing heavy metals is remarkably linked with augmented ROS generation and oxidative damage, worsening AD conditions [80].

Lifestyle Factors

Smoking, lack of movement, and enduring severe psychological distress lead to inflammation of the body as well, in addition to increasing oxidative stress, which trickles down to the brain, worsening the condition of the patient [81].

Pathogen Exposure

Herpes Simplex Virus Type 1 (HSV-1) and a cluster of periodontal bacteria multiply within the brain, leading to heightened oxidative stress and amyloid deposition [82]. These pathogens may worsen oxidative damage by activating neuroinflammatory pathways.

ANTIOXIDANT STRATEGIES IN ALZHEIMER'S DISEASE

Endogenous Antioxidant Defence Systems

The human body possesses various psychosomatic elements that fight against bodily oxidative stress, known as internal defence mechanisms. The body's oxidative defence is enzymatic, and it includes catalase, superoxide dismutase (SOD), and glutathione peroxidase. These are important in combating harmful reactive oxygen species (ROS) [69]. Moreover, cellular redox balance is also maintained by several organic substances like coenzyme Q10 and glutathione, which are classified as non-enzymatic [54]. Research on Alzheimer's disease has shown a reduction of endogenous antioxidants in patients suffering from AD, which notably worsens as the disease progresses [54]. Infusing greater amounts exogenously may help these patients balance the extensive oxidative damage that occurs in the human body and brain.

Dietary Antioxidants and Their Role in AD Prevention

AD models show protective neurological effects when exposed to various dietary antioxidants. The polyphenols found in fruits, vegetables, and tea, including resveratrol and curcumin, show both anti-inflammatory and antioxidant activity according to research by Arnim *et al.*, (1999) [71]. Researchers have carried out extensive studies on vitamin E and vitamin C's ability to lower oxidative stress levels and enhance cognitive function, according to Cristalli *et al.*, (2012) [42]. The antioxidant-rich Mediterranean diet has shown a correlation with reduced Alzheimer's disease risk, according to von Arnim *et al.*, (2012) [72]. Preclinical studies indicate positive results, yet clinical evidence lacks certainty, which requires additional research.

Pharmacological Approaches to Target Oxidative Stress

Most research on Alzheimer's disease (AD) focuses on medications aimed at reducing oxidative stress. Tenoria *et al.*, (2021) found that N-acetylcysteine (NAC) can help lower oxidative damage and boost glutathione levels [83, 84].

MitoQ and SkQ1 are mitochondria-targeted antioxidants that may prevent neuronal death while maintaining mitochondrial function [85]. Furthermore, edaravone, a free radical scavenger, has been studied for its potential neuroprotective effects due to its capacity to prevent lipid peroxidation and oxidative damage to neurons [86]. Similarly, selenium-based antioxidants play a role by enhancing the function of selenium proteins, which are vital for minimizing neuronal degeneration [87]. While initial preclinical findings were promising, problems such as bioavailability, the ability to pass through the blood-brain barrier, and possible adverse reactions will emerge when these treatments are implemented in clinical settings [88]. Thus, more well-structured research and trials are necessary to accurately assess their long-term effectiveness against AD. Additionally, some flavonoid-based compounds appear to offer a combination of antioxidant and anti-inflammatory benefits by altering cellular signalling pathways that are important for neuroprotection [89].

CLINICAL TRIALS AND EFFICACY OF ANTIOXIDANT THERAPIES

Several clinical trials have examined the efficacy of antioxidant treatment for Alzheimer's disease. The Alzheimer's Disease Cooperative Study (ADCS) with vitamin E demonstrated some efficacy in slowing the disease's progression [90]. There have been mixed results when it comes to large-scale studies like polyphenols and flavonoids [91].While cognitive gains have been reported in some studies, no significant effects were reported in other studies, emphasizing the heterogeneity of patient response and the effects of multiple confounding variables.

Scientists are working on mixing different antioxidants as a special kind of treatment to make that therapy work even better. For instance, clinical trials on the combined activity of vitamin E, vitamin C, and coenzyme Q10 have indicated increased antioxidant defence in neuronal cells [92]. In addition, curcumin-containing formulations are being developed with improved bioavailability, demonstrating encouraging initial-phase results in cognitive prevention [93]. Despite these new developments, successfully putting antioxidant therapies to use in clinics still presents tough challenges. Optimal dosing, variability in patient metabolism, variability in disease stage, and restricted permeability of the blood-brain barrier can hinder their efficacy. Future work should focus on personalized medicine approaches, combining antioxidants with treatments that actually modify the disease, to provide maximum benefits to people with AD.

OXIDATIVE STRESS: TARGET FOR THERAPEUTIC INTERVENTION

Oxidative stress has become a key player in the pathogenesis of AD and has been associated with neuronal dysfunction, mitochondrial dysfunction, and protein aggregation. Therefore , suggesting oxidative stress as a target for therapeutic intervention to prevent disease progression and enhance cognition. We discuss the therapeutic opportunities, drug development advancements, and barriers to clinical translation in this section.

THERAPEUTIC STRATEGIES TO MODIFY OXIDATIVE STRESS

This has led to the exploration of multiple strategies to mitigate oxidative stress in AD:

Antioxidative Chemicals

Both natural and synthetic antioxidants (including vitamin E, curcumin, resveratrol, and flavonoids) have been explored for their capability to scavenge reactive oxygen species (ROS) and lessen neuronal damage [94]. However, bioavailability and pharmacokinetic limitations have resulted in inconsistent clinical outcomes [95].

Enhancement of Endogenous Antioxidant Enzymes

Research is currently focused on how to manipulate enzymes like catalase, glutathione peroxidase, and superoxide dismutase (SOD) through gene therapy or pharmacological activators to help restore redox balance [96].

Metal Chelation Treatment

The imbalance of transition metals like copper, iron, and zinc contributes significantly to the oxidative stress linked to AD [97]. Chelating medicines such as PBT2 and deferiprone are being studied for their potential to help restore metal balance and minimise the formation of reactive oxygen species (ROS) [98].

DRUG DEVELOPMENT AND PRECLINICAL RESEARCH

Clinical models of Alzheimer's disease (AD) have shed light on how effective therapies targeting oxidative stress can be. Preclinical studies using transgenic AD animal models have shown that synthetic mimetics of antioxidant enzymes, polyphenols, and edaravone provide neuroprotective benefits, indicating their potential to reduce oxidative damage [99]. Recent breakthroughs in gene therapy have shown how to target processes that control oxidative stress. Scientists focus on the Nrf2/Keap1 pathway to boost cell defenses against oxidative harm [100]. Also, stem cell treatments using mesenchymal stem cells (MSCs) have shown antioxidant and brain-protective effects. These might have an impact on reducing brain cell death caused by oxidative stress [101]. Because Alzheimer's disease (AD) is so complex, researchers are exploring combined therapies. These mix antioxidants with medications that reduce inflammation or target amyloid. The aim is to boost treatment effectiveness. These fresh approaches highlight the importance of ongoing research [102]. They strive to enhance treatment choices and outcomes for AD patients.

CHALLENGES IN TRANSLATING OXIDATIVE STRESS TARGETING TO CLINICAL SETTINGS

Even while early testing seems promising, there are still significant barriers to using antioxidant therapy in hospitals. One major issue is that they do not perform well in real patients. Many antioxidant medicines have not helped significantly in long-term research [103]. This often happens because they can't get through the blood-brain barrier, and different patients react differently. Also, Alzheimer's disease is complicated, which makes things harder [104]. Oxidative stress ties into many parts of the disease, so it's tough to pinpoint its exact effects and create treatments that target it. Another difficulty is a lack of reliable methods for measuring oxidative stress. This makes it difficult to organize patients and determine if therapies are effective [105]. There are also concerns regarding the safety of these medicines and what may happen if patients use them for an extended time. Using antioxidants for too long might mess with normal cell signalling that uses reactive oxygen species (ROS) [106]. This could weaken the immune system and change how the body uses energy. To address these challenges, more research is needed to develop treatment programs and ensure they are both successful and safe to use in hospitals.

New Understandings and Prospects

Recent advancements in the study of neurodegenerative diseases and redox biology have led to the discovery of novelstrategies for treating oxidative stress in AD. This section outlines promising avenues for future investigation.

Novel Antioxidant Compounds and Mechanisms

Molecular Hydrogen Therapy

After exhibiting anti-inflammatory and antioxidative qualities in preclinical studies, molecular hydrogen is currently being studied as a potential therapeutic option [107].

Antioxidants Based on Nanoparticles

By increasing the bioavailability of antioxidants and enabling tailored drug administration, nanotechnology amplifies their neuroprotective advantages [108].

Synthetic Enzyme Mimetics

Mimetics such as catalase and superoxide dismutase (SOD) provide an alternative to conventional antioxidants by imitating the functions of naturalantioxidant enzymes [109].

Redox-Active Metal Complexes

Engineered compounds that combine metal-chelating and reactive oxygen species (ROS)-scavenging properties offer a new strategy for managing oxidative stress in AD [110].

SYNERGY OF OXIDATIVE STRESS AND OTHER PATHOLOGICAL FACTORS IN AD

Neuroinflammation

Oxidative stress worsens inflammatory signalling, leading to neuronal damage [111]. Treatments that address both oxidative stress and inflammation may produce synergistic neuroprotective benefits [112].

Tau and Amyloid Pathology

Oxidative stress promotes tau hyperphosphorylation and the aggregation of amyloid-beta, suggesting that combined antioxidant and anti-amyloid therapies could be advantageous [113].

Mitochondrial Dysfunction

Oxidative damage to mitochondrial components worsens energy deficits in neurons, highlighting the importance of interventions aimed at mitochondrial health [114].

OXIDATIVE STRESS IN EARLY DETECTION AND DISEASE MODULATION

Discovery of Biological Markers

Advanced metabolomics and proteomics help to distinguish oxidative stress-sensitive markers in blood and cerebrospinal fluid (CSF) that help early AD developmentdetection and monitoring [115].

Lifestyle Strategies for Cognitive Health

Lifestyle adjustments such as diet, exercise, and intermittent fasting can delay cognitive decline and lower oxidative stress [116].

Methods of Precision Medicine

Identifying subpopulations of AD patients with high oxidative stress profiles could lead to tailored therapies [117].

CONCLUSION

The development of Alzheimer's disease pathogenesis is advanced by highly oxidative stress due to protein aggregation, mitochondrial impairment, and neuronal dysfunctions. Mixed outcomes have been observed from antioxidant therapies, highlighting the need for more sophisticated methods. Preclinical studies tested the hypothesis. Future work should aim to define patients according to their oxidative stress features so that more effective care can be delivered using precision medicine. Furthermore, even more effective strategies might be attained through combined treatment approaches that include anti-inflammatory, mitochondrial, and disease-modifying oxidative stress response-alleviating treatments. Adjustments to current drug delivery systems require the use highly permeable compounds and nanotechnology to improve the efficacy of antioxidants and bioactive substances and enhance treatment results. Moreover, the study of oxidative stress alterations in the preclinical stages of AD might serve as a novel strategy for delaying the disease's progression. In conclusion, targeting oxidative stress to treat AD remains promising; however, it will take targeted precision medicine, advanced biomarker diagnostics, and new drug targets to achieve translation to clinical practice.

REFERENCES

[1] Bhatia V, Sharma S. Role of mitochondrial dysfunction, oxidative stress and autophagy in progression of Alzheimer's disease. J Neurol Sci 2021; 421: 117253. [http://dx.doi.org/10.1016/j.jns.2020.117253] [PMID: 33476985]

[2] López N, Tormo C, De Blas I, Llinares I, Alom J. Oxidative stress in Alzheimer's disease and mild cognitive impairment with high sensitivity and specificity. J Alzheimers Dis 2013; 33(3): 823-9. [http://dx.doi.org/10.3233/JAD-2012-121528] [PMID: 23076075]

[3] Misrani A, Tabassum S, Yang L. Mitochondrial dysfunction and oxidative stress in alzheimer's disease. Front Aging Neurosci 2021; 13: 617588. [http://dx.doi.org/10.3389/fnagi.2021.617588] [PMID: 33679375]

[4] Lee KW, Kim JB, Seo JS, *et al.* Behavioral stress accelerates plaque pathogenesis in the brain of Tg2576 mice *via* generation of metabolic oxidative stress. J Neurochem 2009; 108(1): 165-75. [http://dx.doi.org/10.1111/j.1471-4159.2008.05769.x] [PMID: 19012747]

[5] Huang WJ, Zhang X, Chen WW. Role of oxidative stress in Alzheimer's disease. Biomed Rep 2016; 4(5): 519-22. [http://dx.doi.org/10.3892/br.2016.630] [PMID: 27123241]

[6] Katzman R, Saitoh T. Advances in Alzheimer's disease. FASEB J 1991; 5(3): 278-86. [http://dx.doi.org/10.1096/fasebj.5.3.2001787] [PMID: 2001787]

[7] Butterfield DA. β-Amyloid-associated free radical oxidative stress and neurotoxicity: implications for Alzheimer's disease. Chem Res Toxicol 1997; 10(5): 495-506. [http://dx.doi.org/10.1021/tx960130e] [PMID: 9168246]

[8] Markesbery WR. Oxidative stress hypothesis in Alzheimer's disease. Free Radic Biol Med 1997; 23(1): 134-47. [http://dx.doi.org/10.1016/S0891-5849(96)00629-6] [PMID: 9165306]

[9] Zhao Y, Zhao B. Oxidative stress and the pathogenesis of Alzheimer's disease. Oxid Med Cell Longev 2013; 2013: 1-10. [http://dx.doi.org/10.1155/2013/316523] [PMID: 23983897]

[10] Kurz A, Perneczky R. Novel insights for the treatment of Alzheimer's disease. Prog Neuropsychopharmacol Biol Psychiatry 2011; 35(2): 373-9. [http://dx.doi.org/10.1016/j.pnpbp.2010.07.018] [PMID: 20655969]

[11] Hardy J, Selkoe DJ. The amyloid hypothesis of Alzheimer's disease: progress and problems on the road to therapeutics. Science 2002; 297(5580): 353-6. [http://dx.doi.org/10.1126/science.1072994] [PMID: 12130773]

[12] Kempuraj D, Mentor S, Thangavel R, *et al.* Mast cells in stress, pain, blood-brain barrier, neuroinflammation and alzheimer's disease. Front Cell Neurosci 2019; 13: 54. [http://dx.doi.org/10.3389/fncel.2019.00054] [PMID: 30837843]

[13] Sweeney MD, Sagare AP, Zlokovic BV. Blood–brain barrier breakdown in Alzheimer disease and other neurodegenerative disorders. Nat Rev Neurol 2018; 14(3): 133-50. [http://dx.doi.org/10.1038/nrneurol.2017.188] [PMID: 29377008]

[14] Tönnies E, Trushina E. Oxidative stress, synaptic dysfunction, and alzheimer's disease. J Alzheimers Dis 2017; 57(4): 1105-21. [http://dx.doi.org/10.3233/JAD-161088] [PMID: 28059794]

[15] Cioffi F, Adam RHI, Broersen K. Molecular mechanisms and genetics of oxidative stress in alzheimer's disease. J Alzheimers Dis 2019; 72(4): 981-1017. [http://dx.doi.org/10.3233/JAD-190863] [PMID: 31744008]

[16] Wojsiat J, Zoltowska KM, Laskowska-Kaszub K, Wojda U. Oxidant/antioxidant imbalance in Alzheimer's disease: therapeutic and diagnostic prospects. Oxid Med Cell Longev. 2018; 2018: 6435861. [http://dx.doi.org/10.1155/2018/6435861]

[17] Kamat PK, Kalani A, Rai S, *et al.* Mechanism of oxidative stress and synapse dysfunction in the pathogenesis of alzheimer's disease: Understanding the therapeutics strategies. Mol Neurobiol 2016; 53(1): 648-61. [http://dx.doi.org/10.1007/s12035-014-9053-6] [PMID: 25511446]

[18] Cecchi C, Fiorillo C, Sorbi S, *et al.* Oxidative stress and reduced antioxidant defenses in peripheral cells from familial Alzheimer's patients. Free Radic Biol Med 2002; 33(10): 1372-9. [http://dx.doi.org/10.1016/S0891-5849(02)01049-3] [PMID: 12419469]

[19] Teixeira JP, de Castro AA, Soares FV, da Cunha EFF, Ramalho TC. Future therapeutic perspectives into the alzheimer's disease targeting the oxidative stress hypothesis. Molecules 2019; 24(23): 4410. [http://dx.doi.org/10.3390/molecules24234410] [PMID: 31816853]

[20] Kim GH, Kim JE, Rhie SJ, Yoon S. The role of oxidative stress in neurodegenerative diseases. Exp Neurobiol 2015; 24(4): 325-40. [http://dx.doi.org/10.5607/en.2015.24.4.325] [PMID: 26713080]

[21] Ahmadinejad F, Geir Møller S, Hashemzadeh-Chaleshtori M, Bidkhori G, Jami MS. Molecular mechanisms behind free radical scavengers function against oxidative stress. Antioxidants 2017; 6(3): 51. [http://dx.doi.org/10.3390/antiox6030051] [PMID: 28698499]

[22] Salim S. Oxidative stress and the central nervous system. J Pharmacol Exp Ther 2017; 360(1): 201-5. [http://dx.doi.org/10.1124/jpet.116.237503] [PMID: 27754930]

[23] John A, Reddy PH. Synaptic basis of Alzheimer's disease: Focus on synaptic amyloid beta, P-tau and mitochondria. Ageing Res Rev 2021; 65: 101208. [http://dx.doi.org/10.1016/j.arr.2020.101208] [PMID: 33157321]

[24] Liu Z, Li T, Li P, *et al.* The ambiguous relationship of oxidative stress, tau hyperphosphorylation, and autophagy dysfunction in alzheimer's disease. Oxid Med Cell Longev 2015; 2015: 1-12. [http://dx.doi.org/10.1155/2015/352723] [PMID: 26171115]

[25] Roy RG, Mandal PK, Maroon JC. Oxidative stress occurs prior to amyloid aβ plaque formation and tau phosphorylation in alzheimer's disease: Role of glutathione and metal ions. ACS Chem Neurosci 2023; 14(17): 2944-54. [http://dx.doi.org/10.1021/acschemneuro.3c00486] [PMID: 37561556]

[26] Wang X, Wang W, Li L, Perry G, Lee H gon, Zhu X. Oxidative stress and mitochondrial dysfunction in Alzheimer's disease. Biochim Biophys Acta BBA - Mol Basis Dis. 2014 Aug; 1842(8): 1240–7.

[27] Santos RX, Correia SC, Zhu X, *et al.* Mitochondrial DNA oxidative damage and repair in aging and Alzheimer's disease. Antioxid Redox Signal 2013; 18(18): 2444-57. [http://dx.doi.org/10.1089/ars.2012.5039] [PMID: 23216311]

[28] Kaur D, Sharma V, Deshmukh R. Activation of microglia and astrocytes: A roadway to neuroinflammation and Alzheimer's disease. Inflammopharmacology 2019; 27(4): 663-77. [http://dx.doi.org/10.1007/s10787-019-00580-x] [PMID: 30874945]

[29] Simpson DSA, Oliver PL. ROS generation in microglia: Understanding oxidative stress and inflammation in neurodegenerative disease. Antioxidants 2020; 9(8): 743. [http://dx.doi.org/10.3390/antiox9080743] [PMID: 32823544]

[30] Chen X, Li M, Wang S, Zhu H, Xiong Y, Liu X. Pittsburgh compound B retention and progression of cognitive status: a meta-analysis. Eur J Neurol 2014; 21(8): 1060-7. [http://dx.doi.org/10.1111/ene.12398] [PMID: 24612390]

[31] Zhang S, Smailagic N, Hyde C, Noel-Storr AH, Takwoingi Y, McShane R. ^{11}C-PIB-PET for the early diagnosis of Alzheimer's disease dementia and other dementias in people with mild cognitive impairment (MCI). Cochrane Database Syst Rev. 2013; (2): CD010386. [http://dx.doi.org/10.1002/14651858.CD010386.pub2]

[32] Mao P. Oxidative stress and its clinical applications in dementia. J Neurodegener Dis 2013; 2013: 1-15. [http://dx.doi.org/10.1155/2013/319898] [PMID: 26316986]

[33] Thanan R, Oikawa S, Hiraku Y, *et al.* Oxidative stress and its significant roles in neurodegenerative diseases and cancer. Int J Mol Sci 2014; 16(1): 193-217. [http://dx.doi.org/10.3390/ijms16010193] [PMID: 25547488]

[34] Barrera G. Oxidative stress and lipid peroxidation products in cancer progression and therapy. ISRN Oncol 2012; 2012: 1-21. [http://dx.doi.org/10.5402/2012/137289] [PMID: 23119185]

[35] Reed TT. Lipid peroxidation and neurodegenerative disease. Free Radic Biol Med 2011; 51(7): 1302-19. [http://dx.doi.org/10.1016/j.freeradbiomed.2011.06.027] [PMID: 21782935]

[36] Serra JA, Domínguez RO, de Lustig ES, *et al.* Parkinson's disease is associated with oxidative stress: comparison of peripheral antioxidant profiles in living Parkinson's, Alzheimer's and vascular dementia patients. J Neural Transm (Vienna) 2001; 108(10): 1135-48. [http://dx.doi.org/10.1007/s007020170003] [PMID: 11725816]

[37] Bourdel-Marchasson I, Delmas-Beauvieux MC, Peuchant E, *et al.* Antioxidant defences and oxidative

stress markers in erythrocytes and plasma from normally nourished elderly Alzheimer patients. Age Ageing 2001; 30(3): 235-41.
[http://dx.doi.org/10.1093/ageing/30.3.235] [PMID: 11443025]

[38] Jeandel C, Nicolas MB, Dubois F, Nabet-Belleville F, Penin F, Cuny G. Lipid peroxidation and free radical scavengers in Alzheimer's disease. Gerontology 1989; 35(5-6): 275-82.
[http://dx.doi.org/10.1159/000213037] [PMID: 2630382]

[39] Casado Á, Encarnación López-Fernández M, Concepción Casado M, de La Torre R. Lipid peroxidation and antioxidant enzyme activities in vascular and Alzheimer dementias. Neurochem Res 2008; 33(3): 450-8.
[http://dx.doi.org/10.1007/s11064-007-9453-3] [PMID: 17721818]

[40] Schrag M, Mueller C, Zabel M, *et al.* Oxidative stress in blood in Alzheimer's disease and mild cognitive impairment: A meta-analysis. Neurobiol Dis 2013; 59: 100-10.
[http://dx.doi.org/10.1016/j.nbd.2013.07.005] [PMID: 23867235]

[41] Aybek H, Ercan F, Aslan D, Şahiner T. Determination of malondialdehyde, reduced glutathione levels and APOE4 allele frequency in late-onset Alzheimer's disease in Denizli, Turkey. Clin Biochem 2007; 40(3-4): 172-6.
[http://dx.doi.org/10.1016/j.clinbiochem.2006.09.005] [PMID: 17069783]

[42] Cristalli DO, Arnal N, Marra FA, de Alaniz MJT, Marra CA. Peripheral markers in neurodegenerative patients and their first-degree relatives. J Neurol Sci 2012; 314(1-2): 48-56.
[http://dx.doi.org/10.1016/j.jns.2011.11.001] [PMID: 22113180]

[43] Bermejo P, Gómez-Serranillos P, Santos J, Pastor E, Gil P, Martín-Aragón S. Determination of malonaldehyde in Alzheimer's disease: a comparative study of high-performance liquid chromatography and thiobarbituric acid test. Gerontology 1997; 43(4): 218-22.
[http://dx.doi.org/10.1159/000213853] [PMID: 9222750]

[44] Ceballos-Picot I, Merad-Boudia M, Nicole A, *et al.* Peripheral antioxidant enzyme activities and selenium in elderly subjects and in dementia of Alzheimer's type—Place of the extracellular glutathione peroxidase. Free Radic Biol Med 1996; 20(4): 579-87.
[http://dx.doi.org/10.1016/0891-5849(95)02058-6] [PMID: 8904299]

[45] Gironi M, Bianchi A, Russo A, *et al.* Oxidative imbalance in different neurodegenerative diseases with memory impairment. Neurodegener Dis 2011; 8(3): 129-37.
[http://dx.doi.org/10.1159/000319452] [PMID: 20838029]

[46] McGrath LT, McGleenon BM, Brennan S, McColl D, McILroy S, Passmore AP. Increased oxidative stress in Alzheimer's disease as assessed with 4-hydroxynonenal but not malondialdehyde. QJM 2001; 94(9): 485-90.
[http://dx.doi.org/10.1093/qjmed/94.9.485] [PMID: 11528012]

[47] Ozcankaya R, Delibas N. Malondialdehyde, superoxide dismutase, melatonin, iron, copper, and zinc blood concentrations in patients with Alzheimer disease: cross-sectional study. Croat Med J 2002; 43(1): 28-32.
[PMID: 11828555]

[48] Aksenov MY, Aksenova MV, Butterfield DA, Geddes JW, Markesbery WR. Protein oxidation in the brain in Alzheimer's disease. Neuroscience 2001; 103(2): 373-83.
[http://dx.doi.org/10.1016/S0306-4522(00)00580-7] [PMID: 11246152]

[49] Castegna A, Thongboonkerd V, Klein JB, Lynn B, Markesbery WR, Butterfield DA. Proteomic identification of nitrated proteins in Alzheimer's disease brain. J Neurochem 2003; 85(6): 1394-401.
[http://dx.doi.org/10.1046/j.1471-4159.2003.01786.x] [PMID: 12787059]

[50] Conrad CC, Marshall PL, Talent JM, Malakowsky CA, Choi J, Gracy RW. Oxidized proteins in Alzheimer's plasma. Biochem Biophys Res Commun 2000; 275(2): 678-81.
[http://dx.doi.org/10.1006/bbrc.2000.3356] [PMID: 10964722]

[51] Aldred S, Bennett S, Mecocci P. Increased low-density lipoprotein oxidation, but not total plasma protein oxidation, in Alzheimer's disease. Clin Biochem 2010; 43(3): 267-71. [http://dx.doi.org/10.1016/j.clinbiochem.2009.08.021] [PMID: 19733555]

[52] Cai Z you, Yan Y, Yan L, *et al.* Serum level of MMP-2, MMP-9 and Ox-LDL in Alzheimer's disease with hyperlipoidemia. J Med Coll PLA. 2007 Dec; 22(6): 352–6.

[53] Puertas MC, Martínez-Martos JM, Cobo MP, Carrera MP, Mayas MD, Ramírez-Expósito MJ. Plasma oxidative stress parameters in men and women with early stage Alzheimer type dementia. Exp Gerontol 2012; 47(8): 625-30. [http://dx.doi.org/10.1016/j.exger.2012.05.019] [PMID: 22664577]

[54] Sultana R, Poon HF, Cai J, *et al.* Identification of nitrated proteins in Alzheimer's disease brain using a redox proteomics approach. Neurobiol Dis 2006; 22(1): 76-87. [http://dx.doi.org/10.1016/j.nbd.2005.10.004] [PMID: 16378731]

[55] Castegna A, Aksenov M, Aksenova M, *et al.* Proteomic identification of oxidatively modified proteins in alzheimer's disease brain. part I: creatine kinase BB, glutamine synthase, and ubiquitin carboxy-terminal hydrolase L-1. Free Radic Biol Med 2002; 33(4): 562-71. [http://dx.doi.org/10.1016/S0891-5849(02)00914-0] [PMID: 12160938]

[56] Korolainen MA, Pirttilä T. Cerebrospinal fluid, serum and plasma protein oxidation in Alzheimer's disease. Acta Neurol Scand 2009; 119(1): 32-8. [http://dx.doi.org/10.1111/j.1600-0404.2008.01057.x] [PMID: 18547271]

[57] Choi J, Malakowsky CA, Talent JM, Conrad CC, Gracy RW. Identification of oxidized plasma proteins in Alzheimer's disease. Biochem Biophys Res Commun 2002; 293(5): 1566-70. [http://dx.doi.org/10.1016/S0006-291X(02)00420-5] [PMID: 12054695]

[58] Korolainen MA, Nyman TA, Nyyssönen P, Hartikainen ES, Pirttilä T. Multiplexed proteomic analysis of oxidation and concentrations of cerebrospinal fluid proteins in Alzheimer disease. Clin Chem 2007; 53(4): 657-65. [http://dx.doi.org/10.1373/clinchem.2006.078014] [PMID: 17289803]

[59] Polidori MC, Stahl W, Eichler O, Niestroj I, Sies H. Profiles of antioxidants in human plasma. Free Radic Biol Med 2001; 30(5): 456-62. [http://dx.doi.org/10.1016/S0891-5849(00)00345-2] [PMID: 11182517]

[60] Carantoni M, Zuliani G, Munari MR, D'Elia K, Palmieri E, Fellin R. Alzheimer disease and vascular dementia: relationships with fasting glucose and insulin levels. Dement Geriatr Cogn Disord 2000; 11(3): 176-80. [http://dx.doi.org/10.1159/000017232] [PMID: 10765049]

[61] Kim TS, Pae CU, Yoon SJ, *et al.* Decreased plasma antioxidants in patients with Alzheimer's disease. Int J Geriatr Psychiatry 2006; 21(4): 344-8. [http://dx.doi.org/10.1002/gps.1469] [PMID: 16534775]

[62] Maesaka JK, Wolf-Klein G, Piccione JM, Ma CM. Hypouricemia, abnormal renal tubular urate transport, and plasma natriuretic factor(s) in patients with Alzheimer's disease. J Am Geriatr Soc 1993; 41(5): 501-6. [http://dx.doi.org/10.1111/j.1532-5415.1993.tb01885.x] [PMID: 8486882]

[63] Rinaldi P, Polidori MC, Metastasio A, *et al.* Plasma antioxidants are similarly depleted in mild cognitive impairment and in Alzheimer's disease. Neurobiol Aging 2003; 24(7): 915-9. [http://dx.doi.org/10.1016/S0197-4580(03)00031-9] [PMID: 12928050]

[64] Jiménez-Jiménez FJ, de Bustos F, Molina JA, *et al.* Cerebrospinal fluid levels of alpha-tocopherol (vitamin E) in Alzheimer's disease. J Neural Transm (Vienna) 1997; 104(6-7): 703-10. [http://dx.doi.org/10.1007/BF01291887] [PMID: 9444569]

[65] Rivière S, Birlouez-Aragon I, Nourhashémi F, Vellas B. Low plasma vitamin C in Alzheimer patients despite an adequate diet. Int J Geriatr Psychiatry 1998; 13(11): 749-54.

[http://dx.doi.org/10.1002/(SICI)1099-1166(199810)13:11<749::AID-GPS860>3.0.CO;2-T] [PMID: 9850871]

[66] Iuliano L, Monticolo R, Straface G, *et al.* Vitamin E and enzymatic/oxidative stress-driven oxysterols in amnestic mild cognitive impairment subtypes and Alzheimer's disease. J Alzheimers Dis 2010; 21(4): 1383-92.
[http://dx.doi.org/10.3233/JAD-2010-100780] [PMID: 21504117]

[67] Schippling S, Kontush A, Arlt S, *et al.* Increased lipoprotein oxidation in alzheimer's disease. Free Radic Biol Med 2000; 28(3): 351-60.
[http://dx.doi.org/10.1016/S0891-5849(99)00247-6] [PMID: 10699746]

[68] Glasø M, Nordbø G, Diep L, Bøhmer T. Reduced concentrations of several vitamins in normal weight patients with late-onset dementia of the Alzheimer type without vascular disease. J Nutr Health Aging 2004; 8(5): 407-13.
[PMID: 15359361]

[69] Sinclair AJ, Bayer AJ, Johnston J, Warner C, Maxwell SRJ. Altered plasma antioxidant status in subjects with Alzheimer's disease and vascular dementia. Int J Geriatr Psychiatry 1998; 13(12): 840-5.
[http://dx.doi.org/10.1002/(SICI)1099-1166(199812)13:12<840::AID-GPS877>3.0.CO;2-R] [PMID: 9884908]

[70] Foy CJ, Passmore AP, Vahidassr MD, Young IS, Lawson JT. Plasma chain-breaking antioxidants in Alzheimer's disease, vascular dementia and Parkinson's disease. QJM 1999; 92(1): 39-45.
[http://dx.doi.org/10.1093/qjmed/92.1.39] [PMID: 10209671]

[71] von Arnim CAF, Herbolsheimer F, Nikolaus T, *et al.* Dietary antioxidants and dementia in a population-based case-control study among older people in South Germany. J Alzheimers Dis 2012; 31(4): 717-24.
[http://dx.doi.org/10.3233/JAD-2012-120634] [PMID: 22710913]

[72] Mecocci P, Polidori MC, Cherubini A, *et al.* Lymphocyte oxidative DNA damage and plasma antioxidants in Alzheimer disease. Arch Neurol 2002; 59(5): 794-8.
[http://dx.doi.org/10.1001/archneur.59.5.794] [PMID: 12020262]

[73] Wiener HW, Perry RT, Chen Z, Harrell LE, Go RCP. A polymorphism in *SOD2* is associated with development of Alzheimer's disease. Genes Brain Behav 2007; 6(8): 770-6.
[http://dx.doi.org/10.1111/j.1601-183X.2007.00308.x] [PMID: 17376152]

[74] Qu XX, He JH, Cui ZQ, Yang T, Sun XH. PPAR-α agonist GW7647 protects against oxidative stress and iron deposit *via* GPx4 in a transgenic mouse model of alzheimer's diseases. ACS Chem Neurosci 2022; 13(2): 207-16.
[http://dx.doi.org/10.1021/acschemneuro.1c00516] [PMID: 34965724]

[75] Massaad CA, Pautler RG, Klann E. Mitochondrial superoxide: a key player in Alzheimer's disease. Aging (Albany NY) 2009; 1(9): 758-61.
[http://dx.doi.org/10.18632/aging.100088] [PMID: 20157564]

[76] Butterfield DA, Mattson MP. Apolipoprotein E and oxidative stress in brain with relevance to Alzheimer's disease. Neurobiol Dis 2020; 138: 104795.
[http://dx.doi.org/10.1016/j.nbd.2020.104795] [PMID: 32036033]

[77] Faraji P, Kühn H, Ahmadian S. Multiple roles of apolipoprotein E4 in oxidative lipid metabolism and ferroptosis during the pathogenesis of alzheimer's disease. J Mol Neurosci 2024; 74(3): 62.
[http://dx.doi.org/10.1007/s12031-024-02224-4] [PMID: 38958788]

[78] Huang YWA, Zhou B, Nabet AM, Wernig M, Südhof TC. Differential signaling mediated by ApoE2, ApoE3, and ApoE4 in human neurons parallels alzheimer's disease risk. J Neurosci 2019; 39(37): 7408-27.
[http://dx.doi.org/10.1523/JNEUROSCI.2994-18.2019] [PMID: 31331998]

[79] Scarmeas N, Luchsinger JA, Mayeux R, Stern Y. Mediterranean diet and Alzheimer disease mortality.

Neurology 2007; 69(11): 1084-93.
[http://dx.doi.org/10.1212/01.wnl.0000277320.50685.7c] [PMID: 17846408]

[80] Calderón-Garcidueñas L, González-Maciel A, Kulesza RJ, *et al.* Air pollution, combustion and friction derived nanoparticles, and alzheimer's disease in urban children and young adults. J Alzheimers Dis 2019; 70(2): 343-60.
[http://dx.doi.org/10.3233/JAD-190331] [PMID: 31256139]

[81] Pizzino G, Irrera N, Cucinotta M, *et al.* Oxidative stress: Harms and benefits for human health. Oxid Med Cell Longev 2017; 2017(1): 8416763.
[http://dx.doi.org/10.1155/2017/8416763] [PMID: 28819546]

[82] You R, Ho YS, Chang RCC. The pathogenic effects of particulate matter on neurodegeneration: A review. J Biomed Sci 2022; 29(1): 15.
[http://dx.doi.org/10.1186/s12929-022-00799-x] [PMID: 35189880]

[83] Fernandes MA, Proenca MT, Nogueira AJ, *et al.* Influence of apolipoprotein E genotype on blood redox status of Alzheimer's disease patients 1999.http://www.spandidos-publications.com/10.3892/ijmm.4.2.179
[http://dx.doi.org/10.3892/ijmm.4.2.179]

[84] Tenório MCS, Graciliano NG, Moura FA, Oliveira ACM, Goulart MOF. N-acetylcysteine (NAC): Impacts on human health. Antioxidants 2021; 10(6): 967.
[http://dx.doi.org/10.3390/antiox10060967]

[85] Sacks B, Onal H, Martorana R, *et al.* Mitochondrial targeted antioxidants, mitoquinone and SKQ1, not vitamin C, mitigate doxorubicin-induced damage in H9c2 myoblast: pretreatment *vs.* co-treatment. BMC Pharmacol Toxicol 2021; 22(1): 49.
[http://dx.doi.org/10.1186/s40360-021-00518-6] [PMID: 34530934]

[86] Wang GH, Jiang ZL, Li YC, *et al.* Free-radical scavenger edaravone treatment confers neuroprotection against traumatic brain injury in rats. J Neurotrauma 2011; 28(10): 2123-34.
[http://dx.doi.org/10.1089/neu.2011.1939] [PMID: 21732763]

[87] Zhang F, Li X, Wei Y. Selenium and selenoproteins in health. Biomolecules 2023; 13(5): 799.
[http://dx.doi.org/10.3390/biom13050799] [PMID: 37238669]

[88] Fock EM, Parnova RG. Protective effect of mitochondria-targeted antioxidants against inflammatory response to lipopolysaccharide challenge: A review. Pharmaceutics 2021; 13(2): 144.
[http://dx.doi.org/10.3390/pharmaceutics13020144] [PMID: 33499252]

[89] Zahra M, Abrahamse H, George BP. Flavonoids: Antioxidant powerhouses and their role in nanomedicine. Antioxidants 2024; 13(8): 922.
[http://dx.doi.org/10.3390/antiox13080922] [PMID: 39199168]

[90] Farina N, Isaac MGEKN, Clark AR, Rusted J, Tabet N. Vitamin E for Alzheimer's dementia and mild cognitive impairment 2012.https://doi.wiley.com/10.1002/14651858.CD002854.pub3
[http://dx.doi.org/10.1002/14651858.CD002854.pub3]

[91] Dysken MW, Sano M, Asthana S, *et al.* Effect of vitamin E and memantine on functional decline in Alzheimer disease: the TEAM-AD VA cooperative randomized trial. JAMA 2014; 311(1): 33-44.
[http://dx.doi.org/10.1001/jama.2013.282834] [PMID: 24381967]

[92] Tippairote T, Bjørklund G, Gasmi A, *et al.* Combined supplementation of coenzyme Q_{10} and other nutrients in specific medical conditions. Nutrients 2022; 14(20): 4383.
[http://dx.doi.org/10.3390/nu14204383] [PMID: 36297067]

[93] Salehi B, Calina D, Docea A, *et al.* Curcumin's nanomedicine formulations for therapeutic application in neurological diseases. J Clin Med 2020; 9(2): 430.
[http://dx.doi.org/10.3390/jcm9020430] [PMID: 32033365]

[94] Ponnampalam EN, Kiani A, Santhiravel S, Holman BWB, Lauridsen C, Dunshea FR. The importance of dietary antioxidants on oxidative stress, meat and milk production, and their preservative aspects in

farm animals: antioxidant action, animal health, and product quality—invited review. Animals (Basel) 2022; 12(23): 3279.
[http://dx.doi.org/10.3390/ani12233279] [PMID: 36496798]

[95] Andrés CMC, Pérez de la Lastra JM, Juan CA, Plou FJ, Pérez-Lebeña E. Antioxidant metabolism pathways in vitamins, polyphenols, and selenium: Parallels and divergences. Int J Mol Sci 2024; 25(5): 2600.
[http://dx.doi.org/10.3390/ijms25052600] [PMID: 38473850]

[96] Zhan CD, Sindhu RK, Pang J, Ehdaie A, Vaziri ND. Superoxide dismutase, catalase and glutathione peroxidase in the spontaneously hypertensive rat kidney. J Hypertens 2004; 22(10): 2025-33.
[http://dx.doi.org/10.1097/00004872-200410000-00027] [PMID: 15361776]

[97] Barman Balfour JA, Foster RH. Deferiprone. Drugs 1999; 58(3): 553-78.
[http://dx.doi.org/10.2165/00003495-199958030-00021] [PMID: 10493280]

[98] Faux NG, Ritchie CW, Gunn A, *et al.* PBT2 rapidly improves cognition in Alzheimer's Disease: additional phase II analyses. J Alzheimers Dis 2010; 20(2): 509-16.
[http://dx.doi.org/10.3233/JAD-2010-1390] [PMID: 20164561]

[99] Drummond E, Wisniewski T. Alzheimer's disease: experimental models and reality. Acta Neuropathol 2017; 133(2): 155-75.
[http://dx.doi.org/10.1007/s00401-016-1662-x] [PMID: 28025715]

[100] Su H, Wang Z, Zhou L, Liu D, Zhang N. Regulation of the Nrf2/HO-1 axis by mesenchymal stem cells-derived extracellular vesicles: implications for disease treatment. Front Cell Dev Biol 2024; 12: 1397954.
[http://dx.doi.org/10.3389/fcell.2024.1397954] [PMID: 38915448]

[101] Gordon J, Lockard G, Monsour M, Alayli A, Borlongan CV. The role of concomitant Nrf2 targeting and stem cell therapy in cerebrovascular disease. Antioxidants 2022; 11(8): 1447.
[http://dx.doi.org/10.3390/antiox11081447] [PMID: 35892653]

[102] Iwatsubo T, Irizarry MC, Lewcock JW, Carrillo MC. Alzheimer's Targeted Treatments: Focus on Amyloid and Inflammation. J Neurosci 2023; 43(47): 7894-8.
[http://dx.doi.org/10.1523/JNEUROSCI.1576-23.2023] [PMID: 37968119]

[103] Steinhubl SR. Why have antioxidants failed in clinical trials? Am J Cardiol 2008; 101(10): S14-9.
[http://dx.doi.org/10.1016/j.amjcard.2008.02.003] [PMID: 18474268]

[104] Iqbal I, Saqib F, Mubarak Z, *et al.* Alzheimer's disease and drug delivery across the blood–brain barrier: approaches and challenges. Eur J Med Res 2024; 29(1): 313.
[http://dx.doi.org/10.1186/s40001-024-01915-3] [PMID: 38849950]

[105] Antoniades C, Tousoulis D, Tentolouris C, Toutouzas P, Stefanadis C. Oxidative stress, antioxidant vitamins, and atherosclerosis. From basic research to clinical practice. Herz 2003; 28(7): 628-38.
[http://dx.doi.org/10.1007/s00059-003-2417-8] [PMID: 14689123]

[106] Forman HJ, Zhang H. Targeting oxidative stress in disease: promise and limitations of antioxidant therapy. Nat Rev Drug Discov 2021; 20(9): 689-709.
[http://dx.doi.org/10.1038/s41573-021-00233-1] [PMID: 34194012]

[107] Ohsawa I, Ishikawa M, Takahashi K, *et al.* Hydrogen acts as a therapeutic antioxidant by selectively reducing cytotoxic oxygen radicals. Nat Med 2007; 13(6): 688-94.
[http://dx.doi.org/10.1038/nm1577] [PMID: 17486089]

[108] Ichihara M, Sobue S, Ito M, Ito M, Hirayama M, Ohno K. Beneficial biological effects and the underlying mechanisms of molecular hydrogen - comprehensive review of 321 original articles -. Med Gas Res 2015; 5(1): 12.
[http://dx.doi.org/10.1186/s13618-015-0035-1] [PMID: 26483953]

[109] López-Espinosa J, Park P, Holcomb M, Godin B, Villapol S. Nanotechnology-driven therapies for neurodegenerative diseases: a comprehensive review. Ther Deliv 2024; 15(12): 997-1024.

[http://dx.doi.org/10.1080/20415990.2024.2401307] [PMID: 39297726]

[110] Zamora PL, Villamena FA. Pharmacological approaches to the treatment of oxidative stress-induced cardiovascular dysfunctions. Future Med Chem 2013; 5(4): 465-78. [http://dx.doi.org/10.4155/fmc.13.15] [PMID: 23495692]

[111] Heneka MT, Carson MJ, Khoury JE, *et al.* Neuroinflammation in Alzheimer's disease. Lancet Neurol 2015; 14(4): 388-405. [http://dx.doi.org/10.1016/S1474-4422(15)70016-5] [PMID: 25792098]

[112] Mecocci P, Tinarelli C, Schulz RJ, Polidori MC. Nutraceuticals in cognitive impairment and Alzheimer's disease. Front Pharmacol. 2014; 5: 147. [http://dx.doi.org/10.3389/fphar.2014.00147]

[113] Butterfield DA, Swomley AM, Sultana R. Amyloid *β*-peptide (1-42)-induced oxidative stress in Alzheimer disease: importance in disease pathogenesis and progression. Antioxid Redox Signal 2013; 19(8): 823-35. [http://dx.doi.org/10.1089/ars.2012.5027] [PMID: 23249141]

[114] Barberger-Gateau P, Lambert JC, Féart C, *et al.* From genetics to dietetics: The contribution of epidemiology to understanding Alzheimer's disease. J Alzheimers Dis. 2013; 33(Suppl 1): S457-S463. [http://dx.doi.org/10.3233/JAD-2012-129019]

[115] Di Domenico F, Tramutola A, Butterfield DA. Role of 4-hydroxy-2-nonenal (HNE) in the pathogenesis of alzheimer disease and other selected age-related neurodegenerative disorders. Free Radic Biol Med 2017; 111: 253-61. [http://dx.doi.org/10.1016/j.freeradbiomed.2016.10.490] [PMID: 27789292]

[116] Kivipelto M, Mangialasche F, Ngandu T. Lifestyle interventions to prevent cognitive impairment, dementia and Alzheimer disease. Nat Rev Neurol 2018; 14(11): 653-66. [http://dx.doi.org/10.1038/s41582-018-0070-3] [PMID: 30291317]

[117] Sagar R, Pathak P, Pandur B, Kim SJ, Li J, Mahairaki V. Biomarkers and precision medicine in Alzheimer's disease. In: Vlamos P, editor. GeNeDis 2020. Adv Exp Med Biol. 2021; 1339: 403-408. [http://dx.doi.org/10.1007/978-3-030-78787-5_50]

CHAPTER 6

The Role of MicroRNAs in the Onset and Progression of Alzheimer's Disease: An Explicative Overview

Sinjini Sarkar[1,*]

[1] *Department of Pharmaceutical Technology, Shobhaben Pratapbhai Patel School of Pharmacy and Technology Management, SVKM's Narsee Monjee Institute of Management Studies, Mumbai, Maharashtra, India*

Abstract: MicroRNAs (miRs) are a class of small non-coding RNAs that harness immense potential in influencing disease pathogenesis by regulating gene expression. Given their abundance in the biological fluids, their ease of detection and quantification, miRs are being extensively studied as diagnostic biomarkers and therapeutic targets in various diseases. It is reported thatmiRs have significant roles in neuroinflammation, amyloid-β accumulation and metabolism, tau protein phosphorylation, and neuronal plasticity, which cumulatively precipitate Alzheimer's disease (AD). This chapter briefly describes the epigenetic landscape of AD, followed by the biogenesis of miRs and their major functionality in gene silencing. Furthermore, it elaborates the roles of different miRs identified in AD pathology, for developing early diagnostic markers and identifying druggable targets. Recent advances in miRNA-based therapeutics, including the use of miRNA mimics, inhibitors, and nanoparticle-mediated delivery systems, offer new possibilities for intervention. The chapter concludes by highlighting the challenges, such as targeted delivery, stability, and immunogenicity, along with the aspects for miRNA-guided drug development to transform AD treatment strategies.

Keywords: Alzheimer's disease, Biomarkers, RNA-binding proteins, Gene silencing, Gene expression, MicroRNAs.

INTRODUCTION

Alzheimer's disease (AD) is a morbid condition characterized by progressive neuronal degeneration usually in the entorhinal cortex and hippocampus. It leads to dementia and cognitive decline. The incidence of AD increased more than 145% in the United States between 2000 and 2021, making it the 7th leading

* **Corresponding author Sinjini Sarkar:** Department of Pharmaceutical Technology, Shobhaben Pratapbhai Patel School of Pharmacy and Technology Management, SVKM's Narsee Monjee Institute of Management Studies, Mumbai, Maharashtra, India; E-mail: sinjini.sarkar@nmims.edu

Swarupananda Mukherjee, Souvik Roy & Dipanjan Karati (Eds.)

cause of death in 2021 [1]. For decades, cholinesterase inhibitors like Galantamine, Memantine, Rivastigmine, and Donepezil have been the mainstays of AD treatment. In 2023, the FDA approved a humanized monoclonal antibody (mAb), Lecanemab, as an anti-amyloid treatment that binds to soluble Amyloid β (Aβ) protofibrils, inhibiting their transformation to insoluble plaques and reducing Aβ burden in the brain. This treatment is indicated for patients with mild AD and mild cognitive impairment caused by AD [2]. However, all these interventions have limited efficacy owing to molecular complexities at different stages of the disease and significant side effects. Thus, to date, there is no cure for AD. The most important pathological characteristic and therapeutic target of AD is the deposition of Aβ plaques, Tau protein, and neurofibrillary tangles (NFT). These plaques are formed due to the imbalance in expression or non-clearance of Aβ. BACE1 (β-site amyloid precursor protein (APP) cleaving enzyme 1) is required to cleave APP to produce monomeric Aβ [3]. Functionally, SCARA-1 to 5, namely scavenger receptor class A members, are involved in the uptake of soluble Aβ, and RAGE (receptor for advanced glycated end products) is responsible for pro-inflammatory signaling following Aβ binding and microglial activation [4, 5].

Along with genetic involvement, epigenetic changes are also investigated thoroughly in recent times, and alteration of gene expression patterns influences the key pathological events like neuroinflammation, oxidative stress, and neuronal plasticity. MicroRNAs (miRNAs/ miRs) are most investigated owing to their activity involving the regulation of multiple gene expressions. Their presence in almost all biological fluids makes them an ideal candidate for diagnostic, prognostic, and therapeutic biomarkers in several neurological diseases. MiRs are non-coding, small RNAs, typically around 22 nucleotides long. They primarily function to suppress gene expression by binding to the 3′ UTR (untranslated region) of target mRNAs (messenger RNAs), but they are also capable of interacting with other regions, *i.e.*, the 5′ UTR, coding sequences, and gene promoters. With multifaceted roles, such as neuroinflammation, Aβ processing and accumulation, tau phosphorylation and synaptic functions, miRNA plays a central role in AD pathogenesis. This chapter briefly describes the epigenetic landscape of AD while focusing on microRNAs. It aims to highlight major miRs with clinical utility in the development of early disease markers and targeted therapeutic strategies.

EPIGENETIC LANDSCAPE UNDERLYING AD

The epigenetic landscape of AD is complex, and key changes like histone modifications and non-coding RNAs are vital players in the development and progression of AD. Hypomethylation and hypermethylation of crucial genes involved in amyloid protein processing (APP and BACE) and neuronal plasticity are observed in AD pathology [6 - 8]. In chromatin, a nucleosome is formed by DNA wrapped around histone proteins. The posttranslational modifications of histone in the amino-terminal regulate their interactions with DNA, thereby influencing gene expression. The histone tails are susceptible to undergo acetylation, ubiquitylation, methylation, glycosylation, ADP-ribosylation, and SUMOylation [9]. Histone acetylation changes memory processes and synaptic plasticity. Hyperacetylation and hypoacetylation of the cerebellum and hippocampus in AD patients were reported [10]. However, the use of HDAC (Histone Deacetylase) inhibitors was not as successful due to notable side effects and non-selective pharmacological effects [11]. On the other hand, histone methyltransferases were considerably more site-specific than acetyltransferases. This makes it more important to identify methylation on specific site and their relevance to pathology. For example, methylation of H2B K108 and H4 R55 and ubiquitination of H2B K120 were reported in the frontal cortexes of patients, which bear significance in the pathology of the disease. However, they are yet to be therapeutically targeted [12].

Tau aggregation, neurodegeneration, and reduction in autophagy that contribute to the AD neuropathology can be attributed to methylation of genes and alteration of histone methylations [13, 14]. In addition, phosphorylation of histone H3 was found to increase in the frontal cortex, and phosphorylation of Ser 47 of histone H4 (H4S47p) was a disease-specific modification, and shares a positive correlation with disease progression [6]. The ubiquitination of K120 on H2B increased by 91% in the frontal cortex of AD cases, as reported by Anderson and Turko. Dysregulated expressions of long non-coding RNA (lncRNA) have been observed post-transcriptomic analysis of brain tissues from animals and AD patients. X inactive specific transcript (XIST) is a widely investigated lncRNA that is correlated with pathological Aβ-mediated neuroinflammation and BACE expression [15, 16]. The ATP-dependent chromatin remodeling complexes are found to be dysregulated, as well as histone-modifying enzymes, leading to abnormal transcription of genes involved in AD pathology. Given that the loss of DEK (Drosophila, Erythrocyte protein band 4.1, and Kidney) protein induces brain aging-related phenotypes such as DNA damage and apoptosis [17].

BIOGENESIS OF MIRNAS

MiRNA Biogenesis: The Canonical Pathway

Predominantly, the canonical biogenesis pathway is utilized for miRNA biosynthesis (Fig. **1**). The pathway involves processing of the pri-miRNA, transcribed from their respective genes within the nucleus, into pre-miRNAs by a microprocessor complex. This microprocessor complex comprises DGCR8

(DiGeorge Syndrome Critical Region 8), an RNA-binding protein, and Drosha, a ribonuclease III enzyme. The DGCR8 recognizes a few motifs and an N6-methyladenylated GGAC sequence within the pri-miRNA, and Drosha cleaves the pri-miRNA base at the characteristic hairpin structure, resulting in the formation of a 2 nt 3′ overhang on the pre-miRNA [18 - 20]. An exportin 5 (XPO5)/RanGTP complex subsequently exports the produced pre-miRNAs to the cytoplasm, where they are further processed by the RNase III endonuclease Dicer. By removing the terminal loop, this step creates a mature miRNA duplex. The designation of the mature miRNA form depends on the strand's directionality. The 5p and 3p strands are derived from the 5′ and 3′ ends of the pre-miRNA hairpin, respectively. In an ATP-dependent mechanism, both strands of the mature miRNA duplex are integrated into the Argonaute (AGO) family of proteins (AGO1-4 in humans). Depending on the type and environment of the cell, near equal proportions or either of the 5p and 3p strands are loaded into the AGO. The thermodynamic stability of the 5′ ends of the miRNA duplex or a 5′ U at nucleotide position 1, plays a crucial part as well, while loading in AGO, and lower 5′ stability or 5′ uracil is generally preferred. The guide strand is the one loaded into AGO, and the unloaded strand is the passenger strand, deemed to be unwound from the guide on the degree of complementarity through various mechanisms. AGO cleaves the passenger strand with no mismatches, which is then degraded by cellular mechanisms [21 - 23].

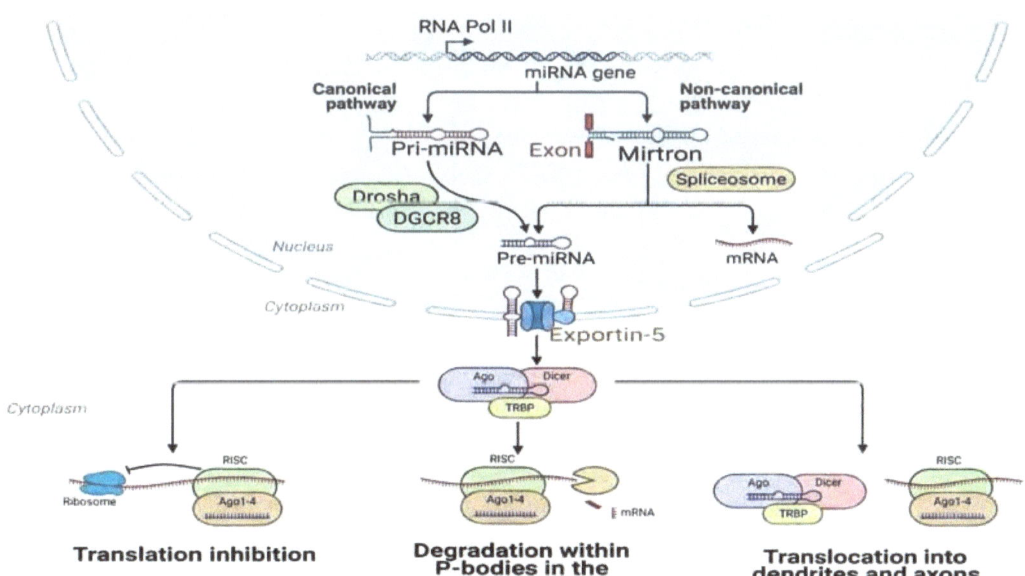

Fig. (1). MiRNA biogenesis.

MiRNA Biogenesis: Non-canonical

Many non-canonical miRNA biogenesis pathways were discovered, which use different key proteins in combinations from the canonical pathway, such as Drosha, Dicer, exportin 5, and AGO2. They are typically divided into two categories of pathways: Drosha/DGCR8-independent and Dicer-independent (Fig. 1). The Drosha/DGCR8-independent pathways produce pre-miRNAs resembling substrates of Dicer. Examples include *Mirtrons* that are generated from mRNA introns at the time of splicing, and 7-methylguanosine (m7G)-capped pre-miRNAs, which bypasses cleaving by Drosha and are exported by exportin 1 directly to the cytoplasm. Mirtrons can also be cleaved by Spliceosome (a ribonucleoprotein complex) during pre-mRNA processing. The m7G cap often causes a bias toward 3p strand incorporation into Argonaute [24 - 26]. Dicer-independent miRs are formed from endogenous short hairpin RNAs (shRNAs) processed by Drosha. These pre-miRNAs are too short for the enzyme Dicer to process, so they rely on AGO2 for their maturation. The full pre-miRNA is loaded into AGO2, where the 3p strand is sliced, and the 5p strand is subsequently trimmed to finalize the maturation process [27].

BIOLOGICAL FUNCTIONS OF MIRNAS

As reported by several studies, miRNAs target a specific sequence of 3'UTR to bind and induce mRNA deadenylation, decapping, and translational repression. MiRs can bind to the 5′ UTR and coding sequencesas well, within promoter regions, which can have silencing effects on a specific gene. In addition, miRNA interaction with the promoter region can also induce transcription, but such mechanisms are not fully elucidated. Under specific conditions, like during amino acid starvation and cell cycle arrest, miRNAs may upregulate gene expression by the activation of translation through AGO2 and Fragile-x-mental retardation related protein 1 (FXR1) [28 - 31].

Gene Silencing

The miRISCor minimal miRNA-induced silencing complex is composed of a guide strand and an AGO.TAR RNA-binding protein (TRBP) plays a vital role in the assembly and function of the RISC during the miRNA and RNA interference (RNAi) pathways. Specifically, TRBP facilitates the loading of miRNA duplexes onto Argonaute (AGO) proteins, a critical step in the formation of the active RISC. The complementary sequences within the target messenger RNAs are called the miRNA response elements (MREs), which interact with MiRISC. The extent of complementarity between MRE and a MiRNA determines the outcome of Argonaute 2 (AGO2) activity on the target mRNA. Full complementarity of the miRNA: MRE pairing activates AGO2's endonuclease function, leading to the cleavage of the target mRNA, whereas partial complementarity leads to translational repression and mRNA degradation through miRISC mechanisms. Interestingly, a fully complementary interaction can also weaken the binding between AGO and the3′ end of the miR, making the latter more susceptible to degradation. In animal cells, most MiRNA interactions are only partially complementary, with MREs typically having central mismatches, which prevents AGO2's endonuclease activity. RNA interference by AGO2 is mediated primarily in a manner identical to the non-endonucleolytic AGO family of proteins (AGO1, AGO3, and AGO4 in humans). Functional miRNA interactions are often established through the 5′ seed region (nucleotides 2–8), though additional pairing at the 3′ end enhances both the stability and specificity of these interactions [32 - 36].

The GW182 protein family (including TNRC6A, with glycine-tryptophan (GW) repeats) is recruited to form the silencing miRISC complex. GW182 acts as a scaffold to bring in other effector proteins or complexes likePAN2-PAN3 (poly(A)-deadenylase complexes) and CCR4-NOT, enabling the miRNA to bind with the target mRNA. The mRNA's poly(A) tail removal process is started by PAN2-PAN3 and completed by the CCR4-NOT complex. To enhance this process, GW182's tryptophan repeats interact with poly(A)-binding protein C (PABPC). Then the decapping takes place with the aid of decapping protein 2 (DCP2) and related proteins, which causes exoribonuclease 1 (XRN1) to degrade 5′-to-3′.

MiRNA machinery is present throughout the cytoplasm. MiRISC also associates with polysomes, which enhances translational inhibition and mRNA degradation. On the endoplasmic reticulum (ER), miRISC facilitates miRNA-mediated repression, with mRNA degradation continuing in endosomes and multivesicular bodies (MVBs) before miRISC is recycled. MiRISC dynamically samples target mRNAs based on their MREs, allowing for rapid regulatory responses in the cell. The presence of multiple MREs on a single mRNA can enhance miRNA activity through cooperative binding. This synergy allows for increased RNAi activity, particularly when miRNAs bind to adjacent MREs on a target mRNA, which increases the retention of the miRISC on the mRNA. Maintaining an equilibrium between unbound and bound states of miRISC is critical for efficient mRNA regulation.

MiRNA cooperation is essential for biological processes like neurogenesis and stem cell differentiation, where combined miRNA effects enhance regulation. When more MREs are present (*e.g.*, from gene upregulation), miRNAs spread across targets, lowering their availability for other mRNAs. Competing endogenous RNAs (ceRNAs), like circular RNAs (circRNAs), can influence this balance by binding miRNAs and reducing their repression of target mRNAs. Additionally, miRNA activity depends on their subcellular localization, as seen in neurons where miRNAs act mainly at synapses [36].

Translational, Transcriptional, and Post-transcriptional regulation

In serum-starved and quiescent cells, like oocytes, and during cell cycle arrest, Fragile-X-mental retardation-related protein 1 (FXR1) and AGO2, which are part of the miRNA-protein complex (microRNPs), activate translation and enhance gene expression. This translation activation relies on AGO2 and FXR1, rather than GW182. In proliferating cells, they inhibit translation [37 - 40].

Nuclear miRISC associates with euchromatin at active gene sites, and affects both the transcription and post-transcriptional regulation of mRNA. Human AGO2 binds to TNRC6A and travels to the cytoplasm from the nucleus *via* Exportin-1 or Importin-8 [41 - 43].

Secretion and Uptake of MicroRNAs

Extracellular miRs, once thought to be by-products of cellular processes, are now recognized as regulated molecules with significant roles in intercellular communication. Studies have shown that exosomalmiR secretion occurs through pathways like ceramide-dependent mechanisms and can influence cell growth in target cells. For example, miR-126-3p is released from endothelial cells under shear stress and regulates smooth muscle cell activity, while in neuroendocrine cells, miRNAs are released *via* exocytosis in a calcium-dependent process. Additionally, extracellular miRNAs can be secreted in response to signaling molecules such as docosahexaenoic acid (DHA) and interleukin-4 (IL-4), influencing cancer invasiveness and angiogenesis, respectively. Extracellular miR-105 from metastatic breast cancer cells promotes metastasis by disrupting endothelial barriers, and miR-21-3p from umbilical cord blood exosomes enhances wound healing [44 - 49]. MiRs also bind to TLRs (Toll-like receptors), triggering pathways involved in tumor growth, metastasis, and even neurodegeneration [50 - 53].

The mechanisms underlying extracellular MiRNA uptake by recipient cells are yet to be entirely understood. Studies suggest that vesicle-associated miRs enter cells through endocytosis, micropinocytosis, or direct membrane fusion, while vesicle-free miRNAs may interact with specific receptors like HDL receptor and SR-BI [54, 55]. Different cell types appear to use distinct pathways for miRNA uptake, and further research will be required to determine the factors driving the specificity of these interactions.

MicroRNAs in the Biological Fluids

Extracellular miRs are detected in CSF, plasma, serum, tears, saliva, colostrum, breast milk, bronchial lavage, peritoneal fluid, urine, and other biological fluids like seminal fluid and ovarian follicular fluid. Unlike cellular RNA, extracellular miRNAs are exceptionally stable, maintaining their integrity up to 4 days at room temperature and even under extreme environments such as boiling, multiple freeze-thaw cycles, and extreme pH levels. In biological fluids, extracellular miRNAs exist in two forms: one encapsulated within vesicles like apoptotic bodies, exosomes, and microvesicles, and others are associated with proteins, primarily AGO2 [36].

ROLE IN ALZHEIMER'S DISEASE

Apparently, miRs have gathered attention as newer therapeutic targets and diagnostic markers for neurodegeneration. MiRNA profiling in the brains reported significantly altered expressions in AD as compared to healthy controls. While the exact impact of these alterations on disease onset and progression remains unclear, evidence suggests that they are involved in driving certain pathological cascades.

MiRNAs and Aβ Processing

Multiple miRs regulate both APP and BACE1 expressions. For instance, miR-106a/520c, miR-20 family, miR-101, miR-153, and miR-16 were identified as negative regulators of APP expression. Additionally, miRNAs such as miR-29 family, miR-107, miR-298/328, and miR-195 have been found to regulate BACE1 expression. MiR-125b also regulates both APP and BACE1 expression, which implicates a potential role in Aβ production. However, conflicting results have been reported, suggesting either upregulation or downregulation of the said miR. The expression of miR-132/212, miR-98-5p, miR-34a, and miR–335–5p was significantly lower in the AD brain tissues when compared to healthy people, regulating various pathways involved in Aβ generation, processing, and clearance. Another study also identified a differentially expressed set of miRs in the blood, CSF, and AD brains of patients compared to healthy controls [55]. Notably, miR-342-3p expression was significantly elevated in the AD hippocampus, contributing to increased Aβ accumulation. Several other miRNAs, including miR-374b-5p, miR-433, miR-148a-3p, and miR-193a-3p, were downregulated in the serum of AD patients. Increasing the levels of these downregulated miRNAs reduced Aβ accumulation in AD cell models. Further research revealed that miR-193a-3p and miR-148a-3p played roles in resistance to AD by targeting JNK3 and ROCK1, respectively, while miR-433 alleviated Aβ-induced neuronal activity inhibition by targeting the JAK2/STAT3 signaling pathway [56 - 62].

MiRs in Diseased Brain as Diverse Regulators

MiRNAs respond to neuroinflammation, oxidative stress, and processes of protein aggregation, leading to alterations in neuronal connectivity and plasticity. Brain tissue analysis is challenging but provides valuable insights. Despite the invasive nature of obtaining brain tissue samples, studies have revealed altered miRNA expression in various regions of AD-affected brains. MiR-140, miR-155-5p, miR-142-5p, miR-455-5p, and miR-146-5p were upregulated, while the hippocampal expression of miR-143-3p was downregulated. MiRNA expression profiles vary depending on AD stage, brain region, and study design [63]. MiR-191-5p expression was found to be lower in the microglia and hippocampal tissues of APP/PS1 mice exposed to Aβ1-42 [64]. The implication of miR-455-5p in AD reports CPED1 as its target, affecting AMPA receptor expression and cognitive function. However, its role remains complex, as overexpression can have both beneficial and detrimental effects. SORL1, an AD risk gene that is involved in APP processing, is targeted by miR-1229. This is an example of a genetic association with non-coding RNA, which requires functional validation. MiR-132, consistently downregulated in AD, is associated with Tau and amyloid aggregation as it bimodally regulates both Tau phosphorylation and amyloidosis. MiR-203 is another example of a miRNA with multilayered roles in AD. It regulates synaptic/neuronal and microglial/inflammatory signals in mouse models of tautopathy. Meta-analysis studies have identified 10 commonly deregulated MiRNA signatures with neuroimmune functions. This report suggested that miRNAs are common downstream regulators of various molecular pathways in neurodegenerative disorders. MiR-191-5p is downregulated in AD and may regulate microglial function as it targets DAPK1 and can reduce Aβ production and neuronal cell death [65]. Another study suggests that miR-375-3p inhibits autophagy by promoting mTOR phosphorylation under normal conditions. However, in early Alzheimer's disease (AD), it promotes autophagy and enhances neural repair by suppressing presenilin 1. Additionally, co-treatment with microRNA-375-3p and Rapamycin synergistically boosted autophagy and microglial activation, helping in neuroprotection by clearing Aβ accumulation, nerve damage repair, improved cognition, and memory deficits in APP/PS1 transgenic mice [66].

Blood and CSF-based miRNA Biomarkers for AD

Studies identified altered expression profiles of miRs that could serve as diagnostic and monitoring biomarkers. Expression patterns vary across blood components, and only a few of the miRNAs, such as miR-107 and miR-125a-5p, show consistent expression in whole blood and plasma. MiR-107 is downregulated in AD, which may be involved in blood coagulation, while it also targets BACE1 [67, 68]. MiR-125a-5p regulates platelet function and blood clotting and is downregulated in acute myocardial infarction, and also plays a suggested potential role in AD pathogenesis [69, 70]. Let-7d-5p, miR-191-5p, miR-384, miR-24-3p, miR-342-3p, miR-30b-5p, and miR-342-5p showed decreased levels in both serum and plasma. A 12 miRNA signature has been proposed in blood that can distinguish between phosphorylated Tau protein concentrations of normal and AD patient cohorts [71]. This data is yet to be incorporated into the clinical pipeline. CognimiR, recently branded by DiamiR, is a diagnostic panel of 24 miRNAs in blood that are brain-enriched, have inflammatory associations, and are capable of distinguishing mild cognitive impairment (MCI) and asymptomatic AD patients from controls, with 90% accuracy. It is currently in Phase I of the clinical trial. Hummingbird Diagnostics developed another miRNA-based diagnostic test for AD, yet to undergo clinical validation [72].

Four miRNAs, let-7b, miR-146a, miR-125b, and miR-29a, were consistently reported to be deregulated in CSF of AD. However, there is variability in their expression patterns across studies. Let-7b levels in the CSF correlate with AD progression: high levels of let-7b were associated with more advanced stages of AD [73]. A three-MiRNA combination and three piwi-interacting RNAs (piRNAs) were isolated from exosomes within CSF, showing significant alterations in AD patients compared to controls. Incorporating this miRNA/piRNA signature alongside Aβ40/42 ratio values and CSF pTAU enhanced the classification accuracy from 83% to 98% for AD patients [74]. Other miRNAs, such as miR-146a and miR-29a, were also associated with AD. Their specific functions and mechanisms of action are still being investigated.

AD patients have higher levels of miR-206 in their nasal mucosa and elevated miR-200b-5p levels in their tear fluid compared to healthy individuals [75, 76]. If confirmed in larger populations, these findings could pave the way for novel, non-invasive methods for early diagnosis of AD and highlight the significance of miRNAs in biomarker-driven drug development for the disease. Future large-scale studies involving diverse patient cohorts are essential to establish these observations.

Therapeutic Potential of miRNA Targeting

MiR-regulated molecular pathways may interfere with early-stage pathology, and functional evidence suggests that modifying miRNA expression may help counteract AD pathology. For example, lentiviral constructs expressing miR-18-5p were administered by intracerebral infusion in 5xFAD mice that improved memory deficits in T-maze tests, restored dendritic spine density, and contextual fear conditioning [77]. Similarly, restoring miR-132 levels in various AD mouse models (APP/PS1, 3xTg AD, APPNL-G-F) using synthetic miRNA mimics reduced amyloid-beta (Aβ40-42) levels, tau phosphorylation, and detrimental cognition and deficits in hippocampal neurogenesis [78]. Additionally, miR-33--5p lentiviral delivery lowered BACE1 protein quantity, reduced Aβ42, and rescued neuroinflammation, and spatial memory deficits in the Morris water maze test [79].

Synthetic miR-146 antisense oligonucleotides (ASO) were administered non-invasively by nose-to-brain delivery in APP/PS1 mice, improved amyloid and tau pathology, reduced neuroinflammation, and improved memory. Similarly, studies show that adjusting miRNA levels in Alzheimer's disease mouse models can reduce these pathologies and symptoms, supporting the therapeutic potential of miRNA-based treatments [80]. This provides proof-of-concept for the therapeutic potential of miRNA-based interventions.

Reports from *in vitro* studies or transgenic mouse models might not fully capture the complexity of miRNA-mediated effects in AD. Increasing miRNA levels in tissues where they are not normally expressed may have unpredictable effects. Precise dose titration is essential to determine the optimal therapeutic window, as both very high and very low levels of miRNAs can be detrimental [81, 82]. Overall, miRNA regulation of gene expression is a finely tuned process that involves multiple layers of complexity, including miRNA abundance, MRE load, subcellular localization, and synergistic interactions, all of which have implications for both normal cellular function and disease states. Understanding the mechanisms through which miRNAs contribute to disease pathogenesis is crucial for developing effective therapeutic strategies.

FUTURE PERSPECTIVES

MiR-based therapeutics focus on either restoring endogenous miRNA levels with synthetic miRNAs (miRNA mimics) or reducing available miRNA with antisense inhibitors (antamiRs/antagomiRs). Genome editing tools like CRISPR/Cas9 offer potential for precise miRNA target validation. Clinical application requires comprehensive mapping of miRNA targets through techniques such as proteomics and single-cell transcriptomics. Preclinical studies have introduced a "miRNA pharmacodynamic signature" to evaluate dose-dependent target engagement. Key challenges include efficient delivery and cellular uptake to minimize side effects and reduce systemic exposure and dosage [65]. These advancements are essential for integrating miRNA-based approaches into clinical development.

Nanoparticle encapsulation offers a promising method for controlled, cell-typ--specific miRNA delivery to the brain, either systemically or *via* direct CNS administration. Benefits include enhanced molecular stability, protection from nucleases, and targeted delivery [83]. Lipid nanoparticles, widely studied and FDA-approved for siRNA delivery to the liver, are key candidates. Intranasal delivery of nanoparticle-encapsulated miR-132 mimics in an Alzheimer's mouse model showed feasibility, though broad target engagement remains to be validated. Challenges include nonspecific uptake, nanoparticle immunogenicity, and rapid clearance by macrophages, peripheral toxicity, and poor stability within cells, hindering clinical development [84 - 88]. Gemfibrozil, an FDA-approved cholesterol-lowering drug, was tested in a phase I clinical trial (NCT02045056) for its potential to increase miR-107 levels in cognitively healthy and MCI individuals to prevent Alzheimer's disease. The trial, involving 48 control and 24 MCI participants, found gemfibrozil to be safe and capable of altering plasma miR-107 levels. Although secondary parameters (CSF Aβ42, pTau, brain atrophy, *etc.*) showed favorable trends, they were not statistically significant [89]. While promising, the study does not directly evaluate the efficacy or toxicity of miRNA-based oligonucleotides in AD, highlighting the need for further trials with greater statistical power.

CONCLUSION

The traditional "one target – one disease" approach is shifting towards a more complex "multiple targets – multiple pathways" strategy, particularly in addressing multigenic disorders like Alzheimer's disease (AD). Multi-modal therapies and network biology/pharmacology are gaining attention in research for AD, with miRNA-targeted therapeutics showing promise due to their ability to regulate multiple molecular pathways relevant to disease phenotypes.

The development of miRNA therapeutics is progressing alongside other oligonucleotide-based therapies (such as siRNA and ASO). However, further investigation is needed to better understand miRNA-targeting mechanisms and to map potential toxic effects. Challenges like targeted brain delivery and assessing the safety of miRNA supplementation or inhibition must also be addressed. Despite the growing interest within the major pharmaceutical firms, the application of miRNA therapeutics in AD lags behind other disease areas, particularly oncology, which sees far more active clinical trials. Increased investment and technological advancements are essential to translating promising miRNA research into clinical applications for AD. Over the coming years, ongoing preclinical, clinical, and screening studies will determine how close miRNA-based treatments are to clinical practice and whether the numerous miRNA targets are manageable for effective therapeutic use.

ACKNOWLEDGEMENT

I would like to express my appreciation for the opportunity to contribute to this book and for the ongoing inspiration and support provided by Dr. Swarupananda Mukherjee, Editor and Associate Professor, NSHM College of Pharmaceutical Technology, Kolkata, India 700058.

REFERENCES

[1] Alzheimer's Association. 2023 Alzheimer's disease facts and figures: At a glance [Internet]. 2023. Available from: https://www.alz.org/media/Documents/Facts-And-Figures-2023-At-A-Glanc--Stats-Fact-Sheet.pdf

[2] van Dyck CH, Swanson CJ, Aisen P, *et al.* Lecanemab in early Alzheimer's disease. N Engl J Med 2023; 388(1): 9-21. [http://dx.doi.org/10.1056/NEJMoa2212948] [PMID: 36449413]

[3] Cole S, Vassar R. BACE1 structure and function in health and Alzheimer's disease. Curr Alzheimer Res 2008; 5(2): 100-20. [http://dx.doi.org/10.2174/156720508783954758] [PMID: 18393796]

[4] von Bernhardi R, Cornejo F, Parada GE, Eugenín J. Role of TGFβ signaling in the pathogenesis of Alzheimer's disease. Front Cell Neurosci 2015; 9: 426. [http://dx.doi.org/10.3389/fncel.2015.00426] [PMID: 26578886]

[5] Sarkar S. Pathological role of RAGE underlying progression of various diseases: its potential as biomarker and therapeutic target. Naunyn Schmiedebergs Arch Pharmacol 2024. [http://dx.doi.org/10.1007/s00210-024-03595-6] [PMID: 39589529]

[6] Rao JS, Keleshian VL, Klein S, Rapoport SI. Epigenetic modifications in frontal cortex from Alzheimer's disease and bipolar disorder patients. Transl Psychiatry 2012; 2(7): e132. [http://dx.doi.org/10.1038/tp.2012.55] [PMID: 22760556]

[7] Bakulski KM, Dolinoy DC, Sartor MA, *et al.* Genome-wide DNA methylation differences between late-onset Alzheimer's disease and cognitively normal controls in human frontal cortex. J Alzheimers Dis 2012; 29(3): 571-88. [http://dx.doi.org/10.3233/JAD-2012-111223] [PMID: 22451312]

[8] Wang SC, Oelze B, Schumacher A. Age-specific epigenetic drift in late-onset Alzheimer's disease. PLoS One 2008; 3(7): e2698. [http://dx.doi.org/10.1371/journal.pone.0002698] [PMID: 18628954]

[9] DesJarlais R, Tummino PJ. Role of Histone-Modifying Enzymes and Their Complexes in Regulation of Chromatin Biology. Biochemistry 2016; 55(11): 1584-99. [http://dx.doi.org/10.1021/acs.biochem.5b01210] [PMID: 26745824]

[10] Santana DA, Bedrat A, Puga RD, *et al.* The role of H3K9 acetylation and gene expression in different brain regions of Alzheimer's disease patients. Epigenomics 2022; 14(11): 651-70. [http://dx.doi.org/10.2217/epi-2022-0096] [PMID: 35588246]

[11] He X, Hui Z, Xu L, *et al.* Medicinal chemistry updates of novel HDACs inhibitors (2020 to present). Eur J Med Chem 2022; 227: 113946. [http://dx.doi.org/10.1016/j.ejmech.2021.113946] [PMID: 34775332]

[12] Anderson KW, Turko IV. Histone post-translational modifications in frontal cortex from human donors with Alzheimer's disease. ClinProteom. 2015;12:26Balmik, A.A.; Chinnathambi, S. Methylation as a key regulator of Tau aggregation and neuronal health in Alzheimer's disease. Cell Commun Signal 2021; 19: 51.

[13] Persico G, Casciaro F, Amatori S, *et al.* Histone H3 Lysine 4 and 27 Trimethylation Landscape of

Human Alzheimer's Disease. Cells 2022; 11(4): 734.
[http://dx.doi.org/10.3390/cells11040734] [PMID: 35203383]

[14] Yan XW, Liu HJ, Hong YX, Meng T, Du J, Chang C. lncRNA XIST induces Aβ accumulation and neuroinflammation by the epigenetic repression of NEP in Alzheimer's disease. J Neurogenet 2022; 36(1): 11-20.
[http://dx.doi.org/10.1080/01677063.2022.2028784] [PMID: 35098860]

[15] Yue D, Guanqun G, Jingxin L, *et al.* Silencing of long noncoding RNA XIST attenuated Alzheimer's disease□related BACE1 alteration through miR□124. Cell Biol Int 2020; 44(2): 630-6.
[http://dx.doi.org/10.1002/cbin.11263] [PMID: 31743528]

[16] Greene AN, Parks LG, Solomon MB, Privette Vinnedge LM. Loss of DEK Expression Induces Alzheimer's Disease Phenotypes in Differentiated SH-SY5Y Cells. Front Mol Neurosci 2020; 13: 594319.
[http://dx.doi.org/10.3389/fnmol.2020.594319] [PMID: 33304240]

[17] Denli AM, Tops BBJ, Plasterk RHA, Ketting RF, Hannon GJ. Processing of primary microRNAs by the Microprocessor complex. Nature 2004; 432(7014): 231-5.
[http://dx.doi.org/10.1038/nature03049] [PMID: 15531879]

[18] Alarcón CR, Lee H, Goodarzi H, Halberg N, Tavazoie SF. N6-methyladenosine marks primary microRNAs for processing. Nature 2015; 519(7544): 482-5.
[http://dx.doi.org/10.1038/nature14281] [PMID: 25799998]

[19] Han J, Lee Y, Yeom KH, Kim YK, Jin H, Kim VN. The Drosha-DGCR8 complex in primary microRNA processing. Genes Dev 2004; 18(24): 3016-27.
[http://dx.doi.org/10.1101/gad.1262504] [PMID: 15574589]

[20] Yoda M, Kawamata T, Paroo Z, *et al.* ATP-dependent human RISC assembly pathways. Nat Struct Mol Biol 2010; 17(1): 17-23.
[http://dx.doi.org/10.1038/nsmb.1733] [PMID: 19966796]

[21] Meijer HA, Smith EM, Bushell M. Regulation of miRNA strand selection: follow the leader? Biochem Soc Trans 2014; 42(4): 1135-40.
[http://dx.doi.org/10.1042/BST20140142] [PMID: 25110015]

[22] Khvorova A, Reynolds A, Jayasena SD. Functional siRNAs and miRNAs exhibit strand bias. Cell 2003; 115(2): 209-16.
[http://dx.doi.org/10.1016/S0092-8674(03)00801-8] [PMID: 14567918]

[23] Ruby JG, Jan CH, Bartel DP. Intronic microRNA precursors that bypass Drosha processing. Nature 2007; 448(7149): 83-6.
[http://dx.doi.org/10.1038/nature05983] [PMID: 17589500]

[24] Babiarz JE, Ruby JG, Wang Y, Bartel DP, Blelloch R. Mouse ES cells express endogenous shRNAs, siRNAs, and other Microprocessor-independent, Dicer-dependent small RNAs. Genes Dev 2008; 22(20): 2773-85.
[http://dx.doi.org/10.1101/gad.1705308] [PMID: 18923076]

[25] Xie M, Li M, Vilborg A, *et al.* Mammalian 5′-capped microRNA precursors that generate a single microRNA. Cell 2013; 155(7): 1568-80.
[http://dx.doi.org/10.1016/j.cell.2013.11.027] [PMID: 24360278]

[26] Yang JS, Maurin T, Robine N, *et al.* Conserved vertebrate *mir-451* provides a platform for Dicer-independent, Ago2-mediated microRNA biogenesis. Proc Natl Acad Sci USA 2010; 107(34): 15163-8.
[http://dx.doi.org/10.1073/pnas.1006432107] [PMID: 20699384]

[27] Ipsaro JJ, Joshua-Tor L. From guide to target: molecular insights into eukaryotic RNA-interference machinery. Nat Struct Mol Biol 2015; 22(1): 20-8.
[http://dx.doi.org/10.1038/nsmb.2931] [PMID: 25565029]

[28] Xu W, San Lucas A, Wang Z, Liu Y. Identifying microRNA targets in different gene regions. BMC

Bioinformatics 2014; 15(S7) (Suppl. 7): S4.
[http://dx.doi.org/10.1186/1471-2105-15-S7-S4] [PMID: 25077573]

[29] Forman JJ, Legesse-Miller A, Coller HA. A search for conserved sequences in coding regions reveals that the *let-7* microRNA targets Dicer within its coding sequence. Proc Natl Acad Sci USA 2008; 105(39): 14879-84.
[http://dx.doi.org/10.1073/pnas.0803230105] [PMID: 18812516]

[30] Zhang J, Zhou W, Liu Y, Liu T, Li C, Wang L. Oncogenic role of microRNA-532□5p in human colorectal cancer *via* targeting of the 5'UTR of *RUNX3*. Oncol Lett 2018; 15(5): 7215-20.
[http://dx.doi.org/10.3892/ol.2018.8217] [PMID: 29849790]

[31] Dharap A, Pokrzywa C, Murali S, Pandi G, Vemuganti R. MicroRNA miR-324-3p induces promoter-mediated expression of RelA gene. PLoS One 2013; 8(11): e79467.
[http://dx.doi.org/10.1371/journal.pone.0079467] [PMID: 24265774]

[32] Jonas S, Izaurralde E. Towards a molecular understanding of microRNA-mediated gene silencing. Nat Rev Genet 2015; 16(7): 421-33.
[http://dx.doi.org/10.1038/nrg3965] [PMID: 26077373]

[33] Ellwanger DC, Büttner FA, Mewes HW, Stümpflen V. The sufficient minimal set of miRNA seed types. Bioinformatics 2011; 27(10): 1346-50.
[http://dx.doi.org/10.1093/bioinformatics/btr149] [PMID: 21441577]

[34] Behm-Ansmant I, Rehwinkel J, Doerks T, Stark A, Bork P, Izaurralde E. mRNA degradation by miRNAs and GW182 requires both CCR4:NOT deadenylase and DCP1:DCP2 decapping complexes. Genes Dev 2006; 20(14): 1885-98.
[http://dx.doi.org/10.1101/gad.1424106] [PMID: 16815998]

[35] Christie M, Boland A, Huntzinger E, Weichenrieder O, Izaurralde E. Structure of the PAN3 pseudokinase reveals the basis for interactions with the PAN2 deadenylase and the GW182 proteins. Mol Cell 2013; 51(3): 360-73.
[http://dx.doi.org/10.1016/j.molcel.2013.07.011] [PMID: 23932717]

[36] O'Brien J, Hayder H, Zayed Y, Peng C. Overview of MicroRNA Biogenesis, Mechanisms of Actions, and Circulation. Front Endocrinol (Lausanne) 2018; 9: 402.
[http://dx.doi.org/10.3389/fendo.2018.00402] [PMID: 30123182]

[37] Vasudevan S, Steitz JA. AU-rich-element-mediated upregulation of translation by FXR1 and Argonaute 2. Cell 2007; 128(6): 1105-18.
[http://dx.doi.org/10.1016/j.cell.2007.01.038] [PMID: 17382880]

[38] Truesdell SS, Mortensen RD, Seo M, *et al.* MicroRNA-mediated mRNA translation activation in quiescent cells and oocytes involves recruitment of a nuclear microRNP. Sci Rep 2012; 2(1): 842.
[http://dx.doi.org/10.1038/srep00842] [PMID: 23150790]

[39] Bukhari SIA, Truesdell SS, Lee S, *et al.* A specialized mechanism of translation mediated by FXR1a-associated microRNP in cellular quiescence. Mol Cell 2016; 61(5): 760-73.
[http://dx.doi.org/10.1016/j.molcel.2016.02.013] [PMID: 26942679]

[40] Nishi K, Nishi A, Nagasawa T, Ui-Tei K. Human TNRC6A is an Argonaute-navigator protein for microRNA-mediated gene silencing in the nucleus. RNA 2013; 19(1): 17-35.
[http://dx.doi.org/10.1261/rna.034769.112] [PMID: 23150874]

[41] Benhamed M, Herbig U, Ye T, Dejean A, Bischof O. Senescence is an endogenous trigger for microRNA-directed transcriptional gene silencing in human cells. Nat Cell Biol 2012; 14(3): 266-75.
[http://dx.doi.org/10.1038/ncb2443] [PMID: 22366686]

[42] Pitchiaya S, Heinicke LA, Park JI, Cameron EL, Walter NG. Resolving subcellular miRNA trafficking and turnover at single-molecule resolution. Cell Rep 2017; 19(3): 630-42.
[http://dx.doi.org/10.1016/j.celrep.2017.03.075] [PMID: 28423324]

[43] Zhu JJ, Liu YF, Zhang YP, *et al.* VAMP3 and SNAP23 mediate the disturbed flow-induced

endothelial microRNA secretion and smooth muscle hyperplasia. Proc Natl Acad Sci USA 2017; 114(31): 8271-6.
[http://dx.doi.org/10.1073/pnas.1700561114] [PMID: 28716920]

[44] Gümürdü A, Yildiz R, Eren E, *et al.* MicroRNA exocytosis by large dense-core vesicle fusion. Sci Rep 2017; 7(1): 45661.
[http://dx.doi.org/10.1038/srep45661] [PMID: 28358390]

[45] Yang M, Chen J, Su F, *et al.* Microvesicles secreted by macrophages shuttle invasion-potentiating microRNAs into breast cancer cells. Mol Cancer 2011; 10(1): 117.
[http://dx.doi.org/10.1186/1476-4598-10-117] [PMID: 21939504]

[46] Hannafon BN, Carpenter KJ, Berry WL, Janknecht R, Dooley WC, Ding WQ. Exosome-mediated microRNA signaling from breast cancer cells is altered by the anti-angiogenesis agent docosahexaenoic acid (DHA). Mol Cancer 2015; 14(1): 133.
[http://dx.doi.org/10.1186/s12943-015-0400-7] [PMID: 26178901]

[47] Zhou W, Fong MY, Min Y, *et al.* Cancer-secreted miR-105 destroys vascular endothelial barriers to promote metastasis. Cancer Cell 2014; 25(4): 501-15.
[http://dx.doi.org/10.1016/j.ccr.2014.03.007] [PMID: 24735924]

[48] Hu Y, Rao SS, Wang ZX, *et al.* Exosomes from human umbilical cord blood accelerate cutaneous wound healing through miR-21-3p-mediated promotion of angiogenesis and fibroblast function. Theranostics 2018; 8(1): 169-84.
[http://dx.doi.org/10.7150/thno.21234] [PMID: 29290800]

[49] Sakha S, Muramatsu T, Ueda K, Inazawa J. Exosomal microRNA miR-1246 induces cell motility and invasion through the regulation of DENND2D in oral squamous cell carcinoma. Sci Rep 2016; 6(1): 38750.
[http://dx.doi.org/10.1038/srep38750] [PMID: 27929118]

[50] Fabbri M. MicroRNAs and miRceptors: a new mechanism of action for intercellular communication. Philos Trans R Soc Lond B Biol Sci 2018; 373(1737): 20160486.
[http://dx.doi.org/10.1098/rstb.2016.0486] [PMID: 29158315]

[51] Fabbri M, Paone A, Calore F, *et al.* MicroRNAs bind to Toll-like receptors to induce prometastatic inflammatory response. Proc Natl Acad Sci USA 2012; 109(31): E2110-6.
[http://dx.doi.org/10.1073/pnas.1209414109] [PMID: 22753494]

[52] Lehmann SM, Krüger C, Park B, *et al.* An unconventional role for miRNA: let-7 activates Toll-like receptor 7 and causes neurodegeneration. Nat Neurosci 2012; 15(6): 827-35.
[http://dx.doi.org/10.1038/nn.3113] [PMID: 22610069]

[53] Vickers KC, Palmisano BT, Shoucri BM, Shamburek RD, Remaley AT. MicroRNAs are transported in plasma and delivered to recipient cells by high-density lipoproteins. Nat Cell Biol 2011; 13(4): 423-33.
[http://dx.doi.org/10.1038/ncb2210] [PMID: 21423178]

[54] Tabet F, Vickers KC, Cuesta Torres LF, *et al.* HDL-transferred microRNA-223 regulates ICAM-1 expression in endothelial cells. Nat Commun 2014; 5(1): 3292.
[http://dx.doi.org/10.1038/ncomms4292] [PMID: 24576947]

[55] Takousis P, Sadlon A, Schulz J, *et al.* Differential expression of microRNAs in Alzheimer's disease brain, blood, and cerebrospinal fluid. Alzheimers Dement 2019; 15(11): 1468-77.
[http://dx.doi.org/10.1016/j.jalz.2019.06.4952] [PMID: 31495604]

[56] Fu Y, Hu X, Zheng C, *et al.* Intrahippocampal miR-342-3p inhibition reduces β-amyloid plaques and ameliorates learning and memory in Alzheimer's disease. Metab Brain Dis 2019; 34(5): 1355-63.
[http://dx.doi.org/10.1007/s11011-019-00438-9] [PMID: 31134481]

[57] Zhang H, Liu W, Ge H, Li K. Aberrant expression of miR-148a-3p in Alzheimer's disease and its protective role against amyloid-β induced neurotoxicity. Neurosci Lett 2021; 756: 135953.

[http://dx.doi.org/10.1016/j.neulet.2021.135953] [PMID: 33979697]

[58] Liu S, Fan M, Zheng Q, Hao S, Yang L, Xia Q, Qi C, Ge J. MicroRNAs in Alzheimer's disease: potential diagnostic markers and therapeutic targets. Biomedicine & Pharmacotherapy. 2022 Apr 1; 148: 112681.

[59] Zhang J, Wang R. Deregulated lncRNA MAGI2-AS3 in Alzheimer's disease attenuates amyloid-β induced neurotoxicity and neuroinflammation by sponging miR-374b-5p. Exp Gerontol 2021; 144: 111180.
[http://dx.doi.org/10.1016/j.exger.2020.111180] [PMID: 33279663]

[60] Cao F, Liu Z, Sun G. Diagnostic value of miR-193a-3p in Alzheimer's disease and miR-193a-3p attenuates amyloid-β induced neurotoxicity by targeting PTEN. Exp Gerontol 2020; 130: 110814.
[http://dx.doi.org/10.1016/j.exger.2019.110814] [PMID: 31857133]

[61] Hernandez-Rapp J, Rainone S, Goupil C, *et al.* microRNA-132/212 deficiency enhances Aβ production and senile plaque deposition in Alzheimer's disease triple transgenic mice. Sci Rep 2016; 6(1): 30953.
[http://dx.doi.org/10.1038/srep30953] [PMID: 27484949]

[62] Wang R, Zhang J. Clinical significance of miR-433 in the diagnosis of Alzheimer's disease and its effect on Aβ-induced neurotoxicity by regulating JAK2. Exp Gerontol 2020; 141: 111080.
[http://dx.doi.org/10.1016/j.exger.2020.111080] [PMID: 32871216]

[63] Abidin SZ, Mat Pauzi NA, Mansor NI, Mohd Isa NI, Hamid AA. A new perspective on Alzheimer's disease: microRNAs and circular RNAs. Front Genet 2023; 14: 1231486.
[http://dx.doi.org/10.3389/fgene.2023.1231486] [PMID: 37790702]

[64] Wu W, Liu G, Li X, Liu Y, Wang Y, Pan H, *et al.* MiR-191-5p alleviates microglial cell injury by targeting Map3k12 to inhibit MAPK signaling pathway in Alzheimer's disease. Bioengineered 2021; 12: 12678-90.
[http://dx.doi.org/10.1080/21655979.2021.2008638] [PMID: 34818971]

[65] Walgrave H, Zhou L, De Strooper B, Salta E. The promise of microRNA-based therapies in Alzheimer's disease: challenges and perspectives. Mol Neurodegener 2021; 16(1): 76.
[http://dx.doi.org/10.1186/s13024-021-00496-7] [PMID: 34742333]

[66] Wang Y, Xiao Z, Yin H, *et al.* miRNA375-3p/rapamycin mediates the mTOR pathway by decreasing PS1, enhances microglial cell activity to regulate autophagy in Alzheimer's disease. Heliyon 2024; 10(19): e37589.
[http://dx.doi.org/10.1016/j.heliyon.2024.e37589] [PMID: 39386837]

[67] Wang D, Fei Z, Luo S, Wang H. MiR-335-5p inhibits β-amyloid accumulation to attenuate cognitive deficits through targeting c-jun-N-terminal kinase 3 in Alzheimer's disease. Curr Neurovasc Res 2020; 17(1): 93-101.
[http://dx.doi.org/10.2174/1567202617666200128141938] [PMID: 32003672]

[68] Gatsiou A, Boeckel JN, Randriamboavonjy V, Stellos K. MicroRNAs in platelet biogenesis and function: implications in vascular homeostasis and inflammation. Curr Vasc Pharmacol 2012; 10(5): 524-31.
[http://dx.doi.org/10.2174/157016112801784611] [PMID: 22338566]

[69] Bhatlekar S, Manne BK, Basak I, *et al.* miR-125a-5p regulates megakaryocyte proplatelet formation *via* the actin-bundling protein L-plastin. Blood 2020; 136(15): 1760-72.
[http://dx.doi.org/10.1182/blood.2020005230] [PMID: 32844999]

[70] Leidinger P, Backes C, Deutscher S, *et al.* A blood based 12-miRNA signature of Alzheimer disease patients. Genome Biol 2013; 14(7): R78.
[http://dx.doi.org/10.1186/gb-2013-14-7-r78] [PMID: 23895045]

[71] Doecke JD, Pérez-Grijalba V, Fandos N, *et al.* Total Aβ42/Aβ40 ratio in plasma predicts amyloid-PET status, independent of clinical AD diagnosis. Neurology. 2020; 94(15)–e1591.

[http://dx.doi.org/10.1212/WNL.0000000000009240]

[72] Liu Y, He X, Li Y, Wang T. Cerebrospinal fluid CD4+ T lymphocyte-derived miRNA-let-7b can enhances the diagnostic performance of Alzheimer's disease biomarkers. Biochem Biophys Res Commun 2018; 495(1): 1144-50. [http://dx.doi.org/10.1016/j.bbrc.2017.11.122] [PMID: 29170128]

[73] Jain G, Stuendl A, Rao P, *et al.* A combined miRNA–piRNA signature to detect Alzheimer's disease. Transl Psychiatry 2019; 9(1): 250. [http://dx.doi.org/10.1038/s41398-019-0579-2] [PMID: 31591382]

[74] Moon J, Lee ST, Kong IG, *et al.* Early diagnosis of Alzheimer's disease from elevated olfactory mucosal miR-206 level. Sci Rep 2016; 6(1): 20364. [http://dx.doi.org/10.1038/srep20364] [PMID: 26842588]

[75] Kenny A, Jiménez-Mateos EM, Zea-Sevilla MA, *et al.* Proteins and microRNAs are differentially expressed in tear fluid from patients with Alzheimer's disease. Sci Rep 2019; 9(1): 15437. [http://dx.doi.org/10.1038/s41598-019-51837-y] [PMID: 31659197]

[76] Lee K, Kim H, An K, *et al.* Replenishment of microRNA-188-5p restores the synaptic and cognitive deficits in 5XFAD Mouse Model of Alzheimer's Disease. Sci Rep 2016; 6(1): 34433. [http://dx.doi.org/10.1038/srep34433] [PMID: 27708404]

[77] Salta E, Sierksma A, Vanden Eynden E, De Strooper B. miR-132 loss de-represses ITPKB and aggravates amyloid and TAU pathology in Alzheimer's brain. EMBO Mol Med 2016; 8(9): 1005-18. [http://dx.doi.org/10.15252/emmm.201606520] [PMID: 27485122]

[78] Qian Q, Zhang J, He FP, *et al.* Down-regulated expression of microRNA-338-5p contributes to neuropathology in Alzheimer's disease. FASEB J 2019; 33(3): 4404-17. [http://dx.doi.org/10.1096/fj.201801846R] [PMID: 30576233]

[79] Mai H, Fan W, Wang Y, *et al.* Intranasal administration of miR-146a agomir rescues the pathological process and cognitive impairment in an AD mouse model. Mol Ther Nucleic Acids 2019; 18: 681-95. [http://dx.doi.org/10.1016/j.omtn.2019.10.002] [PMID: 31707205]

[80] Walgrave H, Balusu S, Snoeck S, *et al.* Restoring miR-132 expression rescues adult hippocampal neurogenesis and memory deficits in Alzheimer's disease. Cell Stem Cell 2021; 28(10): 1805-1821.e8. [http://dx.doi.org/10.1016/j.stem.2021.05.001] [PMID: 34033742]

[81] Hansen KF, Karelina K, Sakamoto K, Wayman GA, Impey S, Obrietan K. miRNA-132: a dynamic regulator of cognitive capacity. Brain Struct Funct 2013; 218(3): 817-31. [http://dx.doi.org/10.1007/s00429-012-0431-4] [PMID: 22706759]

[82] Lee SWL, Paoletti C, Campisi M, *et al.* MicroRNA delivery through nanoparticles. J Control Release 2019; 313: 80-95. [http://dx.doi.org/10.1016/j.jconrel.2019.10.007] [PMID: 31622695]

[83] Chandler RJ, LaFave MC, Varshney GK, *et al.* Vector design influences hepatic genotoxicity after adeno-associated virus gene therapy. J Clin Invest 2015; 125(2): 870-80. [http://dx.doi.org/10.1172/JCI79213] [PMID: 25607839]

[84] Kulkarni JA, Witzigmann D, Chen S, Cullis PR, van der Meel R. Lipid nanoparticle technology for clinical translation of siRNA therapeutics. Acc Chem Res 2019; 52(9): 2435-44. [http://dx.doi.org/10.1021/acs.accounts.9b00368] [PMID: 31397996]

[85] Boraschi D, Italiani P, Palomba R, *et al.* Nanoparticles and innate immunity: new perspectives on host defence. Semin Immunol 2017; 34: 33-51. [http://dx.doi.org/10.1016/j.smim.2017.08.013] [PMID: 28869063]

[86] Zhou Y, Peng Z, Seven ES, Leblanc RM. Crossing the blood-brain barrier with nanoparticles. J Control Release 2018; 270: 290-303. [http://dx.doi.org/10.1016/j.jconrel.2017.12.015] [PMID: 29269142]

[87] Samaridou E, Walgrave H, Salta E, *et al.* Nose-to-brain delivery of enveloped RNA - cell permeating peptide nanocomplexes for the treatment of neurodegenerative diseases. Biomaterials 2020; 230: 119657.
[http://dx.doi.org/10.1016/j.biomaterials.2019.119657] [PMID: 31837821]

[88] Jicha GA, Kryscio RJ, Beech BF, *et al.* Modulation of microRNA pathways by gemfibrozil in predementia Alzheimer disease: a randomized, placebo-controlled, double-blind clinical trial. Alzheimers Dement. 2019; 15(Suppl): P910.
[http://dx.doi.org/10.1016/j.jalz.2019.06.4682]

[89] O'Carroll D, Schaefer A. General principals of miRNA biogenesis and regulation in the brain. Neuropsychopharmacology 2013; 38(1): 39-54.
[http://dx.doi.org/10.1038/npp.2012.87] [PMID: 22669168]

CHAPTER 7

Clinical Indication of the Role of Inflammation in Alzheimer's Disease

Arvind Kumar[1,*], **Nilanjan Sarkar**[1], **Moumita Kundu**[2,3], **Vishal Singh**[4] and **Debankini Dasgupta**[5]

[1] *Department of Pharmaceutical Technology, NSHM Knowledge Campus Kolkata – Group of Institutions, Kolkata, West Bengal, India*

[2] *Department of Pharmaceutical Technology, JIS University, Kolkata, West Bengal, India*

[3] *Department of Pharmacology, Anand College of Pharmacy, Midnapore, West Bengal, India*

[4] *Department of Pharmaceutical Technology, Exemed Pharmaceuticals, Vadodara, Gujarat, India*

[5] *Department of Pharmaceutical Technology, MGM College of Pharmacy, Patna, Bihar, India*

Abstract: Considerable evidence gained over the past decade has supported the conclusion that neuroinflammation is associated with Alzheimer's disease (AD) pathology. Inflammatory components related to AD neuroinflammation include brain cells such as microglia and astrocytes, the classic and alternate pathways of the complement system, the pentraxin acute-phase proteins, neuronal-type nicotinic acetylcholine receptors (AChRs), peroxisomal proliferator-activated receptors (PPARs), as well as cytokines and chemokines. The microglia and astrocytes have been shown to generate beta-amyloid protein (Aβ), one of the main pathologic features of AD. Aβ itself has been shown to act as a pro-inflammatory agent, causing the activation of many of the inflammatory components. Further substantiation for the role of neuroinflammation in AD has come from studies that demonstrate patients who took non-steroidal anti-inflammatory drugs had a lower risk of AD than those who did not. These same results have led to increased interest in pursuing anti-inflammatory therapy for AD, but with poor results. On the other hand, an increasing amount of data suggests that AChRs and PPARs are involved in AD-induced neuroinflammation. In this regard, future therapy may focus on their specific targeting in the AD brain.

Keywords: Acetylcholine receptors, Food and drug administration, Peroxisomal proliferators-activated receptors, Non-steroidal anti-inflammatory drugs.

INTRODUCTION

Alzheimer's disease (AD) is a progressive neurodegenerative disorder characterized by cognitive decline, memory loss, and behavioral changes. While

* **Corresponding author Kumar Arvind:** Department of Pharmaceutical Technology, NSHM Knowledge Campus Kolkata – Group of Institutions, Kolkata, West Bengal, India; E-mail: arvindkumarssm161@gmail.com

the exact mechanisms underlying AD remain unclear, a growing body of evidence highlights the auspicious role of neuroinflammation in its pathogenesis. Inflammation, typically a protective response of the immune system to injury or infection, becomes dysregulated in AD, contributing to disease progression.

In the context of AD, neuroinflammation is primarily mediated by the brain's resident immune cells, microglia, and astrocytes. These cells become activated in response to the accumulation of pathological hallmarks, such as amyloid-beta (aβ) plaques and tau protein tangles. However, instead of resolving the issue, this activation often leads to a chronic inflammatory state. This persistent inflammation exacerbates neuronal damage and synaptic dysfunction. Research also suggests that systemic inflammation, driven by comorbidities like infections, metabolic disorders, or lifestyle factors, may influence the progression of AD by breaching the blood-brain barrier and amplifying neuroinflammatory responses. Genetic factors, such as mutations in the APOE gene, further modulate the inflammatory processes associated with the disease. Understanding the role of inflammation in AD opens new avenues for therapeutic interventions [1]. AD is the most prevalent neurodegenerative disorder, currently impacting an estimated 20 to 30 million individuals globally. It comprises the majority of dementia cases diagnosed in individuals over the age of 60. In the United States alone, approximately 4 million patients are affected. The incidence of AD exhibits a significant age-related increase: around 1% to 3% of the population in their 60s are diagnosed, escalating to 3% to 12% among those aged 70 to 80, and reaching as high as 25% to 35% in older adults [2].

INFLAMMATORY PATHWAYS IN THE AD BRAIN

A key feature of AD is neuroinflammation, which is primarily mediated by microglia and astrocytes. Here's an overview of the inflammatory pathways in the AD brain:

Activation of Microglia and Astrocytes

Microglia and astrocytes are the primary immune cells of the central nervous system, playing crucial roles in maintaining brain homeostasis. In AD, these cells become activated in response to pathological stimuli such as amyloid-beta (Aβ) plaques and tau tangles.

Microglia are among the first responders to amyloid-beta (Aβ) deposition. Upon activation, microglia seek to clear Aβ plaques through phagocytosis. However, long-term activation can lead to the production of pro-inflammatory cytokines. Similarly, astrocytes, which support neuronal function and maintain the blood-brain barrier, become reactive in AD. Persistent activation of these glial cells exacerbates neuroinflammation [3].

NLRP3 Inflammasome Activation

The NLRP3 inflammasome is a multiprotein complex that is activated in response to Aβ accumulation in the AD brain. Once activated, the NLRP3 inflammasome leads to the release of IL-1β, a potent pro-inflammatory cytokine (Fig. **1**). Chronic activation of the inflammasome in microglia promotes a sustained inflammatory environment, contributing to neurodegeneration. Additionally, tau pathology has been shown to further activate the inflammasome, creating a vicious cycle of inflammation and neuronal injury [3, 4].

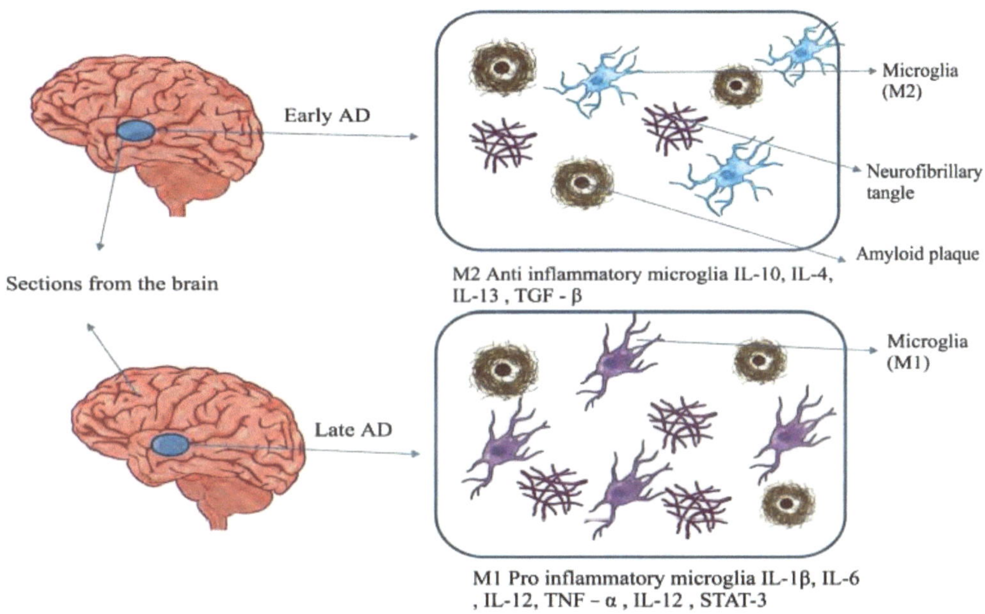

Fig. (1). NLRP3 inflammasome activation.

Toll-like Receptors (TLRs)

Toll-like receptors are expressed in numerous cell types in the brain. In AD, TLRs, particularly TLR2, TLR4, and TLR9, are upregulated in response to the accumulation of amyloid-beta (Aβ) and tau protein aggregates. These receptors recognize Aβ plaques as damage-associated molecular patterns (DAMPs) and initiate an inflammatory response, which is meant to clear the pathological proteins but often leads to chronic neuroinflammation [5, 6].

Complement System

The complement system, a part of the innate immune response, is activated in the AD brain. Components such as C1q, C3, and C4 are found deposited around Aβ plaques and tau tangles. The activation of the complement cascade leads to the formation of the membrane attack complex (MAC), which can cause direct neuronal injury (Fig. **2**). Moreover, complement activation attracts microglia to plaques and tangles, where they can become over-activated and exacerbate inflammation [7, 8].

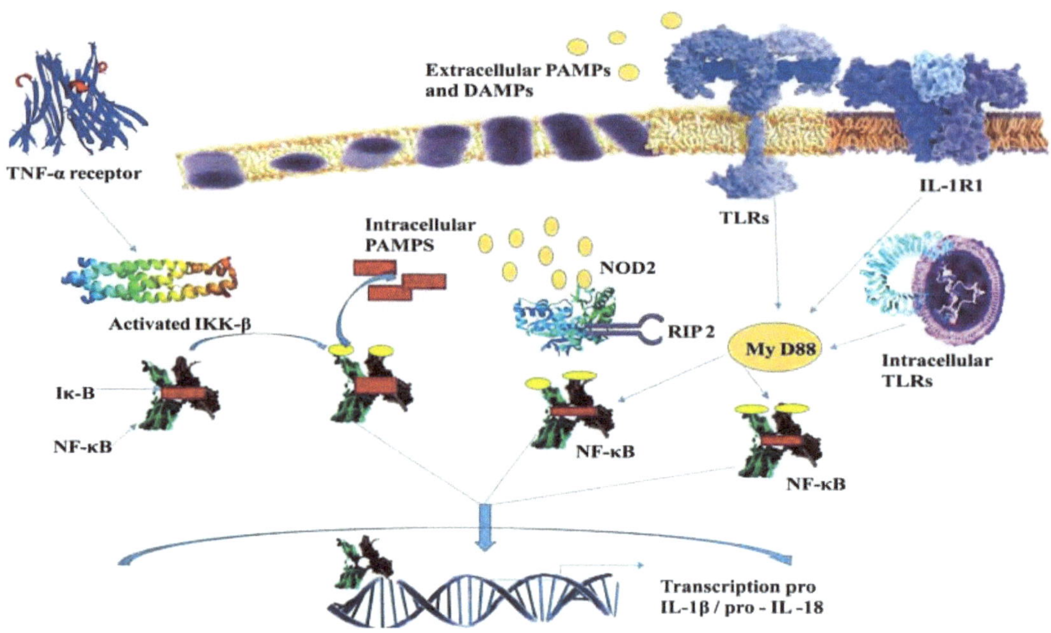

Fig. (2). Complement system.

Cytokine and Chemokine Signalling

Pro-inflammatory **cytokines** amplify the inflammatory response by recruiting more immune cells to the site of pathology and further activating microglia. Chemokines, including CCL2 and CXCL10, also play a role in attracting peripheral immune cells into the brain, thereby exacerbating neuroinflammation (Fig. **3**). This sustained inflammatory response can lead to synaptic dysfunction and neurological death, contributing to cognitive decline [9, 10].

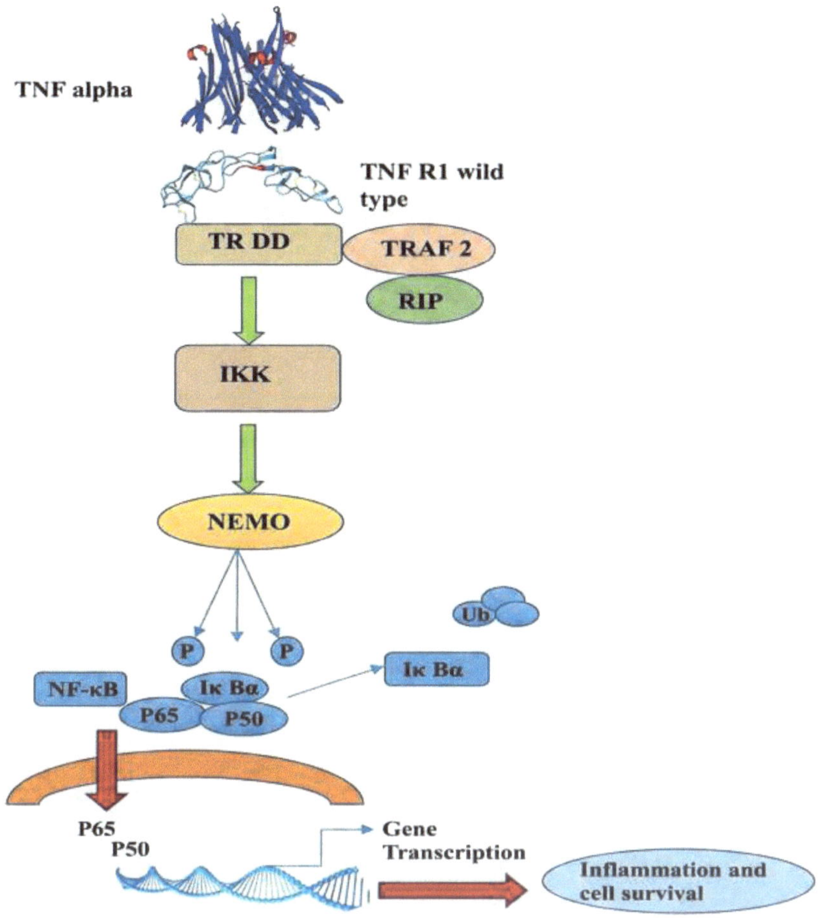

Fig. (3). Cytokine and chemokine signalling pathway.

NF-κB Pathway

The NF-κB (nuclear factor kappa-light-chain-enhancer of activated B cells) pathway is a central regulator of inflammation in the Alzheimer's disease (AD) brain. Activated by amyloid-beta (Aβ), oxidative stress, and pro-inflammatory cytokines such as TNF-α, the NF-κB pathway is predominantly active in microglia and astrocytes. Upon activation, NF-κB translocates to the nucleus, where it induces the transcription of various pro-inflammatory genes. This shows a chronic inflammatory state that inflames neurological damage, promotes tau phosphorylation, and facilitates further Aβ accumulation. The persistent stimulation of the NF-κB contributes to a vicious cycle of neuroinflammation, synaptic dysfunction, and neurodegeneration, making it a crucial driver of AD pathology and a target for potential therapeutic interventions [11].

JAK/STAT Pathway

Phosphorylated STATs dimerize and translocate to the nucleus, where they drive the expression of inflammatory genes. In AD, chronic activation of the JAK/STAT pathway contributes to sustained neuroinflammation, astrogliosis, and exacerbation of amyloid-beta (Aβ) and tau pathologies. This persistent inflammatory response not only accelerates neuronal damage but also impairs synaptic function and promotes cognitive decline, making the JAK/STAT pathway a significant contributor to AD progression and a potential target for therapeutic intervention [12].

MAPK Pathway

The MAPK (Mitogen-Activated Protein Kinase) pathway is a crucial signalling cascade involved in the regulation of inflammation in the Alzheimer's disease (AD) brain. Activated by various extracellular stimuli, including amyloid-beta (Aβ) oligomers, oxidative stress, and pro-inflammatory cytokines, the MAPK pathway encompasses three main kinases: ERK, JNK, and p38 MAPK. In AD, the activation of JNK and p38 MAPK, in particular, has been linked to the promotion of neuroinflammation through the upregulation of pro-inflammatory cytokines. These cytokines contribute to the chronic inflammatory state observed in AD, exacerbating neuronal damage. Additionally, the sustained activation of the MAPK pathway in microglia and astrocytes perpetuates a cycle of inflammation and neurodegeneration, which drives disease development [13].

THE ROLE OF TREM2 IN ALZHEIMER'S DISEASE PATHOLOGY

TREM2 (Triggering Receptor Expressed on Myeloid Cells 2) plays a significant role in the pathology of AD [14, 16]. TREM2 is involved in microglial activation, survival, proliferation, and their ability to respond to brain damage. TREM2 activation interacts with its co-receptor, DNAX-activating protein of 12 kDa (DAP12), triggering intracellular signaling pathways that regulate microglial functions [17, 18]. Mutations in the TREM2 gene (*e.g.*, R47H and R62H) are associated with an increased risk of late-onset Alzheimer's disease. These mutations impair TREM2's function, reducing its ability to interact with ligands and impairing microglial responses to amyloid-beta (Aβ) plaques and other pathological stimuli [19, 20]. TREM2 plays a crucial role in microglial response to amyloid-beta plaques. TREM2 facilitates microglial clustering around Aβ plaques, limiting their spread and associated damage. It enhances the ability of microglia to phagocytose Aβ, reducing plaque burden.TREM2 signaling helps regulate inflammatory responses to Aβ, balancing the protective and damaging effects of inflammation [21, 22]. Emerging evidence suggests that TREM2 is involved in tau pathology, as microglia expressing TREM2 are associated with regions of tau accumulation. Dysregulated TREM2 signaling may impair microglial ability to respond effectively to tau aggregates, contributing to neurodegeneration. TREM2 modulates microglial inflammatory responses, promotes anti-inflammatory phenotypes in microglia, and mitigates neuroinflammation. Mutations in TREM2 result in hyperactive or insufficient inflammatory responses, exacerbating neuronal damage. TREM2 plays a role in lipid metabolism, critical for microglial survival and function. Impaired TREM2 signaling disrupts lipid sensing and handling, leading to dysfunctional microglia in AD [23, 24]. TREM2's role in AD is a promising therapeutic target. TREM2 Agonists help to enhance microglial activity and improve responses to Aβ and tau. Gene Therapy approaches to restore normal TREM2 function in individuals with mutations. The biomarker potential of TREM2 levels in cerebrospinal fluid (CSF) and plasma is being explored for monitoring Alzheimer's disease (AD) progression and treatment response [23, 25]. TREM2 is a critical regulator of microglial function in Alzheimer's disease. Its role in amyloid and tau pathology, as well as neuroinflammation, makes it a pivotal player in disease progression. Understanding TREM2 signaling pathways offers opportunities to develop novel treatments to slow or halt AD progression [26, 27]. Genetic association with AD variants in the TREM2 gene has been identified as a significant risk factor for late-onset AD. The R47H variant of TREM2 is one of the most notable mutations associated with a 2-4 times increased risk of AD.

This genetic link underscores the importance of TREM2 in modulating disease susceptibility [23]. TREM2 is a critical regulator of microglial activity in the brain. It influences key processes related to AD pathology, like TREM2, which is required for the stimulation of microglia in response to brain damage or the presence of Aβ plaques. It promotes the clearance of Aβ aggregates and apoptotic cells, preventing the buildup of toxic materials in the brain. TREM2 enhances microglial energy metabolism, allowing these cells to function effectively in the high-stress AD environment [23, 27].

TREM2 deficiency impairs microglial clustering around Aβ plaques, leading to increased plaque burden and toxicity. Microglia with functional TREM2 form protective barriers around plaques, mitigating the spread of toxic Aβ species into surrounding tissues [27]. Emerging evidence suggests that TREM2 also modulates microglial responses to tau pathology, another hallmark of AD.

TREM2 deficiency exacerbates tau-related neurodegeneration by reducing microglial-mediated clearance and increasing inflammation [28]. TREM2 acts as a regulator of neuroinflammatory responses. While activation of TREM2 can suppress excessive inflammation, its dysfunction or deficiency may lead to uncontrolled inflammatory responses, contributing to neuronal damage [29 - 31].

TREM2 Agonists: Targeting TREM2 signaling with agonists is a promising therapeutic strategy to enhance microglial protective functions.

Biomarkers: Soluble TREM2 (sTREM2), a cleavage product of the receptor, is being investigated as a biomarker for microglial activation and disease progression in AD [32].

Therapeutic approaches targeting TREM2 hold the potential to mitigate disease progression by enhancing the brain's immune defense mechanisms [33]. TREM2 is a transmembrane receptor expressed on microglia in the central nervous system (CNS) and on macrophages in peripheral tissues. Its role in AD involves regulating immune responses to amyloid-beta (Aβ) plaques and tau aggregates [34]. TREM2 is activated upon binding to ligands such as lipids, Aβ, apolipoprotein E (ApoE), and debris from damaged cells. TREM2 signals *via* the adaptor protein DAP12, which contains an immune receptor tyrosine-based activation motif (ITAM). Ligand binding leads to DAP12 phosphorylation, activating SYK (spleen tyrosine kinase) and triggering pathways like PI3K/AKT and ERK, which regulate cell survival, metabolism, and phagocytic activity. REM2 supports microglial clustering around Aβ plaques.

It enhances phagocytosis, facilitating the clearance of Aβ aggregates and apoptotic neurons. TREM2 activation induces a metabolic shift in microglia, enabling energy-demanding responses to neurodegenerative stress [35]. TREM2 expression in macrophages contributes to clearing peripheral debris and modulating inflammatory responses. Peripheral macrophages may also infiltrate the CNS during AD and complement microglial functions in clearing Aβ and tau aggregates. Mutations in the TREM2 gene (*e.g.*, R47H) impair signaling, reducing microglial/macrophage responses. Deficient TREM2 activity results in impaired phagocytosis of Aβ and tau aggregates, increased neuroinflammation due to ineffective resolution of damage, and enhanced neuronal vulnerability to toxic protein accumulations.

NEUROINFLAMMATION IN ALZHEIMER'S DISEASE: STRUCTURAL AND FUNCTIONAL IMPLICATIONS

Neuroinflammation in AD leads to both functional and structural consequences that significantly contribute to the progression and severity of the disease. Understanding these consequences is essential for developing therapeutic strategies to mitigate the impact of neuroinflammation in AD.

Functional Consequences

Synaptic Dysfunction

Synaptic dysfunction is a key feature of neuroinflammation in AD, significantly contributing to cognitive decline. Neuroinflammation, driven by activated microglia and astrocytes, leads to the release of pro-inflammatory cytokines like TNF-α, IL-1β, and IL-6, which disrupt synaptic signalling and plasticity. These cytokines can impair long-term potentiation (LTP), a process crucial for learning and memory, by altering neurotransmitter release, receptor function, and dendritic spine structure. Moreover, neuroinflammatory mediators exacerbate amyloid-beta (Aβ) and tau pathology, which further disrupts synaptic function. The resulting synaptic loss and dysfunction give rise to the characteristic amnesia and cognitive decline detected in AD, making the interplay between neuroinflammation and synaptic dysfunction a critical aspect of the disease's progression [3].

Neuronal Excitotoxicity

Neuronal excitotoxicity is an analytic consequence of neuroinflammation in AD, contributing to neuronal injury and death. In the AD brain, chronic neuroinflammation leads to the excessive release of glutamate, an excitatory neurotransmitter. This excessive glutamate release overstimulates NMDA (N-methyl-D-aspartate) receptors on neurons, resulting in prolonged calcium influx. Elevated intracellular calcium levels trigger a cascade of events, including mitochondrial dysfunction, oxidative stress, and activation of cell death pathways, ultimately leading to neuronal apoptosis. Excitotoxicity is further exacerbated by the inflammatory milieu, where pro-inflammatory cytokines such as TNF-α and IL-1β enhance glutamate release and impair glutamate reuptake by astrocytes. This process contributes significantly to synaptic dysfunction, neuronal loss, and cognitive decline in AD [36].

Impaired Neurogenesis

Impaired neurogenesis is a significant effect of neuroinflammation in AD, contributing to the progressive cognitive decline associated with the disease. In the AD brain, chronic neuroinflammation, characterized by the sustained mobilization of microglia and astrocytes, leads to the release of IL-1β, TNF-α, and IL-6. These cytokines negatively affect the neurogenic niches in the hippocampus, particularly the subgranular zone of the dentate gyrus, where they inhibit the proliferation, differentiation, and survival of neural progenitor cells. The impaired neurogenesis results in reduced hippocampal plasticity and decreased integration of new neurons into existing circuits, which are crucial for learning and memory. This disruption of neurogenesis exacerbates the cognitive deficits seen in AD, linking neuroinflammation directly to the neurodegenerative processes [37].

Altered Neural Connectivity

Altered neural connectivity is an afflictive consequence of neuroinflammation in Alzheimer's disease (AD), significantly contributing to the cognitive decline observed in the disease. In AD, chronic neuroinflammation, driven by activated microglia and astrocytes, disrupts the structural and functional integrity of neural networks. Pro-inflammatory cytokines interfere with synaptic function and ductility. This altered connectivity manifests as impaired communication between brain regions, particularly in networks associated with memory and cognition, such as the default mode network (DMN) and the hippocampal-prefrontal cortex circuitry. The breakdown in these connections results in deficits in memory, attention, and executive function, which are characteristic of AD. Thus, neuroinflammation-induced changes in neural connectivity play a central role in the progression of cognitive impairment in AD [38].

Structural Consequences

Neuronal Loss

The structural consequences of neuronal loss due to neuroinflammation in AD are marked by significant brain atrophy. Chronic neuroinflammation, driven by persistent activation of microglia and astrocytes, leads to the release of pro-inflammatory cytokines like IL-1β and TNF-α, which contribute to neuronal death through mechanisms including oxidative stress and excitotoxicity. This neuronal loss results in a reduction of gray matter volume, cortical thinning, and ventricular enlargement. These structural changes correlate with the severity of cognitive decline in AD, as the loss of neurons disrupts neural circuits essential for memory, learning, and executive function. The resulting brain atrophy is a hallmark of AD progression and is associated with the worsening of clinical symptoms over time [39].

White Matter Damage

White matter damage in Alzheimer's disease (AD) leads to significant structural changes that impair cognitive function. In AD, the degeneration of white matter, which consists of myelinated axons connecting different brain regions, is driven by amyloid-beta (Aβ) accumulation, tau pathology, and vascular changes. This damage is evident as white matter lesions, reduced white matter volume, and decreased integrity of white matter tracts, particularly in regions like the corpus callosum and frontal lobes. These structural alterations disrupt communication between brain regions, leading to a breakdown in the neural networks essential for memory, attention, and executive functions. The resulting disconnection between brain areas contributes to the cognitive decline and behavioural symptoms characteristic of AD, making white matter damage a critical aspect of the disease's pathology [40].

Blood-brain Barrier (BBB) Disruption

Blood-brain barrier (BBB) disruption is a significant pathological feature of Alzheimer's disease (AD), contributing to the progression of neurodegeneration. The BBB, which normally regulates the passage of molecules between the bloodstream and the brain, becomes compromised in AD due to chronic neuroinflammation, amyloid-beta (Aβ) accumulation, and vascular dysfunction. This disruption is characterized by increased permeability, allowing harmful substances such as toxins, pathogens, and immune cells to enter the brain. The leakage of blood-derived proteins like fibrinogen into the brain parenchyma further exacerbates inflammation and promotes neuronal injury. Additionally, impaired clearance of Aβ across the BBB leads to its accumulation, aggravating amyloid pathology. The breakdown of the BBB thus accelerates neuroinflammatory processes, neuronal damage, and cognitive decline in AD [41].

Astrocyte and Microglia Activation

The activation of astrocytes and microglia in Alzheimer's disease (AD) leads to significant structural consequences that contribute to neurodegeneration and cognitive decline. In AD, these glial cells become chronically activated in response to amyloid-beta (Aβ) plaques, tau tangles, and other pathological stimuli. Activated astrocytes and microglia release a variety of pro-inflammatory cytokines, chemokines, and reactive oxygen species (ROS), which induce neuronal damage and apoptosis. This glial activation also disrupts the homeostatic functions of astrocytes, including their roles in maintaining the blood-brain barrier (BBB), regulating synaptic function, and clearing extracellular glutamate and Aβ. The resulting structural changes include synaptic loss, white matter damage, and cortical thinning, all of which impair neural connectivity and brain function. The persistent activation of astrocytes and microglia thus accelerates the structural degeneration of the brain in AD, driving disease progression [42, 43].

ANTI-INFLAMMATORY DRUG STUDIES

Chronic neuroinflammation is a hallmark of Alzheimer's disease, driven by the activation of microglia and astrocytes, as well as the release of pro-inflammatory cytokines in response to amyloid-beta (Aβ) plaques and tau tangles. Anti-inflammatory drugs aim to modulate this neuroinflammatory response, potentially slowing disease progression and alleviating symptoms. Anti-inflammatory drugs target pathways involved in inflammation to reduce neuronal damage. These mechanisms include inhibiting pro-inflammatory cytokines such as IL-1β, IL-6, and TNF-α, which are elevated in AD. Certain drugs promote a shift from a pro-inflammatory to a more protective microglial state. Anti-inflammatory agents may also alleviate inflammation-induced oxidative damage [44].

Anti-inflammatory drugs have been studied as therapeutic scaffolds for AD due to the recognized role of neuroinflammation in its pathogenesis. Here are some key studies and findings related to anti-inflammatory drug studies in AD:

Non-steroidal Anti-inflammatory Drugs (NSAIDs)

Non-steroidal anti-inflammatory drugs (NSAIDs) have been explored as a probable treatment for AD due to their capability to reduce inflammation. Some epidemiological studies have suggested that long-term use of NSAIDs may be associated with a reduced risk of developing AD. However, clinical trials have yielded mixed results, with most showing no significant cognitive benefit in patients with established AD. A notable example is the ADAPT (Alzheimer's Disease Anti-Inflammatory Prevention Trial), which indicated that NSAIDs like naproxen and celecoxib did not slow cognitive decline in patients with mild cognitive impairment or early AD. The current understanding is that while NSAIDs may offer some protective effect if taken before the onset of AD symptoms, they are not effective as a treatment for those already diagnosed with the disease [45, 46].

Corticosteroids

Corticosteroids, known for their potent anti-inflammatory and immunosuppressive properties, have been explored as a potential treatment for Alzheimer's disease (AD) due to the role of neuroinflammation in AD pathogenesis. The rationale is that corticosteroids might reduce the inflammatory processes associated with amyloid-beta accumulation and tau pathology, key features of AD. However, clinical studies and trials have largely shown that corticosteroids, such as prednisone and dexamethasone, do not provide significant cognitive benefits in AD patients. Corticosteroids may even worsen outcomes due to their side effects, including cognitive impairment, mood changes, and increased risk of infections and osteoporosis. For example, a study by Aisen *et al.* (2000) found that low-dose prednisone did not improve cognitive function and was associated with adverse effects, suggesting that corticosteroids are not a viable therapeutic option for AD [47].

Disease-modifying Anti-rheumatic Drugs (DMARDs)

Disease-modifying anti-rheumatic drugs (DMARDs), primarily used to treat inflammatory and autoimmune conditions like rheumatoid arthritis, have gained interest as potential treatments for Alzheimer's disease (AD) due to their anti-inflammatory and immunomodulatory effects. Given that neuroinflammation is a critical component of AD pathology, researchers have hypothesized that DMARDs might mitigate the inflammatory responses contributing to neuronal damage in AD. Studies investigating drugs like methotrexate, hydroxychloroquine, and leflunomide have yielded mixed results. A study showed that methotrexate could reduce neuroinflammation and improve cognitive outcomes in animal models of AD. However, clinical trials in humans are limited, and the available evidence does not yet support the routine use of DMARDs in AD patients. The varying mechanisms of different DMARDs and their side effects necessitate further investigation to determine their potential role in AD management [48].

Immunomodulatory Agents

Immunomodulatory agents have emerged as a promising approach for the treatment of Alzheimer's disease (AD) due to their potential to modulate neuroinflammation, a key factor in AD pathogenesis. These agents work by altering the immune response to reduce the chronic inflammation that contributes to amyloid-beta accumulation and tau protein hyperphosphorylation, which are hallmarks of AD. Drugs such as fingolimod, a sphingosine-1-phosphate receptor modulator, and azathioprine have shown some promise in preclinical studies for their ability to reduce neuroinflammatory markers and improve cognitive function in animal models of AD. For instance, studies on fingolimod have demonstrated its neuroprotective effects by reducing microglial activation and promoting neurogenesis. However, while these preliminary findings are encouraging, clinical trials in humans are still in their early stages, and the safety, efficacy, and long-term effects of immunomodulatory agents in AD patients require further evaluation [49].

Microglial Inhibitors

Microglial inhibitors are being explored as potential therapeutic agents for AD. Activated microglia can release interleukins and other neurotoxic factors that contribute to amyloid-beta plaque formation and tau pathology, key features of AD. Inhibitors targeting microglial activation, such as minocycline and PLX3397 (a CSF1R inhibitor), aim to reduce this inflammatory response and protect neurons from damage. Studies have shown that minocycline can decrease microglial activation and boost impartial function in animal models of AD.

Similarly, PLX3397 has demonstrated the ability to deplete microglia, reduce amyloid-beta accumulation, and mitigate synaptic loss in preclinical studies. However, while these findings are promising, clinical trials are needed to establish the safety, efficacy, and appropriate use of microglial inhibitors in AD patients [50].

Peroxisome Proliferator-activated Receptor (PPAR) Agonists

Peroxisome proliferator-activated receptor (PPAR) agonists have been investigated as potential therapeutic agents for Alzheimer's disease (AD) due to their anti-inflammatory, neuroprotective, and metabolic-modulating properties. PPARs are nuclear receptors that regulate gene expression involved in inflammation, glucose metabolism, and lipid homeostasis, processes that are disrupted in AD. Agonists such as pioglitazone (a PPAR-γ agonist) and fenofibrate (a PPAR-α agonist) have been shown to reduce amyloid-beta accumulation, tau phosphorylation, and neuroinflammation in preclinical studies. For instance, pioglitazone has demonstrated the ability to enhance mitochondrial function and reduce cognitive decline in animal models of AD. However, while some early clinical trials suggested potential cognitive benefits, larger trials like the TOMMORROW study have not confirmed significant efficacy in delaying the onset of mild cognitive impairment or AD. Consequently, while PPAR agonists show promise in preclinical models, further studies are needed to clarify their therapeutic potential and optimal use in AD [51, 52]

Cytokine Modulators

Cytokine modulators are being studied as potential therapies for Alzheimer's disease (AD) because of their ability to regulate the inflammatory responses that contribute to AD pathogenesis. In AD, pro-inflammatory cytokines like tumour necrosis factor-alpha (TNF-α), interleukin-1 beta (IL-1β), and interleukin-6 (IL-6) are elevated, promoting neuroinflammation and neuronal damage. Cytokine modulators, such as etanercept (a TNF-α inhibitor) and tocilizumab (an IL-6 receptor antagonist), aim to reduce this harmful inflammation. For example, preclinical studies have shown that etanercept can reduce amyloid-beta accumulation, neuroinflammation, and synaptic dysfunction in animal models of AD. However, while these findings are encouraging, clinical trials in humans are still limited, and results have been mixed. Further research is required to evaluate the efficacy, safety, and appropriate patient selection for cytokine modulators in AD treatment [53].

THE FUTURE DIRECTIONS OF CLINICAL RESEARCH ON THE EFFECTS OF INFLAMMATION IN AD

The future directions of clinical research on the role of inflammation in AD aim to deepen understanding, improve therapeutic strategies, and refine treatment approaches. These are as follows:

Understanding the Molecular and Cellular Mechanisms of Inflammation in AD

One of the major future directions involves deepening our understanding of the molecular and cellular mechanisms that underlie neuroinflammation in AD. Research will focus on recognizing specific inflammatory pathways and immune cell types involved in the progression of AD. For example, microglia and astrocytes, the resident immune cells of the central nervous system (CNS), play pivotal roles in neuroinflammatory responses. Studies will likely delve deeper into how these cells interact with amyloid-beta (Aβ) plaques and tau tangles, and how this interplay contributes to disease progression. Emerging evidence suggests that distinct subtypes of microglia and astrocytes may either exacerbate or protect against neurodegeneration, suggesting a nuanced role of these cells that warrants further exploration [3, 54].

Biomarker Discovery and Validation for Early Diagnosis and Monitoring

Another promising direction is the discovery and validation of inflammatory biomarkers for the early diagnosis and monitoring of AD. Inflammatory cytokines, chemokines, and other immune-related molecules could serve as potential biomarkers that reflect disease activity and progression. Advances in high-throughput technologies, such as proteomics and transcriptomics, are expected to play a crucial role in identifying novel biomarkers. Furthermore, combining these biomarkers with existing imaging and cerebrospinal fluid (CSF) biomarkers may improve the sensitivity and specificity of early AD diagnosis [55, 56].

Targeting Inflammatory Pathways for Therapeutic Interventions

Targeting inflammatory pathways as a therapeutic strategy is a rapidly evolving area of AD research. Recent clinical trials have explored the use of anti-inflammatory drugs, such as non-steroidal anti-inflammatory drugs (NSAIDs), monoclonal antibodies targeting pro-inflammatory cytokines, and inhibitors of the NLRP3 inflammasome pathway. Future trials are likely to focus on more selective and targeted approaches to modulate neuroinflammation, potentially reducing adverse effects and improving therapeutic efficacy. Additionally, repurposing existing drugs with anti-inflammatory properties is an area of active investigation [57, 58].

Role of the Gut-brain Axis in Neuroinflammation and AD

The gut-brain axis and its role in neuroinflammation are an emerging field of interest in AD research. The gut microbiome influences systemic and CNS inflammation, and dysbiosis has been linked to neurodegenerative diseases, including AD. Future research may investigate how specific microbial metabolites and ingredients, such as short-chain fatty acids and lipopolysaccharides, modulate neuroinflammatory processes. Clinical trials may also explore interventions like probiotics, prebiotics, or dietary modifications to alter the gut microbiota composition, potentially reducing neuroinflammation and slowing AD progression [59, 60].

Exploring the Impact of Lifestyle Interventions on Neuroinflammation

Lifestyle interventions, such as physical exercise, dietary changes, and cognitive training, have been shown to have anti-inflammatory effects and may influence the course of AD. Future clinical trials will likely examine how these interventions can modulate neuroinflammatory markers and cognitive decline in AD patients. Understanding the molecular mechanisms behind these benefits may lead to the development of personalized lifestyle interventions as a part of a multi-targeted strategy against AD [61, 62].

Gene-environment Interactions and Personalized Medicine Approaches

Lastly, understanding gene-environment interactions is crucial for developing personalized medicine approaches in AD treatment. Genetic predispositions, such as variations in the APOE gene, influence an individual's risk of developing AD and their response to therapies. Future studies will likely explore how these genetic factors interact with environmental factors, such as diet, stress, and infections, to influence neuroinflammatory responses. This knowledge could pave the way for personalized interventions targeting inflammation based on an individual's genetic and environmental risk profile [63, 64].

CONCLUSION

The exploration of inflammation's role in AD has significantly deepened our understanding of the disease's pathogenesis and opened new avenues for potential therapeutic interventions. Here are the key takeaways:

- **Therapeutic Potential of Anti-inflammatory Approaches**

Despite mixed results in clinical trials, there is a promising potential for anti-inflammatory drugs in AD treatment. Targeted therapies, personalized medicine approaches, and combination therapies may enhance the efficacy and safety of these treatments [54].

- **Advances in Biomarker Development**

The development of reliable biomarkers for neuroinflammation is crucial for early diagnosis, monitoring disease progression, and assessing treatment responses. Advances in imaging techniques and blood-based biomarkers hold promise for improving the clinical management of AD [56].

- **Importance of Early and Preventive Interventions**

Early intervention and preventive strategies targeting inflammation in high-risk individuals could delay or prevent the onset of AD. Longitudinal studies are necessary to evaluate the long-term benefits of these approaches [65].

- **Mechanistic Understanding and Research Directions**

Continued research is needed to elucidate the precise mechanisms by which inflammation drives AD pathology. Investigating the roles of specific inflammatory pathways, the gut-brain axis, and systemic inflammation will provide deeper insights and guide therapeutic development [42].

- **Collaborative Efforts and Data Sharing**

Collaborative research between academic institutions, pharmaceutical companies, and regulatory agencies is essential to accelerate progress in this field. Promoting data sharing and integration across studies will enhance the understanding of inflammation in AD and improve the design of future clinical trials [66].

- **Patient-centred Research**

Patient-centered research in AD focuses on integrating the perspectives, needs, and preferences of patients and their caregivers to improve care and outcomes. This approach involves developing personalized interventions that consider individual differences, incorporating patient-reported outcomes (PROs) in clinical trials to ensure meaningful endpoints, and fostering shared decision-making among patients, caregivers, and healthcare providers. Digital health tools, such as mobile applications and telemedicine, are also being leveraged to enhance patient engagement and monitoring. Furthermore, engaging patients and caregivers in the design and implementation of research studies ensures that research questions and methodologies are aligned with patient priorities, enhancing the relevance and acceptability of the research [67].

The recognition of inflammation as an important factor in AD has transformed our approach to understanding and treating this complex condition. While challenges remain, the integration of anti-inflammatory strategies with other therapeutic approaches, advancements in biomarker development, and personalized medicine hold promise for improving outcomes for individuals affected by AD. Continued efforts to understand and modulate the inflammatory response in AD are likely to yield significant advancements in the prevention, diagnosis, and treatment of this devastating disease. By focusing on early intervention, targeted therapies, and collaborative research, the field moves closer to achieving meaningful progress in combating AD.

REFERENCES

[1] Akiyama H, Barger S, Barnum S, *et al.* Inflammation and Alzheimer's disease. Neurobiol Aging 2000; 21(3): 383-421.
[http://dx.doi.org/10.1016/S0197-4580(00)00124-X] [PMID: 10858586]

[2] Zhang Q, Yu JT, Zhu QX, *et al.* Complement receptor 1 polymorphisms and risk of late-onset Alzheimer's disease. Brain Res 2010; 1348: 216-21.
[http://dx.doi.org/10.1016/j.brainres.2010.06.018] [PMID: 20558149]

[3] Lee CY, Landreth GE. The role of microglia in amyloid clearance from the AD brain. J Neural Transm (Vienna). 2010 Aug; 117(8): 949-60.

[4] Ising C, Venegas C, Zhang S, *et al.* NLRP3 inflammasome activation drives tau pathology. Nature 2019; 575(7784): 669-73.
[http://dx.doi.org/10.1038/s41586-019-1769-z] [PMID: 31748742]

[5] García Bueno B, Caso JR, Madrigal JLM, Leza JC. Innate immune receptor Toll-like receptor 4 signalling in neuropsychiatric diseases. Neurosci Biobehav Rev 2016; 64: 134-47.
[http://dx.doi.org/10.1016/j.neubiorev.2016.02.013] [PMID: 26905767]

[6] Walter S, Letiembre M, Liu Y, *et al.* Role of the toll-like receptor 4 in neuroinflammation in Alzheimer's disease. Cell Physiol Biochem 2007; 20(6): 947-56.
[http://dx.doi.org/10.1159/000110455] [PMID: 17982277]

[7] Eikelenboom P, Veerhuis R. The role of complement and activated microglia in the pathogenesis of Alzheimer's disease. Neurobiol Aging 1996; 17(5): 673-80.
[http://dx.doi.org/10.1016/0197-4580(96)00108-X] [PMID: 8892339]

[8] Tenner A. Complement in Alzheimer's disease: opportunities for modulating protective and pathogenic events. Neurobiol Aging 2001; 22(6): 849-61.
[http://dx.doi.org/10.1016/S0197-4580(01)00301-3] [PMID: 11754992]

[9] Swardfager W, Lanctôt K, Rothenburg L, Wong A, Cappell J, Herrmann N. A meta-analysis of cytokines in Alzheimer's disease. Biol Psychiatry 2010; 68(10): 930-41.
[http://dx.doi.org/10.1016/j.biopsych.2010.06.012] [PMID: 20692646]

[10] Stolp HB, Dziegielewska KM. Review: Role of developmental inflammation and blood–brain barrier dysfunction in neurodevelopmental and neurodegenerative diseases. Neuropathol Appl Neurobiol 2009; 35(2): 132-46.
[http://dx.doi.org/10.1111/j.1365-2990.2008.01005.x] [PMID: 19077110]

[11] Kaltschmidt B, Czaniera NJ, Schulten W, Kaltschmidt C. NF-κB in alzheimer's disease: Friend or foe? opposite functions in neurons and glial cells. Int J Mol Sci 2024; 25(21): 11353.
[http://dx.doi.org/10.3390/ijms252111353] [PMID: 39518906]

[12] Jain M, Singh MK, Shyam H, *et al.* Role of JAK/STAT in the neuroinflammation and its association with neurological disorders. Ann Neurosci 2021; 28(3-4): 191-200.
[http://dx.doi.org/10.1177/09727531211070532] [PMID: 35341232]

[13] Munoz L, Ammit AJ. Targeting p38 MAPK pathway for the treatment of Alzheimer's disease. Neuropharmacology 2010; 58(3): 561-8.
[http://dx.doi.org/10.1016/j.neuropharm.2009.11.010] [PMID: 19951717]

[14] Zhu X, Lee H, Raina AK, Perry G, Smith MA. The role of mitogen-activated protein kinase pathways in Alzheimer's disease. Neurosignals 2002; 11(5): 270-81.
[http://dx.doi.org/10.1159/000067426] [PMID: 12566928]

[15] Paloneva J, Mandelin J, Kiialainen A, *et al.* DAP12/TREM2 deficiency results in impaired osteoclast differentiation and osteoporotic features. J Exp Med 2003; 198(4): 669-75.
[http://dx.doi.org/10.1084/jem.20030027] [PMID: 12925681]

[16] Paloneva J, Kestilä M, Wu J, *et al.* Loss-of-function mutations in TYROBP (DAP12) result in a presenile dementia with bone cysts. Nat Genet 2000; 25(3): 357-61.
[http://dx.doi.org/10.1038/77153] [PMID: 10888890]

[17] Kaneko M, Sano K, Nakayama J, Amano N. Nasu-Hakola disease: The first case reported by Nasu and review. Neuropathology 2010; 30(5): 463-70.
[http://dx.doi.org/10.1111/j.1440-1789.2010.01127.x] [PMID: 20500450]

[18] Sessa G, Podini P, Mariani M, *et al.* Distribution and signaling of TREM2/DAP12, the receptor system mutated in human polycystic lipomembraneous osteodysplasia with sclerosing leukoencephalopathy dementia. Eur J Neurosci 2004; 20(10): 2617-28.
[http://dx.doi.org/10.1111/j.1460-9568.2004.03729.x] [PMID: 15548205]

[19] Guerreiro R, Wojtas A, Bras J, *et al.* TREM2 variants in Alzheimer's disease. N Engl J Med 2013; 368(2): 117-27.
[http://dx.doi.org/10.1056/NEJMoa1211851] [PMID: 23150934]

[20] Jonsson T, Stefansson H, Steinberg S, *et al.* Variant of TREM2 associated with the risk of Alzheimer's disease. N Engl J Med 2013; 368(2): 107-16.
[http://dx.doi.org/10.1056/NEJMoa1211103] [PMID: 23150908]

[21] Saunders AM, Strittmatter WJ, Schmechel D, *et al.* Association of apolipoprotein E allele ϵ 4 with late-onset familial and sporadic Alzheimer's disease. Neurology 1993; 43(8): 1467-72.
[http://dx.doi.org/10.1212/WNL.43.8.1467] [PMID: 8350998]

[22] Corder EH, Saunders AM, Strittmatter WJ, *et al.* Gene dose of apolipoprotein E type 4 allele and the risk of Alzheimer's disease in late onset families. Science 1993; 261(5123): 921-3.
[http://dx.doi.org/10.1126/science.8346443] [PMID: 8346443]

[23] Jay TR, Miller CM, Cheng PJ, *et al.* TREM2 deficiency eliminates TREM2+ inflammatory macrophages and ameliorates pathology in Alzheimer's disease mouse models. J Exp Med 2015; 212(3): 287-95.
[http://dx.doi.org/10.1084/jem.20142322] [PMID: 25732305]

[24] Henjum K, Almdahl IS, Årskog V, Minthon L, Hansson O, Fladby T, Nilsson LN. Cerebrospinal fluid soluble TREM2 in aging and Alzheimer's disease. Alzheimer's research & therapy. 2016 Apr 27; 8(1): 17.

[25] Suárez-Calvet M, Kleinberger G, Araque Caballero MÁ, Brendel M, Rominger A, Alcolea D, Fortea J, Lleó A, Blesa R, Gispert JD, Sánchez-Valle R. sTREM2 cerebrospinal fluid levels are a potential biomarker for microglia activity in early-stage Alzheimer's disease and associate with neuronal injury markers. EMBO molecular medicine. 2016 May 1; 8(5): 466-76.

[26] Tan YJ, Ng ASL, Vipin A, *et al.* Higher peripheral trem2 mrna levels relate to cognitive deficits and hippocampal atrophy in alzheimer's disease and amnestic mild cognitive impairment. J Alzheimers Dis 2017; 58(2): 413-23.
[http://dx.doi.org/10.3233/JAD-161277] [PMID: 28453482]

[27] Hu N, Tan MS, Yu JT, *et al.* Increased expression of TREM2 in peripheral blood of Alzheimer's disease patients. J Alzheimers Dis 2013; 38(3): 497-501.
[http://dx.doi.org/10.3233/JAD-130854] [PMID: 24002183]

[28] Gratuze M, Schlachetzki JC, Albanus RD, *et al.* TREM2-independent microgliosis promotes tau-mediated neurodegeneration in the presence of ApoE4. Neuron. 2023 111(2): 202-19.

[29] Yu H, Zhang L, Song B, Ren K, *et al.* TREM2-mediated regulation of microglial activity: a promising target for the treatment of ischemic stroke. J Transl Med. 2025 Jul 11; 23(1): 782.

[30] Cantoni C, Bollman B, Licastro D, *et al.* TREM2 regulates microglial cell activation in response to demyelination *in vivo*. Acta Neuropathol 2015; 129(3): 429-47.
[http://dx.doi.org/10.1007/s00401-015-1388-1] [PMID: 25631124]

[31] Poliani PL, Wang Y, Fontana E, *et al.* TREM2 sustains microglial expansion during aging and response to demyelination. J Clin Invest 2015; 125(5): 2161-70.
[http://dx.doi.org/10.1172/JCI77983] [PMID: 25893602]

[32] Ewers M, Biechele G, Suárez-Calvet M, *et al.* Higher CSF sTREM2 and microglia activation are associated with slower rates of beta-amyloid accumulation. EMBO Mol Med. 2020 Sep 7; 12(9): e12308.

[33] Ma YN, Hu X, Karako K, Song P, Tang W, Xia Y. The potential and challenges of TREM2-targeted therapy in Alzheimer's disease: Insights from the INVOKE-2 study. Front Aging Neurosci. 2025; 17: 1576020.
[http://dx.doi.org/10.3389/fnagi.2025.1576020]

[34] Leyns CEG, Ulrich JD, Finn MB, *et al.* TREM2 deficiency attenuates neuroinflammation and protects against neurodegeneration in a mouse model of tauopathy. Proc Natl Acad Sci USA 2017; 114(43): 11524-9.
[http://dx.doi.org/10.1073/pnas.1710311114] [PMID: 29073081]

[35] Shi Q, Gutierrez RA, Bhat MA. Microglia, Trem2, and Neurodegeneration. Neuroscientist. 2025 Apr; 31(2): 159-176.

[36] Dong X, Wang Y, Qin Z. Molecular mechanisms of excitotoxicity and their relevance to pathogenesis of neurodegenerative diseases. Acta Pharmacol Sin 2009; 30(4): 379-87.
[http://dx.doi.org/10.1038/aps.2009.24] [PMID: 19343058]

[37] Monje ML, Toda H, Palmer TD. Inflammatory blockade restores adult hippocampal neurogenesis. Science 2003; 302(5651): 1760-5.
[http://dx.doi.org/10.1126/science.1088417] [PMID: 14615545]

[38] Wang K, Liang M, Wang L, *et al.* Altered functional connectivity in early Alzheimer's disease: A resting-state fMRI study. Hum Brain Mapp 2007; 28(10): 967-78.
[http://dx.doi.org/10.1002/hbm.20324] [PMID: 17133390]

[39] Jack CR Jr, Knopman DS, Jagust WJ, *et al.* Hypothetical model of dynamic biomarkers of the Alzheimer's pathological cascade. Lancet Neurol 2010; 9(1): 119-28.
[http://dx.doi.org/10.1016/S1474-4422(09)70299-6] [PMID: 20083042]

[40] Braidy N, Muñoz P, Palacios AG, *et al.* Recent rodent models for Alzheimer's disease: clinical

implications and basic research. J Neural Transm (Vienna) 2012; 119(2): 173-95. [http://dx.doi.org/10.1007/s00702-011-0731-5] [PMID: 22086139]

[41] Zlokovic BV. Neurovascular pathways to neurodegeneration in Alzheimer's disease and other disorders. Nat Rev Neurosci 2011; 12(12): 723-38. [http://dx.doi.org/10.1038/nrn3114] [PMID: 22048062]

[42] Salter MW, Stevens B. Microglia emerge as central players in brain disease. Nat Med 2017; 23(9): 1018-27. [http://dx.doi.org/10.1038/nm.4397] [PMID: 28886007]

[43] Deng Q, Wu C, Parker E, Liu TCY, Duan R, Yang L. Microglia and astrocytes in alzheimer's disease: significance and summary of recent advances. Aging Dis 2023; 15(4): 0. [http://dx.doi.org/10.14336/AD.2023.0907] [PMID: 37815901]

[44] Martyn C. Anti-inflammatory drugs and Alzheimer's disease. BMJ 2003; 327(7411): 353-4. [http://dx.doi.org/10.1136/bmj.327.7411.353] [PMID: 12919966]

[45] Imbimbo BP, Solfrizzi V, Panza F. Are NSAIDs useful to treat Alzheimer's disease or mild cognitive impairment? Front Aging Neurosci 2010; 2: 19. [http://dx.doi.org/10.3389/fnagi.2010.00019] [PMID: 20725517]

[46] Martin BK, Szekely C, Brandt J, *et al.* Cognitive function over time in the Alzheimer's Disease Anti-inflammatory Prevention Trial (ADAPT): results of a randomized, controlled trial of naproxen and celecoxib. Arch Neurol 2008; 65(7): 896-905. [http://dx.doi.org/10.1001/archneur.2008.65.7.nct70006] [PMID: 18474729]

[47] Aisen PS, Davis KL, Berg JD, *et al.* A randomized controlled trial of prednisone in Alzheimer's disease. Neurology 2000; 54(3): 588-93. [http://dx.doi.org/10.1212/WNL.54.3.588] [PMID: 10680787]

[48] Judge A, Garriga C, Arden NK, *et al.* Protective effect of antirheumatic drugs on dementia in rheumatoid arthritis patients. Alzheimers Dement (N Y) 2017; 3(4): 612-21. [http://dx.doi.org/10.1016/j.trci.2017.10.002] [PMID: 29201995]

[49] Ransohoff RM. How neuroinflammation contributes to neurodegeneration. Science 2016; 353(6301): 777-83. [http://dx.doi.org/10.1126/science.aag2590] [PMID: 27540165]

[50] Heneka MT, Golenbock DT, Latz E. Innate immunity in Alzheimer's disease. Nat Immunol 2015; 16(3): 229-36. [http://dx.doi.org/10.1038/ni.3102] [PMID: 25689443]

[51] Sastre M, Dewachter I, Landreth GE, *et al.* Nonsteroidal anti-inflammatory drugs and peroxisome proliferator-activated receptor-γ agonists modulate immunostimulated processing of amyloid precursor protein through regulation of β-secretase. J Neurosci 2003; 23(30): 9796-804. [http://dx.doi.org/10.1523/JNEUROSCI.23-30-09796.2003] [PMID: 14586007]

[52] Risner ME, Saunders AM, Altman J F B, *et al.* Efficacy of rosiglitazone in a genetically defined population with mild-to-moderate Alzheimer's disease. Pharmacogenomics J 2006; 6(4): 246-54. [http://dx.doi.org/10.1038/sj.tpj.6500369] [PMID: 16446752]

[53] Decourt B, Lahiri DK, Sabbagh MN. Targeting tumor necrosis factor alpha for alzheimer's disease. Curr Alzheimer Res 2017; 14(4): 412-25. [http://dx.doi.org/10.2174/1567205013666160930110551] [PMID: 27697064]

[54] Vandenbark AA, Offner H, Matejuk S, Matejuk A. Microglia and astrocyte involvement in neurodegeneration and brain cancer. J Neuroinflammation. 2021 Dec 23; 18(1): 298.

[55] Park JC, Han SH, Mook-Jung I. Peripheral inflammatory biomarkers in Alzheimer's disease: a brief review. BMB Rep 2020; 53(1): 10-9. [http://dx.doi.org/10.5483/BMBRep.2020.53.1.309] [PMID: 31865964]

[56] Hampel H, O'Bryant SE, Castrillo JI, *et al.* Precision medicine—The golden gate for detection, treatment and prevention of Alzheimer's disease. J Prev Alzheimers Dis. 2016; 3(4): 243-259. [http://dx.doi.org/10.14283/jpad.2016.112]

[57] Bronzuoli MR, Iacomino A, Steardo L, Scuderi C. Targeting neuroinflammation in Alzheimer's disease. J Inflamm Res 2016; 9: 199-208. [http://dx.doi.org/10.2147/JIR.S86958] [PMID: 27843334]

[58] Heneka MT, Kummer MP, Stutz A, *et al.* NLRP3 is activated in Alzheimer's disease and contributes to pathology in APP/PS1 mice. Nature 2013; 493(7434): 674-8. [http://dx.doi.org/10.1038/nature11729] [PMID: 23254930]

[59] Vogt NM, Kerby RL, Dill-McFarland KA, *et al.* Gut microbiome alterations in Alzheimer's disease. Sci Rep 2017; 7(1): 13537. [http://dx.doi.org/10.1038/s41598-017-13601-y] [PMID: 29051531]

[60] Zhuang ZQ, Shen LL, Li WW, *et al.* Gut microbiota is altered in patients with alzheimer's disease. J Alzheimers Dis 2018; 63(4): 1337-46. [http://dx.doi.org/10.3233/JAD-180176] [PMID: 29758946]

[61] Quigley A, MacKay-Lyons M, Eskes G. Effects of Exercise on Cognitive Performance in Older Adults: A Narrative Review of the Evidence, Possible Biological Mechanisms, and Recommendations for Exercise Prescription. J Aging Res 2020; 2020: 1-15. [http://dx.doi.org/10.1155/2020/1407896] [PMID: 32509348]

[62] Gleeson M, Bishop NC, Stensel DJ, Lindley MR, Mastana SS, Nimmo MA. The anti-inflammatory effects of exercise: mechanisms and implications for the prevention and treatment of disease. Nat Rev Immunol 2011; 11(9): 607-15. [http://dx.doi.org/10.1038/nri3041] [PMID: 21818123]

[63] Liu CC, Kanekiyo T, Xu H, Bu G, Bu G. Apolipoprotein E and Alzheimer disease: risk, mechanisms and therapy. Nat Rev Neurol 2013; 9(2): 106-18. [http://dx.doi.org/10.1038/nrneurol.2012.263] [PMID: 23296339]

[64] Migliore L, Coppedè F. Gene–environment interactions in Alzheimer disease: the emerging role of epigenetics. Nat Rev Neurol 2022; 18(11): 643-60. [http://dx.doi.org/10.1038/s41582-022-00714-w] [PMID: 36180553]

[65] Gauthier S, Wu L, Rosa-Neto P, Jia J. Prevention strategies for Alzheimer's disease. Transl Neurodegener 2012; 1(1): 13. [http://dx.doi.org/10.1186/2047-9158-1-13] [PMID: 23210473]

[66] Miao J, Ma H, Yang Y, *et al.* Microglia in Alzheimer's disease: pathogenesis, mechanisms, and therapeutic potentials. Front Aging Neurosci 2023; 15: 1201982. [http://dx.doi.org/10.3389/fnagi.2023.1201982] [PMID: 37396657]

[67] Bethell J, Commisso E, Rostad HM, *et al.* Patient engagement in research related to dementia: A scoping review. Dementia 2018; 17(8): 944-75. [http://dx.doi.org/10.1177/1471301218789292] [PMID: 30373460]

CHAPTER 8

Nanotechnology-based Therapeutic Approach in Alzheimer's Disease

Rajdip Goswami[1], Priyanka Banerjee[1], Saptarshi Sanyal[1], Biswajit Basu[1,*] and Monosiz Rahaman[1]

[1] *Department of Pharmaceutical Technology, School of Health and Medical Sciences, Adamas University, Kolkata, West Bengal, India*

Abstract: Nanotechnology-based newer therapeutic approaches can take care of the numerous shortcomings of the present treatment modalities for Alzheimer's disease (AD). Conventional therapies usually fail at targeting neuronal cells effectively and crossing the Blood Brain Barrier (BBB), leading to a poor drug delivery system and undesirable side effects. So, the use of nanomaterials and nano-carriers such as liposomes, polymeric nanoparticles, and dendrimers can rejuvenate the drug-delivery system. This optimises BBB penetration and thereby specifically targets affected neurons, reducing side effects and increasing drug stability, controlled release, and bioavailability-all of which are crucial in treating neurodegenerative disorders like AD. In this regard, significant advancements have been made in nanoparticle formulations showing great promise in improving the pharmacokinetics and pharmacodynamics of anti-Alzheimer's drugs. For example, liposomal formulations protect drugs from degradation until they reach the brain, whereas polymeric nanoparticles permit sustained drug release so that therapeutic effects can be maintained over a longer duration. Dendrimers serve as a mouldable drug-delivery system due to their hyper-branched construction, capable of co-delivering several therapeutic agents. This review discusses the pharmacological implications of the nanotechnology-based treatment of AD by providing an overview of recent developments and clarifying the mechanisms involved in Action.

Keywords: Alzheimer's disease (AD), Blood brain barrier (BBB), Drug delivery, Nanotechnology, Nano carriers, Neurodegenerative diseases.

INTRODUCTION

Alzheimer's disease (AD) is one of the most difficult and debilitating neurological diseases of our day, with a substantial impact on international healthcare systems. This disorder, which mostly affects the ageing population, is characterised by a

* **Corresponding author Biswajit Basu:** Department of Pharmaceutical Technology, School of Health and Medical Sciences, Adamas University, Kolkata, West Bengal, India; E-mail: bbasu.pharma@gmail.com

Swarupananda Mukherjee, Souvik Roy & Dipanjan Karati (Eds.)

persistent deterioration in cognitive function, memory impairment, and significant behavioural abnormalities. As the illness worsens, people lose their freedom and quality of life, which puts a tremendous amount of emotional and financial strain on families and carers [1]. Remarkably limited is the therapy landscape for AD, despite decades of rigorous research and medical advances. The current therapies do not address the fundamental causes of the illness; instead, they provide momentary symptomatic alleviation. Patients' hope diminishes as the disease progresses because these medications are not able to stop or reverse the progression of AD [2]. The delivery of therapeutic drugs across the BBB, a barrier that selectively restricts the entry of elements into the brain, is one of the most severe obstacles to effective treatment. This has made it challenging to make significant advancements in the treatment of AD, especially in light of the systemic toxicity and restricted effectiveness of conventional medications [3]. The development of nanotechnology has created a new front in the fight against AD in light of these difficulties. With its capacity to modify materials at the molecular and atomic levels, nanotechnology presents previously unheard-of possibilities to transform medicinal strategies completely. Nanoparticles have some unique features: they are very small, have a large surface area, and can be specially designed to target certain areas of the body. These qualities make them useful for improving how medicines are delivered, especially for diseases like Alzheimer's. Scientists are using nanotechnology to find new ways to get drugs into the brain more effectively, reduce side effects, and help patients feel better. This chapter explores how nanotechnology is being used to fight Alzheimer's disease. It looks at the latest research and new materials that could lead to better, more targeted treatments. By studying these developments, we can get a clearer picture of how Alzheimer's might be treated in the future. Nanotechnology could change the way we understand and manage this complex condition [4].

Pathophysiology of Alzheimer's Disease

Among the regions with maximum neuronal loss and/or illness are the entorhinal cortex, hippocampus, amygdala, and cortical association areas of the frontal, temporal, and parietal cortices. The subcortical nuclei such as the serotonergic dorsal raphe, the noradrenergic locus coeruleus, and the cholinergic basal nucleus are also included in this group. The first tangles are found in the entorhinal and trans-entorhinal cortex, in the hippocampus CA1 region, and in cortical association regions, mostly concerning the frontal, parietal, and temporal lobes. When the amyloid plaque is less, the DSM is more tightly linked to the location and extent of tangle formation [5]. Cognitive impairment is hugely correlated with tau protein infarctions and cerebrum shrinkage, especially in the hippocampi. Neuronal death and atrophy occur in the temporofrontal cortex with Alzheimer 's-induced inflammation; amyloid deposits, an abnormal cluster of protein fragments, and twisted fibre bundles. This, in turn, raises the number of monocytes and macrophages in the cerebral cortex along with the activation of parenchymal microglial cells [6]. Fig. (1) illustrates the pathophysiology of AD, with a very detailed visual representation highlighting the processes and mechanisms that are key to the progression of the disease.

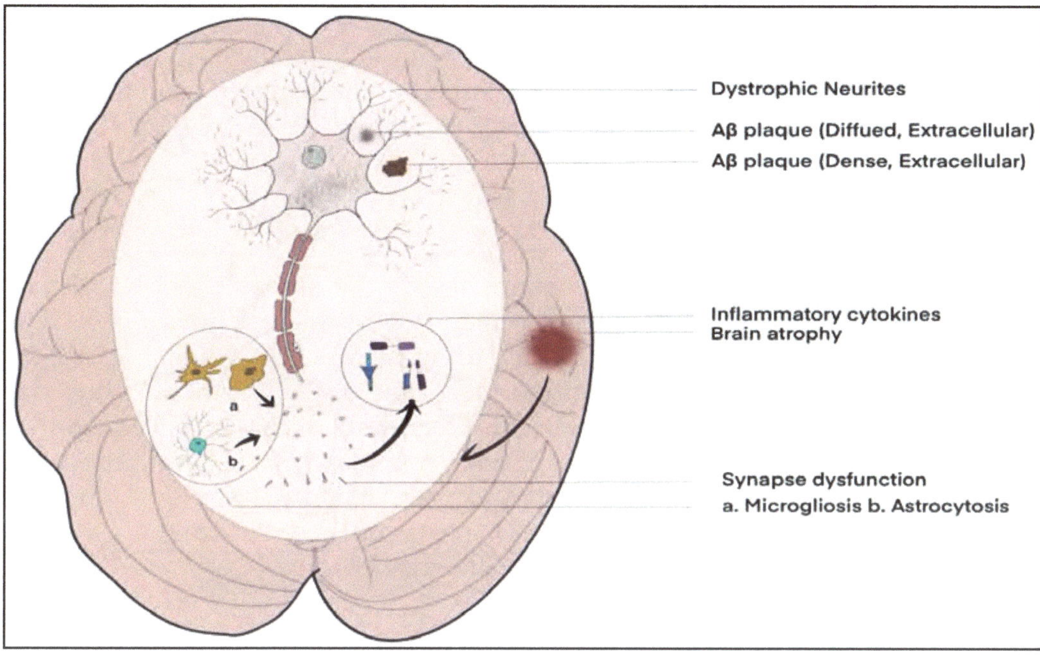

Fig. (1). Pathophysiology of AD

Hyperphosphorylated Tau Protein and Amyloid β Hypothesis

The appearance of senile deposits in the human brain and such accumulations represent one of the major pathogenic features of AD, with the formation of plaques due to amyloid beta (Aβ) depositions. Being subjected to α-α-secretase, β-secretase, and γ-secretase, the amyloid precursor protein (APP) produces small soluble peptides, which are Aβ. These different toxic oligomers- fibrils, plaques, and protofibrils- are generated when there is an imbalance in either clearing or forming β-amyloid (Aβ), depending on the concentration of oligomers. While some factors influencing it include sequence, concentration, and conditions affecting stability, the genuine source of Aβ is still a mystery [7]. Numerous variables, including oxidative stress/mitochondrial dysfunctions, amyloid/tau toxicity, and cholinergic dysfunction, are implicated in the aetiology of AD [8].

Oxidative Stress Hypothesis

Reactive Oxygen Species (ROS) and Reactive Nitrogen Species (RNS) are generated by a range of normal and pathological human processes. They have a dual role in useful cellular signalling pathways and toxic processes that can harm cellular components such as cell membranes, lipids, proteins, and DNA. The brain is particularly vulnerable to oxidative stress because it uses 20% more oxygen than other mitochondrial respiratory tissues. Polyunsaturated fatty acids constitute most of the neurons, the primary building material of the brain. It can initiate lipid peroxidation and molecular death by reacting with ROS. Also, low levels of reduced glutathione in neurons enhance oxidative stress [7].

Metal Ion Hypothesis

Neurodegenerative disorders and cancer are among the illnesses that have metal dyshomeostasis as a contributing factor to their genesis and progression. Several substances used in medicinal research, including metal chelators and ionophore chelators, are known to modify transition metal homeostasis. Not all drugs that aim to balance transition metals are molecules that bind to metals [9]. Concerning the data at hand, it is answered that redox transition metals have been changed in equilibrium, primarily copper, iron, and other trace metals. Brain levels of these metals were observed to be increased in AD. Cu, manganese, aluminium, and zinc are implicated in several neurodegenerative illnesses [10].

Cholinergic Hypothesis

How genotypes affect the therapeutic efficacy of acetylcholinesterase inhibitors administered in AD patients? APOE genotype is the main risk factor, whereas the AChE gene constitutes the mainstay of treatment. Since cholinergic neurones are not the primary targets in AD, the 1976 "Cholinergic Hypothesis" of the disease attempts to explain the absence of the APOE effect. Psychoneurotic symptoms are related to lower receptor binding in the cholinergic systems to certain brain regions, viewed in mild to severe stages of the illness. Poorer receptor binding, on the other hand, may be correlated with processing speed in healthy elderly. Apart from providing links to other important brain changes related to aging, *in vivo* cholinergic receptor binding also offers a promising biological target for therapy. Clinical decline is seen with affected loss of cholinergic neurones produced in the medial forebrain nuclei and decreased acetylcholine-mediated neurotransmission. ChEIs, such as donepezil, have been the mainstay of symptomatic treatment of patients for over 20 years [11].

Symptoms and Progression of AD

AD develops gradually, with progressively deteriorating symptoms: Early-Stage (Mild AD): Common early indicators include mood swings, language problems, memory loss, confusion, trouble with familiar chores and planning, and item misplacing [12, 13]. Middle-Stage (Moderate AD): Confusion, disorientation, and difficulties with day-to-day tasks arise as memory loss intensifies. There may be behavioural shifts, sleep issues, and hallucinations [14]. Late-Stage (Severe AD): This phase is characterised by severe memory loss, a loss of ability to communicate, physical worsening, and total reliance on caretakers. Moreover, incontinence and heightened susceptibility to infections are common [15]. Complete Stages: Physical and verbal abilities fully deteriorate, frequently necessitating hospice care. Although it might vary greatly, the illness usually advances over 8–10 years [16].

Epidemiology of AD

By the middle of the century, there will be 152 million dementia patients worldwide, with low and medium-income nations anticipated to have the largest rise in cases [17]. Facts and numbers on AD for 2020 indicate that by 2050, there might be a significant rise in the number of AD patients (those over 65), from 5.8 million to 13.8 million [18]. Over the last several decades, community-dwelling research conducted in China and Japan has clearly shown an increase in the frequency of AD [19, 20]. In particular, women's age-specific worldwide prevalence was 1.17 times greater than men's, and women's age-standardised death rate was higher than men's, indicating that women's domination was not just due to their longer life spans [21]. AD death increased by 146.2% between 2000 and 2018, placing it sixth among the most common causes of death for the elderly. The emotional impact could be devastating, with mental stress being a product of caring. Thus, the burden of caring for AD populations will become untenable and unsupportable for both the families and society. Well-being is the measure of a good treatment for many cases of AD. The patients affected by AD may suffer from a confusing array of psychosocial problems and symptoms. There is indeed strong evidence from a series of epidemiologic studies that environmental and behavioural factors may be very important in the initiation and course of the disease. As AD cases tend to be accompanied by other age-related diseases than those of normal-aged people, keeping good physical health is important for protecting the intellect. According to the reverse causation theory, a lot of risk factors might be seen as both causes and effects of AD symptoms. An accurate diagnosis is paramount to offering treatment to patients with cognitive deficits. Even though tau and Aβ biomarkers may, on their own, be Morindacitrifolia markers, some cognitively normal individuals with these biomarkers never transform into AD, raising challenges for presymptomatic identification. Future challenges would include the development of less intrusive and more sensitive biomarkers or methods for early screening and diagnosis [22].

LIMITATIONS OF CURRENT THERAPEUTIC APPROACHES

Nanotechnology-based therapeutic approaches for AD hold significant promise, but several limitations persist. One of the primary challenges is the difficulty in achieving effective BBB penetration. While nanocarriers can enhance drug delivery, the BBB is highly selective, making it tough for most nanoparticles to cross it efficiently, limiting drug delivery to the brain [23]. Another issue is the biocompatibility and toxicity of nanoparticles. For example, some metal-based nanoparticles may induce cytotoxic effects, oxidative stress, or inflammatory responses, which pose risks, especially for long-term use [24]. Additionally, there are limitations in drug loading capacity, with many nano-carriers unable to carry sufficient therapeutic doses to achieve optimal efficacy [25]. The clearance of nanoparticles from the body is another concern. Some nanoparticles accumulate in organs and are cleared slowly, which raises potential safety concerns, particularly with non-biodegradable nanoparticles [8]. Moreover, scaling up production for clinical use while ensuring consistency and effectiveness is a significant hurdle, with batch-to-batch variability making regulatory approval more difficult [12]. Nanoparticles can sometimes cause the immune system to react, which might lead the body to remove them too quickly or cause harmful inflammation [9]. Also, because every patient is different due to genetics or how far their disease has progressed, it is hard to create one treatment that works for everyone. People may respond to nanotechnology-based treatments in very different ways [26].

Drug Delivery Challenges

One big challenge in treating Alzheimer's disease is getting drugs to the right parts of the brain. The brain has a special protective barrier called the blood-brain barrier (BBB), which blocks many medicines from getting in. Because of this, traditional drug delivery methods often cannot get enough medicine into the brain, making treatments less effective. Alzheimer's affects different parts of the brain in different ways, which makes it even harder to target drugs where they are needed the most. Regular methods usually regulate the drug all over the brain, instead of focusing on the damaged areas. This can lead to less effective treatment and may require higher doses, which increases the chance of side effects [23, 27 - 29].

Side Effects and Toxicity

Current treatments for Alzheimer's disease often come with serious side effects. Many of the drugs used to manage symptoms or slow down the disease can cause problems for patients. For example, a common type of Alzheimer's medicine called cholinesterase inhibitors can lead to stomach issues like nausea, vomiting, and diarrhea. They can also cause heart-related problems like a slow heart rate and low blood pressure. Taking these drugs for a long time can lead to a build-up of harmful effects in the body. Since Alzheimer's patients usually need several different medications to manage various symptoms, there is a higher risk of side effects from drug interactions. This mix of medications, called polypharmacy, can be complex on both patients and their caregivers, and can reduce the patient's overall quality of life [13].

Limited Efficacy

One of the main problems with current Alzheimer's treatments is that they do not work very well. Most of them only treat the symptoms instead of tackling the root causes of the disease. For example, drugs like cholinesterase inhibitors and NMDA receptor antagonists can help improve memory or thinking for a short time, but they do not stop the disease from getting worse. Creating drugs that can slow down or stop Alzheimer's has been very difficult. Many new drugs that looked promising in early research ended up failing in clinical trials because they did not work well enough or had serious side effects. Since AD is complex and multifactorial, with tau tangles, amyloid plaques, neuro-inflammation, and neuronal loss, it is difficult to develop a single therapy agent that can effectively address each of these elements [30]. In summary, the current therapeutic approaches for Alzheimer's are hindered by significant drug delivery challenges, side effects, toxicity, and limited efficacy. These limitations highlight the urgent need for innovative treatments that can overcome these obstacles and provide more effective and safer options for patients with AD. Certainly, creating a detailed write-up on "Nanotechnology-based Therapeutic Approaches in Alzheimer's" with a focus on the outlined points and within the specified constraints requires careful consideration [31].

INTRODUCTION TO NANOTECHNOLOGY IN MEDICINE

In therapy for most diseases, such as neurodegenerative disorders like AD, nanotechnology has emerged with high potential. Due to the complexity of AD, characterised by tau tangles, amyloid plaques, and relentless neuronal degeneration, new therapeutic approaches are required. An emerging solution is offered by nanotechnology, where medication can be delivered at the molecular and cellular level, enhancing therapy precision and efficiency [32]. The capacity of nanotechnology to get past the obstacles presented by the BBB, which prevents the majority of medications from reaching the brain, is one of the main advantages of nanotechnology in medicine. Therapeutic drugs can be targeted to specific brain regions by using designed nanoparticles that have a higher ability to pass the BBB. Given the diverse nature of Alzheimer's pathology, where different brain regions are afflicted at different stages of the illness, this targeted delivery is essential [23]. Furthermore, nanoparticles can be intended to release drugs in a controlled manner, potentially reducing the side effects associated with traditional therapies that require higher doses [33]. Apart from medication administration, nanotechnology presents benefits for diagnosis. To identify early pathological alterations in the brain and enable early diagnosis and disease progression tracking, nanoparticles can be employed as imaging agents. Because of its dual purpose as a diagnostic and therapeutic tool, nanotechnology presents itself as a flexible means of tackling the complex nature of AD [34].

Historical Perspective

With roots in the mid-20th century, nanotechnology has a long history of manipulating matter at the atomic, molecular, and supramolecular scales. Although Norio Taniguchi initially used the word "nanotechnology" in 1974, the intellectual underpinnings were established much earlier. In his well-known 1959 lecture, "There's Plenty of Room at the Bottom," Richard Feynman described a novel area in which materials might be altered at the atomic level. At first, material sciences and engineering were the main areas of interest for nanotechnology. Its possible uses in medicine, however, quickly became clear. Medical applications were made possible by the development of instruments like the Atomic Force Microscope (AFM) andScanning Tunnelling Microscope (STM) in the 1980s, which allowed scientists to view and work with individual atoms. Significant progress was made in the 1990s in the production of nanoparticles and their applications in medicines, diagnostics, and drug delivery systems. Nanotechnology and medicine started to interact more and more in the early 21st century, leading to the development of nano-medicine. The use of nanoparticles for targeted medicine delivery has drawn attention from researchers because it has the potential to improve treatment outcomes and lessen adverse effects. The goal was to develop "smart" medication delivery devices that would spare healthy tissues by delivering therapeutic substances straight to sick cells. This was especially important for diseases like cancer, where conventional therapies frequently resulted in serious side effects [14].

Fundamental Concepts

Nanotechnology in medicine, or nano-medicine, is built on several fundamental concepts:

Nanoparticles

These are minuscule particles, typically ranging from 1 to 100 nm in size. They can be planned from various materials, including metals, polymers, and lipids. Their minor size allows them to interact with biological molecules and cells in unique ways [35].

Surface Functionalization

Nanoparticles can be modified with specific ligands, antibodies, or other molecules that allow them to target specific cells or tissues. This ability to "decorate" nanoparticles enhances their specificity and efficacy [36].

Drug Delivery

One of the most exciting areas of using nanotechnology is in the medical field, with targeted drug distribution. Nanoparticles can transport therapeutic materials and diminish the maleficent effects that accompany treatment while improving the illness treatment results, aiding in the maleficent effects that accompany treatment.

Imaging and Diagnostics

Nanoparticles can also be used as contrast agents in imaging techniques such as MRI, CT scans, and PET scans. Their unique properties can enhance the resolution and sensitivity of these imaging modalities, aiding in early diagnosis [37].

Therapeutics

Beyond drug delivery, nanoparticles can themselves have therapeutic effects. For example, gold nanoparticles can be used in a treatment called photothermal therapy. In this method, the gold particles absorb light and turn it into heat, which is then used to destroy cancer cells [37].

Biocompatibility and Safety

A key part of using nanomedicine is making sure that the nanoparticles are safe for the body and do not cause harmful immune reactions. To be used in real medical treatments, they have to go through a lot of testing to prove they are safe [37].

Applications in Neurology

Neurological disorders are hard to treat because the brain is very complex, and it has a protective barrier called the blood-brain barrier (BBB) that blocks many medicines from reaching to the brain . Nanotechnology provides new creative ways to overcome these problems and improve treatment [38].

Drug Delivery Across the BBB

One of the biggest challenges in treating brain diseases is the blood-brain barrier (BBB), which acts like a shield and blocks most medicines from getting into the brain. Scientists are designing nanoparticles that can cross this barrier and carry drugs directly to the brain. For example, tiny carriers like liposomes and polymer-based nanoparticles have been studied for their ability to deliver medicine past the BBB [39].

Neuro-protection and Neuro-regeneration

Nanoparticles can be used to deliver medicines that protect brain cells from damage or help repair damaged cells. This is especially useful for diseases like Alzheimer's, Parkinson's, and after a stroke [39].

Imaging and Diagnosis

Nanoparticles can improve the ability to see brain structures, helping doctors diagnose diseases early. For example, iron oxide nanoparticles are used in MRI scans to make brain tumors and other problems easier to spot [39].

Targeted Therapy

In brain diseases, it is important to target specific types of cells or problems in the brain. Nanoparticles can be made to find and attach to amyloid plaques in Alzheimer's, allowing medicine to be delivered directly to the affected areas [39].

Nanotechnology-based Therapeutic Approaches in Alzheimer's

Alzheimer's disease (AD) is a progressive brain disorder that causes memory loss, thinking problems, and changes in behavior. It is linked to the buildup of harmful amyloid plaques and twisted tau protein in the brain. Current treatments do not do much to slow down the disease progression, so there is a strong need for new solutions. Nanotechnology provides some exciting new ways to tackle these problems [39].

Nanoparticles for Amyloid-beta Clearance

One of the main problems in Alzheimer's is the buildup of amyloid-beta plaques in the brain. Scientists can design nanoparticles that target these plaques and help remove them from the brain. Different types of nanoparticles have been tested for this purpose [35].

Nanoparticles for Tau Protein Targeting

In addition to amyloid-beta plaques, the accumulation of tau protein tangles is another hallmark of AD. Nanoparticles can be designed to target and degrade these tangles [35].

Silica Nanoparticles

These nanoparticles can be specially designed with molecules that stick to tau protein, helping to remove it from brain cells.

Dendrimers

These branched polymeric nanoparticles can be used to deliver drugs that inhibit the aggregation of tau protein, potentially slowing the progression of the disease [35].

Drug Delivery Systems

One of the biggest challenges in treating Alzheimer's is getting medicine into the brain. Nanoparticles can help by making it easier for drugs to reach the brain and work more effectively.

Polymeric Micelles

These self-forming nanoparticles can carry water-hating (hydrophobic) drugs, making them easier to dissolve and more stable. Micelles, a type of these particles, can be designed to cross the blood-brain barrier and release the medicine directly in the brain [13].

Solid Lipid Nanoparticles

These nanoparticles can carry both water-loving (hydrophilic) and fat-loving (lipophilic) drugs, making them very flexible for delivering different types of medicine. In lab studies on Alzheimer's, they've been shown to help more medicine reach the brain and improve treatment results [40].

Gene Therapy

Nanoparticles can also carry genetic material, like siRNA or CRISPR/Cas9, into the brain. This could help turn off harmful genes linked to Alzheimer's or even fix genetic problems that cause the disease.

Lipid Nanoparticles

These nanoparticles are often used to carry genetic material, like DNA or RNA. They can be designed to protect it from breaking down and help brain cells absorb it more easily [41].

Polymeric Nanoparticles

Materials like chitosan and polyethylene can be used to make nanoparticles that carry genetic material into the brain. These nanoparticles can be adjusted to make them more stable and better at reaching the right target [41].

Nanoparticles for Neuro-protection

Nanoparticles can carry special medicines that protect brain cells from damage and help them stay alive [41].

Cerium Oxide Nanoparticles

These nanoparticles have antioxidant effects, which means they can help reduce harmful stress in the brain caused by unstable molecules. This stress is a major cause of brain cell damage in Alzheimer's disease [42].

Fullerenes

These carbon-based nanoparticles can remove harmful molecules called free radicals, helping protect brain cells from damage caused by oxidative stress [41].

Liposomes

These round-shaped vesicles can carry drugs or treatments that target amyloid-beta. Liposomes can be designed with antibodies or small proteins that specifically stick to amyloid-beta, making them more effective at reaching the right areas [41].

Polymeric Nanoparticles

Polymers like PLGA (poly (lactic-co-glycolic acid)) can be used to make nanoparticles that carry drugs to the brain. These nanoparticles can be designed to slowly release the medicine over time, providing longer-lasting treatment effects [40].

Gold Nanoparticles

These gold nanoparticles have special properties that allow them to work in a treatment called photo-thermal therapy. When they are exposed to near-infrared light, they produce heat, which can help break down amyloid-beta plaques in the brain [43].

MECHANISM OF NEUROTECHNOLOGY-BASED THERAPEUTIC APPROACHES

Enhanced Permeation and Retention (EPR) Effect

The term "Enhanced Permeation and Retention" (EPR) refers to the way nanoparticles or large drugs can build up in tumor tissues or areas with damaged blood vessels. These areas have leaky blood vessels and poor drainage, which allow large molecules to stay there more easily. While the EPR effect is mostly used in cancer treatment, scientists are also exploring it for brain diseases like Alzheimer's. The idea is that changes in the brain, such as inflammation, could alter the blood-brain barrier, making it easier for nanoparticles or drug carriers to collect in the damaged areas of the brain [13].

Potential EPR-like Mechanisms in AD

Alzheimer's disease (AD) causes long-term inflammation in the brain, which can damage the blood-brain barrier (BBB). This damage could create conditions similar to those found in tumors, making it easier for nanoparticles to reach and stay in the inflamed areas of the brain. Nanoparticles designed to take advantage of this effect can be coated with molecules that specifically target proteins or receptors that are increased in AD, like amyloid plaques or tau tangles. This helps the nanoparticles cross the BBB and gather in the damaged parts of the brain where they are needed most [39].

Applications of the EPR Effect in AD Therapeutics

Different types of nanoparticles, like liposomes, polymer-based particles, and dendrimers, are being studied for their ability to cross the blood-brain barrier and deliver medicine directly to the brain. These nanoparticles can be designed to take advantage of the EPR effect, which may help them gather in brain areas affected by Alzheimer's disease. Because nanoparticles can stay in the body longer and are less likely to be removed by the immune system, they may help deliver drugs more effectively. Nanoparticles can also be used as imaging tools to help see Alzheimer 's-related damage in the brain, such as amyloid plaques. This could help doctors detect the disease earlier and track its progress [44].

Surface Modification and Functionalization

One of the most advanced ways to deliver medicine to the brain for Alzheimer's patients is by using polymeric nanoparticles (NPs). These tiny particles help improve the effectiveness of drugs by ensuring they are properly distributed and processed in the body after being injected [44]. The polymers used to make these nanoparticles include materials like chitosan, albumin, PLA, PLGA, PEG, and PEI. These polymers have special structures that allow them to form three-dimensional networks, either on their own or by reacting with other polymers, creating single or multi-polymer nanoparticles. It can be changed to add new functional groups, which helps customize the nanoparticles for specific drug delivery [45]. This customization allows for controlled release of drugs, proteins, or genetic material to the right areas in the brain or to specific cell types. The drugs can be carried inside these nanoparticles in different ways, such as by bonding them directly, using surface coatings, or preventing them from escaping [46, 47]. Choosing the right polymer is crucial for successfully delivering drugs to specific parts of the brain or certain types of cells. To help these nanoparticles cross the blood-brain barrier (BBB), special molecules (called ligands) can be attached to the surface [48]. These ligands can be used in four ways, which can target specific BBB receptors, attach proteins from the bloodstream improve the particle's charge and ability to interact with the brain, or increase how long the nanoparticles stay in the bloodstream [49].

In addition, NPs can be modified with cationic entities to bolster delivery to the AD-affected brain *via* electrostatic interactions with endothelial cell structures [50, 51]. Orthogonal chemistry represents a pivotal technique employed in the design of NPs, facilitating the selective conjugation of functional groups without the occurrence of side reactions. This approach is instrumental in the development of multifunctional carbon-based systems that closely replicate biological tissues, thereby rendering them appropriate for controlled pharmacological delivery. Methodologies for polymer functionalization and chemo-selective grafting are extensively elaborated upon in the academic literature and are applied in the context of AD therapeutic interventions. Ultimately, beyond their role as carriers for therapeutic pharmacological agents, certain polymers possess the capability to function as therapeutic agents in their own right. For instance, sialic acid-modified selenium NPs, in conjunction with a synthetic peptide, have demonstrated promising therapeutic effects within neuronal cell populations [52].

Targeted Drug Delivery Mechanism

Recent developments in nanotechnology have made it possible to present a fresh option for the treatment of AD. Since they may be controlled in terms of size, shape, hydrophobicity, coating, chemistry, and surface charge, nanoparticle-based methods have been used as potential resources for efficient drugs, since Birrenbach and Speiser's initial discovery of them as carrier materials in the 1970s [53]. Nanoparticles (NPs) are, by definition, minuscule particles that may interact with biological systems and have at least one dimension less than 100 nm. They consist of a layer near the surface that can be equipped with an internal core and several molecules for functionality [54]. Biological barriers and traditional treatment techniques can be overcome by NPs, which enable the encapsulation of medications and their transport into the central nervous system (CNS) without going through the BBB [55]. To enhance their pharmacokinetic and pharmacodynamic profiles, they can be designed and altered using various surface features [56]. In addition to minimal toxicity and immunogenicity response, nano-mediated drug delivery schemes offer high stability, biocompatibility, controlled/sustained drug release, and biodegradability. In addition, nanoparticles can reduce the amount of medicine needed and how often it is given, while also lowering the risk of side effects [57]. The new method for delivering drugs to Alzheimer's patients is shown in Fig. (**2**), which provides a detailed look at the creative ways designed to improve treatment and target the specific causes of the disease.

TYPES OF NANOPARTICLES USED IN ALZHEIMER'S THERAPY

Liposomes

Structure and Composition

Liposomes are round, bubble-like structures that mimic a natural cell membrane and have one or two layers of fats. These liposomes can carry both water-loving (hydrophilic) and water-hating (hydrophobic) drugs, protecting them from breaking down and making it easier for the drugs to spread in the body [4].

Mechanism of Action

Because liposomes are made of fat, they can easily cross the blood-brain barrier (BBB), which is a major challenge in treating brain diseases like Alzheimer's. Once they pass the BBB, liposomes release their medicine directly into the brain, making sure the treatment goes exactly where it is needed [58].

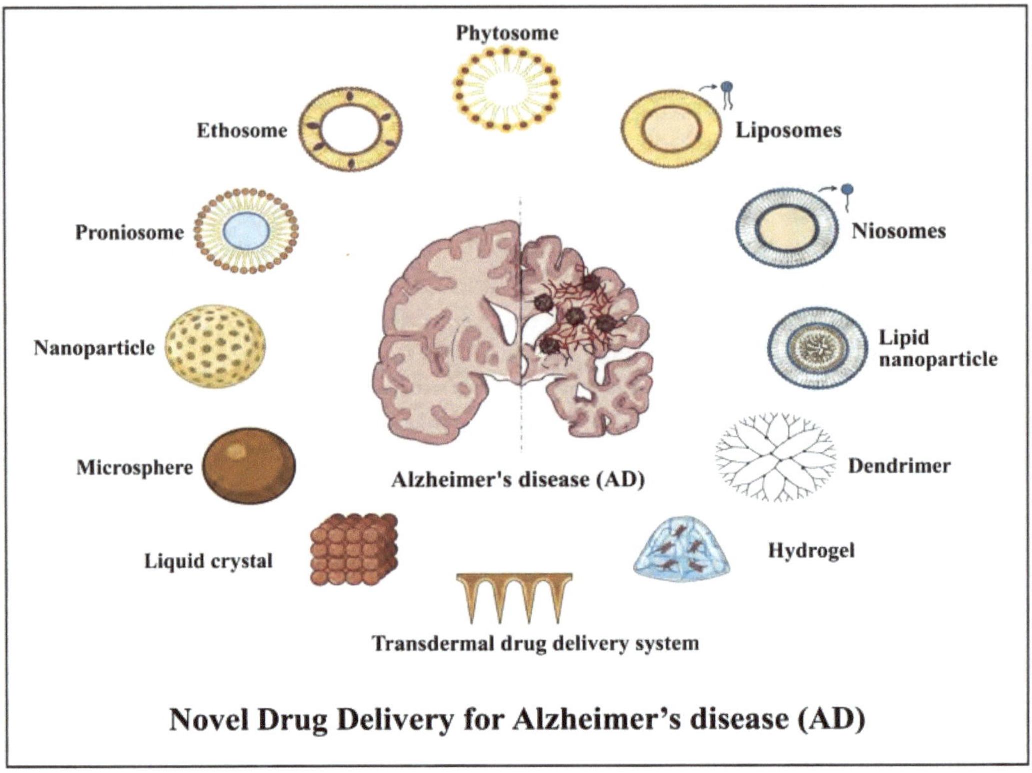

Fig. (2). Novel drug delivery for AD.

Applications in Alzheimer's Therapy

Liposomes are used to deliver different drugs for Alzheimer's, like curcumin and rivastigmine. These drugs become more stable and easier for the body to absorb, which helps improve their effectiveness in treating the disease [58].

Advantages

Liposomes are biocompatible, meaning they are less likely to cause harmful immune reactions, and their structure allows them to carry a variety of treatments. Also, by adding special targeting molecules to their surface, liposomes can be made to specifically deliver medicine to the parts of the brain affected by Alzheimer's [58].

Polymeric Nanoparticles

Structure and Composition

Polymeric nanoparticles are made from biodegradable materials like PLGA, which break down into harmless substances that the body can easily process. These nanoparticles can either carry drugs inside their structure or attach them to their surface [59].

Mechanism of Action

These nanoparticles are made to release medicine slowly and steadily over time, ensuring a continuous effect. This helps keep drug levels stable in the brain, which is important for treating long-term conditions like Alzheimer's [4].

Applications in Alzheimer's Therapy

Polymeric nanoparticles are used to deliver small treatments, like peptides, that can stop amyloid-beta from clumping together, which is a key problem in Alzheimer's disease. By preventing these clumps (amyloid plaques) from forming, these nanoparticles help slow down the progress of the disease [60].

Advantages

Polymeric nanoparticles can be designed to release drugs in a controlled way, reducing the need for frequent doses and making it easier for patients to follow their treatment. Their safety and ability to be customized with specific targeting features also make them a great option for personalized treatments in Alzheimer's therapy [40].

Dendrimers

Structure and Composition

Dendrimers are tree-shaped polymers with a very specific structure. They have many branches on their surface that can be used to attach drugs, imaging tools, or molecules that target specific areas in the body [61].

Mechanism of Action

The special structure of dendrimers lets them carry a lot of drugs and target specific areas precisely, which is important for getting drugs across the blood-brain barrier and delivering them directly to damaged brain cells. Their multiple branches also make it easier for them to interact with and pass through cell membranes [62].

Applications in Alzheimer's Therapy

Dendrimers have shown potential in delivering antioxidants, anti-inflammatory drugs, and other treatments that can help reduce the brain inflammation and stress caused by Alzheimer's. Their ability to target specific areas and deliver these treatments makes them a powerful way to slow the disease down [13].

Advantages

Dendrimers are very versatile in delivering drugs because they have many functional areas on their surface. They can be designed to release drugs only when triggered by certain signals, ensuring the medicine is released exactly where and when it is needed. This targeted approach helps reduce side effects and makes the treatment safer overall [40].

Metallic Nanoparticles

Structure and Composition

Metallic nanoparticles, such as those made from gold, silver, and other metals, have special properties that larger materials do not have. They can be made in different shapes and sizes, and these variations affect how they interact with the body [40].

Mechanism of Action

Metallic nanoparticles can be modified with drugs, targeting molecules, or antibodies to make them more effective at treating specific areas. Their small size helps them pass through the blood-brain barrier and gather in the brain, where they can release the medicine or be used for diagnosis [63].

Applications in Alzheimer's Therapy

In Alzheimer's disease, metallic nanoparticles are being studied for both treatment and diagnosis at the same time—a concept called "theranostics." For example, gold nanoparticles can carry drugs straight to the harmful amyloid plaques in the brain, or they can help doctors see the brain more clearly in scans like MRIs. This helps with early detection and tracking how the disease is progressing [13].

Advantages

Metallic nanoparticles have a large surface area, which means more space to attach drugs or targeting molecules. This makes them very flexible for different treatment needs. Since they can be used for both treating Alzheimer's and tracking the disease in real time, they offer a powerful combined approach to manage the condition [4] better.

Quantum Dots

Structure and Composition

Quantum dots are tiny particles made from semiconductor materials that can glow in different colours depending on their size. This special property makes them useful for both seeing what is happening inside the body (imaging) and for helping treat diseases [13].

Mechanism of Action

Quantum dots glow so that they can be easily tracked inside the body. This makes them great for seeing where drugs go in the brain. Scientists can also attach medicines or targeting molecules to their surface, helping them reach and treat specific areas of the brain [40].

Applications in Alzheimer's Therapy

Quantum dots are mainly used in Alzheimer's research to help with diagnosis. They can show how treatments move through the brain and how well they work. They also have the potential to carry drugs that target the specific problems causing Alzheimer's [43].

Advantages

Quantum dots are more stable and brighter than regular fluorescent dyes, which means they can be used for clearer, longer-lasting imaging. Because they can help both diagnose and treat Alzheimer's at the same time, they are considered a very advanced tool in battling the disease [64].

PHARMACOLOGICAL BENEFITS OF NANOTECHNOLOGY-BASED APPROACHES

Enhanced Drug Bioavailability

Definition and Importance

One big challenge in treating Alzheimer's is getting enough medicine into the brain where it is needed. Nanoparticles help by making the drugs more stable and easier to absorb, so they work better once they get past the brain's protective barrier [63].

Impact on Alzheimer's Therapy

Better bioavailability means the body can use the drug more effectively, even at lower doses. This helps reduce side effects and improves how well the treatment works. It is especially helpful in Alzheimer's, where it is hard for drugs to reach the brain [40].

Improved Drug Stability

Definition and Importance

Nanoparticles work like protective containers for medicine, keeping it safe from being broken down by the body too soon. This helps the medicine stay strong and effective until it reaches the right place in the brain [42].

Impact on Alzheimer's Therapy

In Alzheimer's treatment, there is only a small time frame where the medicine works best. So, keeping the drug stable is very important to make sure it works well. This helps control symptoms better and may even slow down how fast the disease gets worse [13].

Controlled Drug Release

Definition and Importance

Nanoparticles can be designed to release their medicine slowly over time or only when certain conditions are met, like changes in pH or the presence of specific enzymes in the body [13].

Impact on Alzheimer's Therapy

Controlled drug release is important for managing conditions like Alzheimer's, where it is crucial to keep steady levels of medication in the brain. This method reduces how often patients need to take the drug, helps them stick to the treatment plan, and avoids the highs and lows in drug levels that can cause side effects or make the treatment less effective [58].

Reduced Systemic Toxicity

Definition and Importance

Nanoparticles help deliver drugs directly to the intended area, reducing the amount of the drug that affects other parts of the body. This helps lower side effects, which is especially important in treating brain-related diseases where unwanted effects on other organs can cause serious problems [14].

Impact on Alzheimer's Therapy

Nanoparticle-based treatments reduce the risk of harm to other parts of the body, allowing higher doses of medicine to be delivered directly to the brain without causing side effects. This targeted approach is key to maximizing treatment effectiveness and minimizing harm. Using nanotechnology in Alzheimer's treatment could change the way we fight the disease, offering hope for slowing or stopping its progress. The flexibility and accuracy of nanoparticles make them a strong tool in improving care and managing Alzheimer's [35].

Recent Advances

Preclinical Studies

Current therapeutic approaches for neurodegenerative conditions such as AD frequently depend on high molecular weight antibodies, peptides, and proteins, which cannot inherently traverse the BBB independently [65]. Nanoparticles (NPs) present a viable alternative owing to their extensive surface area and the potential for surface modification, which facilitates their ability to penetrate the BBB more efficiently than conventional delivery strategies. Furthermore, NPs can ensure a regulated and gradual release of pharmacological agents into the cerebral milieu, thereby mitigating peripheral toxicity [66]. Notwithstanding their promise, the majority of investigations into NP mediated drug delivery for AD have predominantly been performed in preclinical animal models, resulting in minimal advancement in human clinical trials. Obstacles to the broad implementation of such clinical applications encompass the necessity of ensuring the biocompatibility and safety of NPs, formulating effective mechanisms for cerebral delivery, and optimizing NP characteristics, including composition, dimensions, morphology, and surface alterations. A viable methodology for traversing the BBB entails the modification of the NP surface, such as the conjugation of antibodies that specifically bind to endothelial cell receptors. For instance, chitosan NPs have been successfully linked with antibodies targeting the transferrin receptor (TfR-1) to enhance the delivery of neuroprotective peptides into the cerebral structures of compromised murine models [23]. In a similar vein, poly(butyl-cyanoacrylate) NPs encapsulated with dopamine have demonstrated efficacy in preclinical paradigms of Parkinson's disease and exhibit potential applicability for AD therapeutics. An alternative strategy involves the application of surfactants like T80 to coat NPs, thereby enabling them to mimic lipoproteins and facilitate BBB penetration *via* receptor-mediated endocytosis [67, 68]. This approach has proven effective in augmenting the cerebral uptake of drugs such as rivastigmine in AD experimental models [69]. NPs constructed from hydrophilic polymers or surfactants additionally confer the benefit of prolonged circulation within the bloodstream, as they partially evade the liver's reticuloendothelial system, resulting in enhanced drug availability and sustained release in the brain. In summation, although NPs exhibit considerable potential for the delivery of AD therapeutics across the BBB, further empirical investigation is imperative to resolve issues about safety, efficacy, and the feasibility of large-scale clinical application [30].

Clinical Trials

The creation of novel AD therapies depends heavily on clinical trials. These meticulously planned trials are carried out on human subjects to assess the effectiveness, safety, and possible advantages of novel treatments. An outline of the many stages, difficulties, and most current advancements in AD clinical trials is provided below [40].

Clinical Trial Phases

New treatments for Alzheimer's (AD) go through a careful testing process. First, animal studies and lab tests check if the treatment is safe and works well. In Phase I, a small group of healthy people or AD patients test the safety, dosage, and any side effects of the drug. Phase II involves gathering more information about safety and how well the treatment works at the right dose for more AD patients. Phase III includes a larger group to confirm the treatment's effectiveness, monitor side effects, and compare it to existing treatments, helping to get approval from health authorities. After the treatment is approved, Phase IV studies keep track of its long-term effects on different groups of people [40]. AD clinical trials face challenges such as the complexity of the disease, making it hard to select participants and measure outcomes reliably. Other challenges include finding enough people to join the trials, having reliable tests to diagnose AD early and measure the drug's effectiveness, the influence of placebo effects, and making sure patients understand the risks and give consent. Recent progress in AD treatment includes therapies that target amyloid plaques (like aducanumab and lecanemab) and tau protein tangles, aiming to slow down or stop brain damage. Studies are also exploring anti-inflammatory and neuroprotective therapies, lifestyle interventions, and combination therapies that include nutrition, exercise, and cognitive training. Personalised medicine is gaining traction as understanding of the genetic and molecular basis of AD grows, with clinical trials increasingly focusing on tailoring treatments to individual patient characteristics, including genetic markers like APOE status [61].

Case Studies and Examples

In the field of medication, nanotechnology has become a game-changer, especially in the creation of cutting-edge treatments for AD. The construction of tau tangles and amyloid plaques, along with a steady deterioration in cognitive function, makes this neurodegenerative disease extremely difficult to treat with traditional methods. Recent developments in nanotechnology, however, present encouraging alternatives. This section examines a number of case studies and examples that highlight the creative approaches and successful outcomes used to treat AD using nanotechnology [23, 24, 70 - 72].

Liposomal Delivery Systems

One interesting way nanotechnology is being used in Alzheimer's treatment is with liposomal delivery systems. Liposomes are tiny, round structures made of fat that can carry drugs and help them work better in the body. For example, anti-amyloid drugs like curcumin have been put into liposomes to help prevent the build-up of amyloid plaques in the brain. A study by Sharma, D. M., *et al.*, (2021) tested liposomes loaded with curcumin in a mouse model of Alzheimer's. The results showed that liposomal curcumin was more stable and worked effectively in the body, leading to a noticeable reduction in tau protein build-up and amyloid plaques. This method also helped reduce common side effects of curcumin, like stomach problems [73].

Polymer-based Nanoparticles

Polymeric nanoparticles (NPs) are also being explored for their ability to deliver drugs to the brain, which is a major challenge in Alzheimer's treatment. One example is the use of poly (lactic-co-glycolic acid) (PLGA) nanoparticles to deliver neuroprotective drugs. In a study by Zhou, R. H., *et al*., (2022), PLGA nanoparticles were used to carry the antioxidant resveratrol to the brain. Resveratrol is known to protect the brain, but has trouble crossing the blood-brain barrier on its own. The study showed that PLGA nanoparticles helped resveratrol get into the brain more effectively, improving brain function and memory in a mouse model of Alzheimer's. This method not only made the treatment work better but also reduced side effects in the rest of the body [74].

Dendrimer-based Delivery Systems

Dendrimers, which are highly branched molecules with a precise structure, offer a promising new approach for Alzheimer's treatment. Their unique design allows them to carry multiple drug molecules, targeting agents, or imaging tools. One example is a study by Lee, S. J., *et al*., (2023), where they used PAMAM dendrimers to deliver an anti-tau antibody in Alzheimer's models. The research showed that the dendrimers helped the antibody reach the brain's tau plaques more effectively, leading to better clearance of tau tangles and improved memory and brain function. This study highlights how dendrimers can be used for both targeted treatment and brain imaging in Alzheimer's [75].

Metallic Nanoparticles

Gold and silver nanoparticles are being studied as a new way to treat Alzheimer's. These nanoparticles have special properties that make them useful for both delivering drugs and helping with diagnosis. For example, a study by Park, J. K., *et al*., (2024) looked at how gold nanoparticles (AuNPs) could be used to deliver ibuprofen, an anti-inflammatory drug, to the brain. The research showed that AuNPs were effective in getting ibuprofen into the brain, where it helped reduce inflammation in a mouse model of Alzheimer's. Additionally, the gold nanoparticles were also used to improve MRI imaging, helping doctors see amyloid plaques in the brain and track how the disease is progressing [76].

Hybrid Nanocarriers

Hybrid nanocarriers combine different types of nanomaterials to take advantage of their combined strengths, offering a new way to treat Alzheimer's. One example is the use of magnetic-platinum nanoparticles. In a study by Wang, E. M., *et al*., (2023), these nanoparticles were designed to deliver the anti-amyloid drug donepezil. The magnetic part of the nanoparticles allowed doctors to direct them to specific areas using an external magnetic field, while the platinum part helped release the drug and improved imaging. This combined approach led to more of the drug reaching the amyloid plaque sites in the brain and better cognitive results in animal models [77].

Exosome-based Delivery Systems

Exosomes, which are naturally occurring small particles in the body, have shown great potential as delivery systems for treating Alzheimer's. Because they can cross the blood-brain barrier (BBB) and are compatible with the body, they are well-suited for Alzheimer's treatment. In a study by Zhang, L. F., *et al*., (2024), exosomes were used to deliver small RNA molecules (siRNA) that target amyloid-beta, a key protein involved in Alzheimer's. The study found that using exosomes to deliver siRNA significantly lowered amyloid-beta levels in the brain and improved memory in mouse models of Alzheimer's. This shows that exosomes could be a powerful tool for therapies that target genes, offering new personalized treatment options for Alzheimer's. These case studies highlight the many ways nanotechnology can be used to fight Alzheimer's, such as using liposomes, polymers, dendrimers, metallic nanoparticles, hybrid carriers, and exosomes. While these methods show great potential, more research and clinical testing are needed to fully understand their effectiveness and bring them into real-world treatments for people with Alzheimer's [78]. The mechanisms related to various targeted drug delivery systems in AD are illustrated in Fig. (**3**), providing a comprehensive overview of how these advanced strategies aim to enhance drug specificity, improve therapeutic efficacy, and minimize side effects by targeting disease-specific pathways.

MECHANISMS OF ACTION

Interaction with Amyloid-β Plaques

To elucidate the self-interactions among amyloid-beta (Aβ) molecules, investigators modified a methodology that was previously employed for the examination of the yeast prion [79]. This approach utilizes peptide arrays, wherein the peptides represent a sliding window across a targeted protein. The research team fabricated peptide arrays on a cellulose membrane, systematically scanning the sequence of Aβ1-42. By employing a biotinylated derivative of Aβ1-42 (Biot-Aβ1-42), they executed size exclusion chromatography to discern monomeric and oligomeric conformations of Aβ [80]. Upon exposure of the peptide array to the monomeric variant of Biot-Aβ1-42, no significant binding was observed. Conversely, exposure to the oligomeric form (which was identified in the void volume during chromatography) resulted in pronounced binding in the N-terminal domain of Aβ, particularly within the aggregation-prone regions (APRs). Subsequent experiments monitored the binding affinities of Aβ species at various aggregation stages, demonstrating that early oligomers predominantly interacted with the central APR1 region, whereas later oligomers also engaged with the C-terminal APR2 region [81]. The investigation further delved into the interaction dynamics of "reverse seeds" (fibril fragments produced *via* sonication), which exhibited an interaction pattern analogous to that of late-stage oligomers, implying that these seeds may facilitate the aggregation process by circumventing the rate-limiting phase of amyloid formation. The researchers evaluated the specificity of these interactions through the utilization of control peptides and sequence scrambling. Proline substitutions effectively mitigated binding, underscoring the importance of specific structural characteristics for interaction. Scrambling within the C-terminal region diminished the interaction strength without entirely abolishing it, indicating some degree of non-specific binding within this hydrophobic domain. Collectively, these findings emphasize the significance of APRs in Aβ aggregation and the distinct molecular interactions that transpire at various stages of oligomer formation [79].

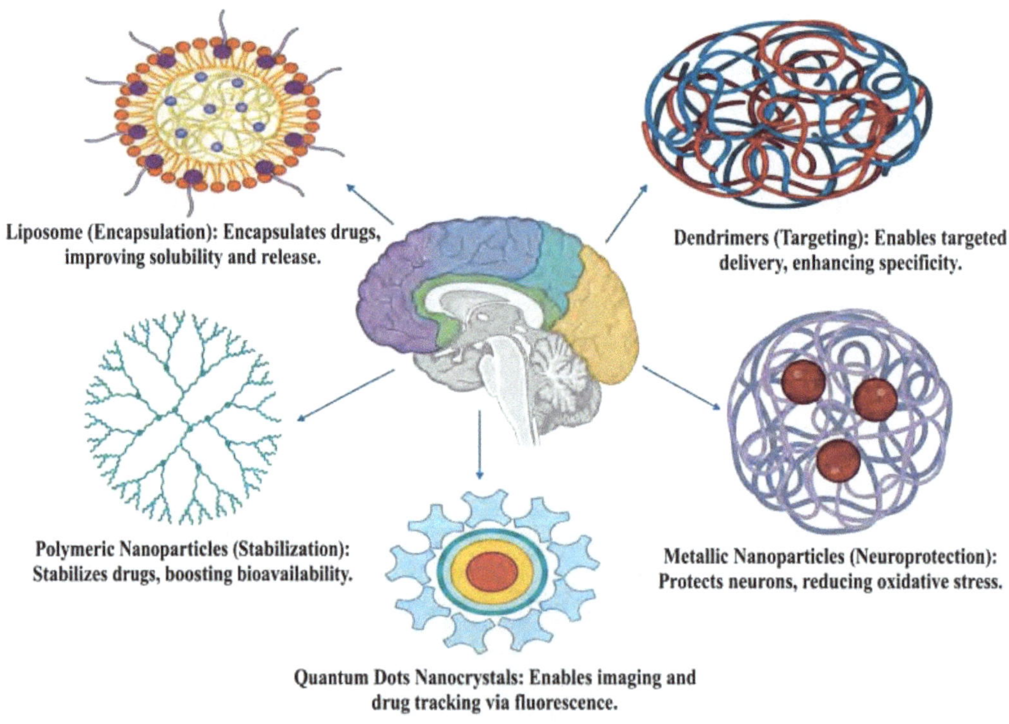

Fig. (3). Mechanism related to the various targeted drug delivery in AD.

Tau Protein Modulation

Tau is part of a tightly controlled class of phosphoproteins with diverse functional roles attributed to axonal transport. Tau regulation is greatly influenced by post-translational modifications (PTMs) such as phosphorylation, dephosphorylation, acetylation, nitration, glycation, sumoylation, ubiquitination, and truncation (proteolytic cleavage) at specific serine, threonine, and tyrosine residues. Thus, these post-translational modifications are vital for controlling Tau's functional characteristics [82]. Phosphorylation and dephosphorylation are major mechanisms that significantly influence the degree of Tau alteration. These processes are regulated by certain protein kinases and phosphatases. The three main classes of protein kinases (PKs) responsible for the phosphorylation of Tau are Proline-Directed Protein Kinases (PDPK), Non-Proline Directed Protein Kinases (Non-PDPK), and Tyrosine Protein Kinases (TPK). Major members of the PDPK family are C-Jun Amino-Terminal Kinase (JNK), Cyclin-Dependent Kinase 5 (cdk5), and Glycogen Synthase Kinase-3 (GSK-3). The Non-PDPK family, however, consists of Tau Protein Kinase I (TPKI) and Tau Protein Kinase II (TPKII), Adenosine Monophosphate Activated Protein Kinase (AMPK), Dual Specificity Tyrosine-Phosphorylation-Regulated Kinase 1A (Dyrk1A), Microtubule-Affinity Regulating Kinases (MARKs), Cyclic AMP (cAMP)-Dependent Protein Kinase (PKA), and Casein Kinase 1 (CK1). Protein Phosphatase 2B (PP2B), Protein Phosphatase 2A (PP2A), Protein Phosphatase 1 (PP1), Protein Phosphatase 5 (PP5), Tissue-Nonspecific Alkaline Phosphatase (TNAP), Calcyclin Binding Protein and Siah-1 Interacting Protein (CacyBP/SIP), and Protein Phosphatase 1 (PP1) are other unique protein phosphatases (PPs). Glycogen synthase kinase 3 (GSK-3), cyclin-dependent kinase 5 (cdk5), and c-Jun N-terminal kinases (JNK) are serine/threonine-specific kinases, and their enzymatic activity is controlled by phosphorylation. A mind map providing the types and categories of the above protein kinases and phosphatases should be detailed. The specific tau protein residues that are targets of the phosphorylation activities that are catalyzed by each kinase are different. Tyrosine 279 (GSK-3α) or tyrosine 216 (GSK-3β) phosphorylation is what activates GSK-3 [36, 60, 83], while cdk5 is activated following phosphorylation at tyrosine 15 [84]. Furthermore, cdk5 necessitates the presence of an activator subunit, which can be either p35 or p25, with the latter exhibiting an extended half-life [39, 85]. In a similar vein, non-proline-directed protein kinases (non-PDPKs) also phosphorylate tau at various residues. For example, the interaction affinity with microtubules is influenced when casein kinase 1 (CK1) phosphorylates tau at Ser202/Thr205 and Ser396/Ser404 [86]. Although dual-specificity tyrosine-regulated kinase 1A (Dyrk1A) phosphorylates tau at numerous sites, the phosphorylation at Thr212, Ser202, and Ser404 is particularly relevant in the context of AD. Notably, in the tau protein, approximately 50% of the phosphorylation sites are adjacent to proline residues. It has been observed that proline-directed protein kinases (PDPKs) significantly contribute to tau phosphorylation and have been implicated in neurodegenerative disorders, such as Pick's Disease, progressive supranuclear palsy, and AD, by facilitating the formation of early tau deposits and tangles within cerebral samples [41, 43, 87].

Moreover, findings from transgenic mouse models reveal that the heightened expression of GSK3 and thc CDK-5 regulatory protein p25 correlates with hyperphosphorylation, which subsequently leads to deficits in spatial learning [39, 42, 88]. Conversely, non-proline sites are phosphorylated by non-PDPKs, including protein kinase A (PKA) and Mark [89]. Consequently, it is imperative to highlight that tau polymerization is modulated by both PDPKs and non-PDPKs synergistically under both physiological and pathological states [90].

NEUROPROTECTION AND ANTI-INFLAMMATORY

AD is characterized by neurodegeneration and chronic inflammation, contributing to cognitive decline. Strategies targeting neuroprotection and inflammation are crucial for mitigating disease progression and improving patient outcomes. Here's a detailed discussion of these aspects [4, 12].

Neuroprotection in AD

AD is associated with increased oxidative stress due to elevated levels of reactive oxygen species (ROS). Neuroprotective strategies aim to counteract oxidative damage by enhancing antioxidant defences, such as using antioxidants (*e.g.*, vitamin E, coenzyme Q10) or promoting endogenous antioxidant systems [13]. Neurotrophic factors, like brain-derived neurotrophic factor (BDNF) and nerve growth factor (NGF), support neuronal survival and function. Therapeutic approaches include enhancing the expression or delivery of these factors to promote neuronal health. Strategies to reduce the accumulation or toxicity of Aβ plaques and tau tangles, such as anti-Aβ antibodies or tau aggregation inhibitors, are central to neuroprotection. These approaches aim to prevent or slow the neurodegenerative processes driven by these pathological hallmarks [14 - 16, 64].

Anti-inflammatory Effect in AD

Although there have been conflicting clinical outcomes, traditional NSAIDs have been studied for their ability to lessen inflammation associated with AD. In preclinical studies, a few DMARDs have demonstrated potential in lowering neuroinflammation. These comprise biologics and small compounds that target cytokines or inflammatory pathways implicated with AD, such as interleukins (*e.g.*, IL-1β) or tumour necrosis factor-alpha (TNF-α) inhibitors [64]. It has been demonstrated that anti-inflammatory lifestyle modifications, including frequent exercise and mental stimulation, as well as anti-inflammatory food therapies like the Mediterranean diet, may have anti-inflammatory properties and may lower the risk or development of AD [35].The gathering of beta-amyloid plaques, the formation of neurofibrillary tangles, BBB leakage, and neuroinflammation, all key features observed in the brain of an Alzheimer's patient, are illustrated in Fig.

(**4**), particularly highlighting their presence in coronal sections at the basal ganglia to provide a detailed visual representation of disease progression.

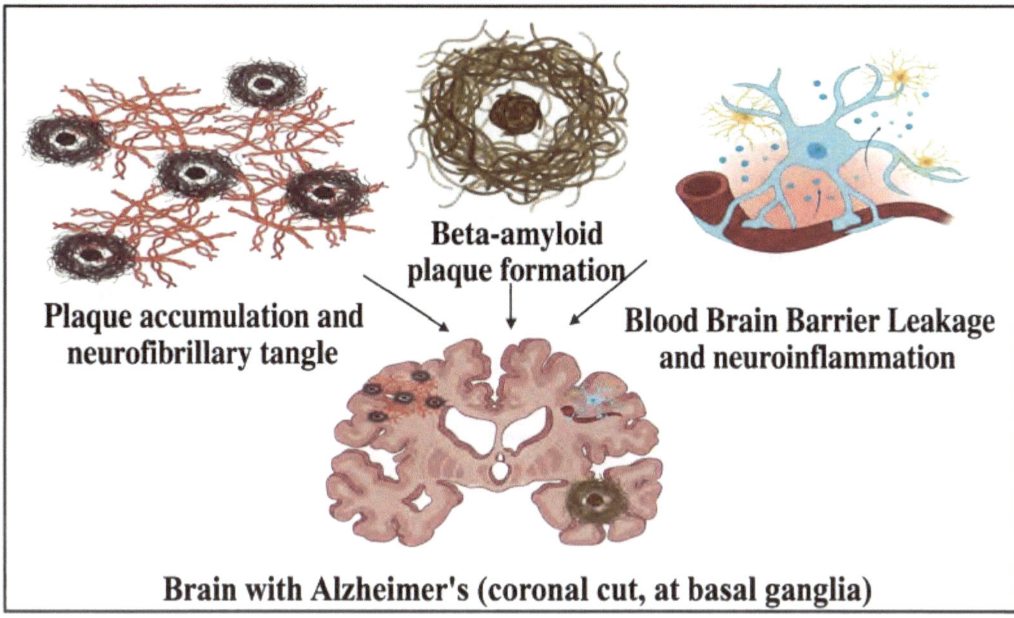

Fig. (4). Beta-amyloid plaque accumulation, neurofibrillary tangle formation, BBB leakage, and neuroinflammation are key features observed in a brain with Alzheimer's, particularly in coronal sections at the basal ganglia.

CHALLENGES, LIMITATIONS, AND FUTURE DIRECTIONS

Potential Toxicity and Biocompatibility Issues

To ensure patient safety when developing therapeutics for AD, it is imperative to consider possible difficulties related to toxicity and biocompatibility [35]. Concerns about toxicity include adverse reactions to anti-amyloid and anti-tau therapies, such as amyloid-related imaging abnormalities (ARIA), as well as side effects from common AD medications, such as gastrointestinal problems from cholinesterase inhibitors and neuropsychiatric effects from NMDA receptor antagonists. Risks associated with nanoparticle-based therapy might include cytotoxicity, inflammation, and long-term organ damage. Biocompatibility concerns include evaluating the long-term effects of chronic exposure, controlling the impact of disruptions to the BBB, and making sure that medication delivery systems employ safe materials. To optimise safety and efficacy, comprehensive preclinical and clinical testing, personalised medical techniques, and cutting-edge technology are necessary for effective risk mitigation [13, 37, 40, 91].

Manufacturing and Scalability

Nanotechnology for AD manufacturing and scalability entails several important issues and concerns. To ensure consistent quality and efficacy, precise control over nanoparticle manufacturing, including size, shape, and surface features, is necessary for the development of nanotechnology-based therapeutics [92]. Production must be scaled up from laboratory to industrial levels, requiring reliable, repeatable manufacturing techniques that can manage high numbers while upholding cost and safety standards. Maintaining the homogeneity of nanoparticles, managing any contamination, and adhering to regulatory requirements are among the difficulties [38, 54]. Advanced manufacturing techniques, like automated systems and microfluidic processes, are essential for making these treatments on a large scale while maintaining high quality. However, to bring these technologies into clinical practice, it's also important to get the necessary approvals, deal with financial challenges, and develop effective ways to distribute and store the treatments [63].

Regulatory and Ethical Considerations

Using nanotechnology in Alzheimer's treatment brings up several ethical and regulatory challenges. To ensure safety and effectiveness, thorough research is needed to check for potential risks and long-term effects. When using nanotechnology for diagnosis, it is important to get patients' informed consent, protect vulnerable groups, and address privacy and security issues [13]. It is also necessary to make sure everyone has equal access to these new treatments. To keep patients' trust and well-being, open communication with everyone involved and a strong focus on ethics are key [63].

PERSONALISED NANO-MEDICINE FOR AD

Personalized nano-medicine for Alzheimer's aims to reduce side effects and improve treatment effectiveness by creating treatments specifically designed for each patient. It uses genetic, biochemical, and imaging information to design drug delivery systems that target the unique features of a patient's Alzheimer's. This approach customizes how the treatment works, based on things like the patient's metabolism, and tracks progress with advanced imaging. The goal is to offer more precise, effective therapies that can better address the differences in how Alzheimer's affects each person, leading to better results for patients [13, 61, 62].

Personalised Nanomedicine for AD

Alzheimer's disease (AD) is a complicated brain disorder where harmful clumps of amyloid-beta plaques and tau tangles build up. Traditional treatments often do not work well because they do not take into account how different the disease can be for each person. This is where nanotechnology comes in as a helpful tool. Nanomedicine uses tiny particles that can be specially designed to target specific markers in the brain, like amyloid-beta plaques or tau tangles. These tiny particles are coated with special molecules that help them stick to the right targets, making sure the drug goes exactly where it is needed. This personalized approach helps avoid side effects and reduces the toxic effects that Alzheimer's drugs can sometimes cause. For example, liposomes, polymer-based particles, and dendrimers can carry drugs and help them cross the blood-brain barrier to reach the damaged parts of the brain. Adding special molecules to these particles improves their ability to target and deliver the drug directly to areas with amyloid or tau buildup [93].

Integration with Other Therapies

Combining nanotechnology with current treatments for Alzheimer's disease (AD) is an important move toward better and more complete care. While nanomedicine is powerful on its own, it works even better when used alongside other treatments—like regular medicines, gene therapy, immune-based treatments, and healthy lifestyle changes such as eating well and staying active. This all-around approach helps tackle different parts of the disease at the same time, making treatment more effective [23, 94 - 96].

Combination with Pharmacological Therapies

Traditional Alzheimer's drugs like donepezil and memantine help manage symptoms, but often do not work as well as they could because they do not reach the brain efficiently and can cause side effects in other parts of the body. Nanotechnology helps solve this problem by packaging these drugs into tiny carriers (like liposomes or nanoparticles) that can cross the blood-brain barrier more easily. This means the drugs can reach the brain better, work more effectively, and cause fewer side effects. For example, a study by Zhang *et al.*, (2022) showed that putting donepezil into nanoparticles helped it get into the brain more efficiently and improve memory in Alzheimer's models better than the regular version of the drug. This shows how nanotechnology can improve current Alzheimer's treatments [97].

Synergy with Immunotherapy

Immunotherapy is a new way to treat Alzheimer's that uses special proteins like antibodies or vaccines to attack the harmful substances in the brain, such as amyloid-beta or tau. However, these treatments have not worked very well yet because they have trouble reaching the brain and can cause side effects in the rest of the body. Nanotechnology can help by acting like a tiny delivery van that brings these treatments straight to the problem areas in the brain. For example, researchers have used tiny gold particles to carry antibodies right to the spots where amyloid builds up. In a study by Chen *et al*., (2021), this method worked better than using the antibodies alone, it cleared more of the harmful amyloid and improved memory in mice with Alzheimer's [98].

Nanotechnology and Gene Therapy

Gene therapy could be a powerful way to treat Alzheimer's by fixing or blocking the faulty genes that help cause the disease. But getting these gene-editing tools, like CRISPR or siRNA, into the brain is very difficult. Nanotechnology can help by acting like a protective vehicle that safely carries these tools across the brain's natural barriers and delivers them exactly where they are needed. For example, in a study by Park *et al*., (2023), scientists used tiny fat-based particles (called lipid nanoparticles) to deliver CRISPR tools that targeted a risky gene linked to Alzheimer's (called APOE ε4). This method worked well; it improved how efficiently the gene was edited in the brain and helped lower the amount of harmful amyloid-beta. This shows how combining gene therapy with nanotechnology could lead to better Alzheimer's treatments [99].

Lifestyle and Non-pharmacological Interventions

Besides using medicines and gene therapies, healthy lifestyle habits like regular exercise, eating well, and brain training can also help slow down Alzheimer's disease. Nanotechnology can support these habits by offering better tools to track how well they are working and how the disease is progressing. For example, scientists have created tiny devices (like nano biosensors) and imaging tools that can detect changes in Alzheimer 's-related substances (like amyloid-beta) in real time. This helps doctors adjust treatments based on how a person is responding to things like diet or exercise. One study by Bhatia *et al*., (2023) showed that a nano biosensor could measure amyloid-beta levels in people with Alzheimer's after they made dietary changes. This gave doctors a clear and fast way to see if the changes were helping [100].

FUTURE PROSPECTS AND INNOVATIONS IN NANOMATERIALS

There are exciting new possibilities for using nanomaterials to improve how we diagnose and treat Alzheimer's disease. Scientists are developing special nanoparticles that can cross the brain's protective barrier more easily and go directly to harmful proteins like tau tangles or amyloid plaques [54, 58]. Some of these new nanoparticles can even do two jobs at once: treat the disease and help doctors track how it is progressing in real time. These advances could make

Alzheimer's treatments work better, cause fewer side effects, and give patients more personalized care [58, 61].

CONCLUSION

Nanotechnology offers a hopeful new way to treat Alzheimer's disease. By using tiny particles called nanoparticles, scientists can create treatments that go straight to the problem areas in the brain. These treatments can be more effective, safer, and better at targeting the root causes of the disease. While significant challenges remain, including ensuring the safety and efficacy of these approaches in humans, the potential benefits make nanotechnology a key area of focus in the quest to combat AD.

LIST OF ABBREVIATIONS

AD	AD
BBB	BBB
NPs	Nanoparticles
ROS	Reactive Oxygen Species
Aβ	Amyloid-beta
NFT	Neurofibrillary Tangles
CNS	Central Nervous System
FDA	Food and Drug Administration
siRNA	Small Interfering RNA
EPR	Enhanced Permeation and Retention
PLGA	Poly(lactic-co-glycolic acid)
PEG	Polyethylene Glycol
MRI	Magnetic Resonance Imaging
GSK-3	Glycogen Synthase Kinase 3
CRISPR	Clustered Regularly Interspaced Short Palindromic Repeats
NMDA	N-methyl-D-aspartate

REFERENCES

[1] Nishida K, Tamura A, Yui N. ER stress-mediated autophagic cell death induction through methylated β-cyclodextrins-threaded acid-labile polyrotaxanes. J Control Release 2018; 275: 20-31. [http://dx.doi.org/10.1016/j.jconrel.2018.02.010] [PMID: 29428200]

[2] Akhter S, Ahmad I, Ahmad MZ, *et al.* Nanomedicines as cancer therapeutics: current status. Curr Cancer Drug Targets 2013; 13(4): 362-78. [http://dx.doi.org/10.2174/1568009611313040002] [PMID: 23517593]

[3] Nasreddine Z, Garibotto V, Kyaga S, Padovani A. The early diagnosis of Alzheimer's disease: a patient-centred conversation with the care team. Neurol Ther. 2023; 12(1): 11-23.

[http://dx.doi.org/10.1007/s40120-022-00428-7]

[4] Barbu E, Molnàr É, Tsibouklis J, Górecki DC. The potential for nanoparticle-based drug delivery to the brain: overcoming the blood–brain barrier. Expert Opin Drug Deliv 2009; 6(6): 553-65. [http://dx.doi.org/10.1517/17425240902939143] [PMID: 19435406]

[5] Kumar A, Singh A, Ekavali . A review on Alzheimer's disease pathophysiology and its management: an update. Pharmacol Rep 2015; 67(2): 195-203. [http://dx.doi.org/10.1016/j.pharep.2014.09.004] [PMID: 25712639]

[6] Mishra S, Palanivelu K. The effect of curcumin (turmeric) on Alzheimer's disease: An overview. Ann Indian Acad Neurol 2008; 11(1): 13-9. [http://dx.doi.org/10.4103/0972-2327.40220] [PMID: 19966973]

[7] Liu Z, Zhang A, Sun H, Han Y, Kong L, Wang X. Two decades of new drug discovery and development for Alzheimer's disease. RSC Advances 2017; 7(10): 6046-58. [http://dx.doi.org/10.1039/C6RA26737H]

[8] Mohamed T, Shakeri A, Rao PPN. Amyloid cascade in Alzheimer's disease: Recent advances in medicinal chemistry. Eur J Med Chem 2016; 113: 258-72. [http://dx.doi.org/10.1016/j.ejmech.2016.02.049] [PMID: 26945113]

[9] Weekley CM, He C. Developing drugs targeting transition metal homeostasis. Curr Opin Chem Biol 2017; 37: 26-32. [http://dx.doi.org/10.1016/j.cbpa.2016.12.011] [PMID: 28040658]

[10] Prakash A, Dhaliwal GK, Kumar P, Majeed ABA. Brain biometals and Alzheimer's disease – boon or bane? Int J Neurosci 2017; 127(2): 99-108. [http://dx.doi.org/10.3109/00207454.2016.1174118] [PMID: 27044501]

[11] Chase TN, Farlow MR, Clarence-Smith K. Donepezil plus solifenacin (CPC-201) treatment for Alzheimer's disease. Neurotherapeutics 2017; 14(2): 405-16. [http://dx.doi.org/10.1007/s13311-016-0511-x] [PMID: 28138837]

[12] Bhaskar S, Tian F, Stoeger T, *et al.* Multifunctional Nanocarriers for diagnostics, drug delivery and targeted treatment across blood-brain barrier: perspectives on tracking and neuroimaging. Part Fibre Toxicol 2010; 7(1): 3. [http://dx.doi.org/10.1186/1743-8977-7-3] [PMID: 20199661]

[13] Fonseca-Santos B, Chorilli M, Palmira Daflon Gremião M. Nanotechnology-based drug delivery systems for the treatment of Alzheimer's disease. Int J Nanomedicine 2015; 10: 4981-5003. [http://dx.doi.org/10.2147/IJN.S87148] [PMID: 26345528]

[14] Chen Y, Liu L. Modern methods for delivery of drugs across the blood–brain barrier. Adv Drug Deliv Rev 2012; 64(7): 640-65. [http://dx.doi.org/10.1016/j.addr.2011.11.010] [PMID: 22154620]

[15] Stöckel T, Wunsch K, Hughes CML. Age-related decline in anticipatory motor planning and its relation to cognitive and motor skill proficiency. Front Aging Neurosci 2017; 9: 283. [http://dx.doi.org/10.3389/fnagi.2017.00283] [PMID: 28928653]

[16] de Lima R, Seabra AB, Durán N. Silver nanoparticles: a brief review of cytotoxicity and genotoxicity of chemically and biogenically synthesized nanoparticles. J Appl Toxicol 2012; 32(11): 867-79. [http://dx.doi.org/10.1002/jat.2780] [PMID: 22696476]

[17] Patterson C. World Alzheimer Report 2018: The state of the art of dementia research: new frontiers. London: Alzheimer's Disease International; 2018. p. 1-48. Available from: https://www.alz.co.uk/news/world-alzheimer-report-2018-state-of-art-of-dementia-research-new-frontiers

[18] Nandi A, Counts N, Bröker J, *et al.* Cost of care for Alzheimer's disease and related dementias in the United States: 2016 to 2060. npj Aging. 2024; 10: 13. [http://dx.doi.org/10.1038/s41514-024-00136-6] [PMID: 38331952]

[19] Ohara T, Hata J, Yoshida D, *et al.* Trends in dementia prevalence, incidence, and survival rate in a Japanese community. Neurology 2017; 88(20): 1925-32. [http://dx.doi.org/10.1212/WNL.0000000000003932] [PMID: 28424272]

[20] Chan KY, Wang W, Wu JJ, *et al.* Epidemiology of Alzheimer's disease and other forms of dementia in China, 1990–2010: a systematic review and analysis. Lancet 2013; 381(9882): 2016-23. [http://dx.doi.org/10.1016/S0140-6736(13)60221-4] [PMID: 23746902]

[21] Nichols E, Szoeke CEI, Vollset SE, *et al.* Global, regional, and national burden of Alzheimer's disease and other dementias, 1990–2016: a systematic analysis for the Global Burden of Disease Study 2016. Lancet Neurol 2019; 18(1): 88-106. [http://dx.doi.org/10.1016/S1474-4422(18)30403-4] [PMID: 30497964]

[22] Livingston G, Huntley J, Sommerlad A, *et al.* Dementia prevention, intervention, and care: 2020 report of the Lancet Commission. Lancet 2020; 396(10248): 413-46. [http://dx.doi.org/10.1016/S0140-6736(20)30367-6] [PMID: 32738937]

[23] Saraiva C, Praça C, Ferreira R, Santos T, Ferreira L, Bernardino L. Nanoparticle-mediated brain drug delivery: Overcoming blood–brain barrier to treat neurodegenerative diseases. J Control Release 2016; 235: 34-47. [http://dx.doi.org/10.1016/j.jconrel.2016.05.044] [PMID: 27208862]

[24] Zielińska A, Costa B, Ferreira MV, *et al.* Nanotoxicology and nanosafety: Safety-by-design and testing at a glance. Int J Environ Res Public Health 2020; 17(13): 4657. [http://dx.doi.org/10.3390/ijerph17134657] [PMID: 32605255]

[25] Hu L, Tao Y, Jiang Y, Qin F. Recent progress of nanomedicine in the treatment of Alzheimer's disease. Front Cell Dev Biol 2023; 11: 1228679. [http://dx.doi.org/10.3389/fcell.2023.1228679] [PMID: 37457297]

[26] Tinkle S, McNeil SE, Mühlebach S, *et al.* Nanomedicines: addressing the scientific and regulatory gap. Ann N Y Acad Sci 2014; 1313(1): 35-56. [http://dx.doi.org/10.1111/nyas.12403] [PMID: 24673240]

[27] Pardridge WM. Drug transport across the blood-brain barrier. J Cereb Blood Flow Metab 2012; 32(11): 1959-72. [http://dx.doi.org/10.1038/jcbfm.2012.126] [PMID: 22929442]

[28] De Strooper B, Karran E. The cellular phase of Alzheimer's disease. Cell 2016; 164(4): 603-15. [http://dx.doi.org/10.1016/j.cell.2015.12.056] [PMID: 26871627]

[29] Banks WA. From blood–brain barrier to blood–brain interface: new opportunities for CNS drug delivery. Nat Rev Drug Discov 2016; 15(4): 275-92. [http://dx.doi.org/10.1038/nrd.2015.21] [PMID: 26794270]

[30] Gaur U, Sahoo SK, De TK, Ghosh PC, Maitra A, Ghosh PK. Biodistribution of fluoresceinated dextran using novel nanoparticles evading reticuloendothelial system. Int J Pharm 2000; 202(1-2): 1-10. [http://dx.doi.org/10.1016/S0378-5173(99)00447-0] [PMID: 10915921]

[31] Sabbagh JJ, Dickey CA. The metamorphic nature of the tau protein: dynamic flexibility comes at a cost. Front Neurosci 2016; 10: 3. [http://dx.doi.org/10.3389/fnins.2016.00003] [PMID: 26834532]

[32] Masoudi Asil S, Ahlawat J, Guillama Barroso G, Narayan M. Nanomaterial based drug delivery systems for the treatment of neurodegenerative diseases. Biomater Sci 2020; 8(15): 4109-28. [http://dx.doi.org/10.1039/D0BM00809E] [PMID: 32638706]

[33] Kreuter J. Drug delivery to the central nervous system by polymeric nanoparticles: What do we know? Adv Drug Deliv Rev 2014; 71: 2-14. [http://dx.doi.org/10.1016/j.addr.2013.08.008] [PMID: 23981489]

[34] Nune SK, Gunda P, Thallapally PK, Lin YY, Laird Forrest M, Berkland CJ. Nanoparticles for biomedical imaging. Expert Opin Drug Deliv 2009; 6(11): 1175-94. [http://dx.doi.org/10.1517/17425240903229031] [PMID: 19743894]

[35] Fang J, Nakamura H, Maeda H. The EPR effect: Unique features of tumor blood vessels for drug delivery, factors involved, and limitations and augmentation of the effect. Adv Drug Deliv Rev 2011; 63(3): 136-51. [http://dx.doi.org/10.1016/j.addr.2010.04.009] [PMID: 20441782]

[36] Giese KP. GSK-3: A key player in neurodegeneration and memory. IUBMB Life 2009; 61(5): 516-21. [http://dx.doi.org/10.1002/iub.187] [PMID: 19391164]

[37] Zabara M, Ren Q, Amenitsch H, Salentinig S. Bioinspired antimicrobial coatings from peptide-functionalized liquid crystalline nanostructures. ACS Appl Bio Mater 2021; 4(6): 5295-303. [http://dx.doi.org/10.1021/acsabm.1c00415] [PMID: 35007010]

[38] Moghimi SM, Hunter AC, Murray JC. Nanomedicine: current status and future prospects. FASEB J 2005; 19(3): 311-30. [http://dx.doi.org/10.1096/fj.04-2747rev] [PMID: 15746175]

[39] Noble W, Olm V, Takata K, *et al.* Cdk5 is a key factor in tau aggregation and tangle formation *in vivo.* Neuron 2003; 38(4): 555-65. [http://dx.doi.org/10.1016/S0896-6273(03)00259-9] [PMID: 12765608]

[40] Deng A, Yang Y, Du S, *et al.* Preparation of a recombinant collagen-peptide (RHC)-conjugated chitosan thermosensitive hydrogel for wound healing. Mater Sci Eng C 2021; 119: 111555. [http://dx.doi.org/10.1016/j.msec.2020.111555] [PMID: 33321619]

[41] Pei JJ, Grundke-Iqbal I, Iqbal K, Bogdanovic N, Winblad B, Cowburn RF. Accumulation of cyclin-dependent kinase 5 (cdk5) in neurons with early stages of Alzheimer's disease neurofibrillary degeneration. Brain Res 1998; 797(2): 267-77. [http://dx.doi.org/10.1016/S0006-8993(98)00296-0] [PMID: 9666145]

[42] de Barreda EG, Pérez M, Ramos PG, *et al.* Tau-knockout mice show reduced GSK3-induced hippocampal degeneration and learning deficits. Neurobiol Dis 2010; 37(3): 622-9. [http://dx.doi.org/10.1016/j.nbd.2009.11.017] [PMID: 20004245]

[43] Ferrer I, Blanco R, Carmona M, *et al.* Phosphorylated map kinase (ERK1, ERK2) expression is associated with early tau deposition in neurones and glial cells, but not with increased nuclear DNA vulnerability and cell death, in Alzheimer disease, Pick's disease, progressive supranuclear palsy and corticobasal degeneration. Brain Pathol 2001; 11(2): 144-58. [http://dx.doi.org/10.1111/j.1750-3639.2001.tb00387.x] [PMID: 11303790]

[44] Allen TM, Cullis PR. Drug delivery systems: entering the mainstream. Science 2004; 303(5665): 1818-22. [http://dx.doi.org/10.1126/science.1095833] [PMID: 15031496]

[45] Kröger APP, Paulusse JMJ. Single-chain polymer nanoparticles in controlled drug delivery and targeted imaging. J Control Release 2018; 286: 326-47. [http://dx.doi.org/10.1016/j.jconrel.2018.07.041] [PMID: 30077737]

[46] Mauri E, Papa S, Masi M, Veglianese P, Rossi F. Novel functionalization strategies to improve drug delivery from polymers. Expert Opin Drug Deliv 2017; 14(11): 1305-13. [http://dx.doi.org/10.1080/17425247.2017.1285280] [PMID: 28103740]

[47] Mauri E, Gori M, Giannitelli SM, *et al.* Nano-encapsulation of hydroxytyrosol into formulated nanogels improves therapeutic effects against hepatic steatosis: An *in vitro* study. Mater Sci Eng C 2021; 124: 112080. [http://dx.doi.org/10.1016/j.msec.2021.112080] [PMID: 33947572]

[48] Petri B, Bootz A, Khalansky A, *et al.* Chemotherapy of brain tumour using doxorubicin bound to surfactant-coated poly(butyl cyanoacrylate) nanoparticles: Revisiting the role of surfactants. J Control

Release 2007; 117(1): 51-8.
[http://dx.doi.org/10.1016/j.jconrel.2006.10.015] [PMID: 17150277]

[49] Choi CHJ, Alabi CA, Webster P, Davis ME. Mechanism of active targeting in solid tumors with transferrin-containing gold nanoparticles. Proc Natl Acad Sci USA 2010; 107(3): 1235-40.
[http://dx.doi.org/10.1073/pnas.0914140107] [PMID: 20080552]

[50] Lu W. Adsorptive-mediated brain delivery systems. Curr Pharm Biotechnol 2012; 13(12): 2340-8.
[http://dx.doi.org/10.2174/138920112803341851] [PMID: 23016640]

[51] Zhu X, Jin K, Huang Y, Pang Z. Brain drug delivery by adsorption-mediated transcytosis. In: Brain Targeted Drug Delivery System: A Focus on Nanotechnology and Nanoparticulates. Elsevier; 2019: 159-183.
[http://dx.doi.org/10.1016/B978-0-12-814001-7.00007-X]

[52] Yin T, Yang L, Liu Y, Zhou X, Sun J, Liu J. Sialic acid (SA)-modified selenium nanoparticles coated with a high blood–brain barrier permeability peptide-B6 peptide for potential use in Alzheimer's disease. Acta Biomater 2015; 25: 172-83.
[http://dx.doi.org/10.1016/j.actbio.2015.06.035] [PMID: 26143603]

[53] Birrenbach G, Speiser PP. Polymerized micelles and their use as adjuvants in immunology. J Pharm Sci 1976; 65(12): 1763-6.
[http://dx.doi.org/10.1002/jps.2600651217] [PMID: 1036442]

[54] Khan I, Saeed K, Khan I. Nanoparticles: Properties, applications and toxicities. Arab J Chem 2019; 12(7): 908-31.
[http://dx.doi.org/10.1016/j.arabjc.2017.05.011]

[55] Loureiro J, Andrade S, Duarte A, *et al.* Resveratrol and grape extract-loaded solid lipid nanoparticles for the treatment of Alzheimer's disease. Molecules 2017; 22(2): 277.
[http://dx.doi.org/10.3390/molecules22020277] [PMID: 28208831]

[56] Leszek J, Md Ashraf G, Tse WH, *et al.* Nanotechnology for Alzheimer disease. Curr Alzheimer Res 2017; 14(11): 1182-9.
[PMID: 28164767]

[57] Wen MM, El-Salamouni NS, El-Refaie WM, *et al.* Nanotechnology-based drug delivery systems for Alzheimer's disease management: Technical, industrial, and clinical challenges. J Control Release 2017; 245: 95-107.
[http://dx.doi.org/10.1016/j.jconrel.2016.11.025] [PMID: 27889394]

[58] Zhou S, Hashida Y, Kawakami S, *et al.* Preparation of immunostimulatory single-walled carbon nanotube/CpG DNA complexes and evaluation of their potential in cancer immunotherapy. Int J Pharm 2014; 471(1-2): 214-23.
[http://dx.doi.org/10.1016/j.ijpharm.2014.05.037] [PMID: 24861942]

[59] Ye T, Li F, Ma G, Wei W. Enhancing therapeutic performance of personalized cancer vaccine *via* delivery vectors. Adv Drug Deliv Rev 2021; 177: 113927.
[http://dx.doi.org/10.1016/j.addr.2021.113927] [PMID: 34403752]

[60] Wang QM, Fiol CJ, DePaoli-Roach AA, Roach PJ. Glycogen synthase kinase-3 beta is a dual specificity kinase differentially regulated by tyrosine and serine/threonine phosphorylation. J Biol Chem 1994; 269(20): 14566-74.
[http://dx.doi.org/10.1016/S0021-9258(17)36661-9] [PMID: 7514173]

[61] Zhu Y, Zhang J, Meng F, *et al.* cRGD-functionalized reduction-sensitive shell-sheddable biodegradable micelles mediate enhanced doxorubicin delivery to human glioma xenografts *in vivo.* J Control Release 2016; 233: 29-38.
[http://dx.doi.org/10.1016/j.jconrel.2016.05.014] [PMID: 27178807]

[62] Altinoglu G, Adali T. Alzheimer's disease targeted nano-based drug delivery systems. Curr Drug Targets 2020; 21(7): 628-46.

[http://dx.doi.org/10.2174/1389450120666191118123151] [PMID: 31744447]

[63] Su M, Yang B, Xi M, Qiang C, Yin Z. Therapeutic effect of pH-Responsive dexamethasone prodrug nanoparticles on acute lung injury. J Drug Deliv Sci Technol 2021; 66: 102738. [http://dx.doi.org/10.1016/j.jddst.2021.102738] [PMID: 36568326]

[64] Liu Y, Xie X, Chen H, *et al.* Advances in next-generation lipid-polymer hybrid nanocarriers with emphasis on polymer-modified functional liposomes and cell-based-biomimetic nanocarriers for active ingredients and fractions from Chinese medicine delivery. Nanomedicine 2020; 29: 102237. [http://dx.doi.org/10.1016/j.nano.2020.102237] [PMID: 32534047]

[65] Mukherjee S, Madamsetty VS, Bhattacharya D, Roy Chowdhury S, Paul MK, Mukherjee A. Recent advancements of nanomedicine in neurodegenerative disorders theranostics. Adv Funct Mater 2020; 30(35): 2003054. [http://dx.doi.org/10.1002/adfm.202003054]

[66] Zhang W, Wang W, Yu DX, Xiao Z, He Z. Application of nanodiagnostics and nanotherapy to CNS diseases. Nanomedicine (Lond) 2018; 13(18): 2341-71. [http://dx.doi.org/10.2217/nnm-2018-0163] [PMID: 30088440]

[67] Kreuter J, Shamenkov D, Petrov V, *et al.* Apolipoprotein-mediated transport of nanoparticle-bound drugs across the blood-brain barrier. J Drug Target 2002; 10(4): 317-25. [http://dx.doi.org/10.1080/10611860290031877] [PMID: 12164380]

[68] Koffie RM, Farrar CT, Saidi LJ, William CM, Hyman BT, Spires-Jones TL. Nanoparticles enhance brain delivery of blood–brain barrier-impermeable probes for *in vivo* optical and magnetic resonance imaging. Proc Natl Acad Sci USA 2011; 108(46): 18837-42. [http://dx.doi.org/10.1073/pnas.1111405108] [PMID: 22065785]

[69] Wilson B, Samanta MK, Santhi K, Kumar KPS, Paramakrishnan N, Suresh B. Poly(n-butylcyanoacrylate) nanoparticles coated with polysorbate 80 for the targeted delivery of rivastigmine into the brain to treat Alzheimer's disease. Brain Res 2008; 1200: 159-68. [http://dx.doi.org/10.1016/j.brainres.2008.01.039] [PMID: 18291351]

[70] Ahmad J, Akhter S, Rizwanullah M, *et al.* Nanotechnology based theranostic approaches in alzheimer's disease management: Current status and future perspective. Curr Alzheimer Res 2017; 14(11): 1164-81. [PMID: 28482786]

[71] Wen CJ, Yen TC, Al-Suwayeh SA, Chang HW, Fang JY. *In vivo* real-time fluorescence visualization and brain-targeting mechanisms of lipid nanocarriers with different fatty ester:oil ratios. Nanomedicine (Lond) 2011; 6(9): 1545-59. [http://dx.doi.org/10.2217/nnm.11.46] [PMID: 22077462]

[72] Behera A, Sa N, Pradhan SP, Swain S, Sahu PK. Metal nanoparticles in alzheimer's disease. J Alzheimers Dis Rep 2023; 7(1): 791-810. [http://dx.doi.org/10.3233/ADR-220112] [PMID: 37662608]

[73] Blanco E, Shen H, Ferrari M. Principles of nanoparticle design for overcoming biological barriers to drug delivery. Nat Biotechnol 2015; 33(9): 941-51. [http://dx.doi.org/10.1038/nbt.3330] [PMID: 26348965]

[74] Cunha A, Gaubert A, Latxague L, Dehay B. PLGA-based nanoparticles for neuroprotective drug delivery in neurodegenerative diseases. Pharmaceutics 2021; 13(7): 1042. [http://dx.doi.org/10.3390/pharmaceutics13071042] [PMID: 34371733]

[75] Milazzo FM, Chaves-Sanjuan A, Minenkova O, *et al.* Spike mutation resilient scFv76 antibody counteracts SARS-CoV-2 lung damage upon aerosol delivery. Mol Ther 2023; 31(2): 362-73. [http://dx.doi.org/10.1016/j.ymthe.2022.09.010] [PMID: 36114671]

[76] Nag OK, Delehanty JB. Active cellular and subcellular targeting of nanoparticles for drug delivery. Pharmaceutics 2019; 11(10): 543.

[http://dx.doi.org/10.3390/pharmaceutics11100543] [PMID: 31635367]

[77] Domingues I, Michalowski CB, Marotti V, *et al.* Exploiting the biological effect exerted by lipid nanocapsules in non-alcoholic fatty liver disease. J Control Release 2023; 356: 542-53. [http://dx.doi.org/10.1016/j.jconrel.2023.03.012] [PMID: 36907563]

[78] Alvarez-Erviti L, Seow Y, Yin H, Betts C, Lakhal S, Wood MJA. Delivery of siRNA to the mouse brain by systemic injection of targeted exosomes. Nat Biotechnol 2011; 29(4): 341-5. [http://dx.doi.org/10.1038/nbt.1807] [PMID: 21423189]

[79] Tessier PM, Lindquist S. Prion recognition elements govern nucleation, strain specificity and species barriers. Nature 2007; 447(7144): 556-61. [http://dx.doi.org/10.1038/nature05848] [PMID: 17495929]

[80] Chang WP, Downs D, Huang XP, Da H, Fung KM, Tang J. Amyloid-beta reduction by memapsin 2 (beta-secretase) immunization. FASEB J 2007; 21(12): 3184-96. [http://dx.doi.org/10.1096/fj.06-7993com] [PMID: 17494994]

[81] Dobson CM. Protein misfolding, evolution and disease. Trends Biochem Sci 1999; 24(9): 329-32. [http://dx.doi.org/10.1016/S0968-0004(99)01445-0] [PMID: 10470028]

[82] Mietelska-Porowska A, Wasik U, Goras M, Filipek A, Niewiadomska G. Tau protein modifications and interactions: their role in function and dysfunction. Int J Mol Sci 2014; 15(3): 4671-713. [http://dx.doi.org/10.3390/ijms15034671] [PMID: 24646911]

[83] Bhat RV, Shanley J, Correll MP, *et al.* Regulation and localization of tyrosine ^{216} phosphorylation of glycogen synthase kinase-3β in cellular and animal models of neuronal degeneration. Proc Natl Acad Sci USA 2000; 97(20): 11074-9. [http://dx.doi.org/10.1073/pnas.190297597] [PMID: 10995469]

[84] Lee M, Kwon YT, Li M, Peng J, Friedlander RM, Tsai LH. Neurotoxicity induces cleavage of p35 to p25 by calpain. Nature 2000; 405(6784): 360-4. [http://dx.doi.org/10.1038/35012636] [PMID: 10830966]

[85] Cruz JC, Tseng HC, Goldman JA, Shih H, Tsai LH. Aberrant Cdk5 activation by p25 triggers pathological events leading to neurodegeneration and neurofibrillary tangles. Neuron 2003; 40(3): 471-83. [http://dx.doi.org/10.1016/S0896-6273(03)00627-5] [PMID: 14642273]

[86] Li G, Yin H, Kuret J. Casein kinase 1 delta phosphorylates tau and disrupts its binding to microtubules. J Biol Chem 2004; 279(16): 15938-45. [http://dx.doi.org/10.1074/jbc.M314116200] [PMID: 14761950]

[87] Ferrer I, Barrachina M, Puig B. Glycogen synthase kinase-3 is associated with neuronal and glial hyperphosphorylated tau deposits in Alzheimer's disease, Pick's disease, progressive supranuclear palsy and corticobasal degeneration. Acta Neuropathol 2002; 104(6): 583-91. [http://dx.doi.org/10.1007/s00401-002-0587-8] [PMID: 12410379]

[88] Li B, Ryder J, Su Y, *et al.* Overexpression of GSK3betaS9A resulted in tau hyperphosphorylation and morphology reminiscent of pretangle like neurons in the brain of PDGSK3β transgenic mice. Transgenic Res 2004; 13(4): 385-96. [http://dx.doi.org/10.1023/B:TRAG.0000040039.44899.6f] [PMID: 15517997]

[89] Dolan PJ, Johnson GVW. The role of tau kinases in Alzheimer's disease. Curr Opin Drug Discov Devel 2010; 13(5): 595-603. [PMID: 20812151]

[90] Martin L, Latypova X, Wilson CM, *et al.* Tau protein kinases: Involvement in Alzheimer's disease. Ageing Res Rev 2013; 12(1): 289-309. [http://dx.doi.org/10.1016/j.arr.2012.06.003] [PMID: 22742992]

[91] Song Z, Jia G, Ma P, Cang S. Exosomal miR-4443 promotes cisplatin resistance in non-small cell lung carcinoma by regulating FSP1 m6A modification-mediated ferroptosis. Life Sci 2021; 276: 119399.

[http://dx.doi.org/10.1016/j.lfs.2021.119399] [PMID: 33781830]

[92] Peers S, Montembault A, Ladavière C. Chitosan hydrogels for sustained drug delivery. J Control Release 2020; 326: 150-63.
[http://dx.doi.org/10.1016/j.jconrel.2020.06.012] [PMID: 32562854]

[93] Brambilla D, Le Droumaguet B, Nicolas J, *et al.* Nanotechnologies for Alzheimer's disease: diagnosis, therapy, and safety issues. Nanomedicine 2011; 7(5): 521-40.
[http://dx.doi.org/10.1016/j.nano.2011.03.008] [PMID: 21477665]

[94] Alghamdi MA, Fallica AN, Virzì N, Kesharwani P, Pittalà V, Greish K. The promise of nanotechnology in personalized medicine. J Pers Med 2022; 12(5): 673.
[http://dx.doi.org/10.3390/jpm12050673] [PMID: 35629095]

[95] Cummings J, Lee G, Ritter A, Sabbagh M, Zhong K. Alzheimer's disease drug development pipeline: 2019. Alzheimers Dement (N Y) 2019; 5(1): 272-93.
[http://dx.doi.org/10.1016/j.trci.2019.05.008] [PMID: 31334330]

[96] Sahni JK, Doggui S, Ali J, Baboota S, Dao L, Ramassamy C. Neurotherapeutic applications of nanoparticles in Alzheimer's disease. J Control Release 2011; 152(2): 208-31.
[http://dx.doi.org/10.1016/j.jconrel.2010.11.033] [PMID: 21134407]

[97] La Barbera L, Mauri E, D'Amelio M, Gori M. Functionalization strategies of polymeric nanoparticles for drug delivery in Alzheimer's disease: Current trends and future perspectives. Front Neurosci 2022; 16: 939855.
[http://dx.doi.org/10.3389/fnins.2022.939855] [PMID: 35992936]

[98] Liu W, Dong X, Liu Y, Sun Y. Photoresponsive materials for intensified modulation of Alzheimer's amyloid-β protein aggregation: A review. Acta Biomater 2021; 123: 93-109.
[http://dx.doi.org/10.1016/j.actbio.2021.01.018] [PMID: 33465508]

[99] Bhardwaj S, Kesari KK, Rachamalla M, *et al.* CRISPR/Cas9 gene editing: New hope for Alzheimer's disease therapeutics. J Adv Res 2022; 40: 207-21.
[http://dx.doi.org/10.1016/j.jare.2021.07.001] [PMID: 36100328]

[100] Carneiro P, Morais S, Pereira MC. Nanomaterials towards biosensing of alzheimer's disease biomarkers. Nanomaterials (Basel) 2019; 9(12): 1663.
[http://dx.doi.org/10.3390/nano9121663] [PMID: 31766693]

CHAPTER 9

Treatment Using Anti-Amyloid Antibodies for Alzheimer's Disease

Soumyadeep Chatterjee[1], **Sakuntala Gayen**[1] and **Souvik Roy**[1,*]

[1] *Department of Pharmacy, NSHM Knowledge Campus Kolkata – Group of Institutions, Kolkata, West Bengal, India*

Abstract: This chapter critically examines the latest advancements in novel antibody therapies targeting amyloid-β for Alzheimer's disease, as jointly endorsed by the European Association of Neurology and the European Psychiatric Association. Following numerous setbacks in the pursuit of disease-modifying treatments, compelling and consistent evidence now underscores the clinical efficacy of monoclonal antibodies against amyloid-β. Recent trials have not only succeeded in decelerating disease progression over several months but have also demonstrated positive secondary clinical outcomes and a reduction in amyloid-β levels, as shown through positron emission tomography scans. Collectively, these findings represent a significant breakthrough, confirming that reducing amyloid-β yields tangible clinical benefits beyond mere biomarker changes. As these new-generation drugs become more widely utilized, it remains to be seen whether their statistical efficacy will translate into clinically meaningful improvements. This could indeed mark the dawn of a new era in Alzheimer's disease therapeutics.

Keywords: Anti-amyloid immunotherapy, Cognitive decline treatment, Dementia, Fluid and imaging biomarkers, Mild cognitive impairment, Monoclonal antibodies.

INTRODUCTION

Alzheimer's disease (AD), a chronic and progressive neurodegenerative disorder, is the most prevalent form of dementia, afflicting millions of elderly individuals with cognitive decline and behavioral impairments, responsible for up to 70% of all cases. Its prevalence surges with age, affecting roughly 10% of those over 65 and up to 50% of individuals past 85 [1]. The disease's hallmark pathology includes the accumulation of amyloid-β (Aβ) plaques and neurofibrillary tangles,

* **Corresponding author Souvik Roy:** Department of Pharmacy, NSHM Knowledge Campus Kolkata – Group of Institutions, Kolkata, West Bengal, India; E-mail: souvikroy35@gmail.com; souvik.roy@nshm.com

Swarupananda Mukherjee, Souvik Roy & Dipanjan Karati (Eds.)

formed from hyperphosphorylated tau protein, which disrupts neuronal communication, ultimately leading to neuronal death and cognitive decline [2]. Historically, no treatments could modify the disease course, but in 2021, remarkable progress has been made in the treatment of AD, with the U.S. FDA approving five cognitive-enhancing drugs, one agent aimed at reducing agitation, and two disease-modifying therapies (DMTs). All approved DMTs for AD are currently anti-amyloid monoclonal antibodies (mAbs) [3]. The approval of Aducanumab (Aduhelm®), the first Aβ-targeting antibody, marked a breakthrough in AD treatment, offering a glimpse of hope in the development of disease-modifying therapies. Before this, the FDA had approved only a few drugs aimed at symptomatic relief, such as acetylcholine esterase inhibitors and NMDA receptor modulators, often discontinued due to adverse effects and limited efficacy [4]. The success of aducanumab, followed by the approval of Lecanumab (Leqembi®), a next-generation Aβ antibody, underscores the potential of Aβ-targeted therapies. The two approved therapies, Aducanumab and Lecanemab, have received approval based on their significant reduction of β-amyloid (Aβ) plaques, a hallmark of AD, as evidenced by amyloid positron emission tomography (PET). Donanemab, another promising agent, is under review for standard approval following phase II and III clinical trial data (Fig. **1**) [5]. While all anti-amyloid mAbs share a common mechanism of action—targeting high molecular weight fibrillar Aβ aggregates and inducing significant Aβ clearance—they also exhibit distinct characteristics. These differences lie in the specific amyloid species they target, as well as their pharmacokinetic profiles, including half-life, infusion frequency, and titration schedules [6]. Notably, these mAbs have been tested in populations with early AD, though the criteria for early AD, in terms of severity, vary across trials, potentially influencing patient selection for treatment. This chapter delves into the mechanisms of action of these mAbs, summarizes preclinical data, and highlights key features of their phase I, II, and III clinical trials [7]. We also explore how the similarities and differences among these agents may shape their use in clinical practice. Additionally, we discuss other drugs in development, including Remternetug, currently in a phase III trial, and Gantenerumab, whose development was halted after negative phase III results [8]. It is crucial to interpret the efficacy and safety of these drugs with caution, as direct comparisons can only be made if the agents are tested in equivalent arms within the same clinical trial, considering the variations in entry criteria, trial sites, investigators, and participant profiles [9].

THE CHRONICLE OF AMYLOID CASCADE HYPOTHESIS

In 1984, the discovery of amyloid-beta (Aβ) as the main component of extracellular plaques marked a pivotal moment in Alzheimer's disease (AD) research, highlighting a distinct pathological hallmark of the condition [10]. This breakthrough laid the foundation for the "amyloid cascade hypothesis," proposed by Hardy and Higgins in 1992, which posits that Aβ deposition is the initial trigger for AD pathogenesis, leading to tau tangles, neuronal loss, and cognitive decline. Since then, extensive genetic and non-genetic research has reinforced this hypothesis [11, 12]. For instance, Down syndrome, associated with APP gene triplication, and APP mutations in early-onset Alzheimer's disease (EOAD) both elevate Aβ production and alter the Aβ42/40 ratio, accelerating plaque formation and cognitive deterioration. Furthermore, key genetic risk factors for late-onset Alzheimer's disease (LOAD), such as APOE and Clusterin (CLU), have been found to significantly influence Aβ aggregation and clearance [13].

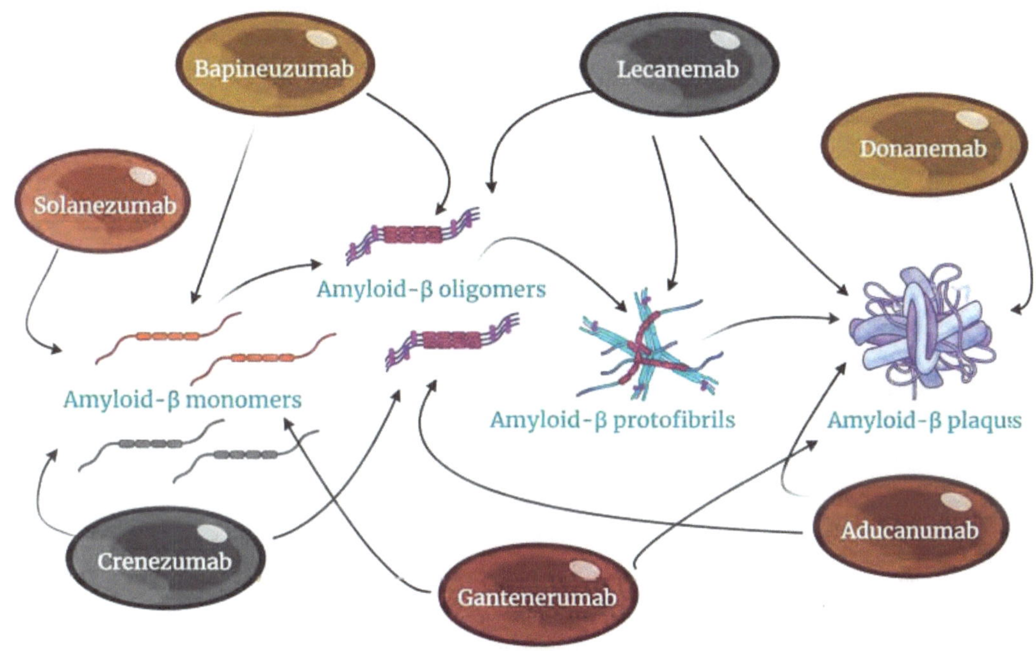

Fig. (1). Advancements in Alzheimer's therapies: mechanisms, trials, and implications of anti-amyloid monoclonal antibodies.

Aβ Aggregate Morphology

Amyloid-beta (Aβ) aggregation is a pivotal event in the pathogenesis of Alzheimer's disease (AD). After its secretion, Aβ transitions from soluble forms into structured cross-β-sheet fibrils, ultimately forming amyloid plaques [14]. These plaques manifest in two distinct types: classical and diffuse. Classical plaques feature a dense Aβ core surrounded by a clear zone and a corona comprising degenerating neurites, reactive astrocytes, and microglia. In contrast, diffuse plaques are more scattered, lacking a concentrated core, and their Aβ deposits are dispersed throughout the brain tissue. Recent research highlights that it is the classical plaques, marked by their association with inflammatory cells, rather than diffuse plaques, that are closely linked to cognitive decline in AD [15].

Amyloid-beta (Aβ) aggregates, after secretion, initially form soluble species that eventually undergo a conformational shift into cross-β-sheet fibrils, culminating in plaque formation. Two distinct types of amyloid plaques have been identified: classical and diffuse. Classical plaques are defined by a dense Aβ core surrounded by an optically clear zone and an outer corona, comprising neuronal and glial components, including degenerating neuronal processes, reactive astrocytes, and microglia. In contrast, diffuse plaques are characterized by small, often star-shaped assemblies scattered throughout brain tissue [16]. The term "diffuse" refers to the widespread and scattered nature of Aβ accumulation rather than its concentration. Notably, recent research has shown that cognitive impairment in Alzheimer's disease is more strongly associated with classical plaques containing inflammatory cells than with diffuse plaques. The amyloid cascade hypothesis has been the prevailing framework for understanding Alzheimer's disease (AD) pathogenesis, though it has evolved. Initially, this hypothesis focused on large, insoluble Aβ fibrils as the primary culprits behind neuronal damage. However, growing evidence now suggests that Aβ oligomers, which are soluble and ligand-like, also play a significant role in neurotoxicity, acting independently of mature fibrils. The amyloid-beta oligomer (AβO) hypothesis posits that these soluble Aβ oligomers are the primary drivers of AD pathogenesis [17].

Aβ aggregates can directly interact with the lipid and cholesterol components of cell membranes, compromising membrane integrity and permeability. This disruption facilitates the influx of calcium ions (Ca^{2+}) into the cell, inhibiting long-term potentiation (LTP) and ultimately resulting in neuronal death. Aβ oligomers can bind to specific molecules such as sialic acid-containing GM1 gangliosides on the cell membrane, triggering further impairment of LTP [18]. Cholesterol-rich lipid rafts also create an environment that enhances Aβ synthesis and strengthens the interaction between Aβ and the membrane. Elevated cholesterol levels within these rafts increase the activity of enzymes involved in amyloidogenic pathways while inhibiting those in non-amyloidogenic pathways. It is well established that cholesterol-enriched membranes facilitate Aβ seeding and aggregation, and reducing cholesterol levels in cellular compartments like endosomes or lysosomes has been shown to alleviate Aβ aggregation and its associated toxicity in mouse models [19]. Disrupted synaptic function is recognized as an early and crucial hallmark of Alzheimer's disease, with synapse loss closely linked to the cognitive decline observed in affected individuals. Aβ oligomers alter the structure and density of synapses, leading to compromised synaptic plasticity. As key glutamate receptors, NMDARs are vital for regulating synapse formation and plasticity; however, Aβ oligomers directly disrupt NMDAR activity, impairing signaling pathways that lead to synaptic loss and reduced spine density. Additionally, Aβ oligomers interfere with glutamate recycling at the synapse by increasing glutamate release, decreasing glutamate uptake, and impairing glutamate transporters. This disruption results in the overactivation of extra-synaptic NMDARs, ultimately causing suppression of LTP, enhancement of long-term depression (LTD), and synaptic loss [20].

Moreover, Aβ oligomers induce the ubiquitination and degradation of AMPA receptors (AMPARs), leading to their loss and suppression of synaptic transmission. Recent studies have revealed that intracellular administration of Aβ oligomers alters synaptic transmission and fast axonal transport through the activation of casein kinase 2 (CK-2) [21]. Additionally, Aβ aggregates inhibit LTP and enhance LTD, resulting in dendritic spine shrinkage through actin remodeling. Aβ aggregates also synergize with hyperphosphorylated tau protein to impair synaptic function, inducing tau hyperphosphorylation and accumulation in dendritic spines, which further exacerbates synaptic loss and dysfunction. Pathological tau interacts with presynaptic components, inhibiting synaptic vesicle mobility and release, thereby contributing to Alzheimer's disease progression [22]. Mislocalized tau proteins at postsynaptic terminals interact with AMPAR and NMDAR subunits, leading to excessive activation of glutamate receptors, increased Ca2+ influx, impaired LTP, and enhanced LTD. Interestingly, the absence of tau proteins has been shown to prevent Aβ-induced LTP impairment in mouse models, suggesting that Aβ-induced synaptic toxicity is at least partially dependent on pathological tau proteins [23].

Aβ-induced Tauopathy

Neurofibrillary tangles (NFTs) composed of hyperphosphorylated tau, alongside amyloid-beta (Aβ) plaques, are central features of Alzheimer's disease pathology. Over the past decade, a growing body of evidence has underscored the pivotal role of the interaction between Aβ and tau in the pathogenesis of Alzheimer's disease [24]. In triple transgenic mice (3xTg-AD), the accumulation of extracellular Aβ in the neocortex and hippocampus occurs before tau aggregates into fibrillar tangles. In experimental models, the injection of Aβ aggregates into the brains of P301L mutant tau transgenic mice results in a five-fold increase in NFTs within the amygdala [25]. Clinically, neuroimaging studies of sporadic Alzheimer's patients show that elevated cortical tau-PET ligand retention is observed only in the presence of Aβ accumulation, which correlates with cortical atrophy in Alzheimer's disease. Moreover, longitudinal studies have demonstrated that early Aβ aggregation is a reliable predictor of subsequent tau changes in the inferior temporal cortex. As an upstream factor, Aβ triggers the hyperphosphorylation of tau proteins, with both elements synergistically contributing to neuronal damage and cognitive deficits.

Aβ facilitates tau hyperphosphorylation through the activation of cyclin-dependent kinase 5 (CDK5) and glycogen synthase kinase 3 (GSK-3). GSK-3β, which is closely associated with Aβ production and accumulation, is a key driver of tau phosphorylation and exacerbates Aβ-induced tau toxicity. CDK5-P25 phosphorylates tau at specific sites, including Thr181, Ser199, Ser202, Thr205, Thr212, Ser214, Ser217, Thr231, Ser235, Ser396, and Ser404 [26]. As a result, inhibitors of GSK-3β or CDK5, such as AZD1080 and roscovitine, significantly reduce tau phosphorylation levels and prevent further tau aggregation. Additional studies have highlighted the role of mitogen-activated protein kinases (MAPKs), including ERK1/2, SAPKs, and p38, in Aβ-induced formation of paired helical filament (PHF)-tau in Alzheimer's disease. The cellular prion protein (PrPC) has been identified as a receptor for toxic Aβ oligomers, leading to long-term potentiation (LTP) loss and cognitive impairment in Alzheimer's disease model mice. PrPC has also been detected in Aβ plaques in Alzheimer's patients, where it activates Fyn kinase, which subsequently phosphorylates tau *via* the GluN2B subunit of NMDARs [27]. Beyond promoting tau phosphorylation, Aβ also influences tau oligomerization and tangle formation. Aβ initiates caspase-3 (CASP3)-induced cleavage of tau at Asp421, producing an N-terminal fragment that self-aggregates and forms neurotoxic oligomers. These tau oligomers not only induce neuronal damage but also bind to astrocytes and microglia, triggering neuroinflammation. In hippocampal neurons, Aβ also activates calpain-1, generating a 17-kDa tau fragment that leads to neurite degeneration and neuronal death [28]. Simultaneously, the toxic state of tau proteins also influences Aβ production. For example, knocking out tau genes in APP/PS1 mice inhibits the amyloidogenic pathway of amyloid precursor protein (APP) processing, thereby reducing Aβ production and amyloid plaque formation. Furthermore, the neurotoxic effects of Aβ are dependent on the presence of tau. The absence of tau on NMDARs in dendritic spines effectively prevents the toxic effects induced by Aβ binding to these receptors. A recent study suggests that tau phosphorylation at Tyr18 by Fyn kinase also mitigates Aβ toxicity. Aβ enhances the phosphorylation and activation of Fyn kinase, which then translocates into dendritic spines, leading to synaptic impairment. Tau mediates Aβ toxicity by interacting with Fyn kinase through its amino-terminal projection domain (PD) [29]. As a result, inhibiting Fyn has been shown to improve cognitive deficits in transgenic mice with Aβ and tau deposits. PET and CSF studies further reveal the synergistic interaction between Aβ and tau, contributing to brain dysfunction and cognitive decline. Intriguingly, Aβ and tau also exhibit antagonistic effects on neural circuits, with tau significantly silencing circuits by blocking Aβ-induced hyperactivity in the cortex [30].

Inducing an Inflammatory Response

Neuroinflammation, primarily driven by activated microglia and astrocytes, plays a significant role in Alzheimer's disease (AD) pathology. This chronic inflammation within the central nervous system (CNS) results in the production of pro-inflammatory cytokines, which are often found near amyloid-beta (Aβ) plaques in AD brain [31]. Microglia, the CNS's resident immune cells, become activated in response to Aβ and attempt to clear these plaques through phagocytosis. However, prolonged microglial activation leads to impaired Aβ clearance, sustained inflammation, and further neuronal damage [32, 33]. Astrocytes, another type of glial cell, also become reactive near Aβ plaques, releasing cytokines that exacerbate inflammation and Aβ accumulation. Mitochondrial dysfunction, triggered by Aβ, further contributes to AD by disrupting energy production and increasing oxidative stress, which damages neurons and promotes Aβ aggregation [34]. Additionally, Aβ disrupts neurotransmission, impairing synaptic plasticity and contributing to cognitive decline [35]. As the disease progresses, significant disruptions occur in neural networks, particularly in the default mode and salience networks, correlating with cognitive deficits and brain atrophy. Current diagnostic methods focus on detecting Aβ through cerebrospinal fluid analysis, PET imaging, and emerging blood-based biomarkers, aiming for early detection and improved disease management [36].

ALZHEIMER'S DISEASE'S CURRENT BIOMARKERS AND AMYLOID-B AS A TREATMENT TARGET

The accumulation of amyloid-beta (Aβ) plaques within the brain is postulated to serve as an incipient event in the pathogenesis of Alzheimer's disease (AD), preceding the aberrant hyperphosphorylation of tau protein. These pathological hallmarks collectively disrupt neuronal homeostasis, instigate neuroinflammation, and ultimately culminate in neuronal demise [37]. Although the fundamental features of AD pathology are extensively documented, their precise role in disease progression remains a subject of active scientific inquiry. It remains uncertain whether the deposition of Aβ plaques and tau aggregates constitutes a primary etiological factor or merely a downstream consequence of the disease. Nevertheless, despite this ambiguity, therapeutic strategies predominantly focus on mitigating Aβ accumulation as a means of developing disease-modifying interventions for AD [38].

The diagnosis of AD presents considerable challenges due to its symptomatic overlap with other dementias and the initial clinical manifestations that closely resemble normative cognitive aging. Historically, AD diagnosis has been predicated on clinical criteria, including progressive memory deterioration and impairments in daily functioning [39]. However, these diagnostic approaches are inherently fallible, as studies indicate that nearly 20% of clinically diagnosed AD cases lack definitive AD pathology. To improve diagnostic precision and facilitate longitudinal disease monitoring, various biomarkers have been developed [40]. Currently available biomarkers encompass cerebrospinal fluid quantification of Aβ and tau proteins, as well as Aβ and tau positron emission tomography (PET) imaging. These modalities exhibit promise in detecting AD-related pathology even during its prodromal phase. However, their invasive nature and challenges associated with scalability significantly hinder widespread clinical implementation [41].

THE MECHANISM OF ANTI-AMYLOID MONOCLONAL ANTIBODIES

The groundbreaking anti-Aβ monoclonal antibody, bapineuzumab, was the first of its class to advance into phase 3 clinical trials in the early 2000s. Engineered to selectively bind the N-terminus of Aβ and facilitate the clearance of amyloid plaques from the brain, it initially demonstrated promise. However, subsequent trials failed to yield substantial clinical benefits, likely due to complexities associated with dosing strategies and patient stratification [42]. Another investigational antibody, solanezumab, designed to target the mid-region of Aβ and hinder its aggregation, produced mixed clinical outcomes. While certain studies suggested a deceleration of cognitive decline in individuals with mild Alzheimer's disease, others failed to substantiate a significant therapeutic advantage [43].

Aducanumab, a monoclonal antibody that preferentially binds aggregated forms of Aβ, particularly the fibrillar constituents of amyloid plaques, exhibited a dose-dependent reduction in plaque burden and an associated attenuation of cognitive decline in early-stage trials. Notably, its phase 3 trials were prematurely halted following a pre-specified futility analysis. However, a subsequent re-evaluation of the data prompted its accelerated approval by the U.S. Food and Drug Administration (FDA) in June 2021, based on its biomarker efficacy, though the extent of its clinical utility remains a topic of ongoing debate [44]. In contrast, the European Medicines Agency (EMA) opted against approval, resulting in the withdrawal of its marketing authorization application within the European Union. Lecanemab (BAN2401), a humanized derivative of murine mAb158 targeting Aβ protofibrils, emerged as a key therapeutic candidate following the CLARITY-AD phase 3 trial in September 2022. This pivotal study successfully met its primary endpoint by demonstrating a significant attenuation of disease progression, alongside achieving all secondary endpoints, including enhancements in quality of life metrics and reductions in caregiver burden [45]. Nonetheless, concerns regarding its safety profile, particularly the incidence of amyloid-related imaging abnormalities (ARIA), including cerebral hemorrhages, necessitate meticulous patient selection and vigilant monitoring. Lecanemab was granted faster FDA approval in January 2023, with full regulatory endorsement anticipated following a favorable advisory panel vote in June 2023. Gantenerumab, another anti-Aβ antibody directed against aggregated Aβ species, initially failed to demonstrate significant clinical efficacy in its phase 3 trial. However, a post hoc analysis suggested potential benefits in patients with milder forms of Alzheimer's disease. Despite subsequent trials employing higher dosing regimens, the therapy did not meet its primary endpoints, culminating in the discontinuation of further development [46]. Donanemab, an antibody engineered to recognize an early conformational state of Aβ preceding overt plaque deposition, demonstrated compelling efficacy in phase 2 trials, effecting substantial reductions in Aβ burden and a measurable deceleration of cognitive decline. Encouraging phase 3 results, disclosed in May 2023, reported a 35% reduction in clinical deterioration and a 40% decrease in the rate of functional decline in activities of daily living, reinforcing the notion that its therapeutic impact is most pronounced in the earliest stages of Alzheimer's disease [47].

ANTI-AB MONOCLONAL ANTIBODIES AS IMMUNOTHERAPIES FOR AD PATIENTS

The progression of amyloid pathology in Alzheimer's disease (AD) unfolds through a cascade of events, beginning with the aggregation of Aβ monomers, advancing to the formation of dimers and trimers, evolving into oligomers, protofibrils, and fibrils, and culminating in the deposition of insoluble amyloid plaques [48]. Monoclonal antibodies (mAbs) against Aβ target various stages of this intricate process, promoting the clearance of Aβ. Recently, the FDA approved two such mAbs, aducanumab and Lecanemab, marking significant strides in AD treatment. Another promising candidate, Donanemab, has also made headway, having submitted a marketing application to the FDA and secured priority review from the Center for Drug Evaluation (CDE) in China as of November 2023. The following sections delve into the therapeutic mechanisms and clinical progress of these antibodies, alongside an exploration of other mAbs poised for future approval [49].

Aducanumab

Aducanumab, a monoclonal antibody designed to target residues 3–7 in the Aβ N-terminus, received accelerated FDA approval in June 2021, marking a significant milestone in Alzheimer's disease (AD) treatment [50]. Despite its low monovalent affinity, aducanumab exhibits strong avidity for epitope-rich aggregates, enabling it to bind to Aβ oligomeric or fibrillar aggregates selectively. This interaction activates microglia, promoting the clearance of Aβ from the brain. Phase I clinical trials (NCT01397539) indicated that doses up to 30 mg/kg were generally well-tolerated with no severe adverse events reported [51]. The subsequent phase Ib trial (PRIME, NCT01677572) demonstrated that a dose range of 3 to 10 mg/kg effectively reduced amyloid plaques, paving the way for the Phase III EMERGE (NCT02484547) and ENGAGE (NCT02477800) trials, both initiated in 2015. However, these trials, along with a Phase II safety trial (EVOLVE, NCT03639987), were prematurely halted after an interim futility analysis suggested a lack of efficacy [52]. In October 2019, Biogen announced that this interim analysis was flawed. A more comprehensive analysis revealed that high-dose aducanumab in the EMERGE trial met its primary endpoint, although the low-dose did not show significant benefits compared to placebo. While the ENGAGE trial did not meet its primary endpoint, participants who received 10 or more doses of 10 mg/kg experienced a slower cognitive decline, similar to those in the EMERGE trial [53]. The difference in outcomes between the two trials likely stemmed from variations in exposure duration to high-dose aducanumab. Safety data revealed that approximately one-third of aducanumab-treated participants developed amyloid-related imaging abnormalities (ARIA), with a quarter of these cases being symptomatic and 3% classified as severe [54]. ARIA-E (vasogenic edema) and ARIA-H (microhemorrhages and hemosiderosis) were commonly observed in patients receiving 10 mg/kg, with incidence rates of 19.1% and 35%, respectively. Notably, APOE ε4 carriers had a higher incidence of ARIA compared to non-carriers. ARIA is a known phenomenon associated with anti-Aβ immunotherapies, likely due to the antibody's role in disaggregating amyloid plaques into soluble forms, triggering glial cell-mediated neuroinflammation, and potentially leading to vascular pathology [55]. Despite ongoing controversies, aducanumab's accelerated approval, based on its ability to reduce Aβ, represents a significant breakthrough in AD therapeutics. It embodies the culmination of nearly 25 years of research into the amyloid hypothesis, heralding a new era in AD treatment. However, access remains limited, as the Centers for Medicare & Medicaid Services (CMS) currently restricts coverage for aducanumab outside of approved clinical trials. Post-approval studies are still necessary to confirm its clinical benefits [56].

Lecanumab

Lecanemab, a humanized IgG1 monoclonal antibody derived from the murine mAb158, was granted accelerated approval by the U.S. Food and Drug Administration (FDA) in January 2023, followed by full approval in July 2023, for the treatment of mild cognitive impairment (MCI) and mild dementia associated with Alzheimer's disease (AD). Notably, Lecanemab exhibits an extraordinary binding affinity for soluble amyloid-beta (Aβ) aggregates—specifically oligomers and protofibrils—demonstrating an affinity nearly 1,000-fold higher than for Aβ monomers and 10–15 times greater than for insoluble fibrils. A Phase I clinical investigation (NCT01230853) comprising 80 individuals with mild-to-moderate AD established the agent's favorable safety, tolerability, and pharmacokinetic profile across all tested doses, with a maximum regimen of 10 mg/kg administered biweekly over four months [57]. Importantly, the incidence of amyloid-related imaging abnormalities (ARIA-E and ARIA-H) remained comparable to that observed in the placebo cohort. Furthermore, pharmacokinetic assessments revealed a dose-proportional response at doses equal to or exceeding 10 mg/kg, with a serum elimination half-life of approximately seven days. Subsequently, a Phase IIb clinical trial (NCT01767311), enrolling 856 participants, aimed to delineate the optimal dosage and therapeutic efficacy of Lecanemab. Although the study did not meet its primary endpoint at the 12-month mark, it was extended to an 18-month duration. The findings demonstrated that individuals receiving 10 mg/kg of Lecanemab biweekly exhibited a statistically significant attenuation of cognitive decline at 6, 12, and 18 months [58]. Notably, this regimen resulted in a profound 93% reduction in cerebral amyloid plaque burden, a 47% deceleration in cognitive deterioration as assessed by the Alzheimer's Disease Assessment Scale-Cognitive Subscale (ADAS-Cog), and a 30% mitigation in decline as measured by the Alzheimer's Disease Composite Score (ADCOMS). The pivotal Phase III CLARITY AD trial (NCT03887455), encompassing 1,795 individuals diagnosed with early-stage AD, provided further validation of Lecanemab's therapeutic potential. Participants were randomly assigned to receive either a placebo or biweekly 10 mg/kg Lecanemab, with stratification based on clinical presentation (MCI or mild AD) and concomitant administration of approved symptomatic AD treatments [59]. The primary efficacy endpoint, evaluated using the Clinical Dementia Rating-Sum of Boxes (CDR-SB), revealed a pronounced reduction in the trajectory of clinical decline among the Lecanemab-treated cohort. Additionally, treatment was associated with a significant deceleration in cognitive and functional deterioration over 18 months, accompanied by a marked decrease in amyloid plaque burden, a 24% reduction in disease progression, and a 37% slower decline in activities of daily living.

Although ARIA-E, ARIA-H, and infusion-related reactions—primarily mild to moderate in severity, with most occurring following the initial dose—were among the most frequently observed adverse events, the overall safety profile of Lecanemab remained favorable [60]. Collectively, these findings underscore Lecanemab's emergence as a highly promising disease-modifying therapy for early-stage AD, characterized by substantial amyloid clearance and attenuation of cognitive decline, with a relatively lower incidence of ARIA-E. Nevertheless, despite its moderate therapeutic efficacy and improved safety profile, Lecanemab failed to exhibit clinically meaningful benefits in individuals with advanced or prodromal dementia. Consequently, further investigations are warranted to comprehensively delineate its long-term efficacy and safety [61].

Donanemab

Donanemab, a humanized IgG1 monoclonal antibody, is meticulously designed to selectively target the pyroglutamated form of amyloid-beta (N3pG-Aβ), a particularly neurotoxic and hydrophobic variant that exhibits a propensity for rapid aggregation into amyloid plaques. By preferentially binding to these stable plaques, Donanemab effectively circumvents the challenges associated with soluble Aβ species, which often impede the targeted recognition of deposited amyloid aggregates [62]. In November 2023, Donanemab was granted priority review by the Center for Drug Evaluation (CDE), positioning it as a strong candidate to become the third monoclonal antibody (mAb) to receive regulatory approval from the U.S. Food and Drug Administration (FDA). The clinical development of Donanemab commenced with a Phase Ia trial (NCT01837641), wherein a range of intravenous doses (0.3–10 mg/kg) was evaluated alongside a subcutaneous administration group. Findings from this study revealed that a monthly intravenous dose of 10 mg/kg facilitated a 40-50% reduction in amyloid plaque burden. Advancing to Phase Ib (NCT02624778), a cohort of 61 participants received either single or multiple intravenous doses ranging from 10 to 40 mg/kg, all of whom exhibited substantial reductions in cerebral amyloid levels over a 72-week period [63].

A critical milestone was achieved in Phase II TRAILBLAZER-ALZ trial (NCT03367403), which enrolled 272 individuals diagnosed with early symptomatic Alzheimer's disease (AD), confirmed *via* tau and amyloid biomarkers. Participants received either Donanemab or a placebo through intravenous infusions every four weeks for a duration of up to 72 weeks. The primary efficacy endpoint, assessed *via* changes in the Integrated Alzheimer's Disease Rating Scale (iADRS) at 76 weeks, underscored Donanemab's capacity to attenuate cognitive and functional decline [64]. Notably, the therapeutic intervention elicited profound reductions in amyloid plaque deposition and global tau burden relative to placebo, with near-complete clearance of amyloid-beta plaques observed within six months. The Phase III TRAILBLAZER-ALZ 2 trial (NCT04437511), encompassing 1,736 patients, further corroborated Donanemab's efficacy, demonstrating a 35.1% reduction in the risk of disease progression in individuals with early AD and low-to-moderate tau pathology, as measured by iADRS scores at 76 weeks [65, 66]. Remarkably, 47% of treated patients remained cognitively stable after one year of therapy, compared to only

29% in the placebo cohort. Despite these promising findings, Donanemab administration was associated with amyloid-related imaging abnormalities (ARIA), occurring in approximately 40% of participants in the treatment arm, with 26.1% exhibiting symptomatic manifestations. Notably, symptomatic ARIA-E was observed in only 0.8% of placebo recipients. Given its compelling therapeutic potential, Donanemab has been granted breakthrough therapy designation by the FDA, paving the way for its forthcoming application for full regulatory approval [67].

Gantenerumab

Gantenerumab (RO4909832; R1450), a pioneering fully human monoclonal IgG1 antibody targeting the amyloid-beta (Aβ) peptide, was designed to recognize both the N-terminal and central regions of Aβ. This dual recognition facilitates the recruitment of microglia for cell-mediated clearance of amyloid plaques. Derived from a synthetic human combinatorial antibody library (HuCAL®; MorphoSys, Germany), gantenerumab exhibited strong affinity for aggregated cerebral Aβ plaques and demonstrated an ability to cross the blood-brain barrier (BBB) [68]. Preclinical studies indicated that gantenerumab could neutralize oligomer toxicity in rat brains and, in APP751(Swedish)xPS2(N141I) transgenic mice, it significantly reduced Aβ plaques while preventing the formation of new ones through cell-mediated mechanisms. In a Phase I single ascending dose (SAD) trial (NCT02711423), the safety, tolerability, and pharmacokinetics (PK) of subcutaneous gantenerumab were assessed in healthy male volunteers. Although primary measures focused on adverse events (AEs) up to 12 weeks from baseline, the results of this trial remain unpublished [69]. A subsequent Phase I multiple ascending dose (MAD) trial (NCT00531804) involving participants with probable Alzheimer's disease (AD) revealed a dose-dependent reduction in Aβ levels, observed *via* Pittsburgh Compound B amyloid PET imaging. However, two participants with the APOE ε4/ε4 genotype in the higher dose group experienced amyloid-related imaging abnormalities (ARIA-E), which were transient [70]. These findings prompted more conservative dosing strategies in later studies to mitigate the risk of ARIA. The Phase II/III Scarlet RoAD trial (NCT01224106) employed a cautious dosing regimen over two years in participants with prodromal AD. Although ARIA-E was more prevalent in higher dose cohorts, the trial was discontinued early due to a lack of efficacy in both primary and secondary clinical endpoints. Subsequent analysis suggested that higher doses with extended titration schedules might be necessary to achieve therapeutic benefits [71]. A Phase II/III trial (DIAN-TU-001, NCT01760005) is ongoing, investigating gantenerumab in dominantly inherited Alzheimer's disease (DIAD). This study, with a four-year treatment duration and a target dose of 1200 mg, aims to assess cognitive efficacy. Early results indicated the presence of ARIA-E in 10 of 52 participants, but the trial continues due to the unique context of DIAD. The GRADUATE I and II Phase III studies (NCT03444870 and NCT03443973) were large-scale trials investigating gantenerumab in prodromal to mild AD, with over 1900 participants [72]. Despite a carefully designed titration schedule aimed at balancing efficacy and safety, the trials failed to meet their primary endpoints, leading to the discontinuation of gantenerumab's development. These outcomes underscored the critical importance of reducing Aβ to a sufficient threshold for clinical benefit, highlighting the complexities of anti-amyloid monoclonal antibody therapies in AD [73].

Remternetug

Remternetug (LY3372993) is an innovative N3pG-AB monoclonal antibody specifically designed to target pyroglutamate Aβ, making it a potent candidate for addressing Aβ plaques. In a completed phase I clinical trial (NCT03720548), the safety and tolerability of remternetug were evaluated in a randomized, double-blind, placebo-controlled study involving 36 healthy participants [74]. The trial featured a single- and multiple-dose escalation design, where participants received monthly doses of 250, 700, 1400, or 2800 mg of remternetug *via* intravenous infusion, compared against a placebo. Additionally, a titration group that escalated from 700 to 1400 mg was included. The study spanned six months of dosing followed by a one-year extension period. The primary outcome focused on the occurrence of serious adverse events (SAEs), while secondary outcomes involved pharmacokinetic (PK) and pharmacodynamic (PD) assessments, including changes in Aβ burden as measured by PET scans. Results revealed a dose-dependent reduction in Aβ plaques, with participants receiving the highest dose of 2800 mg experiencing a dramatic decrease of up to 100 centroids, with Aβ levels dropping below 24 centroids within three months. However, safety data related to ARIA-E and ARIA-H remain blinded, preventing direct comparisons between remternetug and placebo [75]. A subsequent phase I trial is currently recruiting 224 participants to further investigate the safety and tolerability of remternetug in a two-part study (NCT04451408). Part A will involve non-Japanese individuals with Alzheimer's disease (AD), selected based on criteria such as gradual memory decline and a Mini-Mental State Examination (MMSE) score of ≥16. Part B will focus on healthy participants of first-generation Japanese origin, with a BMI ranging from 18 to 32 kg/m^2. Remternetug will be administered either intravenously or subcutaneously, in single or multiple doses, over approximately 61 weeks. The primary outcome measure is the incidence of SAEs, with secondary outcomes including Aβ changes on PET scans for Part A and PK/PD assessments for Part B [76].

A pivotal phase III clinical trial (NCT05463731) is now underway, aiming to enroll 600 participants with early symptomatic AD. Eligibility criteria include progressive cognitive decline, an MMSE score between 20 and 28, plasma p-tau levels indicative of Aβ presence, and a positive amyloid PET scan. Participants will receive one or two doses of remternetug or a placebo, administered either intravenously or subcutaneously, over a 52-week period. The primary outcome is the percentage of participants achieving Aβ plaque clearance as determined by PET imaging [77]. Secondary outcomes will assess changes in Aβ plaque burden from baseline, the time taken to achieve plaque clearance, PK measurements of trough serum concentration, and the incidence of treatment-emergent anti-drug antibodies. Following the initial study period, participants will be offered an additional 52-week extension where those originally on placebo will receive remternetug, and vice versa. Additionally, an open-label safety cohort will enroll 640 participants with early AD, who will receive remternetug *via* intravenous or subcutaneous administration [78].

ANTI-AB ANTIBODY IMMUNOTHERAPY FOR ALZHEIMER'S

Despite various theories like increased tau phosphorylation and neuroinflammation, Aβ plaque remains a prominent pathological hallmark and a key driver of Alzheimer's disease (AD). The imbalance between Aβ accumulation and clearance is considered a significant contributor to the formation of these plaques. Thus, targeting the production of Aβ at its source appears to be a promising strategy to reduce its levels in the brain [79]. Two main enzymes, beta-site amyloid precursor protein cleaving enzyme 1 (BACE1) and γ-secretase, play pivotal roles in the amyloidogenic cleavage of the transmembrane amyloid precursor protein (APP). Among these, BACE1 is particularly critical, serving as a rate-limiting factor in Aβ production. Its high enzymatic activity correlates with elevated Aβ levels, underscoring its importance in the progression of AD. Consequently, numerous inhibitors have been developed to lower Aβ concentrations in patients. However, due to the structural similarity of BACE1 with other aspartyl proteases and its widespread presence in the brain, designing inhibitors that are both highly selective and capable of efficiently crossing the blood-brain barrier (BBB) with minimal off-target effects is essential [80].

In recent years, pharmaceutical companies have developed various BACE1 inhibitors, including 13 small molecules, to target Alzheimer's disease (AD). These inhibitors are classified into peptidomimetic and non-peptidomimetic types based on their structure. Peptidomimetic inhibitors like OM99-2 initially showed potential but faced poor brain permeability and low bioavailability, limiting their effectiveness. Non-peptidomimetic inhibitors, such as verubecestat, demonstrated better properties, including crossing the blood-brain barrier (BBB) and reducing

Aβ levels. However, clinical trials often failed due to side effects and lack of efficacy, leading to the abandonment of these inhibitors [81]. The safety of BACE1 inhibition remains a concern, as excessive inhibition can lead to adverse effects like epilepsy and nerve damage. Recent studies suggest that moderate inhibition may avoid these side effects, but determining the correct dosage is critical. Beyond small-molecule inhibitors, siRNA therapies targeting BACE1 have emerged as promising alternatives, offering good targeting ability and lower side effects [82]. Advanced nanocarriers are being developed to enhance BBB penetration and improve brain targeting to overcome delivery challenges, showing potential in preclinical studies. Immunotherapy targeting Aβ in Alzheimer's disease (AD) includes both active and passive approaches. Unlike passive immunotherapy, which requires frequent re-administration, vaccination as an active form of immunotherapy induces the body to produce antibodies against Aβ, making it more cost-effective and enhancing patient compliance [83]. The first vaccine, AN-1792, showed promise in clearing Aβ plaques but was halted due to adverse effects in phase II trials. However, newer vaccines like CAD106 and UB-311 have improved safety and efficacy by targeting specific Aβ fragments to minimize side effects. Recent research has also identified N-terminally truncated Aβ peptides, such as pE3-Aβ, as potential targets for vaccines. These peptides accumulate early in AD and are major components of toxic plaques. New vaccine strategies, like the one developed by Ghochikyan and his colleagues, have successfully reduced levels of pE3-Aβ and full-length Aβ in animal models. Despite these advances, further work is needed to optimize target selection and delivery methods to develop safer and more effective AD immunotherapies [84].

THE EVOLUTION OF ANTI-AB THERAPY

Four of these medications are classified as cholinesterase inhibitors (CIs): tacrine, donepezil, rivastigmine, and galantamine. While most are approved for treating mild-to-moderate Alzheimer's disease (AD), donepezil is unique in its approval for use in patients with severe or late-stage AD [85]. However, tacrine has been discontinued in the US due to its severe hepatotoxicity. In contrast to these CIs, memantine functions as an N-methyl-D-aspartate (NMDA) receptor antagonist, offering neuroprotective effects by inhibiting glutamate activity. Despite their efficacy in alleviating symptoms, these drugs do not modify the course of the disease, underscoring the urgent need for effective disease-modifying therapies for AD [86]. As of March 2023, according to ALZFORUM, 298 AD therapies are in clinical trials, with 76 targeting the amyloid-beta (Aβ) peptide or its aggregates. These therapies include small molecules and immunotherapies, classified into four categories: (1) reducing Aβ generation, (2) enhancing the degradation and clearance of Aβ and its aggregates, (3) neutralizing soluble Aβ monomers or their toxicity, and (4) directly inhibiting Aβ aggregation. Notably, the FDA has approved two antibody-based drugs, aducanumab and lecanemab [87].

BACE1 Inhibitors

In 1999, BACE1 was identified as a critical enzyme necessary for amyloid-beta (Aβ) production, prompting extensive research into BACE1 inhibitors as a potential strategy to halt the amyloid cascade in Alzheimer's disease [88]. LY2886721, the first BACE inhibitor to advance to Phase 2 clinical trials, demonstrated improved brain penetrance over earlier compounds. In 2012, Eli Lilly reported promising Phase 1 results, showing reduced cerebrospinal fluid (CSF) levels of Aβ40 and Aβ42, along with increased sAPPα levels (P3-359, Alzheimer's Association International Conference, 2012). However, the Phase 2 trials were terminated due to abnormal liver biochemistry in four participants, a side effect deemed unrelated to BACE1 inhibition but likely due to off-target effects (The 11th International Conference on Alzheimer's & Parkinson's Disease, 2013) [89].

Other BACE1 inhibitors, such as atabecestat (Phase 2/3), elenbecestat (Phase 3), lanabecestat (Phase 2/3), and umibecestat (Phase 2/3), have also reached advanced stages of clinical trials but failed to achieve market approval [90]. The development of effective BACE1 inhibitors has encountered significant challenges, primarily due to BACE1's structural similarity to other aspartyl proteases, such as BACE2, pepsin, renin, cathepsin D, and cathepsin E. This similarity complicates efforts to create inhibitors that are selective for BACE1 without off-target effects. Additionally, the relatively large size of the BACE1 active site, which includes catalytic aspartic acid residues, a flap, and a 10S loop, presents another obstacle for small-molecule inhibitors to block BACE1 activity effectively [91].

γ-secretase Inhibitors/Modulators

γ-secretase inhibitors (GSIs) have been explored extensively as potential treatments for Alzheimer's disease (AD) due to their ability to inhibit amyloid-beta (Aβ) production. However, existing GSIs have broad activity, leading to significant side effects by also inhibiting the processing of other proteins, such as Notch, a key transmembrane receptor involved in cell fate decisions [92]. This lack of specificity has driven efforts to develop more selective γ-secretase inhibitors that specifically target Aβ production without affecting other pathways. Avagacestat, an arylsulfonamide γ-secretase inhibitor, was developed with high selectivity for amyloid precursor protein (APP) over Notch [93]. While it successfully reduced cerebrospinal fluid (CSF) Aβ levels in animal models without inducing Notch-related toxicity, it was ultimately discontinued in Phase 2 clinical trials due to gastrointestinal and dermatological side effects. These setbacks have shifted focus toward γ-secretase modulators (GSMs) as a more refined approach. GSMs modulate rather than completely inhibit γ-secretase activity. For example, SGSM-36 was shown to lower toxic Aβ42 levels without altering Notch signaling or the proteolytic processing of APP by α- and β-secretases [94]. Similarly, EVP-0962 reduced Aβ42 levels while increasing Aβ38 levels, without impacting Notch signaling, and improved memory deficits in AD model mice. Despite their initial promise, all these compounds were eventually discontinued in clinical trials [95].

Immunotherapy, one of the most promising strategies for modifying the progression of Alzheimer's disease (AD), involves designing synthetic peptides or monoclonal antibodies (mAbs) to reduce brain amyloid-beta (Aβ) load and slow disease progression. The first AD vaccine tested in clinical trials, AN1792, was a synthetic full-length Aβ42 peptide [96]. Although it showed some therapeutic benefits, such as slowing cognitive decline, the trials were terminated due to the development of aseptic meningoencephalitis in 6% of participants. This adverse effect may have been due to the induction of T helper 2 (Th2) cell responses by the excipients used in producing the C-terminus region of Aβ peptides. To mitigate this risk, subsequent vaccines have excluded this region of Aβ peptides [97].

Vanutide cridificar (ACC-001) was designed as a safer alternative, consisting of a conjugate of multiple short Aβ fragments. Despite promising preclinical data showing it could induce N-terminal anti-Aβ antibodies and improve cognitive impairment in AD animal models, all clinical trials were discontinued following a serious adverse event. Another innovative approach, Lu AF20513, combined three repeats of the first 12 amino acids of the Aβ peptide with sequences from the tetanus toxin to stimulate a B-cell response and produce polyclonal antibodies against Aβ [98]. While it successfully removed brain amyloid deposits in preclinical studies, its clinical trials were halted due to a lack of efficacy. Currently, several vaccines are under investigation in clinical trials. ALZ-101, now in Phase 1B, targets soluble Aβ oligomers rather than Aβ monomers or fibrils. ACI-24, a liposome vaccine based on Aβ1-15 sequences, has begun Phase 2 trials and is the first anti-Aβ vaccine being evaluated for treating AD in Down syndrome patients. ABvac40, targeting the C-terminus of Aβ peptides, is also in Phase 2 trials. UB-311, comprising Aβ1-14 peptides combined with a T helper cell epitope, has shown promise in preclinical studies and Phase 2 trials for enhancing plaque clearance and generating Aβ antibodies in 96% of patients with mild AD [99]. UB-311 has been granted fast-track designation by the FDA and is moving into Phase 3 clinical testing. In contrast, passive immunotherapy utilizes mAbs directly targeting various forms of Aβ peptides—monomers, oligomers, and fibrils—to prevent toxic aggregate formation. These mAbs bind to Fc-γ receptors on microglia through their Fc domains, promoting the phagocytosis of the Aβ-mAb complex and inducing complement-dependent cytotoxicity to lyse target cells. Additionally, in the bloodstream, mAbs interact with Aβ to lower its concentration, creating a gradient that facilitates Aβ efflux from the brain. Bapineuzumab, a humanized version of the mouse anti-Aβ monoclonal 3D6 antibody targeting the N-terminal region of Aβ, was the first mAb tested in clinical trials. Humanized antibodies are engineered to closely resemble natural human antibody variants, reducing immunogenicity and potential adverse reactions [100].

THE PRIMARY CHALLENGE OF ANTI-AB THERAPY

Amyloid-beta (Aβ) peptides are ubiquitously present in both the cerebral and circulatory compartments throughout an individual's lifespan. While aggregated forms of Aβ have conventionally been implicated in neurotoxicity, physiological concentrations of soluble Aβ peptides are increasingly recognized for their diverse neuroprotective and homeostatic roles [101]. These include the facilitation of long-term potentiation (LTP), induction of neuronal differentiation, promotion of post-injury cerebral repair, attenuation of oxidative stress, antimicrobial activity, and potential tumor-suppressive functions. These findings necessitate a nuanced approach when designing therapeutic strategies to modulate Aβ levels in Alzheimer's disease (AD), ensuring the selective targeting of pathogenic conformations such as fibrils, protofibrils, or oligomers, while preserving the physiological monomeric forms of Aβ [102].

The influence of Aβ peptides on synaptic modulation is multifaceted. While oligomeric Aβ species are known to disrupt synaptic plasticity by inhibiting LTP and enhancing long-term depression (LTD), emerging evidence suggests that physiological concentrations of Aβ contribute to synaptic integrity and cognitive function. Notably, the KLVFF sequence (amino acids 16-20) within Aβ peptides has been shown to confer neuroprotection against excitotoxic insults, thereby preventing neuronal apoptosis [103]. Additionally, both synthetic and endogenous Aβ42 monomers, at nanomolar concentrations, potentiate the activation of cyclic adenosine monophosphate (cAMP) response element-binding protein (CREB) and brain-derived neurotrophic factor (BDNF), which are pivotal regulators of neuronal survival and synaptic plasticity in the healthy brain [104].

Furthermore, the depletion of endogenous Aβ *via* anti-Aβ antibody administration or genetic ablation leads to pronounced deficits in LTP and memory, which can be ameliorated upon supplementation with human Aβ42 [105]. This underscores the critical role of Aβ in synaptic modulation, learning, and memory. Intriguingly,

Aβ monomers have been found to enhance astrocytic-mediated glutamate clearance, mitigating excitotoxic neuronal damage. Additionally, synaptic release of Aβ facilitates neurotransmitter secretion, including acetylcholine, and activates α7-nicotinic acetylcholine receptors (α7-nAChRs), thereby enhancing LTP [106]. Nicotinic acetylcholine receptors (nAChRs) are expressed in both neuronal and non-neuronal cells within the central nervous system and function as ligand-gated ion channels that permit the influx of Na+, K+, and Ca2+ upon activation. Among the various isoforms, α7-nAChRs exhibit the highest permeability to Ca2+ [107]. Aβ-mediated activation of α7-nAChRs is postulated to involve intracellular signaling disruptions, leading to elevated calcium influx. These receptors are integral to neurotransmission, synaptic plasticity, and neurogenesis. In AD, the depletion of nAChRs in Aβ42-positive neurons correlates with disease progression, with an increased presence of Aβ/nAChR-like complexes observed in carriers of the APOE ε4 allele, a known genetic risk factor for late-onset AD (LOAD) [108]. Notably, Aβ selectively interacts with distinct nAChR subtypes to exert either physiological or deleterious effects on cholinergic neurons. Under normal conditions, low Aβ levels engage the α7-nAChR subtype *via* the nitric oxide/cGMP/protein kinase G pathway, thereby modulating synaptic function. Interestingly, α7-nAChR knockout mice exhibit compensatory increases in Aβ levels and develop AD-like neuropathologies by 12 months of age [109]. The inhibition of amyloid precursor protein (APP) expression perturbs the synaptic architecture by altering the expression of critical postsynaptic proteins, such as the GluA1 subunit of AMPA receptors, underscoring the role of APP in synaptic formation [110]. Reduced LTP has been reported in hippocampal neurons with APP knockdown. Similarly, conditional deletion of presenilin 1 (PSEN1) and presenilin 2 (PSEN2), which diminishes Aβ production, results in profound synaptic and cognitive deficits in animal models. Conversely, the administration of synthetic Aβ at nanomolar concentrations enhances cognitive and memory function in mice, though these concentrations exceed physiological picomolar Aβ levels [111]. More recent studies employing picomolar concentrations of Aβ peptides have corroborated their role in improving synaptic plasticity and memory formation, reinforcing the notion that monomeric Aβ is essential for normal synaptic function, whereas aggregated forms mediate neurotoxicity [112].

Accumulating evidence suggests that the transient surge in Aβ expression following cerebral injury confers neuroprotection. Elevated Aβ levels observed post-traumatic brain injury (TBI) may reflect either a pathological response or a compensatory mechanism for neuroprotection. Notably, intracerebroventricular administration of Aβ40 in TBI-afflicted BACE1–/– mice significantly ameliorates motor memory deficits, emphasizing its protective capacity. Conversely, pharmacological or genetic reduction of endogenous Aβ impairs functional recovery in spinal cord injury (SCI) models [113]. Beyond TBI, Aβ also exhibits neuroprotective effects in ischemic stroke models. Overexpression of human amyloid precursor protein (hAPP695) reduces cortical infarct volumes in ischemic mice [114]. Additionally, in experimental autoimmune encephalomyelitis (EAE), an inflammatory demyelinating disorder, Aβ treatment suppresses pathogenic T-helper cell responses (TH1 and TH17) and associated cytokines (IL-6, IFN-γ, and IL-17), thereby alleviating disease severity. Conversely, APP deletion exacerbates EAE pathology, further supporting the neuroprotective role of Aβ [115]. Emerging evidence underscores the antimicrobial properties of Aβ peptides. Transgenic mice expressing human Aβ exhibit enhanced resistance to bacterial and viral infections. Moreover, AD patients' brain tissues demonstrate greater antimicrobial activity relative to age-matched controls, correlating with Aβ burden [116]. Aβ entraps pathogens by forming a fibrillar mesh, corroborated by the presence of viral and bacterial DNA within AD amyloid plaques [117]. Aβ has also been shown to aggregate viral particles, facilitating their uptake by leukocytes and stimulating type I interferon (IFN) responses, further enhancing antimicrobial defense [118 - 120]. Additionally, AD patients exhibit a lower incidence of various malignancies, including skin, lung, breast, and bladder cancers, suggesting an anti-tumorigenic role for Aβ. *In vitro* and *in vivo* studies demonstrate that Aβ inhibits tumor proliferation and induces apoptosis *via* upregulation of p53 and oxidative stress-mediated downregulation of anti-apoptotic proteins such as XIAP and Bcl-2, while concurrently enhancing pro-apoptotic Bax expression [121, 122]. Furthermore, Aβ peptides exhibit antioxidant properties by chelating redox-active metals and reducing reactive oxygen species (ROS) production. In physiological concentrations, Aβ prevents lipid peroxidation in cerebrospinal fluid and plasma, while its absence exacerbates oxidative stress [123, 124]. Lastly, Aβ influences neurogenesis by modulating neural stem/progenitor cell (NSPC) proliferation and differentiation. While Aβ40 promotes neuronal differentiation, Aβ42 preferentially enhances gliogenesis [125 - 127]. Additionally, Aβ may reinforce blood-brain barrier integrity by acting as a protective seal against neuroinflammation [128, 129]. These findings highlight the multifaceted physiological roles of Aβ, necessitating precise therapeutic strategies that target pathogenic Aβ species while preserving its essential functions.

CONCLUSION

Although the failure of numerous clinical trials has ignited discourse regarding the validity of the amyloid hypothesis and raised concerns about the strategic direction of Alzheimer's disease research, these setbacks have nonetheless yielded valuable insights into disease pathogenesis and therapeutic development. The following principles and pragmatic approaches may prove instrumental in advancing the next generation of Aβ-targeted interventions [130]. Contemporary therapeutic strategies, including BACE inhibitors and γ-secretase inhibitors/modulators, are designed to impede Aβ synthesis, an early-stage event in the amyloid cascade. While these inhibitors have demonstrated efficacy in attenuating plaque formation, they have been largely ineffective in eradicating pre-existing Aβ aggregates or mitigating the neurotoxicity induced by these deposits [131]. Consequently, the integration of combination therapy should be considered in Alzheimer's disease management, mirroring its success in other conditions such as rheumatoid arthritis and HIV/AIDS. Increasing evidence suggests that Aβ accumulation precipitates tau hyperphosphorylation, leading to the formation of neurofibrillary tangles and subsequent neurodegeneration [132]. Hence, therapeutic regimens incorporating tau kinase inhibitors, agents that disrupt tau aggregation, or compounds that facilitate the disassembly of tau aggregates may yield additional benefits. Furthermore, both APP and Aβ can translocate into mitochondria, where they perturb mitochondrial function, impair ATP synthesis, and exacerbate oxidative stress. As a result, antioxidants such as lipoic acid, vitamin E, vitamin C, and β-carotene hold potential as adjunctive therapies in Alzheimer's treatment [133]. Aβ's involvement in synaptic modulation has garnered significant attention, with neurotoxic soluble Aβ oligomers implicated in synaptic dysfunction and impaired plasticity across various animal models of Alzheimer's disease. Accordingly, targeting synaptic integrity and function may constitute an effective therapeutic strategy. Once the pathological cascade is initiated, a combinatorial approach addressing multiple facets of Alzheimer's pathology is likely to surpass the efficacy of monotherapies targeting isolated pathological factors [134].

Mounting evidence suggests that elevated cerebral Aβ levels in Alzheimer's disease may stem from upstream dysregulations, including neurovascular dysfunction, impaired glucose metabolism, aberrant cell cycle control, and chronic inflammation. Autophagy, a fundamental component of the lysosomal degradation system, is instrumental in the clearance of toxic protein aggregates and dysfunctional organelles [135]. The autophagic process comprises distinct phases—sequestration, elongation, maturation, fusion, and degradation—culminating in the delivery of cellular debris and misfolded proteins to lysosomes for degradation. The process is initiated with the formation of a phagophore, which subsequently elongates and encapsulates the cargo to form an autophagosome. The autophagosome may then directly merge with a lysosome to generate an autolysosome or first fuse with late endosomes to form amphisomes, which subsequently interact with lysosomes. Dysfunction of the autophagy-lysosomal system has been implicated as a pivotal factor in neurodegenerative diseases characterized by amyloid protein deposition [136]. Defective autophagy is intrinsically linked to Aβ metabolism and accumulation in Alzheimer's disease, influencing its synthesis, secretion, and clearance. Aβ peptides are produced *via* the proteolytic cleavage of amyloid precursor protein (APP) by β-secretase

(BACE1) and γ-secretase, and ATG5-dependent autophagy has been found to modulate APP degradation. Additionally, the presence of APP and the γ-secretase complex within autophagosomes underscores the role of autophagy in Aβ biogenesis [137]. Furthermore, autophagy influences Aβ secretion, as evidenced by murine models deficient in ATG7, which exhibit reduced extracellular Aβ plaque burden and heightened intraneuronal Aβ accumulation, indicative of compromised Aβ secretion due to impaired autophagic function. Autophagy is also critical for Aβ degradation; for instance, the lysosomal protease cathepsin B (CatB) plays a crucial role in the breakdown of autophagic substrates. Genetic ablation of CatB markedly exacerbates Aβ42 deposition and accelerates amyloid aggregation in Alzheimer's models, whereas CatB overexpression significantly attenuates amyloid burden. Notably, the accumulation of immature autophagosomes within dystrophic neurites has been observed in the brains of Alzheimer's patients, likely attributable to defective axonal transport of autophagosomes [138]. Thus, autophagy modulation has emerged as a compelling therapeutic avenue for Alzheimer's disease. Rapamycin, a well-established autophagy activator, inhibits the mTOR pathway by interacting with immunophilin FK506-binding protein (FKBP12). Studies have demonstrated that 3xTg-AD mice exhibit heightened mTOR activity in the hippocampus and neocortex—regions characterized by extensive Aβ plaque accumulation. Administration of rapamycin significantly augments autophagic activity, leading to profound reductions in both intracellular and extracellular Aβ deposition, concomitant with amelioration of cognitive impairments in Alzheimer's models [139]. Therapeutic interventions targeting these pathological pathways are expected to yield maximal efficacy when initiated during the preclinical stage of Alzheimer's disease. Traditional Chinese Medicine (TCM), a cornerstone of Eastern medical practice for millennia, is predominantly derived from natural compounds and is characterized by a multi-target, multi-pathway approach with minimal adverse effects [140]. TCM has demonstrated prophylactic and therapeutic efficacy in diverse chronic conditions, including cancer, allergic disorders, diabetes, and infections, through mechanisms such as cellular growth regulation, anti-inflammatory activity, and improved carbohydrate metabolism. Several TCM-derived compounds, including morroniside, rutin, resveratrol, triptolide, and berberine, have exhibited neuroprotective effects against Alzheimer's disease [141].

Human pluripotent stem cell (hPSC)-derived three-dimensional brain organoids offer significant advantages in modeling neurodegenerative disorders, including autism, microcephaly, and Parkinson's disease. Three principal methodologies have been established to recapitulate Alzheimer's phenotypes in brain organoids: (i) exposure to Aftin-5, an Aβ42 agonist that enhances Aβ42 production; (ii) derivation of brain organoids from familial Alzheimer's patient-induced pluripotent stem cells (iPSCs); and (iii) conversion of APOE3 to APOE4 in patient-derived iPSCs to generate sporadic Alzheimer's brain organoids [142]. Unlike conventional cellular models, Alzheimer's brain organoids are capable of forming a blood-brain barrier (BBB) and establishing inter-organ connectivity, positioning them as an advanced platform for studying Alzheimer's pathogenesis and exploring therapeutic interventions [143]. Furthermore, brain organoid transplantation presents a novel paradigm for restoring neuronal function and reconstructing neural networks following neuronal degeneration in Alzheimer's disease. However, substantial limitations persist, notably the inability to sustain brain organoids beyond six months due to volumetric contraction and cellular apoptosis resulting from inadequate oxygenation and nutrient supply to the inner core. Overcoming this challenge will necessitate the development of vascularized brain organoids [144]. The identification of biomarkers capable of detecting Alzheimer's disease in its earliest stages would substantially enhance the potential for disease-modifying interventions. In addition to conventional pathological markers (*e.g.*, Aβ and tau), molecules implicated in inflammation and synaptic plasticity may serve as highly specific early diagnostic biomarkers. Progranulin, a growth factor expressed in neurons and microglia, modulates neuroinflammation by attenuating microgliosis and astrogliosis [145]. Elevated cerebrospinal fluid (CSF) progranulin levels have been detected up to a decade prior to symptomatic onset in both familial and sporadic Alzheimer's patients. Additionally, neurogranin, a synaptic marker predominantly expressed in the cortex and hippocampus, exhibits heightened CSF levels in Alzheimer's and mild cognitive impairment patients [146].

REFERENCES

[1] Feigin VL, Nichols E, Alam T, *et al.* Global, regional, and national burden of neurological disorders, 1990–2016: a systematic analysis for the Global Burden of Disease Study 2016. Lancet Neurol 2019; 18(5): 459-80.
[http://dx.doi.org/10.1016/S1474-4422(18)30499-X] [PMID: 30879893]

[2] Swanson CJ, Zhang Y, Dhadda S, *et al.* A randomized, double-blind, phase 2b proof-of-concept clinical trial in early Alzheimer's disease with lecanemab, an anti-Aβ protofibril antibody. Alzheimers Res Ther 2021; 13(1): 80.
[http://dx.doi.org/10.1186/s13195-021-00813-8] [PMID: 33865446]

[3] van Dyck CH, Swanson CJ, Aisen P, *et al.* Lecanemab in early Alzheimer's disease. N Engl J Med 2023; 388(1): 9-21.
[http://dx.doi.org/10.1056/NEJMoa2212948] [PMID: 36449413]

[4] Mintun MA, Lo AC, Duggan Evans C, *et al.* Donanemab in early Alzheimer's disease. N Engl J Med 2021; 384(18): 1691-704.
[http://dx.doi.org/10.1056/NEJMoa2100708] [PMID: 33720637]

[5] Sperling RA, Jack CR Jr, Black SE, *et al.* Amyloid-related imaging abnormalities in amyloid-modifying therapeutic trials: Recommendations from the Alzheimer's Association Research Roundtable Workgroup. Alzheimers Dement 2011; 7(4): 367-85.
[http://dx.doi.org/10.1016/j.jalz.2011.05.2351] [PMID: 21784348]

[6] Uddin MS, Lim LW. Glial cells in Alzheimer's disease: From neuropathological changes to therapeutic implications. Ageing Res Rev 2022; 78(101622): 101622. [http://dx.doi.org/10.1016/j.arr.2022.101622] [PMID: 35427810]

[7] Grubman A, Choo XY, Chew G, *et al.* Transcriptional signature in microglia associated with Aβ plaque phagocytosis. Nat Commun 2021; 12(1): 3015. [http://dx.doi.org/10.1038/s41467-021-23111-1] [PMID: 34021136]

[8] Lu L, Zheng X, Wang S, *et al.* Anti-Aβ agents for mild to moderate Alzheimer's disease: systematic review and meta-analysis. J Neurol Neurosurg Psychiatry 2020; 91(12): 1316-24. [http://dx.doi.org/10.1136/jnnp-2020-323497] [PMID: 33046560]

[9] Alzheimer's Association. 2021 Alzheimer's disease facts and figures. Alzheimers Dement 2021; 17(3): 327-406. [http://dx.doi.org/10.1002/alz.12328] [PMID: 33756057]

[10] Hardy J, Selkoe DJ. The amyloid hypothesis of Alzheimer's disease: progress and problems on the road to therapeutics. Science 2002; 297(5580): 353-6. [http://dx.doi.org/10.1126/science.1072994] [PMID: 12130773]

[11] Hardy JA, Higgins GA. Alzheimer's disease: the amyloid cascade hypothesis. Science 1992; 256(5054): 184-5. [http://dx.doi.org/10.1126/science.1566067] [PMID: 1566067]

[12] Zhang Y, Song W. Islet amyloid polypeptide: Another key molecule in Alzheimer's pathogenesis? Prog Neurobiol 2017; 153: 100-20. [http://dx.doi.org/10.1016/j.pneurobio.2017.03.001] [PMID: 28274676]

[13] DeMattos RB, Cirrito JR, Parsadanian M, *et al.* ApoE and clusterin cooperatively suppress Aβ levels and deposition. Neuron 2004; 41(2): 193-202. [http://dx.doi.org/10.1016/S0896-6273(03)00850-X] [PMID: 14741101]

[14] Masters CL, Beyreuther K, Henryk M. Henryk M. Wisniewski and the amyloid theory of Alzheimer's disease. J Alzheimers Dis 2001; 3(1): 83-6. [http://dx.doi.org/10.3233/JAD-2001-3112] [PMID: 12214076]

[15] Serrano-Pozo A, Frosch MP, Masliah E, Hyman BT. Neuropathological alterations in Alzheimer disease. Cold Spring Harb Perspect Med 2011; 1(1): a006189-9. [http://dx.doi.org/10.1101/cshperspect.a006189] [PMID: 22229116]

[16] Duyckaerts C, Delatour B, Potier MC. Classification and basic pathology of Alzheimer disease. Acta Neuropathol 2009; 118(1): 5-36. [http://dx.doi.org/10.1007/s00401-009-0532-1] [PMID: 19381658]

[17] Liu F, Sun J, Wang X, *et al.* Focal-type, but not diffuse-type, amyloid beta plaques are correlated with Alzheimer's neuropathology, cognitive dysfunction, and neuroinflammation in the human hippocampus. Neurosci Bull 2022; 38(10): 1125-38. [http://dx.doi.org/10.1007/s12264-022-00927-5] [PMID: 36028642]

[18] Hong S, Ostaszewski BL, Yang T, *et al.* Soluble Aβ oligomers are rapidly sequestered from brain ISF *in vivo* and bind GM1 ganglioside on cellular membranes. Neuron 2014; 82(2): 308-19. [http://dx.doi.org/10.1016/j.neuron.2014.02.027] [PMID: 24685176]

[19] DelBove CE, Strothman CE, Lazarenko RM, Huang H, Sanders CR, Zhang Q. Reciprocal modulation between amyloid precursor protein and synaptic membrane cholesterol revealed by live cell imaging. Neurobiol Dis 2019; 127: 449-61. [http://dx.doi.org/10.1016/j.nbd.2019.03.009] [PMID: 30885793]

[20] Gimpl G, Fahrenholz F. The oxytocin receptor system: structure, function, and regulation. Physiol Rev 2001; 81(2): 629-83. [http://dx.doi.org/10.1152/physrev.2001.81.2.629] [PMID: 11274341]

[21] Panchal M, Loeper J, Cossec JC, *et al.* Enrichment of cholesterol in microdissected Alzheimer's disease senile plaques as assessed by mass spectrometry. J Lipid Res 2010; 51(3): 598-605. [http://dx.doi.org/10.1194/jlr.M001859] [PMID: 19779135]

[22] Matsuzaki K. Formation of toxic amyloid fibrils by amyloid β-protein on ganglioside clusters. Int J Alzheimers Dis 2011; 2011(1): 956104. [http://dx.doi.org/10.4061/2011/956104] [PMID: 21318142]

[23] Henry S, Bercu NB, Bobo C, Cullin C, Molinari M, Lecomte S. Interaction of Aβ_{1-42} peptide or their variant with model membrane of different composition probed by infrared nanospectroscopy. Nanoscale 2018; 10(3): 936-40. [http://dx.doi.org/10.1039/C7NR07489A] [PMID: 29292465]

[24] Grundke-Iqbal I, Iqbal K, Tung YC, Quinlan M, Wisniewski HM, Binder LI. Abnormal phosphorylation of the microtubule-associated protein tau (tau) in Alzheimer cytoskeletal pathology. Proc Natl Acad Sci USA 1986; 83(13): 4913-7. [http://dx.doi.org/10.1073/pnas.83.13.4913] [PMID: 3088567]

[25] Goedert M, Spillantini MG, Cairns NJ, Crowther RA. Tau proteins of alzheimer paired helical filaments: Abnormal phosphorylation of all six brain isoforms. Neuron 1992; 8(1): 159-68. [http://dx.doi.org/10.1016/0896-6273(92)90117-V] [PMID: 1530909]

[26] Greenberg SG, Davies P, Schein JD, Binder LI. Hydrofluoric acid-treated tau PHF proteins display the same biochemical properties as normal tau. J Biol Chem 1992; 267(1): 564-9. [http://dx.doi.org/10.1016/S0021-9258(18)48531-6] [PMID: 1370450]

[27] Busche MA, Hyman BT. Synergy between amyloid-β and tau in Alzheimer's disease. Nat Neurosci 2020; 23(10): 1183-93. [http://dx.doi.org/10.1038/s41593-020-0687-6] [PMID: 32778792]

[28] Swatton JE, Sellers LA, Faull RLM, Holland A, Iritani S, Bahn S. Increased MAP kinase activity in Alzheimer's and Down syndrome but not in schizophrenia human brain. Eur J Neurosci 2004; 19(10): 2711-9. [http://dx.doi.org/10.1111/j.0953-816X.2004.03365.x] [PMID: 15147305]

[29] Um JW, Nygaard HB, Heiss JK, *et al.* Alzheimer amyloid-β oligomer bound to postsynaptic prion protein activates Fyn to impair neurons. Nat Neurosci 2012; 15(9): 1227-35. [http://dx.doi.org/10.1038/nn.3178] [PMID: 22820466]

[30] Gimbel DA, Nygaard HB, Coffey EE, *et al.* Memory impairment in transgenic Alzheimer mice requires cellular prion protein. J Neurosci 2010; 30(18): 6367-74. [http://dx.doi.org/10.1523/JNEUROSCI.0395-10.2010] [PMID: 20445063]

[31] Roberson ED, Scearce-Levie K, Palop JJ, *et al.* Reducing endogenous tau ameliorates amyloid beta-induced deficits in an Alzheimer's disease mouse model. Science 2007; 316(5825): 750-4. [http://dx.doi.org/10.1126/science.1141736] [PMID: 17478722]

[32] Ransohoff RM. How neuroinflammation contributes to neurodegeneration. Science 2016; 353(6301): 777-83. [http://dx.doi.org/10.1126/science.aag2590] [PMID: 27540165]

[33] Grammas P. Neurovascular dysfunction, inflammation and endothelial activation: Implications for the pathogenesis of Alzheimer's disease. J Neuroinflammation 2011; 8(1): 26. [http://dx.doi.org/10.1186/1742-2094-8-26] [PMID: 21439035]

[34] Griffin WS, Sheng JG, Roberts GW, Mrak RE. Interleukin-1 expression in different plaque types in Alzheimer's disease: significance in plaque evolution. J Neuropathol Exp Neurol 1995; 54(2): 276-81. [http://dx.doi.org/10.1097/00005072-199503000-00014] [PMID: 7876895]

[35] Baik SH, Kang S, Lee W, *et al.* A breakdown in metabolic reprogramming causes microglia dysfunction in Alzheimer's disease. Cell Metab 2019; 30(3): 493-507.e6. [http://dx.doi.org/10.1016/j.cmet.2019.06.005] [PMID: 31257151]

[36] Johansson JU, Woodling NS, Wang Q, *et al.* Prostaglandin signaling suppresses beneficial microglial function in Alzheimer's disease models. J Clin Invest 2015; 125(1): 350-64. [http://dx.doi.org/10.1172/JCI77487] [PMID: 25485684]

[37] Vandenberghe R, Rinne JO, Boada M, *et al.* Bapineuzumab for mild to moderate Alzheimer's disease in two global, randomized, phase 3 trials. Alzheimers Res Ther 2016; 8(1): 18. [http://dx.doi.org/10.1186/s13195-016-0189-7] [PMID: 27176461]

[38] Doody RS, Thomas RG, Farlow M, *et al.* Phase 3 trials of solanezumab for mild-to-moderate Alzheimer's disease. N Engl J Med 2014; 370(4): 311-21. [http://dx.doi.org/10.1056/NEJMoa1312889] [PMID: 24450890]

[39] Sevigny J, Chiao P, Bussière T, *et al.* The antibody aducanumab reduces Aβ plaques in Alzheimer's disease. Nature 2016; 537(7618): 50-6. [http://dx.doi.org/10.1038/nature19323] [PMID: 27582220]

[40] Eisai Co., Ltd. Lecanemab confirmatory phase 3 clarity ad study met primary endpoint, showing highly statistically significant reduction of clinical decline in large global clinical study of 1,795 participants with early Alzheimer's disease [Internet]. Eisai Co., Ltd.

[41] Lord A, Gumucio A, Englund H, *et al.* An amyloid-β protofibril-selective antibody prevents amyloid formation in a mouse model of Alzheimer's disease. Neurobiol Dis 2009; 36(3): 425-34. [http://dx.doi.org/10.1016/j.nbd.2009.08.007] [PMID: 19703562]

[42] Salloway S, Sperling R, Gilman S, *et al.* A phase 2 multiple ascending dose trial of bapineuzumab in mild to moderate Alzheimer disease. Neurology 2009; 73(24): 2061-70. [http://dx.doi.org/10.1212/WNL.0b013e3181c67808] [PMID: 19923550]

[43] Renteros MS, Barreto-Abanto R, Huapaya DC, *et al.* The efficacy of solanezumab in patients with alzheimer's disease: a systematic review and meta-analysis of clinical trials. Pharmaceutics 2025; 17(8): 999. [http://dx.doi.org/10.3390/pharmaceutics17080999]

[44] Salloway S, Sperling R, Fox NC, *et al.* Two phase 3 trials of bapineuzumab in mild-to-moderate Alzheimer's disease. N Engl J Med 2014; 370(4): 322-33. [http://dx.doi.org/10.1056/NEJMoa1304839] [PMID: 24450891]

[45] Rinne JO, Brooks DJ, Rossor MN, *et al.* 11C-PiB PET assessment of change in fibrillar amyloid-β load in patients with Alzheimer's disease treated with bapineuzumab: a phase 2, double-blind, placebo-controlled, ascending-dose study. Lancet Neurol 2010; 9(4): 363-72. [http://dx.doi.org/10.1016/S1474-4422(10)70043-0] [PMID: 20189881]

[46] Alkhalifa AE, Al Mokhlf A, Ali H, *et al.* Anti-amyloid monoclonal antibodies for alzheimer's disease: Evidence, ARIA risk, and precision patient selection. J. Pers. Med 2025; 15(9): 437. [http://dx.doi.org/10.3390/jpm15090437]

[47] Zhang Y, Lee DHS. Sink hypothesis and therapeutic strategies for attenuating Abeta levels. Neuroscientist 2011; 17(2): 163-73. [http://dx.doi.org/10.1177/1073858410381532] [PMID: 21330304]

[48] Mohammed AA, Barale SS, Kamble SA, Paymal SB, Sonawane KD. Molecular insights into the inhibition of early stages of Aβ peptide aggregation and destabilization of Alzheimer's Aβ protofibril by dipeptide D-Trp-Aib: A molecular modelling approach. Int J Biol Macromol 2023; 242(Pt 3): 124880. [http://dx.doi.org/10.1016/j.ijbiomac.2023.124880] [PMID: 37217059]

[49] Shi M, Chu F, Zhu F, Zhu J. Impact of anti-amyloid-β monoclonal antibodies on the pathology and clinical profile of Alzheimer's disease: A focus on aducanumab and lecanemab. Front Aging Neurosci 2022; 14: 870517. [http://dx.doi.org/10.3389/fnagi.2022.870517] [PMID: 35493943]

[50] Brockmann R, Nixon J, Love BL, Yunusa I. Impacts of FDA approval and Medicare restriction on

antiamyloid therapies for Alzheimer's disease: patient outcomes, healthcare costs, and drug development. Lancet Reg Health Am 2023; 20: 100467.
[http://dx.doi.org/10.1016/j.lana.2023.100467] [PMID: 36908502]

[51] Arndt JW, Qian F, Smith BA, *et al.* Structural and kinetic basis for the selectivity of aducanumab for aggregated forms of amyloid-β. Sci Rep 2018; 8(1): 6412.
[http://dx.doi.org/10.1038/s41598-018-24501-0] [PMID: 29686315]

[52] Song C, Shi J, Zhang P, *et al.* Immunotherapy for Alzheimer's disease: targeting β-amyloid and beyond. Transl Neurodegener 2022; 11(1): 18.
[http://dx.doi.org/10.1186/s40035-022-00292-3] [PMID: 35300725]

[53] Budd Haeberlein S, Aisen PS, Barkhof F, *et al.* Two randomized phase 3 studies of aducanumab in early Alzheimer's disease. J Prev Alzheimers Dis 2022; 9(2): 197-210.
[http://dx.doi.org/10.14283/jpad.2022.30] [PMID: 35542991]

[54] Salloway S, Chalkias S, Barkhof F, *et al.* Amyloid-related imaging abnormalities in 2 phase 3 studies evaluating aducanumab in patients with early Alzheimer disease. JAMA Neurol 2022; 79(1): 13-21.
[http://dx.doi.org/10.1001/jamaneurol.2021.4161] [PMID: 34807243]

[55] Barakos J, Purcell D, Suhy J, *et al.* Detection and management of amyloid-related imaging abnormalities in patients with Alzheimer's disease treated with anti-amyloid beta therapy. J Prev Alzheimers Dis 2022; 9(2): 211-20.
[http://dx.doi.org/10.14283/jpad.2022.21] [PMID: 35542992]

[56] Vaz M, Silva V, Monteiro C, *et al.* Role of aducanumab in the treatment of alzheimer's disease: Challenges and opportunities. Clin Interv Aging 2022; 17: 797-810.
[http://dx.doi.org/10.2147/CIA.S325026] [PMID: 35611326]

[57] Jönsson L, Wimo A, Handels R, *et al.* The affordability of lecanemab, an amyloid-targeting therapy for Alzheimer's disease: an EADC-EC viewpoint. Lancet Reg Health Eur 2023; 29(100657): 100657.
[http://dx.doi.org/10.1016/j.lanepe.2023.100657] [PMID: 37251789]

[58] Tucker S, Möller C, Tegerstedt K, *et al.* The murine version of BAN2401 (mAb158) selectively reduces amyloid-β protofibrils in brain and cerebrospinal fluid of tg-ArcSwe mice. J Alzheimers Dis 2015; 43(2): 575-88.
[http://dx.doi.org/10.3233/JAD-140741] [PMID: 25096615]

[59] Logovinsky V, Satlin A, Lai R, *et al.* Safety and tolerability of BAN2401 - a clinical study in Alzheimer's disease with a protofibril selective Aβ antibody. Alzheimers Res Ther 2016; 8(1): 14.
[http://dx.doi.org/10.1186/s13195-016-0181-2] [PMID: 27048170]

[60] Honig LS, Barakos J, Dhadda S, *et al.* ARIA in patients treated with lecanemab (BAN2401) in a phase 2 study in early Alzheimer's disease. Alzheimers Dement (N Y) 2023; 9(1): e12377.
[http://dx.doi.org/10.1002/trc2.12377] [PMID: 36949897]

[61] Bregman N, Nathan T, Shir D, *et al.* Lecanemab in clinical practice: real-world outcomes in early Alzheimer's disease. Alzheimers Res Ther 2025; 17(1): 119.
[http://dx.doi.org/10.1186/s13195-025-01763-1] [PMID: 40437535]

[62] Jawhar S, Wirths O, Bayer TA. Pyroglutamate amyloid-β (Aβ): a hatchet man in Alzheimer disease. J Biol Chem 2011; 286(45): 38825-32.
[http://dx.doi.org/10.1074/jbc.R111.288308] [PMID: 21965666]

[63] Bayer TA. Pyroglutamate Aβ cascade as drug target in Alzheimer's disease. Mol Psychiatry 2022; 27(4): 1880-5.
[http://dx.doi.org/10.1038/s41380-021-01409-2] [PMID: 34880449]

[64] Lowe SL, Willis BA, Hawdon A, *et al.* Donanemab (LY3002813) dose-escalation study in Alzheimer's disease. Alzheimers Dement (N Y) 2021; 7(1): e12112.
[http://dx.doi.org/10.1002/trc2.12112] [PMID: 33614890]

[65] Lowe SL, Duggan Evans C, Shcherbinin S, *et al.* Donanemab (LY3002813) phase 1b study in

Alzheimer's disease: Rapid and sustained reduction of brain amyloid measured by florbetapir F18 imaging. J Prev Alzheimers Dis 2021; 8(4): 414-24.
[http://dx.doi.org/10.14283/jpad.2021.56] [PMID: 34585215]

[66] Shcherbinin S, Evans CD, Lu M, *et al.* Association of amyloid reduction after donanemab treatment with tau pathology and clinical outcomes: The trailblazer-alz randomized clinical trial. JAMA Neurol 2022; 79(10): 1015-1024.
[http://dx.doi.org/10.1001/jamaneurol.2022.2793] [PMID: 36094645]

[67] Yadollahikhales G, Rojas JC. Anti-amyloid immunotherapies for Alzheimer's disease: A 2023 clinical update. Neurotherapeutics 2023; 20(4): 914-31.
[http://dx.doi.org/10.1007/s13311-023-01405-0] [PMID: 37490245]

[68] Rauchenberger R, Borges E, Thomassen-Wolf E, *et al.* Human combinatorial Fab library yielding specific and functional antibodies against the human fibroblast growth factor receptor 3. J Biol Chem 2003; 278(40): 38194-205.
[http://dx.doi.org/10.1074/jbc.M303164200] [PMID: 12842902]

[69] Novakovic D, Feligioni M, Scaccianoce S, *et al.* Profile of gantenerumab and its potential in the treatment of Alzheimer's disease. Drug Des Devel Ther 2013; 7: 1359-64.
[PMID: 24255592]

[70] Cheung D, Fong A, Ding HT, *et al.* A phase 1, randomized study to evaluate safety, tolerability, and pharmacokinetics of GDC-3280, a potential novel anti-fibrotic small molecule, in healthy subjects. Pulm Pharmacol Ther 2021; 69(102051): 102051.
[http://dx.doi.org/10.1016/j.pupt.2021.102051] [PMID: 34166834]

[71] Roche. A multiple ascending dose study of R1450 in patients with Alzheimer disease [Internet]. ClinicalTrials.gov; 2007. Available from: https://clinicaltrials.gov/ct2/show/NCT00531804

[72] Ostrowitzki S, Lasser RA, Dorflinger E, *et al.* A phase III randomized trial of gantenerumab in prodromal Alzheimer's disease. Alzheimers Res Ther 2017; 9(1): 95.
[http://dx.doi.org/10.1186/s13195-017-0318-y] [PMID: 29221491]

[73] Joseph-Mathurin N, Llibre-Guerra JJ, Li Y, *et al.* Amyloid-related imaging abnormalities in the DIAN-TU-001 trial of gantenerumab and solanezumab: Lessons from a trial in dominantly inherited Alzheimer disease. Ann Neurol 2022; 92(5): 729-44.
[http://dx.doi.org/10.1002/ana.26511] [PMID: 36151869]

[74] Cummings J, Osse AML, Cammann D, Powell J, Chen J. Anti-amyloid monoclonal antibodies for the treatment of Alzheimer's disease. BioDrugs 2024; 38(1): 5-22.
[http://dx.doi.org/10.1007/s40259-023-00633-2] [PMID: 37955845]

[75] International conference on alzheimer's and parkinson's diseases. International Conference on Alzheimer's and Parkinson's Diseases 2023; Gothenburg, Sweden; 2023 Mar 28–Apr 1.

[76] Pardridge WM. Blood–brain barrier drug delivery of IgG fusion proteins with a transferrin receptor monoclonal antibody. Expert Opin Drug Deliv 2015; 12(2): 207-22.
[http://dx.doi.org/10.1517/17425247.2014.952627] [PMID: 25138991]

[77] Cummings J, Zhou Y, Lee G, Zhong K, Fonseca J, Cheng F. Alzheimer's disease drug development pipeline: 2023. Alzheimers Dement (N Y) 2023; 9(2): e12385.
[http://dx.doi.org/10.1002/trc2.12385] [PMID: 37251912]

[78] Cummings J. Anti-amyloid monoclonal antibodies are transformative treatments that redefine alzheimer's disease therapeutics. Drugs 2023; 83(7): 569-76.
[http://dx.doi.org/10.1007/s40265-023-01858-9] [PMID: 37060386]

[79] Xiong B, Liu Y, Xu Y, *et al.* Breaking the limitation of polarization multiplexing in optical metasurfaces with engineered noise. Science 2023; 379(6629): 294-9.
[http://dx.doi.org/10.1126/science.ade5140] [PMID: 36656947]

[80] Chen X, Zhu H, Bao K, *et al.* Bis-isatin derivatives: design, synthesis, and biological activity

evaluation as potent dimeric DJ-1 inhibitors. Acta Pharmacol Sin 2021; 42(7): 1160-70. [http://dx.doi.org/10.1038/s41401-020-00600-5] [PMID: 33495517]

[81] Henley D, Raghavan N, Sperling R, Aisen P, Raman R, Romano G. Preliminary results of a trial of atabecestat in preclinical Alzheimer's disease. N Engl J Med 2019; 380(15): 1483-5. [http://dx.doi.org/10.1056/NEJMc1813435] [PMID: 30970197]

[82] Hampel H, Vassar R, De Strooper B, *et al.* The β-secretase BACE1 in Alzheimer's disease. Biol Psychiatry 2021; 89(8): 745-56. [http://dx.doi.org/10.1016/j.biopsych.2020.02.001] [PMID: 32223911]

[83] Endres K, Fahrenholz F, Lotz J, *et al.* Increased CSF APPs-α levels in patients with Alzheimer disease treated with acitretin. Neurology 2014; 83(21): 1930-5. [http://dx.doi.org/10.1212/WNL.0000000000001017] [PMID: 25344383]

[84] Decourt B, Wilson J, Ritter A, *et al.* MCLENA-1: A phase II clinical trial for the assessment of safety, tolerability, and efficacy of lenalidomide in patients with mild cognitive impairment due to Alzheimer's disease. Open Access J Clin Trials 2020; 12: 1-13. [http://dx.doi.org/10.2147/OAJCT.S221914] [PMID: 32123490]

[85] Bakker A, Albert MS, Krauss G, Speck CL, Gallagher M. Response of the medial temporal lobe network in amnestic mild cognitive impairment to therapeutic intervention assessed by fMRI and memory task performance. Neuroimage Clin 2015; 7: 688-98. [http://dx.doi.org/10.1016/j.nicl.2015.02.009] [PMID: 25844322]

[86] Maccecchini ML, Chang MY, Pan C, John V, Zetterberg H, Greig NH. Posiphen as a candidate drug to lower CSF amyloid precursor protein, amyloid-β peptide and τ levels: target engagement, tolerability and pharmacokinetics in humans. J Neurol Neurosurg Psychiatry 2012; 83(9): 894-902. [http://dx.doi.org/10.1136/jnnp-2012-302589] [PMID: 22791904]

[87] Vassar R, Bennett BD, Babu-Khan S, *et al.* Beta-secretase cleavage of Alzheimer's amyloid precursor protein by the transmembrane aspartic protease BACE. Science 1999; 286(5440): 735-41. [http://dx.doi.org/10.1126/science.286.5440.735] [PMID: 10531052]

[88] Madrasi K, Das R, Mohmmadabdul H, *et al.* Systematic *in silico* analysis of clinically tested drugs for reducing amyloid-beta plaque accumulation in Alzheimer's disease. Alzheimers Dement 2021; 17(9): 1487-98. [http://dx.doi.org/10.1002/alz.12312] [PMID: 33938131]

[89] Dorey A, Perret-Liaudet A, Tholance Y, Fourier A, Quadrio I. Cerebrospinal fluid Aβ40 improves the interpretation of Aβ42 concentration for diagnosing alzheimer's disease. Front Neurol. 2015 Nov 27; 6: 247. [http://dx.doi.org/10.3389/fneur.2015.00247] [PMID: 26640457]

[90] Yuan J, Venkatraman S, Zheng Y, McKeever BM, Dillard LW, Singh SB. Structure-based design of β-site APP cleaving enzyme 1 (BACE1) inhibitors for the treatment of Alzheimer's disease. J Med Chem 2013; 56(11): 4156-80. [http://dx.doi.org/10.1021/jm301659n] [PMID: 23509904]

[91] Albright CF, Dockens RC, Meredith JE Jr, *et al.* Pharmacodynamics of selective inhibition of γ-secretase by avagacestat. J Pharmacol Exp Ther 2013; 344(3): 686-95. [http://dx.doi.org/10.1124/jpet.112.199356] [PMID: 23275065]

[92] Coric V, Salloway S, van Dyck CH, *et al.* Targeting prodromal alzheimer disease with avagacestat. JAMA Neurol 2015; 72(11): 1324-33. [http://dx.doi.org/10.1001/jamaneurol.2015.0607] [PMID: 26414022]

[93] Raven F, Ward JF, Zoltowska KM, *et al.* Soluble gamma-secretase modulators attenuate alzheimer's β-amyloid pathology and induce conformational changes in presenilin 1. EBioMedicine 2017; 24: 93-101. [http://dx.doi.org/10.1016/j.ebiom.2017.08.028] [PMID: 28919280]

[94] Rogers K, Felsenstein KM, Hrdlicka L, *et al.* Modulation of γ-secretase by EVP-0015962 reduces amyloid deposition and behavioral deficits in Tg2576 mice. Mol Neurodegener 2012; 7(1): 61. [http://dx.doi.org/10.1186/1750-1326-7-61] [PMID: 23249765]

[95] Fox NC, Black RS, Gilman S, *et al.* Effects of Aβ immunization (AN1792) on MRI measures of cerebral volume in Alzheimer disease. Neurology 2005; 64(9): 1563-72. [http://dx.doi.org/10.1212/01.WNL.0000159743.08996.99] [PMID: 15883317]

[96] Gilman S, Koller M, Black RS, *et al.* Clinical effects of Aβ immunization (AN1792) in patients with AD in an interrupted trial. Neurology 2005; 64(9): 1553-62. [http://dx.doi.org/10.1212/01.WNL.0000159740.16984.3C] [PMID: 15883316]

[97] Ryan JM, Grundman M. Anti-amyloid-beta immunotherapy in Alzheimer's disease: ACC-001 clinical trials are ongoing. J Alzheimers Dis 2009; 17(2): 243. [http://dx.doi.org/10.3233/JAD-2009-1118] [PMID: 19502708]

[98] Ullah R, Park TJ, Huang X, Kim MO. Abnormal amyloid beta metabolism in systemic abnormalities and Alzheimer's pathology: Insights and therapeutic approaches from periphery. Ageing Res Rev 2021; 71: 101451. [http://dx.doi.org/10.1016/j.arr.2021.101451] [PMID: 34450351]

[99] Cirrito JR, Yamada KA, Finn MB, *et al.* Synaptic activity regulates interstitial fluid amyloid-beta levels *in vivo*. Neuron 2005; 48(6): 913-22. [http://dx.doi.org/10.1016/j.neuron.2005.10.028] [PMID: 16364896]

[100] Romani A, Marchetti C, Bianchi D, *et al.* Computational modeling of the effects of amyloid-beta on release probability at hippocampal synapses. Front Comput Neurosci 2013; 7(7): 1. [http://dx.doi.org/10.3389/fncom.2013.00001] [PMID: 23355821]

[101] Li X, Xiao Z, Han J, *et al.* Promotion of neuronal differentiation of neural progenitor cells by using EGFR antibody functionalized collagen scaffolds for spinal cord injury repair. Biomaterials 2013; 34(21): 5107-16. [http://dx.doi.org/10.1016/j.biomaterials.2013.03.062] [PMID: 23591390]

[102] Scott G, Ramlackhansingh AF, Edison P, *et al.* Amyloid pathology and axonal injury after brain trauma. Neurology 2016; 86(9): 821-8. [http://dx.doi.org/10.1212/WNL.0000000000002413] [PMID: 26843562]

[103] Greenberg SM, Bacskai BJ, Hernandez-Guillamon M, Pruzin J, Sperling R, van Veluw SJ. Cerebral amyloid angiopathy and Alzheimer disease — one peptide, two pathways. Nat Rev Neurol 2020; 16(1): 30-42. [http://dx.doi.org/10.1038/s41582-019-0281-2] [PMID: 31827267]

[104] Mannix RC, Zhang J, Berglass J, Qui J, Whalen MJ. Beneficial effect of amyloid beta after controlled cortical impact. Brain Inj 2013; 27(6): 743-8. [http://dx.doi.org/10.3109/02699052.2013.771797] [PMID: 23672448]

[105] Clarke J, Thornell A, Corbett D, Soininen H, Hiltunen M, Jolkkonen J. Overexpression of APP provides neuroprotection in the absence of functional benefit following middle cerebral artery occlusion in rats. Eur J Neurosci 2007; 26(7): 1845-52. [http://dx.doi.org/10.1111/j.1460-9568.2007.05807.x] [PMID: 17897395]

[106] Kontush A, Berndt C, Weber W, *et al.* Amyloid-β is an antioxidant for lipoproteins in cerebrospinal fluid and plasma. Free Radic Biol Med 2001; 30(1): 119-28. [http://dx.doi.org/10.1016/S0891-5849(00)00458-5] [PMID: 11134902]

[107] Kontush A. Amyloid-β: an antioxidant that becomes a pro-oxidant and critically contributes to Alzheimer's disease. Free Radic Biol Med 2001; 31(9): 1120-31. [http://dx.doi.org/10.1016/S0891-5849(01)00688-8] [PMID: 11677045]

[108] Frain L, Swanson D, Cho K, *et al.* Association of cancer and Alzheimer's disease risk in a national cohort of veterans. Alzheimers Dement 2017; 13(12): 1364-70.

[http://dx.doi.org/10.1016/j.jalz.2017.04.012] [PMID: 28711346]

[109] Cai W, Li L, Sang S, Pan X, Zhong C. Physiological roles of β-amyloid in regulating synaptic function: Implications for AD pathophysiology. Neurosci Bull 2023; 39(8): 1289-308. [http://dx.doi.org/10.1007/s12264-022-00985-9] [PMID: 36443453]

[110] Giuffrida ML, Tomasello MF, Pandini G, *et al.* Monomeric ß-amyloid interacts with type-1 insulin-like growth factor receptors to provide energy supply to neurons. Front Cell Neurosci 2015; 9: 297. [http://dx.doi.org/10.3389/fncel.2015.00297] [PMID: 26300732]

[111] Zimbone S, Monaco I, Gianì F, *et al.* Amyloid Beta monomers regulate cyclic adenosine monophosphate response element binding protein functions by activating type-1 insulin-like growth factor receptors in neuronal cells. Aging Cell 2018; 17(1): e12684. [http://dx.doi.org/10.1111/acel.12684] [PMID: 29094448]

[112] Nagahara AH, Tuszynski MH. Potential therapeutic uses of BDNF in neurological and psychiatric disorders. Nat Rev Drug Discov 2011; 10(3): 209-19. [http://dx.doi.org/10.1038/nrd3366] [PMID: 21358740]

[113] Seabrook GR, Smith DW, Bowery BJ, *et al.* Mechanisms contributing to the deficits in hippocampal synaptic plasticity in mice lacking amyloid precursor protein. Neuropharmacology 1999; 38(3): 349-59. [http://dx.doi.org/10.1016/S0028-3908(98)00204-4] [PMID: 10219973]

[114] Puzzo D, Privitera L, Fa' M, *et al.* Endogenous amyloid-β is necessary for hippocampal synaptic plasticity and memory. Ann Neurol 2011; 69(5): 819-30. [http://dx.doi.org/10.1002/ana.22313] [PMID: 21472769]

[115] Kamenetz F, Tomita T, Hsieh H, *et al.* APP processing and synaptic function. Neuron 2003; 37(6): 925-37. [http://dx.doi.org/10.1016/S0896-6273(03)00124-7] [PMID: 12670422]

[116] Ikegaya Y, Matsuura S, Ueno S, *et al.* Beta-amyloid enhances glial glutamate uptake activity and attenuates synaptic efficacy. J Biol Chem 2002; 277(35): 32180-6. [http://dx.doi.org/10.1074/jbc.M203764200] [PMID: 12070161]

[117] Castro NG, Albuquerque EX. alpha-Bungarotoxin-sensitive hippocampal nicotinic receptor channel has a high calcium permeability. Biophys J 1995; 68(2): 516-24. [http://dx.doi.org/10.1016/S0006-3495(95)80213-4] [PMID: 7696505]

[118] Unwin N. Nicotinic acetylcholine receptor and the structural basis of neuromuscular transmission: insights from *Torpedo* postsynaptic membranes. Q Rev Biophys 2013; 46(4): 283-322. [http://dx.doi.org/10.1017/S0033583513000061] [PMID: 24050525]

[119] Dougherty JJ, Wu J, Nichols RA. Beta-amyloid regulation of presynaptic nicotinic receptors in rat hippocampus and neocortex. J Neurosci 2003; 23(17): 6740-7. [http://dx.doi.org/10.1523/JNEUROSCI.23-17-06740.2003] [PMID: 12890766]

[120] Letsinger AC, Gu Z, Yakel JL. α7 nicotinic acetylcholine receptors in the hippocampal circuit: taming complexity. Trends Neurosci 2022; 45(2): 145-57. [http://dx.doi.org/10.1016/j.tins.2021.11.006] [PMID: 34916082]

[121] Cecon E, Dam J, Luka M, *et al.* Quantitative assessment of oligomeric amyloid β peptide binding to α7 nicotinic receptor. Br J Pharmacol 2019; 176(18): 3475-88. [http://dx.doi.org/10.1111/bph.14688] [PMID: 30981214]

[122] Gulisano W, Melone M, Ripoli C, *et al.* Neuromodulatory action of picomolar extracellular Aβ42 oligomers on presynaptic and postsynaptic mechanisms underlying synaptic function and memory. J Neurosci 2019; 39(30): 5986-6000. [http://dx.doi.org/10.1523/JNEUROSCI.0163-19.2019] [PMID: 31127002]

[123] Tropea MR, Li Puma DD, Melone M, *et al.* Genetic deletion of α7 nicotinic acetylcholine receptors induces an age-dependent Alzheimer's disease-like pathology. Prog Neurobiol 2021; 206(102154):

102154.
[http://dx.doi.org/10.1016/j.pneurobio.2021.102154] [PMID: 34453977]

[124] Puzzo D, Privitera L, Leznik E, *et al.* Picomolar amyloid-β positively modulates synaptic plasticity and memory in hippocampus. J Neurosci 2008; 28(53): 14537-45.
[http://dx.doi.org/10.1523/JNEUROSCI.2692-08.2008] [PMID: 19118188]

[125] Pajoohesh-Ganji A, Burns MP, Pal-Ghosh S, *et al.* Inhibition of amyloid precursor protein secretases reduces recovery after spinal cord injury. Brain Res 2014; 1560: 73-82.
[http://dx.doi.org/10.1016/j.brainres.2014.02.049] [PMID: 24630972]

[126] Park JC, Han SH, Mook-Jung I. Peripheral inflammatory biomarkers in Alzheimer's disease: a brief review. BMB Rep 2020; 53(1): 10-9.
[http://dx.doi.org/10.5483/BMBRep.2020.53.1.309] [PMID: 31865964]

[127] Suárez-Calvet M, Capell A, Araque Caballero MÁ, *et al.* CSF progranulin increases in the course of Alzheimer's disease and is associated with sTREM 2, neurodegeneration and cognitive decline. EMBO Mol Med 2018; 10(12): e9712.
[http://dx.doi.org/10.15252/emmm.201809712] [PMID: 30482868]

[128] Guadaño-Ferraz A, Viñuela A, Oeding G, Bernal J, Rausell E. RC3/neurogranin is expressed in pyramidal neurons of motor and somatosensory cortex in normal and denervated monkeys. J Comp Neurol 2005; 493(4): 554-70.
[http://dx.doi.org/10.1002/cne.20774] [PMID: 16304627]

[129] Portelius E, Zetterberg H, Skillbäck T, *et al.* Cerebrospinal fluid neurogranin: relation to cognition and neurodegeneration in Alzheimer's disease. Brain 2015; 138(11): 3373-85.
[http://dx.doi.org/10.1093/brain/awv267] [PMID: 26373605]

[130] Karran E, De Strooper B. The amyloid hypothesis in Alzheimer disease: new insights from new therapeutics. Nat Rev Drug Discov 2022; 21(4): 306-18.
[http://dx.doi.org/10.1038/s41573-022-00391-w] [PMID: 35177833]

[131] Koelsch G. BACE1 function and inhibition: implications of intervention in the amyloid pathway of alzheimer's disease pathology. Molecules 2017; 22(10): 1723.
[http://dx.doi.org/10.3390/molecules22101723] [PMID: 29027981]

[132] Salloway SP, Sevingy J, Budur K, *et al.* Advancing combination therapy for Alzheimer's disease. Alzheimer's & dementia (New York, N. Y.). 2020; 6(1): e12073.
[http://dx.doi.org/10.1002/trc2.12073]

[133] Atayik MC, Çakatay U. Mitochondria-associated cellular senescence mechanisms: Biochemical and pharmacological perspectives. Adv Protein Chem Struct Biol 2023; 136: 117-55.
[http://dx.doi.org/10.1016/bs.apcsb.2023.03.003] [PMID: 37437976]

[134] Zhang H, Jiang X, Ma L, *et al.* Role of Aβ in Alzheimer's-related synaptic dysfunction. Front Cell Dev Biol 2022; 10: 964075.
[http://dx.doi.org/10.3389/fcell.2022.964075] [PMID: 36092715]

[135] Uddin MS, Stachowiak A, Mamun AA, *et al.* Autophagy and alzheimer's disease: from molecular mechanisms to therapeutic implications. Front Aging Neurosci. 2018; 10: 04.

[136] Zhang W, Xu C, Sun J, Shen HM, Wang J, Yang C. Impairment of the autophagy–lysosomal pathway in Alzheimer's diseases: Pathogenic mechanisms and therapeutic potential. Acta Pharm Sin B 2022; 12(3): 1019-40.
[http://dx.doi.org/10.1016/j.apsb.2022.01.008] [PMID: 35530153]

[137] Hung COY, Livesey FJ. Altered γ-secretase processing of APP disrupts lysosome and autophagosome function in monogenic alzheimer's disease. Cell Rep 2018; 25(13): 3647-3660.e2.
[http://dx.doi.org/10.1016/j.celrep.2018.11.095] [PMID: 30590039]

[138] Mançano ASF, Pina JG, Froes BR, Sciani JM. Autophagy-lysosomal pathway impairment and cathepsin dysregulation in Alzheimer's disease. Front Mol Biosci 2024; 11: 1490275.

[http://dx.doi.org/10.3389/fmolb.2024.1490275] [PMID: 39544403]

[139] Xie PL, Zheng MY, Han R, Chen WX, Mao JH. Pharmacological mTOR inhibitors in ameliorating Alzheimer's disease: current review and perspectives. Front Pharmacol 2024; 15: 1366061. [http://dx.doi.org/10.3389/fphar.2024.1366061] [PMID: 38873415]

[140] Matos LC, Machado JP, Monteiro FJ, Greten HJ. Understanding traditional chinese medicine therapeutics: An overview of the basics and clinical applications. Healthcare (Basel) 2021; 9(3): 257. [http://dx.doi.org/10.3390/healthcare9030257] [PMID: 33804485]

[141] Zhang Y, Chen H, Li R, Sterling K, Song W. Amyloid β-based therapy for Alzheimer's disease: challenges, successes and future. Signal Transduct Target Ther 2023; 8(1): 248. [http://dx.doi.org/10.1038/s41392-023-01484-7] [PMID: 37386015]

[142] Bose R, Banerjee S, Dunbar GL. Modeling neurological disorders in 3D organoids using human-derived pluripotent stem cells. Front. Cell Dev. Biol. 2021; 9: 640212. [http://dx.doi.org/10.3389/fcell.2021.640212]

[143] Cerneckis J, Bu G, Shi Y. Pushing the boundaries of brain organoids to study Alzheimer's disease. Trends Mol Med 2023; 29(8): 659-72. [http://dx.doi.org/10.1016/j.molmed.2023.05.007] [PMID: 37353408]

[144] Urrestizala-Arenaza N, Cerchio S, Cavaliere F, Magliaro C. Limitations of human brain organoids to study neurodegenerative diseases: a manual to survive. Front Cell Neurosci 2024; 18: 1419526. [http://dx.doi.org/10.3389/fncel.2024.1419526] [PMID: 39049825]

[145] Rhinn H, Tatton N, McCaughey S, Kurnellas M, Rosenthal A. Progranulin as a therapeutic target in neurodegenerative diseases. Trends Pharmacol Sci 2022; 43(8): 641-52. [http://dx.doi.org/10.1016/j.tips.2021.11.015] [PMID: 35039149]

[146] Liu W, Lin H, He X, *et al.* Neurogranin as a cognitive biomarker in cerebrospinal fluid and blood exosomes for Alzheimer's disease and mild cognitive impairment. Transl Psychiatry 2020; 10: 125. [http://dx.doi.org/10.1038/s41398-020-0801-2]

CHAPTER 10

Small Molecules as Anti-Alzheimer's Scaffolds

Rudradeep Hazra[1], **Souvik Roy**[1,*], **Sakuntala Gayen**[1], **Ankita Parui**[1], **Amima Arshad**[1], **Nipa Roy**[1] and **Asmita Nag Sarkar**[1]

[1] *Department of Pharmacy, NSHM Knowledge Campus Kolkata – Group of Institutions, Kolkata, West Bengal, India*

Abstract: Alzheimer's disease (AD) remains one of the most common diseases in our society. Its prevalence is increasing gradually, particularly in advanced nations, because life expectancy is increasing, and it presents a major worldwide economic burden. Throughout the last decades, all efforts to the development of newer diagnostic and therapeutic approaches have invariably met with failure, understanding that AD is currently irremediable and emphasizing the urgent requirement for innovative strategies. Recently, small molecules have emerged as an optimistic avenue for the cure of AD. These compounds can simultaneously provide diagnostic insights and therapeutic effects, enabling the evaluation of molecular activity, therapeutic responses, and pharmacokinetics. This dual functionality makes them highly promising for advancing AD drug research and their integration into personalized medicine. The small molecule theranostic compounds are the subject of this review article as a possible resource for the development of innovative therapeutic and diagnostic strategies for AD, which may highlight their noteworthy and advantageous influence in upcoming clinical applications.

Keywords: Alzheimer's disease, Dementia, Neurodegeneration, Pathophysiology, Small molecule theranostic agents.

INTRODUCTION

Dementia is a general term used to describe a collection of symptoms linked to cognitive impairment, including memory loss, changes in mood and behavior, difficulty solving problems, and the inability to do daily tasks. Alzheimer's disease (AD) has drawn more attention than other dementia symptoms because of its high incidence (60–80%), which can result in the development of Lewy body disease, hippocampus sclerosis, Parkinson's disease, frontotemporal lobar degeneration, and cardiovascular disease [1]. The most common multifactorial neurodegenerative disease is AD, which is typified by a progressive decline in

* **Corresponding author Souvik Roy:** Department of Pharmacy, NSHM Knowledge Campus Kolkata – Group of Institutions, Kolkata, West Bengal, India; E-mail: souvikroy35@gmail.com; souvik.roy@nshm.com

brain neuronal function. Currently, it is estimated that around 57 million people are affected worldwide, representing a considerable burden. It was predicted that AD will progress markedly to exceed 150 million cases in 2025 [2], demonstrating that AD is a debilitating condition that affects not just patients but also their family members and caregivers, and attesting to its significant influence on our society.

Clinically, AD manifests as cognitive impairment, including mood swings, depression, apathy, behavioural changes, and memory loss with difficulty recalling recent knowledge, leading to the display of physical disabilities with difficulties in speaking, working, and ultimately death [3]. These manifestations appeared in a slight way over a long duration of time, where three stages are generally discriminated, such as moderate cognitive impairment (slight symptoms that do not interfere with everyday work), dementia (symptoms that interfere with daily performance), and asymptomatic or preclinical AD. The asymptomatic symptoms in the preclinical stage do not reveal severe pathogenic mechanisms, while they can be observed in two decades prior to the onset of the symptoms, which is highly significant to search for therapeutic tools for early diagnosis of AD [4, 5]. Despite the numerous studies on AD, the cause of AD progression remains unclear. A few pathways have been found to efficiently target the onset and development of AD. The formation and accumulation of misfolded protein leads to the triggering of the induction of neurodegenerative disorder, which subsequently causes neuronal death. Tau and β-amyloid proteins are two important hallmarks associated with the initiation of AD pathophysiology, and both proteins have an important role in protein misfolding. Additionally, neuroinflammation, oxidative stress, imbalance in cholinergic and glutamatergic transduction, and mitochondrial dysfunction also participate in the progression of AD [6]. Furthermore, some risk factors are also involved in AD pathogenesis, including intrinsic factors, such as genetic factors associated with the amyloid protein precursor APP, γ-secretase – PSEN1 / PSEN2, and apolipoprotein E), aging, diseases like traumatic brain injury, cardiovascular disease, obesity, and diabetes, and external factors, like unhealthy lifestyle, smoking, exposure to metals – aluminium, lead, and cadmium [7, 8].

Only a few medications are authorized to treat AD as acetylcholinesterase inhibitors (AChE), rivastigmine, tacrine, galantamine, and donepezil block the route that suppresses the effects of acetylcholine (ACh). Memantine, an N-methyl-D-aspartate (NMDA) receptor antagonist, comes in fifth. Additionally, a human IgG1 anti-Aβ monoclonal antibody *i.e.*, Aducanumab (Aduhelm), was authorized by the Food and Drug Administration (FDA) in 2021for treating AD, especially to target β-amyloid oligomers and fibrils [9]. The previous review highlighted the relevance of the innovative therapeutic and diagnostic approaches for the treatment of AD. Moreover, the most pertinent developments for the treatment of AD in relation to small-molecule theranostic drugs are critically reviewed in this paper.

PATHOPHYSIOLOGY OF ALZHEIMER'S DISEASE

Neurons in vertebrates share a critical physiological process involving the production and turnover of amyloid-beta (Aβ) (Fig. **1**). Several studies have shown that Aβ monomers play an important role in regulating synaptic activity [10, 11]. Preserving the homeostasis of synaptic Aβ monomer ratios is crucial and requires a very complex procedure. The interaction of the metastable hydrophobic peptide with lipids, vesicles, and membranes is what gives rise to this intricacy. It is difficult to quantify the amounts of metastable Aβ monomers in living animals because intrinsically disordered proteins (IDPs) can take on their structure during extraction. While some progress has been made in characterizing intermediate Aβ species in APP transgenic mice by combining synchrotron-based Fourier transform infrared microspectroscopy with nondenaturing gel electrophoresis [12], it is still very challenging to evaluate nascent Aβ monomer concentration in-vivo. According to certain theories, disruptions in the processes of Aβ synthesis and metabolism are likely the first signs of pathology [12].

Given the importance of preserving physiological Aβ levels at synapses, disruption of the Aβ turnover pathway leads to the early development of misfolded neuropathogenic species. If the proper monomer concentration at the synapse is crucial, losing Aβ monomers necessitates quick replacement. The only ways to restore this are to upregulate BACE and increase Aβ synthesis *via* APP processing. Because of the increased synthesis and turnover of Aβ monomers, this positive feedback loop raises the possibility of Aβ misfolding. Elevated BACE levels in the presynaptic endings of transgenic AD models [13] and the cerebrospinal fluid (CSF) of AD patients [14, 15] are among the most obvious markers of this effect. Mild cognitive impairment (MCI) patients exhibit early biochemical abnormalities in Aβ physiology, such as decreased CSF levels of Aβ42 monomers, even before severe neuronal loss in the advanced stages of AD [16]. Monomeric Aβ is a physiological cofactor that is necessary for the synaptic vesicle cycle (SVC) process and is considered a harmless pre-amyloid peptide.

Presynaptic terminals within the SVC have a significant concentration of Aβ production, which is acknowledged as the major site of Aβ generation [17]. Thus far, the conversation surrounding the function of Aβ monomer in SVC turnover has mainly centred on the pathophysiological function of APP or the precursor molecule itself. Compared to research on synuclein, considering the variations within pathological and physiological isoforms have been better recognized [18], further investigation is needed to elucidate the possible physiological role of Aβ monomer, especially with regard to protein binding during the formation and turnover of synaptic vesicles.

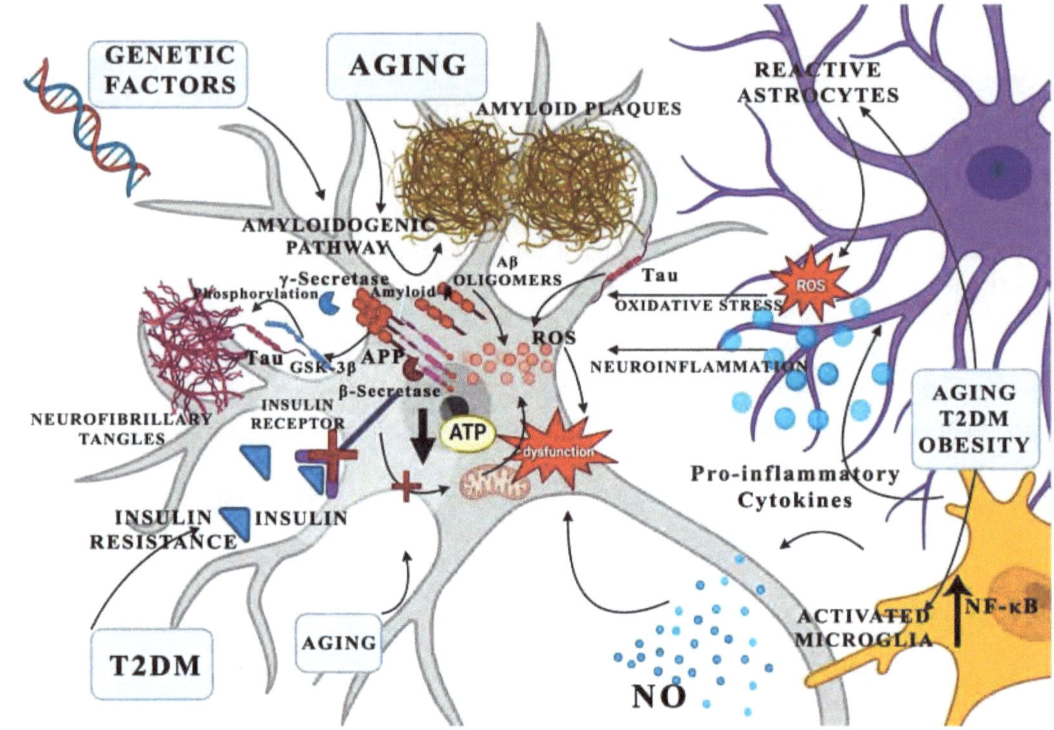

Fig. (1). Pathophysiology of Alzheimer's disease.

The Production and Turnover of Physiological Aβ

There is substantial evidence that Aβ monomers have a physiological role [19]. Human cerebrospinal fluid (CSF) has been found to produce and turn over Aβ at rates of 7.6% and 8.3% per hour, respectively, *in vivo* investigations [20]. The unusually high turnover rates underscore the difficulty of maintaining this protein's proper shape under *in vivo* folding conditions. Stable Isotope Labeling Kinetics (SILK) technology depicted that Aβ turnover is slowed down by about 2.5 times as people age and is altered in AD. At synaptic locations, Aβ concentrations are strictly regulated by carefully regulated gamma- and beta-secretase activities that cooperate to maintain appropriate synaptic Aβ monomer levels in accordance with the particular requirements of neuronal activity [21].

The Initial Pathophysiological Aβ Process

It is now well recognized that cognitive impairments in Alzheimer's disease (AD) occur more than ten years before Aβ pathology, which is characterized by misfolding in the brain [22]. In patients with AD and moderate cognitive impairment (MCI), a decreased level of Aβ monomer 1–42 in the cerebrospinal fluid (CSF) is the first detectable Aβ measure that indicates disease. This decrease serves as an early marker of physiological impairment, occurring when the Aβ monomer begins to partially escape *in vivo* folding control. In familial Alzheimer's disease (FAD), chaperone regulation is probably eventually overpowered by APP mutations or overproduction; in sporadic AD, the causes of oligomer development are yet unknown. Oligomer-selective antibodies can be used to identify Aβx-y oligomers in the first stages of MCI. These oligomers have a unique structure along the standard oligomer folding mechanism [22, 23]. These adhesive molecules can bind to a variety of proteins and cell-surface receptors, including RAGE [24] and PrPc [11]. Additionally, through their interactions with important mitochondrial proteins, oligomers reduce the excessive energy consumption of neurons [25]. Over the past 20 years, the detrimental consequences of Aβ oligomers have been thoroughly examined and documented [26].

Compensatory Mechanisms Deteriorate Pathology

In addition to the synapto-toxic effects of oligomers through potential receptor-mediated pathways, early misfolding of Aβ monomers results in a shortage of Aβ monomers at the synapse. If we consider that the concentration of Aβ monomers associated with neuronal activity is crucial for modulating synaptic function, this implies a need for compensatory mechanisms, such as the upregulation of BACE, to offset Aβ monomer losses. This process can occur within a typical positive feedback loop. Consequently, increased Aβ production leads to a further rise in the misfolding rate. A vicious cycle is thus created, marked by increased Aβ synthesis and turnover, which exacerbates Aβ pathogenesis by increasing oligomer formation and concurrently depleting monomers [27].

Currently, there is no direct evidence confirming that beta-secretase (BACE) upregulation occurs in response to Aβ monomer deficiency. Nonetheless, considerable evidence suggests BACE modulation is a very delicate and primary mechanism that is strongly related to presynaptic APP control. Increased BACE1 activity functions as an early biomarker of Aβ pathology in moderate cognitive impairment (MCI) and early Alzheimer's disease (AD), akin to the decrease of Aβ monomers in cerebrospinal fluid (CSF) [28]. Furthermore, it has been discovered that sporadic AD cases had higher BACE1 gene expression [29]. Within the same vesicles, synaptic BACE1 and APP colocalize [30, 31]. It has been demonstrated that APP processing is influenced by the binding of oligomers to the Nogo-66 receptor 1 (NgR1), providing compelling evidence for an interaction involving Aβ regulation and Aβ oligomers [11].

Reverses Aβ Dysregulation with Early Aβ Oligomer-type Therapy

This idea suggests that the therapeutic approach should focus on promptly eliminating misfolded Aβ species at neuronal sites to reverse the disease. A strong and adequately CNS-penetrant Aβ oligomer-directed selective immunotherapy, either with a particular antibody or a suitable active vaccination regimen, would be the most efficient way to do this (Liu *et al.*, 2023). Normalization of Aβ turnover is anticipated as a result of this intervention, which will also likely result in normalization of the biomarkers BACE and Aβ42 in CSF. A pure gamma-secretase modulator may be used as an additional therapy to raise Aβ38 and Aβ40 levels at the expense of Aβ42 levels, therefore reducing the tendency for Aβ aggregation [32].

Tau in Alzheimer's Disease

Usually categorized as a "natively unfolded" protein, tau is essential for maintaining microtubule stability. Tau has a relatively low tendency for misfolding and aggregation in both intracellular and extracellular environments when it is in its normally mostly unfolded state. But when tau experiences harmful changes, such as "prion-like" dispersions, it can cause aberrant folding and aggregation, which can result in tauopathies, which are neurodegenerative illnesses [33].

While phosphorylation plays a vital role in regulating tau activity in normal physiological conditions, overphosphorylation leads to hyperphosphorylated tau (p-tau), which self-aggregates and is the main characteristic of many tauopathies [34, 35]. Hyperphosphorylation has the potential to modify the charge and conformation of the protein, thereby revealing the microtubule-binding domain. This, in turn, stimulates tau oligomerization and self-aggregation [36 - 38]. Eventually, these clumped tau proteins create neurofibrillary tangles (NFTs). Hyperphosphorylation at the tau C-terminus stimulates tau protein self-assembly, resulting in the production of paired helical filaments (PHFs) prior to the formation of neurofibrillary tangles (NFTs). Axonal transport is disrupted by this aggregated conformation, which also leads to microtubule destabilization [39]. Compared to healthy controls, patients with Alzheimer's disease (AD) present a significantly higher level of abnormal or hyperphosphorylated tau proteins, with an increase of fourfold. Moreover, these misfolded tau proteins lose their primary function of stabilizing microtubules and exhibit heightened aggregation effects, rendering them potential neurotoxins [40 - 44]. Ultimately, the functioning of tau in relation to microtubules is compromised, which adversely affects synaptic plasticity and impairs axonal transport, leading to cognitive deficits. Furthermore, problems with microtubule assembly are exacerbated by hyperphosphorylated tau (p-tau), which activates proteins that break microtubules, such as katanin [45]. One important factor in the development of tau disease is abnormal tau phosphorylation. These pathogenic effects of tau are more intimately linked to the onset and course of AD than Aβ buildup. When phosphorylation and dephosphorylation are abnormal, patients may experience serious pathogenic consequences. The pathogenic effects of tau are mediated by several proteins, such as α-Synuclein, Amyloid-β, Pin1, Fyn Kinase, Heat Shock Proteins, FKBP51 and FKBP52 Immunophilins, and PACSIN1. These proteins play key roles in either the phosphorylation or dephosphorylation of tau [46]. Consequently, the regulation of tau is influenced by two essential factors: post-translational modification and protein interactions. Understanding these factors provides opportunities for therapeutic targeting of tau proteins.

Truncation

In addition to tau hyperphosphorylation, tau truncation is another significant modification linked to tau aggregation. Tau truncation refers to the proteolytic cleavage of tau, which promotes abnormal accumulation. It has been demonstrated that caspase 3 belongs to the cysteine protease caspase family, and participates in the *in-vitro* cleavage of tau at aspartic acid residue 421 (D421) in Alzheimer's disease (AD) brains [47]. More readily than tau at its full length, tau shortened at D421 aggregates [48]. Interestingly, the monoclonal antibody Tau-C3 is capable of detecting the caspase 3 cleavage site. Additionally, there is *in vitro* evidence [49] that phosphorylated tau at serine 422 can prevent caspase cleavage at D421. Moreover, a study discovered that tau truncation also takes place at glutamic acid residue 391 (E391), and that the cleavage site may be identified by antibody MN243 since the MN243 epitope is formed there [50].

Glycosylation

Tau is abnormally glycosylated in Alzheimer's disease (AD) brains, and this is associated with tau aggregation. Studies conducted *in vitro* have shown that tau that has been glycosylated is a more favourable substrate for cAMP-dependent protein kinase than tau that has not been glycosylated. This suggests that tau hyperphosphorylation in AD is encouraged by tau glycosylation. It is probable that glycogen synthase kinase-3 beta (GSK3β) and cyclin-dependent kinase 5 (cdk5) mediate this process at particular phosphorylation sites [51, 52].O-GlcNAcylation, a kind of O-glycosylation, controls tau phosphorylation at particular locations, in contrast to N-glycosylation. Reduced O-GlcNAcylation in AD brains may be the cause of the increased hyperphosphorylation and aggregation of tau. According to research utilizing models of starved mice, reduced glucose absorption or metabolism leads to a decrease in O-GlcNAcylation, which in turn causes tau hyperphosphorylation (Pinho *et al.*, 2018; Park *et al.*, 2020). This implies that there may be a higher chance of AD development in those with diabetes, as they also have impaired glucose metabolism [53].

Glycation

Through the creation of advanced glycation end products (AGEs), glycation is a non-enzymatic post-translational alteration that may aid in tau aggregation. Studies have demonstrated that AGE build-up in paired helical filaments (PHF) causes oxidative stress, which in turn causes neuronal dysfunction in patients with Alzheimer's disease (AD) [54]. Li and associates found that AD brains have higher levels of the reactive carbonyl chemical methylglyoxal (MG). Their research indicates that MG stimulates the synthesis of AGEs, upregulates the receptors for AGEs (RAGE), and activates p38 MAPK and GSK-3β in order to cause tau hyperphosphorylation. Furthermore, another study has shown that MG can promote the *in vivo* formation of tangles, a process that is further accelerated by tau hyperphosphorylation [55].

Nitration

Another alteration that can promote tau aggregation is tau nitration. In neurofibrillary tangles (NFTs) in Alzheimer's disease (AD) brains, abnormal tau nitration has been noted. According to Zhao *et al.*, (2021), the tyrosine residues Tyr18, Tyr29, Tyr197, and Tyr394 are implicated in tau nitration. According to studies, nitrated tau at Tyr197 is found in healthy brains and may be involved in normal bodily functions. The other tyrosine residues, on the other hand, are unique to AD brains. Despite this, it remains unknown how tau nitration contributes to AD pathogenesis. According to Zhang and colleagues, there is a dose-dependent relationship between nitration and oligomerization and tau treatment with peroxynitrite. According to the study, conformational changes in nitrated tau prevent it from linking to microtubules and encourage tau aggregation [56].

Ubiquitination

Tau is known to be ubiquitylated, which aids in its accumulation into filamentous tangles, which in turn cause neuronal death (Lin *et al.*, 2024). Neurodegenerative tauopathies have been associated with ubiquitin ligase dysfunction, namely at the carboxyl terminus of the Hsc-70interacting proteins (CHIP). Studies have demonstrated that tau aggregation can be facilitated by tau ubiquitination, which is facilitated by CHIP's interaction with Hsp70/90. On the other hand, there is a notable decrease in tau levels in mouse models that overexpress inducible Hsp70. These results imply that the Hsp70/CHIP chaperone system is essential for controlling tau ubiquitination and degradation, which in turn prevents tau from aggregating [57].

Oxidative Stress and Neuroinflammation for Alzheimer's Disease

Reactive oxygen species (ROS), cellular homeostasis disruption, and the elevation of Aβ and phosphorylated tau (p-tau) are the three main ways that oxidative stress (OS) has been shown to contribute to the development of Alzheimer's disease (AD) [58]. The redox potential of Aβ metal ions, macromolecule peroxidation, and mitochondrial dysfunction are some of these pathways [59]. In particular, membrane-associated OS that causes lipid peroxidation and the generation of 4-hydroxynonenal (HNE), a neurotoxic aldehyde, is referred to as macromolecule peroxidation. Early in the course of AD, HNE can be discovered, and research has shown a correlation between its levels and the degree of neuronal damage. Furthermore, long-term potentiation and other synaptic processes essential for learning and memory—both of which are compromised in AD brains—may also be hampered by lipid peroxidation [60]. Additionally, research has shown that neuronal copper (Cu^{2+}) and zinc (Zn^{2+}) levels in Alzheimer's disease (AD) brains are raised, up to three times higher than in healthy control brains. These metal cations can attach to the hydrophilic N-terminal ends of Aβ peptides, promoting redox processes that generate substantial levels of reactive oxygen species (ROS) [61]. This creates a positive feedback loop that increases oxidation and raises ROS generation. Moreover, AD patients have pathological copper deposition in their senile plaques, which causes a copper deficiency in their brain cells. Another sign of this disturbance of metal homeostasis is the dysregulation of physiological processes controlled by metalloenzymes [62].

Because ROS-induced oxidative stress is linked to the build-up and deposition of β-amyloid, it is also considered a crucial element in the pathophysiology of AD [63]. The accumulation of β-amyloid can aggravate oxidative stress and result in mitochondrial dysfunction, even in patients who are young in the disease. Research reveals that while antioxidants and their enzymes (*e.g.*, vitamin C) are detected at low levels in Alzheimer's patients, the oxidative stress imbalance generated by β-amyloid leads to elevated quantities of by-products like protein and DNA/RNA oxidation [64].

The pathophysiology of Alzheimer's disease (AD) is increasingly understood to involve neuroinflammation, typified by the activation of immune cells in the brain, particularly astrocytes and microglia, which can have both beneficial and detrimental effects (Thakur *et al.*, 2023). Microglia are activated in response to neurotoxic factors such as tau tangles and amyloid-beta (Aβ) plaques in order to remove these toxic proteins; however, chronic activation results in persistent inflammation, as pro-inflammatory cytokines and reactive oxygen species (ROS) released by activated microglia cause damage to neurons and dysfunction of synapses [63]. In the brains of AD patients, elevated levels of pro-inflammatory cytokines have been found, including interleukin-1 beta (IL-1β), tumor necrosis factor-alpha (TNF-α), and interleukin-6 (IL-6). These cytokines disrupt neuronal signaling and promote tau hyperphosphorylation and Aβ aggregation, which worsen neurodegeneration. Furthermore, persistent neuroinflammation can weaken the blood-brain barrier (BBB), which makes it possible for inflammatory mediators and peripheral immune cells to enter the central nervous system (CNS). This increases local inflammation and raises the risk of neuronal damage and cognitive impairment [65]. This continuous neuroinflammatory process is linked to cognitive impairments, such as learning difficulties and memory loss, and it eventually results in synapse loss and neuronal death [66].

MEDIATORS OF NEURONAL INFLAMMATION

Microglia

Distinct from other tissue-resident macrophages and peripheral ones, microglia function as the immune cells of the central nervous system (CNS). By evaluating synaptic activity, controlling synaptic pruning, removing cell debris, and giving neurons trophic support, microglia are constantly monitoring their surroundings. When the blood-brain barrier (BBB) is breached in pathological circumstances like long-term stress, peripheral hematopoietic cells can enter the brain and contribute to the parenchymal microglia/macrophage population within the brain [67]. Microglia can activate to create pro- or anti-inflammatory substances (M1 phenotype) in response to insults to the central nervous system, such as infection or neuronal injury (M2 phenotype). Maintaining a healthy central nervous system (CNS) requires a delicate balance between pro-inflammatory mediators, which aid in the removal of misfolded proteins and cellular detritus, and anti-inflammatory mediators, which support tissue healing and repair [68]. Microglia undergo activation and emit pro-inflammatory cytokines, such as IL-1β, TNF-α, and IL-6, as aging progresses. Microglia in Alzheimer's disease (AD) take on the M1 phenotype in response to pathogen-associated molecular patterns (PAMPs) or danger-associated molecular patterns (DAMPs), which intensifies inflammation and quickens the course of the disease (Ganz *et al.*, 2022). Initial research indicates a relationship between neuroinflammation and amyloid-beta (Aβ). Neurons with neurofibrillary tangles (NFTs) and extracellular Aβ plaques are surrounded by active microglia in brain slices from AD patients [69]. Aβ is thought to activate microglia, causing them to secrete IL-1β, IL-6, TNF-α, and CCL2/4/11, which draws more astrocytes and microglia to the Aβ locations. Microglia can phagocytize Aβ *via* numerous cellular surface receptors, such as CD-14, TLR-2, TLR-4, β6 integrin, CD47, and scavenger receptors like CD36. The extensive build-up of Aβ in AD is partially caused by microglia's inability to efficiently remove extracellular Aβ; research suggests that microglia near plaques have poorer Aβ absorption [70].

Astrocytes

The most common cell type in the central nervous system (CNS) is the astrocyte, which is crucial to the tripartite synapse. These cells play a crucial role in upholding and controlling neuronal functionality and maturation. Astrocytes can be in different states of activation, and they can show either neurotoxic effects, which can cause neurodegeneration through inflammation, or neuroprotective qualities, which reduce inflammation and promote repair. They may identify aggregated proteins like amyloid-beta (Aβ) and respond to inflammatory cues like cytokines and chemokines [71]. Astrocytes become hypertrophic and express more glial fibrillary acidic protein (GFAP) when they are activated. Reactive astrocytes are a characteristic found in the brains of AD mouse models as well as in the brains of individuals with the condition. AD patients' postmortem brains show severe disruption and shrinkage of intralaminar astrocytes [72]. Atrophic astrocytes are found in the entorhinal cortex as early as 30 days of development in the 3xTg mouse model, which has three mutations linked to familial AD (APP Swedish, MAPT P301L, and PSEN1 M146V). These astrocytes remain until the appearance of amyloid-beta (Aβ) plaques at 12 months of age. Astrocytes derived from both familial and sporadic AD-induced pluripotent stem cells (iPSCs) display an atrophic phenotype *in vitro*. Inhibition of astrogliosis in AD mouse models leads to increased Aβ accumulation and worsens histopathological changes, which are associated with cognitive decline [73]. Due to disruptions in glutamate homeostasis and changes in calcium signaling, this may weaken the blood-brain barrier (BBB) and allow peripheral immune cells to enter the brain, escalating neuroinflammation and causing neurotoxicity [71].

Oligodendrocytes

The primary role of oligodendrocytes is to surround nerve fibers with myelin sheaths, which support and insulate axons. Emerging research indicates they may be important to the pathophysiology and development of Alzheimer's disease

(AD), even if their precise role in the condition is still unclear (Ettle *et al.*, 2016). According to recent studies, oligodendrocytes in AD are markedly degraded; they exhibit localized loss and a reduction in myelin proteins close to amyloid-beta (Aβ) plaques (Blanchand *et al.*, 2022). Aβ not only interferes with the development of the myelin sheath but also has an impact on the survival and maturation of oligodendrocyte progenitor cells (OPCs). Furthermore, oligodendrocyte dysfunction and cell death may be further exacerbated by neuroinflammation and oxidative stress [74].

Genetics and Environmental Factors for Alzheimer's Disease

The complex interactions between genetics, lifestyle, and environmental elements play a critical role in disease progression, particularly in Alzheimer's Disease (AD). The APOE4 allele is a significant genetic risk factor, yet it does not account for all AD cases; some carriers remain unaffected. Relative risks (RR), hazard ratios (HR), and odds ratios (OR) associated with various factors highlight the varied impact of lifestyle choices on AD risk. For instance, alcohol consumption is associated with an HR of 1.45, while cholesterol levels present a RR of 2.96. Conversely, findings related to general pesticide exposure (RR 4.35) and air pollution (RR 4.17) warrant caution due to limited studies and the necessity for further validation [75]. A multifactorial approach that integrates lifestyle, environmental, and genetic factors is essential to understanding individual susceptibility to AD. Gene-environment interactions, which describe how environmental exposures influence disease risk among individuals with different genotypes, remain underexplored in AD research. Given the multifaceted nature of the disease, identifying single genetic risk factors is challenging; most genetic findings, with the exception of APOE, exhibit modest effects. This underscores the need to consider additional risk factors that may interact with the APOE genotype, complicating the etiology of AD [76].

A longitudinal study indicated that increased physical activity correlates with a reduced risk of dementia and AD among older APOE4 carriers. Conversely, those APOE4 carriers with low physical activity exhibited a significantly elevated dementia risk compared to individuals with either factor alone. Additionally, the Honolulu-Asia Aging Study found that smoking significantly increases dementia risk (OR = 2.18) among non-smokers, independent of APOE genotype [77]. Emerging research also highlights a potential relationship between the APOE4 genotype and alcohol consumption. A cohort study indicated that low to moderate alcohol intake is linked to a lower risk of AD in individuals lacking the APOE4 allele, while APOE4 carriers do not benefit from the same protective effect. Similar findings from the Framingham Heart Study suggest that low to moderate alcohol consumption may accelerate cognitive decline in APOE4 carriers [77]. A cross-sectional study emphasized that individuals with the combined risk factors of smoking, alcohol consumption, and the APOE4 genotype experienced AD onset approximately 10 years earlier than those without any risk factors.Beyond lifestyle factors, exposure to environmental toxins such as pesticides (*e.g.*, DDT) and air pollution has been implicated in AD risk. Research indicates significantly elevated serum levels of DDE in AD patients, with cognitive impairments correlated with higher DDE levels. Notably, these associations are influenced by APOE genotype, indicating a genetic predisposition to the neurotoxic effects of environmental contaminants. Air pollution has also been scrutinized, with findings demonstrating an elevated risk for female APOE4 carriers [78]. Experimental models reveal that exposure to particulate matter (PM) increases Aβ oligomers, supporting the notion that environmental exposures can exacerbate AD pathology in genetically susceptible individuals. Despite a wealth of studies examining gene-environment interactions in AD, significant gaps remain regarding the influence of other genetic variants and modifiable risk factors. Existing literature on metal or solvent exposure presents mixed results, indicating a need for further research to elucidate the interplay between these environmental factors and genetic predispositions, especially in the context of aging [79]. Modifiable risk factors like PM exposure have been associated with pro-inflammatory mechanisms, yet their interaction with immunity-related genes remains largely unexplored, representing a promising avenue for future research. This is particularly relevant regarding candidate genes linked to microglial dysfunction, such as TREM2 variants, and their relationship with environmental exposures. Given AD's multifactorial nature, individuals often present with multiple risk factors that collectively predispose them to the disease [80]. Employing a gene-environment interaction approach can reveal associations with AD that may remain hidden when examining individual factors in isolation. The current landscape of AD therapeutics includes 26 drugs in Phase III clinical trials, with 17 designated as disease-modifying treatments (DMTs) [81]. Most of these agents aim to reduce amyloid burden, incorporating immunotherapies, BACE1 inhibitors, and anti-aggregation strategies, while only a minority target tau pathology. The high attrition rate of clinical trials, illustrated by the withdrawal of numerous compounds, highlights the pressing need to explore alternative therapeutic strategies or combinations of DMTs [82]. A significant contributor to the disappointing outcomes of these trials may be the advanced stage of disease at enrolment. Despite promising advances, lifestyle and environmental factors remain largely unaccounted for in emerging models of AD risk assessment. A proposed personalized therapy approach emphasizes identifying multifactorial risk profiles that contribute to individual susceptibility to AD [75]. This model necessitates a comprehensive patient history encompassing demographic data, genetic variants, family histories, and a detailed assessment of modifiable risk factors and environmental exposures. Such an integrative approach could facilitate biomarker analyses, allowing for monitoring of at-risk individuals before clinical symptom onset and enabling earlier therapeutic interventions [83]. For instance, individuals with prior pesticide exposure and the APOE4 gene variant may be more vulnerable to cognitive disruptions caused by pesticide exposure. Thorough assessments of environmental exposure histories and serum measurements for pesticides would provide critical insights into individual risk profiles. It is crucial to acknowledge the challenges inherent in capturing self-reported exposures for newer pesticides, which may require real-time monitoring to ascertain recent contact. As individuals are tracked for amyloid accumulation *via* neuroimaging or biomarker analyses, targeted therapeutic strategies aimed at reducing amyloid levels, such as β-secretase inhibitors or immunotherapies, could be prioritized [77].

SMALL MOLECULES TARGETING AMYLOID BETA

Inhibitors of Amyloid Beta Production

One kind of protein that can undergo structural change and assemble into fibrils with a cross-hatched shape is called an amyloid. Amyloid β plaques are the most common pathogenic characteristic of AD, which makes the disease so unique. The hydrophobic transmembrane section of the amyloid precursor protein (APP) is broken down in the presence of β and γ secretases, resulting in the production of Aβ peptides. They are produced in a variety of isoforms; in particular, the two Aβ40 and Aβ42 isoforms are the main components of the amyloid plaques that are discovered in the brains of AD patients [84]. The hallmark of Alzheimer's disease is the aberrant build-up of the Aβ protein in certain brain areas, which is crucial for memory and cognition. Aβ is a naturally occurring byproduct of the metabolism of cells, originating from the amyloid precursor protein (APP). After being produced in the endoplasmic reticulum (ER), APP is sent to the Golgi complex to finish maturation before being transferred to the plasma membrane [85]. Previous associative studies suggest that amyloid β is a viable target for the development of treatments aimed at decreasing the progression of AD illness. Interestingly, it has been demonstrated that phenserine, a cholinesterase inhibitor presently undergoing clinical trials, inhibits the formation of both amyloid precursor protein (APP) and amyloid β. It has also been demonstrated that phenserine can reduce amyloid β levels *in vivo.* After screening several phenserine analogues in human SH-SY-5Y neuroblastoma cells, eight lipophilic analogues were found to inhibit intracellular and extracellular APP levels as well as amyloid β production in human SK-N-SH cell culture media at concentrations that were basically free of AChE activity [86]. Researchers have treated Phenserine analogues in C57Blk adult male mice, and after 21 days of consecutive treatment, they observed that both doses (2.5 and 7.5 mg/kg i.p. once daily) markedly decreased the brain APP (36% and 38%) and Amyloid β levels by 38% and 30%, respectively [86]. Furthermore, an extract from the Withaniasomnifera plant called Withaferin A (WA) dramatically reduces the synthesis of Aβ. Researchers have treated SH-APP cells with WA, and it was observed that WA significantly reduced Aβ production [87].

BACE1 was discovered to be an enzyme necessary for the synthesis of Aβ [88]. One important strategy for stopping the amyloid cascade is to block BACE1 activity, and the creation of potent BACE1 inhibitors has drawn the attention of numerous clinical trials. The first BACE inhibitor to enter Phase 2 clinical trials was LY2886721 [89]. Eli Lilly declared that Phase 1 tests using LY2886721 showed an expected reduction in amyloid β formation [90]. In addition to LY2886721, numerous other candidates - such as atabecestat (Phase 2/3) [91], elenbecestat (Phase 3) [92], lanabecestat (Phase 2/3) [93], and umibecestat (Phase 2/3) [94] have progressed to the final stages of clinical studies. The overview of amyloid oligomer small molecule inhibitors for Alzheimer's disease treatment has been displayed in Table **1**.

Table 1. An overview of amyloid oligomer small molecule inhibitors used to treat Alzheimer's disease.

Compound Name	Mechanism of Action	Species	Outcome	Refs.
2-Amino-4-chlorophenol	Prevents Aβ oligomerization and fibrillization.	18-day-old rat embryos hippocampi	Approximately 50% inhibition of Aβ oligomer formation.	[95]
4-Aminophenol	Prevents Aβ oligomerization and fibrillization.	18-day-old rat embryos hippocampi	Inhibits 50 to 65% Aβ oligomer formation.	[95]
4-Aminoanisole	Prevents Aβ oligomerization and fibrillization.	18-day-old rat embryos hippocampi	Approximately 50% inhibition of Aβ oligomer formation.	[95]
3,4-Dihydroxybenzoic acid	Prevents Aβ oligomerization and fibrillization.	18-day-old rat embryos hippocampi	Inhibits 50 to 65% Aβ oligomer formation.	[95]
2-Hydroxy-3-ethoxy benzoaldehyde	Prevents Aβ oligomerization and fibrillization	18-day-old rat embryos hippocampi	Inhibits 50 to 65% Aβ oligomer formation.	[95]
Furosemide	Blocks Aβ oligomerization.	Adult female Tg2576 mice	Two-fold elimination of total guanidine extractable $A\beta 1-40$ peptide and $A\beta 1-42$ peptide in the cerebral cortex and hippocampal formation.	[96]

(Table 1) cont.....

Compound Name	Mechanism of Action	Species	Outcome	Refs.
D737	Prevents Aβ production	*Drosophila melanogaster*	Minimizes the cytotoxicity of $Aβ_{42}$, prevents $Aβ_{42}$ formation, and decreases the amount of ROS that builds up inside cells. The most noteworthy effect of D737 is a considerable increase in life span and motor abilities in a transgenic D. melanogaster model of AD.	[97]
Huperzine A	Inhibits the apoptosis caused by the amyloid beta-peptide fragment 25–35	Embryos of pregnant Sprague-Dawley rats	Safeguards neurons against amyloid $β_{25\text{-}35}$ stimulated apoptosis through the blocking of ROS production and caspase-3 activation in cortical neurons.	[98]
Berberine	Decreases extracellular Aβ synthesis and BACE activity without affecting LDH release.	3XTg-AD mice	Berberine reduced the level of BACE1 protein to prevent the generation of Aß and enhanced autophagic clearance of Aß by activating autophagy *via* the class III PI3K/beclin-1 pathway.	[99]
Tanshinone	Its anti-inflammatory and antioxidant properties make it an effective Aβ-peptide inhibitor, reducing AChE-positive fibers.	Adult male Sprague-Dawley rats	It helps with Alzheimer's disease (AD) by reducing the loss of spatial memory, enhancing the expression of inflammatory proteins, and assisting in the removal of senile plaques.	[100]
Idebenone	It blocks the production of Aβ and β-secretase.	Hippocampi of embryonic Sprague-Dawley rats.	Idebenone significantly impacted the rise in LDH release and decrease in neuronal cell count produced by $Aβ_{1\text{-}40}$.	[101]

(Table 1) cont.....

Compound Name	Mechanism of Action	Species	Outcome	Refs.
Acitretin	Encourages α-secretase (ADAM10) expression to reduce Aβ levels and enhanceAPP's nonamyloidogenic processing.	5xFAD Mice	Treatment with Acitretin markedly alleviated behavioural deficits.	[102]

Amyloid Beta Aggregation Inhibitors

Aβ42 agglomerates are a particularly appealing target for inhibitor design because genetic, physiological, and biochemical research indicates a significant correlation between Aβ42 agglomerates and the aetiology of AD [103]. Epigallocatechin gallate (EGCG), a naturally occurring, polyphenolic component obtained in the extract of green tea, has been demonstrated to prevent Aβ aggregation [104]. Myricetin, curcumin, nordihydroguaiaretic acid (NDGA), rosmarinic acid (RA), and ferulic acid (FA) are organic substances that might also have the ability to prevent Aβ40 and Aβ42 aggregation [105]. The synthetic molecule tweezers CLR01 demonstrated responsiveness against amyloid aggregation through the prevention of oligomerization and fibrillization [106].

Turmeric is a rhizomatous plant that thrives throughout Southeast Asia. It is rich in curcumin, also known as (1E,6E)-1,7-bis(4-hydroxy-3-methoxypheny-)-1,6-heptadiene-3,5-dione. It' is a key ingredient in Indian curries [107]. It has been demonstrated that this molecule prevents Aβ aggregation [108].

The primary phenolic component of olive oil, oleeuropein, has been shown to have a number of positive health impacts on humans, the most notable of which are its anti-tumor, anti-inflammatory, and antioxidative properties in addition to its capacity to stop the development of harmful amyloid aggregates (Table **2**). It has been demonstrated that this substance and its aglycone derivative have anti-amyloidogenic properties on Aβ [109].

Table 2. Amyloid β aggregation inhibitors in clinical trials.

Compound Name	Mechanism of Action	Clinical Trial Phase	Clinical Trial Number	Status	Refs.
ALZT-OP1	Inhibits Aβ aggregation and Neuroinflammation.	Phase III	NCT02547818	Ongoing	[110]

(Table 2) cont.....

Compound Name	Mechanism of Action	Clinical Trial Phase	Clinical Trial Number	Status	Refs.
GV-971	Reduces the toxicity of the Aβ peptide.	Phase III	NCT01453569	Completed on October 25, 2018, as a safe, well-tolerated oral medication.	[112]
KHK6640	Inhibits Aβ aggregation	Phase III	NCT02127476	Ongoing	[112]
ELND005	Inhibits Aβ aggregation	Phase II	NCT00568776	Owing to the limited sample sizes, there is not enough data from this Class II trial to confirm or deny ELND005's benefits.	[113]
Posiphen	Reduces Aβ aggregation	Phase II	NCT01072812	Ongoing	[114]
AZD-3293	Inhibits Aβ aggregation	Phase III	NCT02245737 NCT02783573	Two Phase III studies are ongoing	[115]
ALZ-801	Inhibits Aβ aggregation	Phase III	NCT06304883	Ongoing	[116]
Tramiprosate	Inhibits Aβ aggregation	Phase II	-	Failed due to lack of efficacy	[117]
Contraloid	Stabilizes Aβ42 monomers to inhibit its aggregation.	Phase I	NCT06182085	Ongoing	[118]

Clearance Enhancers of Amyloid

In order to eliminate amyloid-β, the brain uses a variety of enzymatic and non-enzymatic processes [119, 120]. Scientists have discovered around 20 amyloid---degrading proteases (AβDPs) in the brain, which cleave and transform amyloid-β proteins into less harmful, shorter forms, including zinc metalloendopeptidase, thiol-dependent metalloendopeptidase, serine/cysteine proteases, and matrix metalloproteinases [121].

Neprilysin (NEP) is a glycoprotein found in plasma membranes, which is a member of the neutral zinc metalloendopeptidase family. Amyloid-β in the brain and periphery may be cleaved into monomeric and oligomeric forms by NEP, a key Aβ-degrading protease [122]. Additionally, NEP and the breakdown or clearance of amyloid-β in AD have been linked in recent research [123]. Combined with the most recent research, it is clear that NEP plays a critical role in the clearance of amyloid-β. A decline in NEP activity is associated with the neurodegenerative disorders, contributing to increased levels of amyloid-β in the brain [123].

Angiotensin-converting enzyme (ACE) is a zinc metalloprotease that is widely distributed throughout the body, including cerebral vasculature and pyramidal neurons of the human brain [124]. Numerous investigations in genetics, biochemistry, and cellular biology revealed that ACE is crucial in controlling amyloid-β metabolism [125]. Studies conducted *in vitro* have shown that ACE can split amyloid-β between Asp7 and Ser8, which inhibits the cytotoxicity, fibril formation, aggregation, and deposition of amyloid-β [126]. Recognizing the contentious function of ACE in clearing amyloid-β in the brain is essential in light of the contradictions that exist now and the conclusions of recent studies [123]. It is highly advised to support more studies in order to resolve these differences and have a better knowledge of the precise role that ACE plays in clearing amyloid-β. These discoveries may be helpful in reducing the brain's development of amyloid-β, which is a hallmark of diseases like Alzheimer's disease [127].

The highly conserved thiol metalloprotease insulin-degrading enzyme (IDE), which is an essential step in the amyloid-β clearance process, is currently one of the enzymes for removing amyloid-β from the brain [128]. Insulin-degrading enzyme (IDE), sometimes referred to as insulinase or insulysin, is a neutral thiol metalloprotease that is present in the brain, testes, skeletal muscle, skin, and tongue [129]. For example, the catalytic function of IDE mutants (cf-E111Q-IDE, a cysteine-free mutant) in amyloid-β proteolysis/degradation was the topic of a recent study, which found that this mutant is very efficient in degrading amyloid-β peptides [130].

It has been documented that certain matrix metalloproteinases (MMPs), such as MMP2 and MMP9, are utilized in the breakdown of amyloid-β in both its monomeric and fibrillar forms [131]. Interestingly, one of the proteases found to be in control of activating MMPs *via* this mechanism is the extracellular matrix metalloproteinase inducer (EMMPRIN; CD147) [132]. There is a substantial correlation between MMPs and AD, according to recent studies [133]. MMP7 has the ability to break down amyloid-β, prevent it from aggregating, and reverse the pathology caused by amyloid-β [134]. Furthermore, a current *in-vitro* study has shown that reducing the MMP9 release from astrocytes decreases the amyloid-β's proteolytic clearance and destruction [135]. MMP activation and upregulation are important processes in the metabolism of amyloid-β. Interestingly, blocking MMPs raises amyloid-β levels, highlighting their importance in the reduction of amyloid-β. As a result, targeting MMPs becomes a viable treatment strategy for conditions where amyloid-β accumulation occurs, namely AD [123].

Serine proteinases are the most prevalent and substantial class of mammalian proteinases, because they have a serine residue in their active sites that is necessary for catalysis. Myelin basic protein (MBP), plasmin, and acyl-peptide hydrolase are well-known members of this proteinase class. As a special kind of chaperone, myelin basic proteins (MBP) effectively degrade amyloid-β peptides and inhibit the formation of amyloid-β fibrillogenesis. Despite these convincing results, little is currently known about MBP's function in the brain's removal of amyloid-β. Therefore, we highly recommend further research endeavours focused on elucidating the exact processes behind MBP-mediated clearance of amyloid-β and devising tactics to augment this mechanism [136]. Among these proteases, only plasmin has been demonstrated to destroy amyloid-β. Amyloid-β is broken down and cleaved at several locations by plasmin, which stops it from aggregating into β-pleated sheets. Additionally, plasmin has the ability to break down both non-aggregate and aggregated amyloid-β. Furthermore, a noteworthy association has been revealed within the proteolytic activity of plasmin and the levels of amyloid-β, suggesting that the proteolytic activity of plasmin encouraged the amyloid-β destruction or clearance, which may be a feasible treatment approach to reduce amyloid-β levels in the brain [137]. Previous research has demonstrated the participation of acylpeptidehydrolase (APH) in the amyloid-β degradation process in SKNMC-neuroblastoma cells, highlighting the significance of this enzyme in this process. Additionally, research conducted *in vitro* showed that APH selectively breaks down amyloid-β in its monomeric and oligomeric forms [138].

Cathepsin B, a well-known member of the cysteine protease family, functions as both an endopeptidase and an exopeptidase, found in lysosomes, and plays a crucial role in protein degradation [139]. In the mouse brain, cathepsin B plays a role in the amyloid-βdegradation. Furthermore, the elimination of oligomeric amyloid-β peptide in microglia depends on lysosomal cathepsin B, and its increased expression promotes the breakdown of amyloid-β in monocytes [140]. Most mammalian cells have the aspartyl protease cathepsin D, which breaks down internalized and endocytosed proteins, such as amyloid-β peptide [141]. Researchers have discovered that in mice lacking the cathepsin D gene, there is a notable build-up of amyloid-β within lysosomes. This suggests that extracellular amyloid-β is transported to lysosomes and that lysosomal AβDPs, such as cathepsin B and D, are necessary for its destruction [142, 143].

SMALL MOLECULES TARGETING TAU PROTEINS

Tau protein, primarily located in neurons of the central nervous system, is a microtubule-associated protein. Its main function is to stabilize microtubules, which are crucial for the neuronal cytoskeleton, offering structural support and aiding in intracellular transport. By binding to microtubules, tau promotes their assembly, ensuring the proper functioning of axonal transport systems vital for neuronal health [144, 145].

In a healthy brain, tau protein undergoes normal phosphorylation, which helps regulate its attachment to microtubules. However, in pathological conditions such as AD, unusual hyperphosphorylation of tau has been seen. This hyperphosphorylated tau removes from the microtubules and assembles into paired helical filaments (PHFs) and neurofibrillary tangles (NFTs), which are hallmark features of AD pathology [146 - 149].

One effective treatment approach for tau-related neurodegenerative illnesses is targeting the tau protein [150]. Among many techniques, the use of small compounds has attracted substantial attention due to their capacity to influence tau pathology at multiple phases, such as blocking tau aggregation, boosting its clearance, and modifying post-translational changes. Because small molecules may easily pass the blood-brain barrier and reach neuronal targets due to their generally low molecular weight, they are favorable [151 - 153].

TAU AGGREGATION INHIBITORS

Tau aggregation is essential to the development of tauopathies, including AD, which is typified by the production of oligomers, fibrils, and eventually neurofibrillary tangles (NFTs) [144, 154]. In these conditions, tau proteins, normally responsible for stabilizing microtubules in neurons, become hyperphosphorylated and dissociate from microtubules, leading to cytoskeletal instability. Once released into the cytoplasm, tau proteins aggregate abnormally, forming toxic oligomers and fibrils that contribute to neurodegeneration [155, 156]. The pathological aggregation of tau is neurotoxic and has been closely linked to the disruption of neuronal function. NFTs, a hallmark of AD and other tauopathies, accumulate within neurons, causing synaptic dysfunction, neuronal death, and ultimately cognitive decline [157]. As tau aggregation is central to the development of these disorders, strategies that inhibit this process have become an important focus in therapeutic research [158].

Targeting tau aggregation with small molecule inhibitors offers a promising approach to treating tauopathies. These inhibitors work by preventing tau monomers from oligomerizing into toxic aggregates, promoting the disassembly of existing aggregates, or enhancing the clearance of pathological tau from neurons [159].By halting or reversing tau aggregation, these treatments aim to slow or prevent the progression of neurodegenerative diseases like AD [160, 161].

Tau aggregation, defined by the development of oligomers, fibrils, and eventually NFTs, has a significant part in the evolution of tauopathies [162, 163]. A dissociative phenotype of hyperphosphorylated tau proteins from microtubules results in an unstable cytoskeleton. Upon liberation within the cytoplasm, tau often forms oligomers and fibrils. Tau aggregates in a pathological way that is neurotoxic and causes neurodegeneration. In recent years, one important treatment approach that has gained traction is the suppression of tau aggregation (Table **3**) [164, 165].

Table 3. Examples of tau aggregation inhibitors.

Compound Name	Structure	Mechanism of Action	Preclinical Data (Species Used)	Clinical Data (Phase, Outcome)	Refs.
Leuco-Methylthioninium (LMTX)	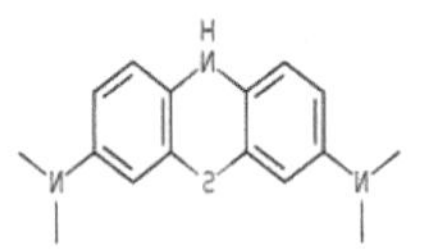	Inhibits tau aggregation and disassembles existing tau aggregates.	Mouse models (transgenic mice expressing human tau).	Phase 3 (negative outcome, no cognitive improvement in Alzheimer's disease patients).	[166, 167]
Methylene Blue	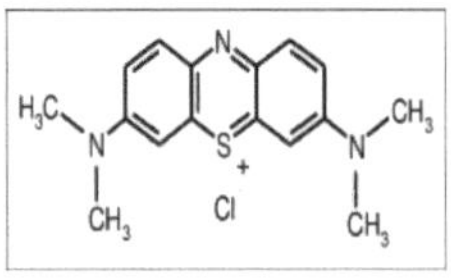	Inhibits tau aggregation and reduces tau hyperphosphorylation.	Mouse models (PS19 tauopathy mouse).	Phase 2: moderate cognitive improvement in AD patients.	[167]
Anle138b	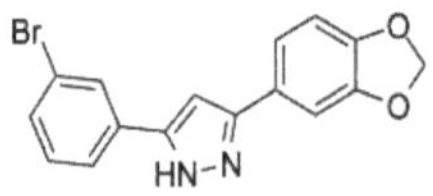	Binds to pathological tau aggregates, preventing aggregation	PS19 tauopathy mice, reduction of tau inclusions, and cognitive improvement.	Preclinical, no clinical trials yet	[168]
Epothilone D	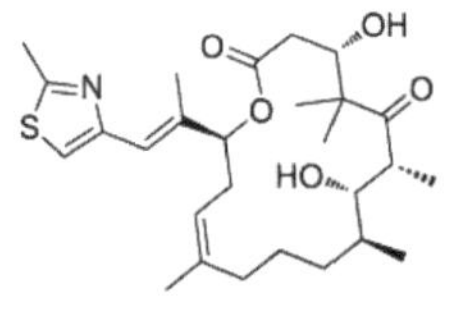	Stabilizes microtubules, prevents tau detachment and aggregation.	Tau transgenic mice, improvement in memory and reduction in tau pathology.	Phase 1: completed, potential cognitive improvement noted.	[169]
Salsalate	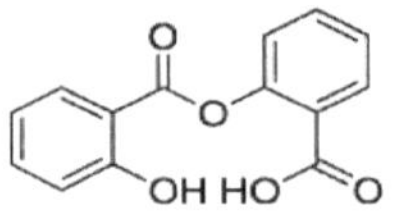	Inhibits tau acetylation, reducing tau aggregation.	3xTg-AD and rTg4510 mouse models, reduction in tau acetylation and tau pathology.	Preclinical only, no human trials yet.	[169]

(Table 3) cont.....

Compound Name	Structure	Mechanism of Action	Preclinical Data (Species Used)	Clinical Data (Phase, Outcome)	Refs.
TRx0237 (Hydromethylthionine)	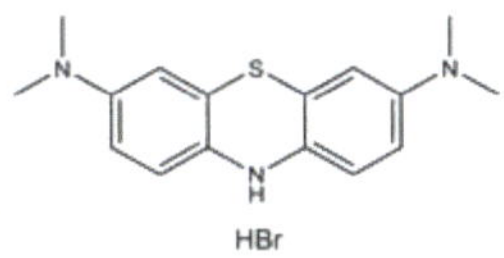	Tau aggregation inhibitor, potential microtubule stabilization.	Transgenic tauopathy mouse models, reduction in tau pathology.	Phase 3 (no cognitive improvement in Alzheimer's).	[166]
P301S Tau Antibody (C2N-8E12)	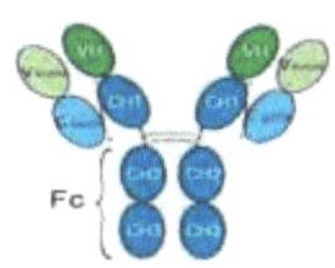	Monoclonal antibody targeting tau aggregates clears pathological tau.	P301S tauopathy mice, reduction of pathological tau.	Phase 1 (safe, well-tolerated, further studies ongoing).	[166]

Tau Aggregation Inhibitors in Clinical Trials

Several tau aggregation inhibitors are currently being evaluated in clinical trials (Table **4**). These drugs aim to reduce tau burden and slow the progression of tau-related diseases like AD, progressive supranuclear palsy (PSP), and other tauopathies.

Table 4. Examples of Tau inhibitors in clinical trials.

Drug Name	Mechanism of Action	Phase	Clinical Trial Date	Refs.
Epi-589 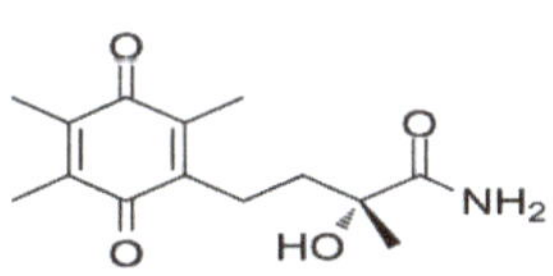	A redox modulator that targets mitochondrial dysfunction and reduces tau aggregation.	Phase 2	2021	[170]
Zagotenemab (LY3303560) 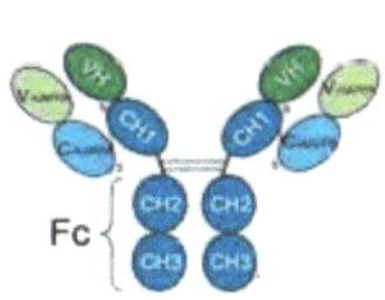	An anti-tau antibody that targets extracellular tau to prevent its proliferation and aggregation.	Phase 2	2019	[171]
BIIB080 (IONIS-MAPTRx)	An antisense oligonucleotide that reduces tau protein production by targeting tau mRNA.	Phase 1/2	2022	[172]
AADvac1	A tau vaccine that induces an immune response against pathological tau, inhibiting its aggregation.	Phase 2	2020	[173]

(Table 4) cont.....

Drug Name	Mechanism of Action	Phase	Clinical Trial Date	Refs.
MK-8719	A small molecule O-GlcNAcase inhibitor that modulates tau phosphorylation and aggregation.	Phase 1	2021	[174]

Tau Phosphorylation Modulators

Hyperphosphorylation of tau proteins is a critical step in the pathogenesis of tauopathies. Modulating tau phosphorylation is a potential therapeutic approach to prevent tau aggregation and neurodegeneration [154, 175, 176]

Therapeutic substances known as tau phosphorylation modulators work to either prevent or return tau to its normal hyperphosphorylated state (Table **5**) [177]. These modulators work by precisely targeting protein kinases and phosphatases, which are enzymes that control tau phosphorylation. Tau requires a balance between the activities of protein kinases and phosphatases to remove and add phosphate groups, respectively, for normal function [178, 179].

Table 5. Examples of tau phosphorylation modulators.

Modulator	Mechanism of Action	Target	Clinical Status	Refs.
Tideglusib 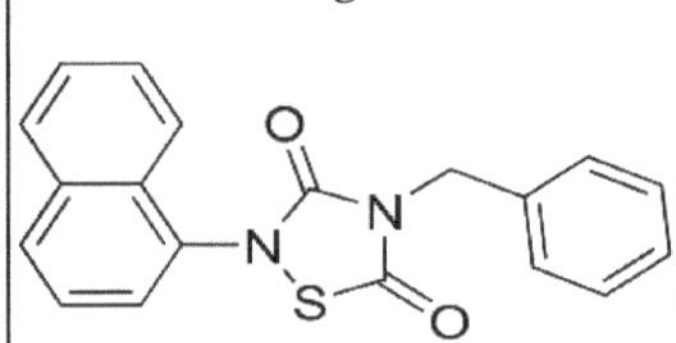	GSK-3β inhibitor that reduces tau phosphorylation and aggregation.	GSK-3β	Phase 2 (AD, PSP)	[180]
Lithium	Inhibits GSK-3β, reducing tau hyperphosphorylation.	GSK-3β	Approved (Bipolar), studied in AD	[181]
Roscovitine 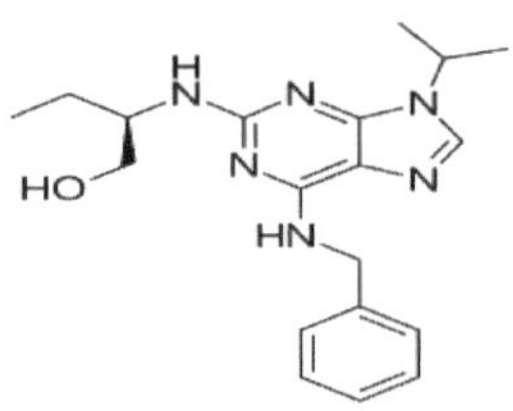	CDK5 inhibitor that prevents tau hyperphosphorylation.	CDK5	Preclinical	[182]

(Table 5) cont.....

Modulator	Mechanism of Action	Target	Clinical Status	Refs.
Sodium selenate 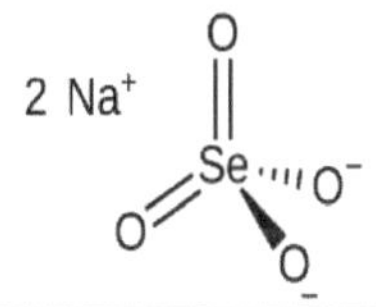	Activates PP2A, promoting tau dephosphorylation.	PP2A	Phase 2 (AD, PSP)	[183]
AUY922 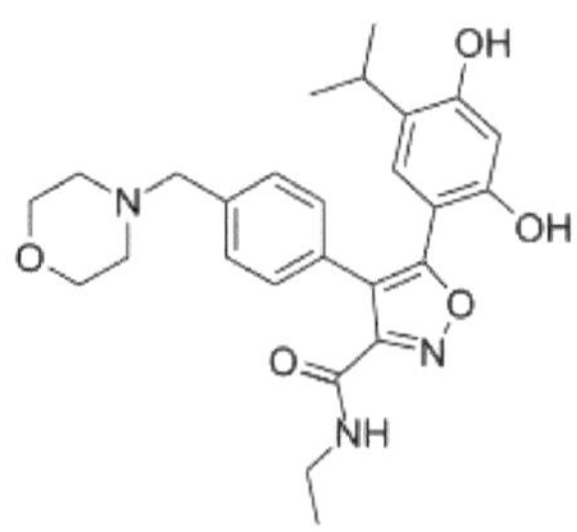	HSP90 inhibitor that reduces tau phosphorylation indirectly.	HSP90	Preclinical	[184]
17-AAG (Tanespimycin) 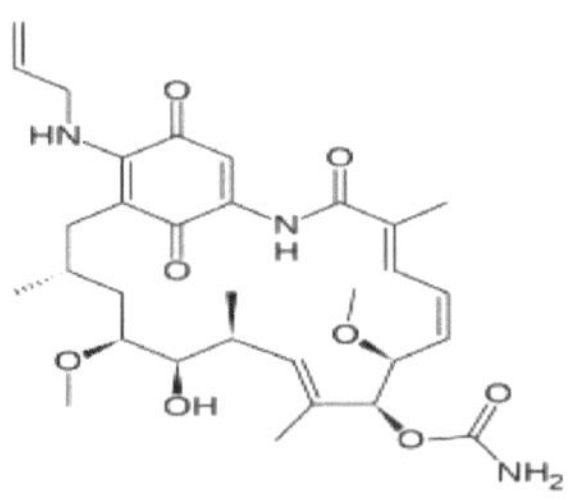	Inhibits HSP90, enhancing tau degradation and reducing hyperphosphorylation.	HSP90	Phase 2 (Cancer), Preclinical in AD	[185]

MICROTUBULE STABILIZER

Microtubules are essential elements of the cytoskeleton, providing structural support and enabling intracellular transportation [186]. These structures are extremely dynamic, constantly assembling and disassembling as a result of tubulin subunit polymerization and depolymerization. Tau proteins play a vital role in stabilizing microtubules by binding to them and promoting their polymerization. However, in tauopathies such as AD, tau proteins become hyperphosphorylated and dissociate from microtubules, leading to their destabilization and contributing to neuronal dysfunction and degeneration [169, 187].

Microtubule stabilizers are compounds that enhance microtubule polymerization or prevent their disassembly, thus preserving microtubule integrity. These stabilizers can help mitigate the detrimental effects of tau dysfunction in tauopathies by compensating for the loss of tau-mediated stabilization. By maintaining the structural integrity of microtubules, these agents can potentially protect neurons from degeneration and promote cellular health [188].

These agents act by directly interacting with tubulin or indirectly modulating the stability of microtubules, thereby reducing the toxic effects of tau hyperphosphorylation and aggregation. Several microtubule stabilizers are being explored as therapeutic agents for neurodegenerative diseases, especially AD and other tauopathies [189]. Microtubule stabilizers play a crucial role in cellular stability by binding to microtubules and preventing their depolymerization. Paclitaxel, commonly known as Taxol, binds to microtubules, stabilizing them to prevent depolymerization [190]. Similarly, Epothilone D enhances microtubule polymerization, compensating for tau dysfunction, crucial in neurodegenerative disease contexts [191]. TPI-287, a taxane derivative with brain penetrance, works by stabilizing microtubules, preventing their disassembly [192]. Dictyostatin also binds directly to microtubules, enhancing their stability and polymerization [193]. Finally, Noscapine, while binding to tubulin, reduces microtubule depolymerization, adding to the stability essential for cellular functions [194].

MODULATING NEUROINFLAMMATION AND OXIDATIVE STRESS WITH SMALL MOLECULES

Modulating neuroinflammation and oxidative stress with antioxidant small molecules is a promising strategy for developing anti-Alzheimer's therapies. Neuroinflammation is a characteristic of AD, distinguished by the activation of microglia and astrocytes, which produce reactive oxygen species (ROS) and pro-inflammatory cytokines. This inflammatory response can accelerate the development of AD and worsen neuronal damage. Oxidative stress occurs when there is an imbalance between the production of ROS and the brain's ability to detoxify these reactive intermediates. This leads to the damage of cellular components, including lipids, proteins, and DNA, which further contributes to neuronal dysfunction and eventually death [195].

Antioxidant Small Molecules

Antioxidant medications decrease the pathophysiology of dementia in AD patients and lessen the harm that free radicals inflict on neuronal cells through hazardous chain reactions. In 1997, a study reported that α-tocopherol therapy, administered at a daily dose of 2000 IU, reduced neuronal death and alleviated the severity of AD in patients with moderate-to-severe disabilities (Table **6**), suggesting a clinical delay in AD-induced deterioration of neuronal function. According to a 2004 study, α-tocopherol reduced the generation of Aβ and senile plaque in animal models and inhibited brain lipid peroxidation when administered before AD. It has been found that patients who take vitamin E supplements live longer than non-users. β-carotene and vitamins C and E work together to prevent lipid peroxidation. Curcumin, a natural compound found in turmeric, has potent anti-inflammatory and antioxidant properties. It inhibits microglia and astrocytesactivation, reducing the generation of ROS and pro-inflammatory cytokines [196]. Resveratrol, present in grapes and red wine, activates antioxidant pathways and reduces oxidative stress. It also has anti-inflammatory effects by modulating signaling pathways involved in neuroinflammation [197]. Nrf2 activators, compounds like sulforaphane (found in cruciferous vegetables) activate the Nrf2 pathway, enhancing the functionality of antioxidant enzymes. This helps in reducing oxidative stress and protecting neurons [198]. The anti-inflammatory antibiotic minocycline decreases the synthesis of pro-inflammatory cytokines and prevents microglial activation. It has shown potential in reducing neuroinflammation in various neurodegenerative diseases [199]. Pyrroloquinoline Quinone (PQQ) has strong antioxidant properties and can protect neurons from oxidative damage. It also promotes mitochondrial biogenesis, which is crucial for maintaining neuronal health [200]. Cinnamic acid derivatives, such as ferulic acid (FA), have been shown to avoid chain-breaking in the oxidation of low-density lipoproteins, related to their hydrogen or electron-donating capacity and the formation of phenoxyl radicals. The direct reducing action of disulfide bonds and its role as a precursor to the powerful antioxidant glutathione account for N-acetylcysteine's (NAC) antioxidant activity. Therefore, after months of ad libitum consumption, rats treated with NAC showed a decrease in the oral intake of ethanol and nicotine, which is consistent with the successful normalization of oxidative stress and inflammation in the rat brain caused by exposure to drugs of abuse like ethanol, nicotine, and methamphetamine [201].

Table 6. Examples of small molecule antioxidants and neurotransmitter modulators used in the treatment of Alzheimer's disease.

Class of Drug	Name of Drug	Mechanism	Preclinical/Clinical	Refs.
Anti-oxidant	Curcumin 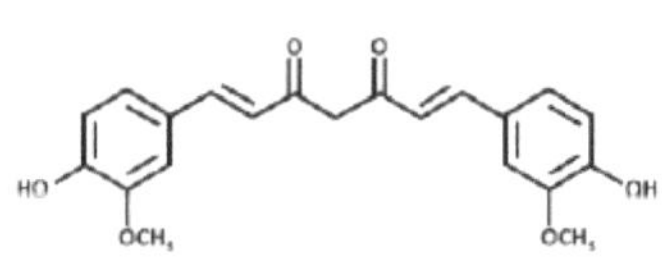	It prevents the activation of microglia and astrocytes, lowers the production of ROS and pro-inflammatory cytokines.	Phase-II	[220]
Anti-oxidant	Resveratrol 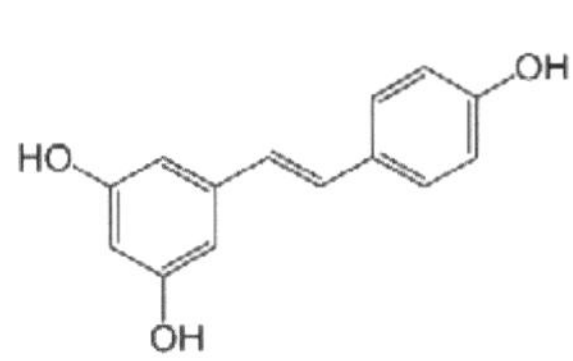	It shows anti-inflammatory effects by modulating signaling pathways involved in neuroinflammation.	Phase-II	[221]

(Table 6) cont.....

Class of Drug	Name of Drug	Mechanism	Preclinical/Clinical	Refs.
Anti-oxidant (Nrf2 Activators)	Sulforaphane 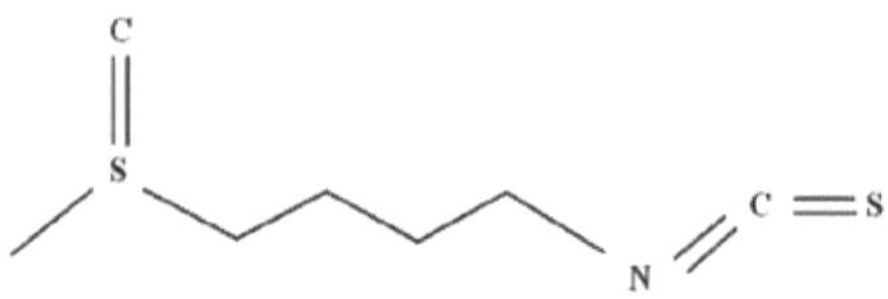	It activates the Nrf2 pathway, enhancing the expression of antioxidant enzymes. This helps in reducing oxidative stress and protecting neurons.	Phase-II	[222]
Anti-oxidant	Minocycline 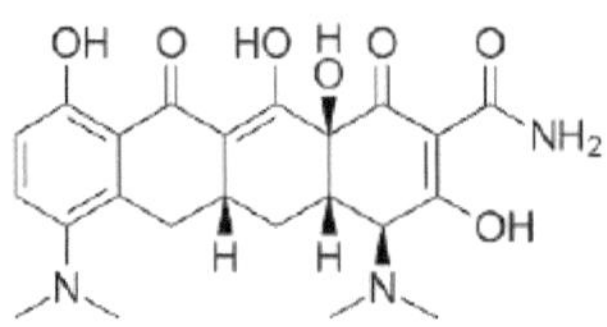	It decreases the microglial activation and prevents pro-inflammatory cytokine production. It has shown potential in reducing neuroinflammation in various neurodegenerative diseases.	Phase-II	[199]
Anti-oxidant	Pyrroloquinoline Quinone 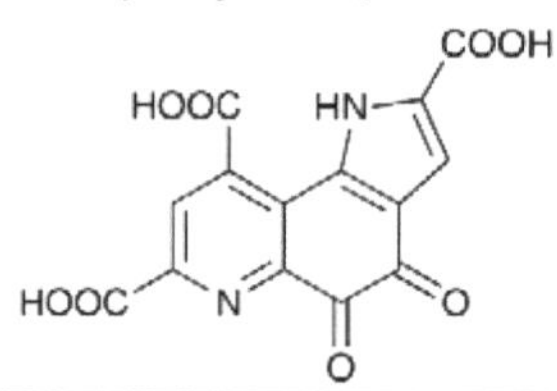	It can protect neurons from oxidative damage and also promotes mitochondrial biogenesis, which is crucial for maintaining neuronal health.	Preclinical trial	[199]
Anti-oxidant (Cinnamic acid derivatives)	Ferulic acid 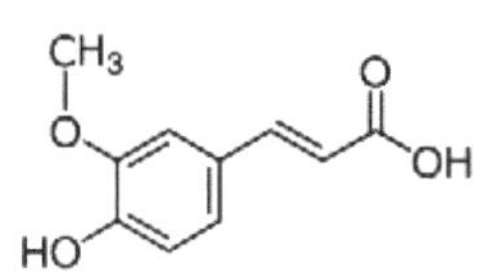	It prevents chain-breaking in low-density lipoprotein, which is associated with the stability of the phenoxyl radicals that are enabled to donate hydrogen or electrons.	Preclinical trial	[201]
Anti-oxidant	N-Acetylcysteine (NAC) 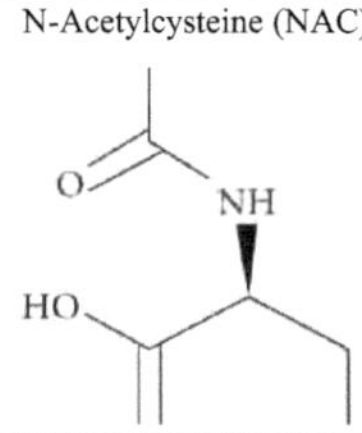	It directly reduces the effects of disulfide bonds and acts as a precursor of glutathione, a powerful antioxidant.	Preclinical trial	[201]
Noradrenaline reuptake inhibitor	DDP-225 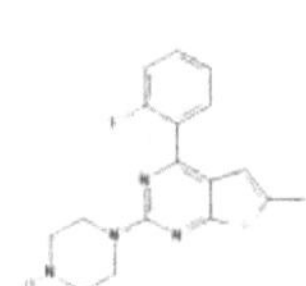	It works by blocking the reuptake of 5-HT3 and noradrenaline.	Phase-II	[202]

(Table 6) cont.....

Class of Drug	Name of Drug	Mechanism	Preclinical/Clinical	Refs.
Cholinesterase inhibitor	Tacrine 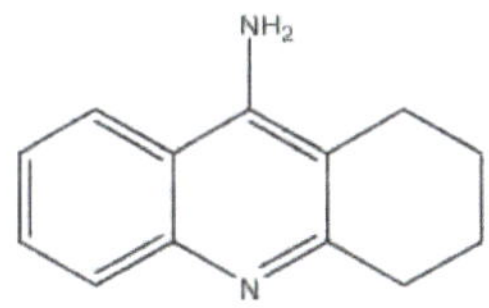	It inhibits MAO activity by inhibition of 5-hydroxytryptamine activation and dopamine neuronal uptake, blocks certain potassium ion channels, and interacts with muscarinic ACh receptors.	Phase-IV	[208]
Cholinesterase inhibitor	Donepezil 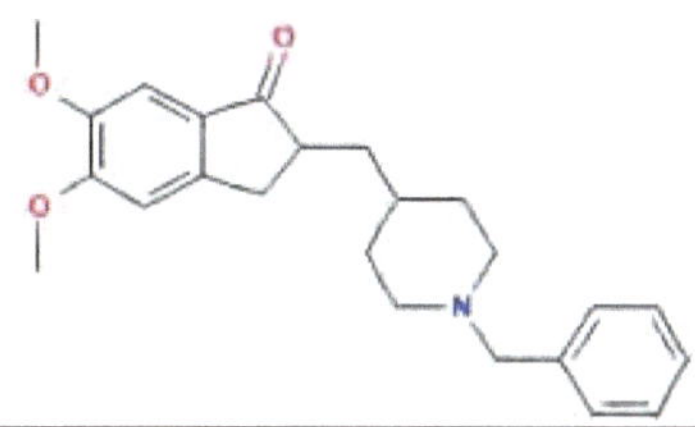	It selectively and reversibly inhibits the enzyme acetylcholinesterase and increases acetylcholine levels.	Phase-III	[223]
Cholinesterase inhibitor	Rivastigmine 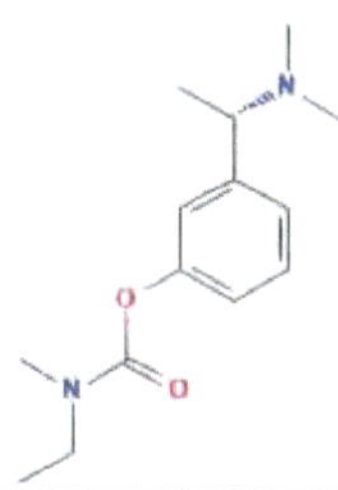	It is a pseudo-irreversible carbamate-type of AChE and BuChE inhibitor, being selective for the CNS compared to peripheral tissues.	Phase-III	[214-216]
Cholinesterase inhibitor	Galantamine 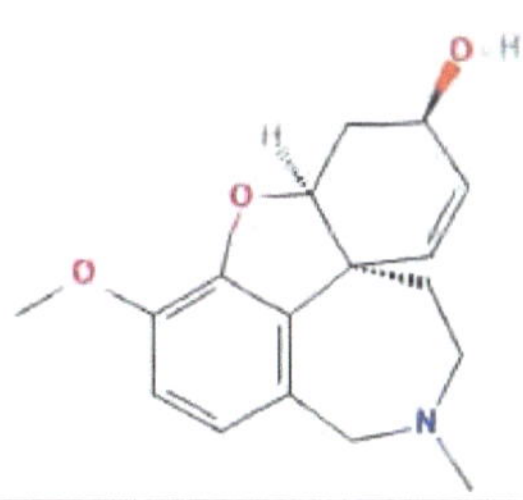	It interacts with the anionic subsite and the aromatic gorge to inhibit AChE in a reversible, competitive, and selective manner. Its activity in inhibiting BuChE is minimal.	Phase-III	[218]

Modulators of Neurotransmitter Systems

The physiology of the gastrointestinal tract (GIT) is regulated by the neurotransmitters serotonin (5-HT3) and noradrenaline (Table **6**). The combination of 5-HT3 antagonist and noradrenaline reuptake inhibition in a single oral medication offers a potential treatment strategy for irritable bowel syndrome (IBS) and other functional GIT disorders. Based on a thieno[2,3-d] pyrimidine backbone, DDP-225 was developed by Mitsubishi Tanabe Pharma in 2003 to treat IBS and GIT problems by preventing 5-HT3 and noradrenalin from being reabsorbed. Preclinical and clinical data pertaining to DDP225, an orally active substance being studied for the treatment of AD and depression, were licensed by Dynogen. The safety and efficacy of DDP-225, a fused thiophene derivative, in the treatment of AD are being evaluated in phase II clinical trials. Olmutinib, which blocks the epidermal growth factor receptor (EGFR), was marketed in South Korea to treat non-small cell lung cancer. In phase I clinical trials, SNS-314, a strong inhibitor of aurora kinases A, B, and C, is being investigated for the treatment of advanced solid cancers. The oral bioavailable drug GDC-0941, sometimes referred to as pictilisib, is a potent phosphatidylinositol 3-kinase (PI3K) inhibitor with acceptable ADME characteristics. Pransugrel, a P2Y12 platelet inhibitor, is used to treat patients with unstable angina, non-ST-elevation myocardial infarction (NSTEMI), and STEMI patients receiving primary or delayed percutaneous coronary intervention (PCI). Ticlopidine is a platelet aggregation inhibitor that is used to prevent thrombi-related conditions such as stroke and transient ischemic episodes (TIA). The clinical research is investigating the effectiveness of tinoridine in treating adult pain and inflammation. Ilorasertib has been investigated as a treatment target for myelodysplasia, solid neoplasms, advanced solid tumors, acute myelogenous leukemia, and advanced malignancies. CRS3123 is a new small chemical that effectively inhibits the methionyl-tRNA synthetase of Clostridium difficile, stopping the bacterium from generating toxins and spores. CRS3123 has been evaluated in a phase I placebo-controlled experiment using different ascending dosages [202]. Shaw and Bentley first described tacrine's pharmacological activities in 1946 [203]. It was initially applied in clinical settings to improve succinylcholine's muscle-relaxing effects and treat delirium brought on by anesthesia. Tacrine was initially believed to help counterbalance the respiratory depression brought on by morphine, but it was later discovered that it also functioned as an inhibitor of Butyryl cholinesterase (BChE) and AChE [204, 205]. Tacrine was the first medication approved in 1993 to treat Alzheimer's disease, but its use was restricted due to its hepatotoxicity [206]. Over time, further effects of tacrine have been identified, such as decreased monoamine oxidase activity, inhibition of dopamine neuronal uptake and 5-hydroxytryptamine receptor, blocking of certain potassium ion channels, and interaction with muscarinic ACh receptors [207 - 209]. As a first-line treatment for AD since 1996, donepezil is frequently prescribed for mild, moderate, and severe cases [210]. It is a mixed inhibitor that is reversible and shows both competitive and non-competitive AChE activity [211, 212]. Donepezil has the ability to concurrently block the AChE CAS and PAS sites [211]. In contrast to other substances like rivastigmine and tacrine, it has selective activity for AChE but only a slight effect on BuChE [213]. Apart from its inhibition of AChE, donepezil exhibits molecular and cellular actions in nearly every step of the pathophysiology of AD. However, negative side effects are possible when using it, and they are more noticeable at larger dosages (10 mg/d) than at lower dosages (5 mg/d). The symptoms may include rhinitis, nausea, vomiting, diarrhea, and loss of appetite. But the most common adverse effects are in the gastrointestinal tract [213]. In 2000, rivastigmine received approval for the treatment of mild to moderate AD. Being selective for the central nervous system (CNS) as opposed to peripheral tissues, it is a pseudo-irreversible carbamate-type inhibitor of AChE and BuChE [214 - 216]. Because it binds to AChE, which cleaves the rivastigmine molecule, it is categorized as a pseudo-irreversible inhibitor. The formation of a covalent carbamoyl-AChE complex inhibits acetylcholine catalysis and temporarily deactivates the enzyme [215]. After gastrointestinal adverse reactions, the transdermal patch was developed to provide a continuous and well-controlled dose of rivastigmine, decreasing variations in plasma levels and causing minimal side effects [213, 216]. The Amaryllidaceae family's galantamine is an alkaloid that was extracted from the Galanthus woronowii plant and is recommended for the treatment of mild to moderate AD [217, 218]. It interacts with the anionic subsite and the aromatic gorge to inhibit AChE in a reversible, competitive, and selective manner. Its activity in inhibiting BuChE is minimal [216, 218]. Galantamine has a minimal impact on peripheral tissues and is selective for the central nervous system. Moreover, it modulates nicotinic acetylcholine receptors (nAChRs) allosterically. Despite being just as effective in clinical settings as donepezil [219], compared to other AChE medications, galantamine appears to have higher adverse effects, particularly gastrointestinal complaints (Table 6) [213].

ANTI-INFLAMMATORY TARGETING SMALL MOLECULES

Numerous independent observational studies have shown that using anti-inflammatory medications is linked to a decreased incidence of AD (Table 7). According to a new prospective population-based study, aged individuals who take non-steroidal anti-inflammatory medicines (NSAIDs) had a 71% lower chance of dying from AD. **ALZT-OP1** is a combination of NSAID (ibuprofen) plus a mast cell stabilizer (cromolyn) that reduces neuroinflammation and encourages the phagocytosis of Aβ to facilitate its clearance. The potential of ALZT-OP1 to slow down, arrest, or counteract the early-stage AD's cognitive and functional decline on the CDR-SB subjects is being evaluated in a phase 3 clinical trial called COGNITE, which is a randomized, double-blinded, placebo-controlled study (NCT02547818) [224]. **Masitinib** is a selective tyrosine kinase inhibitor (TKI) that is recognized for regulating mast cell-mediated neuroinflammation. In 2020, Li *et al.*, showed that in the APP/PS1 mice model of amyloidosis, long-term masitinib therapy might restore synaptic density and spatial learning in the hippocampus. From 2012 to 2020, AB Science® carried out a phase 2b/3 clinical trial in 21 predominantly European countries, comparing the use of masitinib at doses of 4.5 or 6 mg/kg/day with a placebo in 721 verified cases with mild to moderate AD receiving a ChE inhibitor and/or memantine. The business said that the study's main objective was achieved [125, 126]. In a two-year randomized clinical trial, minocycline, a tetracycline derivative with anti-inflammatory properties, did not enhance the cognitive and functional abilities of people with mild AD. The tenable justifications for why this medication did not work in the phase 3 clinical trials were (i) neuroinflammation "may be a reaction to pathologic characteristics of the disease rather than an important factor in neurodegeneration"; (ii) intricate relationship between neurodegeneration and microglial activation and (iii) "minocycline did have some efficacy against AD, but treatment effects were too small to be detectable" [199]. **Pioglitazone** (AD4833), a high-affinity PPAR-γ agonist, is an insulin-sensitizing medication. Together with RXR, it forms a heterodimer that influences the transcription of genes important for lipid and glucose metabolism, as well as the decrease of inflammation. Pioglitazone is helpful in treating AD because of its favourable effects on inflammation, lipid metabolism, and cerebral glucose. Pioglitazone is well-tolerated and harmless, according to a phase II investigation in AD and a prior trial [127, 128]. The administration of pioglitazone to high-risk AD asymptomatic subjects in a Phase III trial called "TOMORROW" showed a different impact on cognitive impairment [129]. Since long-term neuroinflammation is a crucial feature shared by all non-inflammatory diseases (NDs), it has been discovered that using non-steroidal anti-inflammatory medicines (NSAIDs), likefenoprofen, ibuprofen, and indomethacin, lowers the risk of AD. NSAIDs have the ability to prevent COX-1 and COX-2, two of the isoforms of cyclooxygenase (COX). COX-2 has a crucial role when it comes to inflammatory reactions. In mice models of AD and PD, elevated levels of COX-2 expression have been reported. Furthermore, NSAIDs lower A~42 levels, which may have neuroprotective benefits. Epidemiological evidence has also hinted that NSAIDs may slow or even stop the course of Parkinson's disease. Another NSAID that may be helpful in the treatment of NDs is ibuprofen, since daily injection of 50 mg of ibuprofen improved cognitive skills in APP23 AD animal models and people. Remarkably, it was also discovered that R-flurbiprofen reduced AD learning impairments. Furthermore, the maintenance of mitochondrial activity may provide insight into the anti-apoptotic impact of NSAIDs. These compounds reduce ROS production, inhibit the release of cytochrome c, and lessen mitochondrial calcium excess. Another neuroprotective effect of R-flurbiprofen and other anti-inflammatory medications is the increased production of neurotrophins. Still, the results of clinical studies and additional clinical research with the aforementioned NSAIDs are necessary to determine whether or not NSAIDs genuinely have a function in improving neuroprotection and have an impact on cognitive problems. Results using NSAIDS were not encouraging [130].

Table 7. Examples of small molecules acting as anti-inflammatory agents in Alzheimer's disease treatment.

Class of Drug	Name of Drug	Mechanisms	Preclinica/Clinical	Refs.
Anti-inflammatory	ALZT-OP1 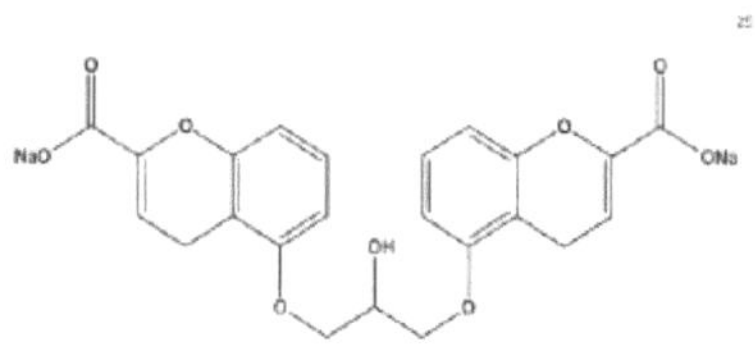	Inhibits the accumulation of amyloid-beta (Aβ) plaques and reduces the release of pro-inflammatory cytokines by brain immune cells likeastrocytes and microglias	Phase 3 clinical trials	[224]
Anti-inflammatory	Masitinib 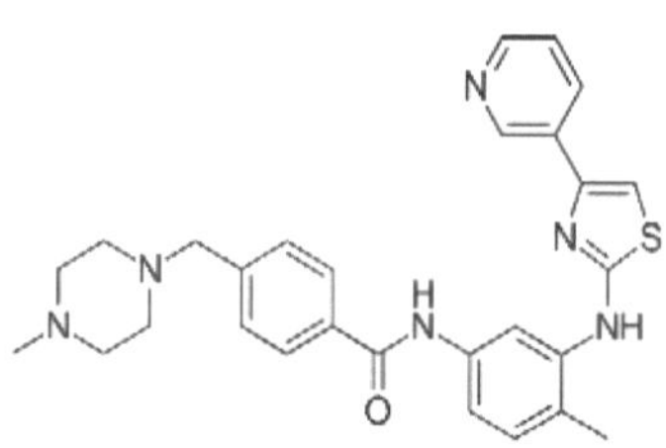	Inhibits tyrosine kinases, which are enzymes responsible for activating many proteins through signal transduction cascades. By targeting these enzymes, masitinib modulates the the activity of mast cells and macrophages/ microglia. This modulation is crucial in treating various conditions, including neuroinflammatory diseases, inflammatory diseases, and certain types of cancer.	Phase 3 clinical trials	[225]
anti-inflammatory	Minocycline 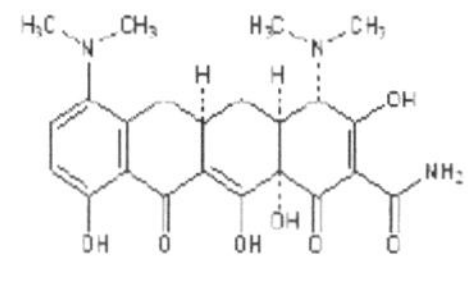	Reduces neuroinflammation by inhibiting the stimulation of microglia, the brain's immune cells. This helps decrease the generation of pro-inflammatory cytokines and other inflammatory mediators.	Phase 3 clinical trials	[230, 231]

(Table 7) cont.....

Class of Drug	Name of Drug	Mechanisms	Preclinica/Clinical	Refs.
Anti-inflammatory	Pioglitazone 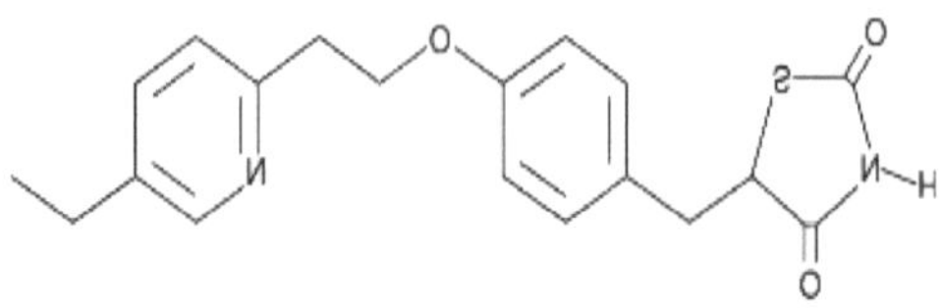	Activates the peroxisome proliferator-activate receptor gamma (PPAR-γ), a nuclear receptor that controls gene transcription. This stimulation helps to reduce inflammation in the brain.	preclinical	[228]

CHALLENGES AND OPPORTUNITIES IN DEVELOPING SMALL MOLECULE THERAPIES

Developing small-molecule therapies for AD presents a unique set of challenges and opportunities. One of the primary challenges lies in the complexity of AD pathology, which involves multiple mechanisms, including β-amyloid aggregation, tau hyperphosphorylation, neuroinflammation, synaptic dysfunction, and oxidative stress. Targeting of these interconnected pathways with small molecules often leads to limited efficacy or unintended side effects [232]. Moreover, there is a lack of predictive preclinical models, as animal models often fail to replicate the multifaceted nature of human AD, resulting in high attrition rates in clinical trials [233]. Hence, identifying biomarkers to track disease progression and therapeutic response remains a critical unmet need, complicating clinical trial design and evaluation.

Despite these challenges, advances in drug discovery technologies, such as structure-based drug designing, high-throughput screening, and artificial intelligence, are enabling the identification of novel small molecules with high specificity and efficacy. Harnessing these opportunities could significantly advance the drug discovery and clinical success of small molecule therapies for AD, which ultimately addresses this devastating neurodegenerative disease.

CONCLUDING REMARKS

In past decades, numerous efforts have been made for the identification of novel therapeutic agents and diagnostic tools that restrain AD pathogenesis. The accumulation of these endeavours has produced several therapeutic agents for both diagnosis and AD therapy. Theranostic strategy utilizing small-molecule scaffolds demonstrates a useful approach that empowers the AD treatment, which previously achieved greater difficulties in prompt diagnosis. This kind of molecule enables the evaluation of molecular activity, therapeutic responses, and pharmacokinetics, expediting the investigation and ensuring these molecules are promising for customized healthcare. Many small molecules have displayed auspicious characteristics as biomarker tracers, including β-amyloid and tau proteins involved in AD pathogenesis, and have shown a number of ways to reverse various processes of AD development. There is no doubt that theranostics will represent a potential approach for the establishment of newer resources for diagnosis and treatment in many health issues, especially for AD.

REFERENCES

[1] Kamatham PT, Shukla R, Khatri DK, Vora LK. Pathogenesis, diagnostics, and therapeutics for Alzheimer's disease: Breaking the memory barrier. Ageing Res Rev 2024; 101: 102481. [http://dx.doi.org/10.1016/j.arr.2024.102481] [PMID: 39236855]

[2] Vitali F, Branigan GL, Brinton RD. Preventing Alzheimer's disease within reach by 2025: Targeted-risk-AD-prevention (TRAP) strategy. Alzheimer's & dementia (New York, N. Y.). 2021; 7(1): e12190.

[3] Botto R, Callai N, Cermelli A, *et al.*, Anxiety and depression in Alzheimer's disease: a systematic review of pathogenetic mechanisms and relation to cognitive decline. Neurol Sci. 2022; 43(7): 4107–4124. [http://dx.doi.org/10.1007/s10072-022-06068-x]

[4] Epelbaum S, Genthon R, Cavedo E, *et al.* Preclinical Alzheimer's disease: A systematic review of the cohorts underlying the concept. Alzheimers Dement 2017; 13(4): 454-67. [http://dx.doi.org/10.1016/j.jalz.2016.12.003] [PMID: 28188032]

[5] Jack CR Jr, Andrews JS, Beach TG, *et al.* Revised criteria for diagnosis and staging of Alzheimer's disease: Alzheimer's Association Workgroup. Alzheimers Dement 2024; 20(8): 5143-69. [http://dx.doi.org/10.1002/alz.13859] [PMID: 38934362]

[6] Yarns BC, Holiday KA, Carlson DM, Cosgrove CK, Melrose RJ. Pathophysiology of Alzheimer's Disease. Psychiatr Clin North Am 2022; 45(4): 663-76. [http://dx.doi.org/10.1016/j.psc.2022.07.003] [PMID: 36396271]

[7] Suresh S, Singh S A, Rushendran R, Vellapandian C, Prajapati B. Alzheimer's disease: the role of extrinsic factors in its development, an investigation of the environmental enigma. Front Neurol 2023; 14: 1303111. [http://dx.doi.org/10.3389/fneur.2023.1303111] [PMID: 38125832]

[8] Liu CC, Kanekiyo T, Xu H, Bu G, Bu G. Apolipoprotein E and Alzheimer disease: risk, mechanisms and therapy. Nat Rev Neurol 2013; 9(2): 106-18. [http://dx.doi.org/10.1038/nrneurol.2012.263] [PMID: 23296339]

[9] Wu W, Ji Y, Wang Z, *et al.* The FDA-approved anti-amyloid-β monoclonal antibodies for the treatment of Alzheimer's disease: a systematic review and meta-analysis of randomized controlled trials. Eur J Med Res 2023; 28(1): 544. [http://dx.doi.org/10.1186/s40001-023-01512-w] [PMID: 38017568]

[10] Duan Y, Lv J, Zhang Z, *et al.* Exogenous $A\beta_{1\text{-}42}$ monomers improve synaptic and cognitive function in Alzheimer's disease model mice. Neuropharmacology 2022; 209: 109002. [http://dx.doi.org/10.1016/j.neuropharm.2022.109002] [PMID: 35196539]

[11] Smith LM, Strittmatter SM. Binding sites for amyloid-β oligomers and synaptic toxicity. Cold Spring Harb Perspect Med 2017; 7(5): a024075. [http://dx.doi.org/10.1101/cshperspect.a024075] [PMID: 27940601]

[12] Klementieva O, Willén K, Martinsson I, *et al.* Pre-plaque conformational changes in Alzheimer's disease-linked Aβ and APP. Nat Commun 2017; 8(1): 14726. [http://dx.doi.org/10.1038/ncomms14726] [PMID: 28287086]

[13] Subramanian J, Savage JC, Tremblay MÈ. Synaptic loss in alzheimer's disease: mechanistic insights provided by two-photon *in vivo* imaging of transgenic mouse models. Front Cell Neurosci 2020; 14: 592607.
[http://dx.doi.org/10.3389/fncel.2020.592607] [PMID: 33408613]

[14] Sun J, Roy S. The physical approximation of APP and BACE-1: A key event in alzheimer's disease pathogenesis. Dev Neurobiol 2018; 78(3): 340-7.
[http://dx.doi.org/10.1002/dneu.22556] [PMID: 29106038]

[15] Decourt B, Sabbagh MN. BACE1 as a potential biomarker for Alzheimer's disease. Journal of Alzheimer's disease: JAD.2011; Suppl 2(Suppl 2): 53–59.
[http://dx.doi.org/10.3233/JAD-2011-110017]

[16] Fagan AM, Head D, Shah AR, *et al.* Decreased cerebrospinal fluid $A\beta_{42}$ correlates with brain atrophy in cognitively normal elderly. Ann Neurol 2009; 65(2): 176-83.
[http://dx.doi.org/10.1002/ana.21559] [PMID: 19260027]

[17] Ovsepian SV, O'Leary VB, Zaborszky L, Ntziachristos V, Dolly JO. Synaptic vesicle cycle and amyloid β: Biting the hand that feeds. Alzheimers Dement 2018; 14(4): 502-13.
[http://dx.doi.org/10.1016/j.jalz.2018.01.011] [PMID: 29494806]

[18] Burré J, Sharma M, Südhof TC. α-Synuclein assembles into higher-order multimers upon membrane binding to promote SNARE complex formation. Proc Natl Acad Sci USA 2014; 111(40): E4274-83.
[http://dx.doi.org/10.1073/pnas.1416598111] [PMID: 25246573]

[19] Copani A. The underexplored question of β-amyloid monomers. Eur J Pharmacol 2017; 817: 71-5.
[http://dx.doi.org/10.1016/j.ejphar.2017.05.057] [PMID: 28577967]

[20] Hampel H, Hardy J, Blennow K, *et al.* The Amyloid-β Pathway in Alzheimer's Disease. Mol Psychiatry 2021; 26(10): 5481-503.
[http://dx.doi.org/10.1038/s41380-021-01249-0] [PMID: 34456336]

[21] Patterson BW, Elbert DL, Mawuenyega KG, *et al.* Age and amyloid effects on human central nervous system amyloid-beta kinetics. Ann Neurol 2015; 78(3): 439-53.
[http://dx.doi.org/10.1002/ana.24454] [PMID: 26040676]

[22] Singh R, Kaur N, Dhingra N, Kaur T. Protein misfolding, ER stress and chaperones: an approach to develop chaperone-based therapeutics for Alzheimer's disease. Int J Neurosci 2023; 133(7): 714-34.
[http://dx.doi.org/10.1080/00207454.2021.1968859] [PMID: 34402740]

[23] Hillen H, Barghorn S, Striebinger A, *et al.* Generation and therapeutic efficacy of highly oligomer-specific beta-amyloid antibodies. J Neurosci 2010; 30(31): 10369-79.
[http://dx.doi.org/10.1523/JNEUROSCI.5721-09.2010] [PMID: 20685980]

[24] Marques CMS, Gomes RN, Pedron T, Batista BL, Cerchiaro G. Cellular prion protein offers neuroprotection in astrocytes submitted to amyloid β oligomer toxicity. Mol Cell Biochem 2023; 478(8): 1847-65.
[http://dx.doi.org/10.1007/s11010-022-04631-w] [PMID: 36576715]

[25] Gonzalez-Garcia M, Fusco G, De Simone A. Membrane interactions and toxicity by misfolded protein oligomers. Front Cell Dev Biol 2021; 9: 642623.
[http://dx.doi.org/10.3389/fcell.2021.642623] [PMID: 33791300]

[26] Cline EN, Bicca MA, Viola KL, Klein WL. The amyloid-β oligomer hypothesis: Beginning of the third decade. J Alzheimers Dis 2018; 64(s1): S567-610.
[http://dx.doi.org/10.3233/JAD-179941] [PMID: 29843241]

[27] Hillen H. The beta amyloid dysfunction (BAD) hypothesis for alzheimer's disease. Front Neurosci 2019; 13: 1154.
[http://dx.doi.org/10.3389/fnins.2019.01154] [PMID: 31787864]

[28] Maia MA, Sousa E. BACE-1 and γ-secretase as therapeutic targets for alzheimer's disease.

Pharmaceuticals (Basel) 2019; 12(1): 41.
[http://dx.doi.org/10.3390/ph12010041] [PMID: 30893882]

[29] Shen Y, Wang H, Sun Q, *et al.* Increased plasma beta-secretase 1 may predict conversion to alzheimer's disease dementia in individuals with mild cognitive impairment. Biol Psychiatry 2018; 83(5): 447-55.
[http://dx.doi.org/10.1016/j.biopsych.2017.02.007] [PMID: 28359566]

[30] Roselli S, Satir TM, Camacho R, *et al.* APP-BACE1 interaction and intracellular localization regulate Aβ production in iPSC-derived cortical neurons. Cell Mol Neurobiol 2023; 43(7): 3653-68.
[http://dx.doi.org/10.1007/s10571-023-01374-0] [PMID: 37355492]

[31] Deng M, He W, Tan Y, *et al.* Increased expression of reticulon 3 in neurons leads to reduced axonal transport of β site amyloid precursor protein-cleaving enzyme 1. J Biol Chem 2013; 288(42): 30236-45.
[http://dx.doi.org/10.1074/jbc.M113.480079] [PMID: 24005676]

[32] Nordvall G, Lundkvist J, Sandin J. Gamma-secretase modulators: a promising route for the treatment of Alzheimer's disease. Front Mol Neurosci 2023; 16: 1279740.
[http://dx.doi.org/10.3389/fnmol.2023.1279740] [PMID: 37908487]

[33] Clavaguera F, Duyckaerts C, Haïk S. Prion-like properties of Tau assemblies. Curr Opin Neurobiol 2020; 61: 49-57.
[http://dx.doi.org/10.1016/j.conb.2019.11.022] [PMID: 31923760]

[34] González A, Singh SK, Churruca M, Maccioni RB. Alzheimer's disease and tau self-assembly: in the search of the missing link. Int J Mol Sci 2022; 23(8): 4192.
[http://dx.doi.org/10.3390/ijms23084192] [PMID: 35457009]

[35] Liu M, Sui D, Dexheimer T, *et al.* Hyperphosphorylation renders tau prone to aggregate and to cause cell death. Mol Neurobiol 2020; 57(11): 4704-19.
[http://dx.doi.org/10.1007/s12035-020-02034-w] [PMID: 32780352]

[36] Alonso AD, Cohen LS, Corbo C, *et al.* Hyperphosphorylation of tau associates with changes in its function beyond microtubule stability. Front Cell Neurosci 2018; 12: 338.
[http://dx.doi.org/10.3389/fncel.2018.00338] [PMID: 30356756]

[37] Iqbal K, Gong CX, Liu F. Hyperphosphorylation-induced tau oligomers. Front Neurol 2013; 4: 112.
[http://dx.doi.org/10.3389/fneur.2013.00112] [PMID: 23966973]

[38] Moszczynski AJ, Gohar M, Volkening K, Leystra-Lantz C, Strong W, Strong MJ. Thr175-phosphorylated tau induces pathologic fibril formation *via* GSK3β-mediated phosphorylation of Thr231 *in vitro*. Neurobiol Aging 2015; 36(3): 1590-9.
[http://dx.doi.org/10.1016/j.neurobiolaging.2014.12.001] [PMID: 25573097]

[39] Berth SH, Lloyd TE. Disruption of axonal transport in neurodegeneration. J Clin Invest 2023; 133(11): e168554.
[http://dx.doi.org/10.1172/JCI168554] [PMID: 37259916]

[40] Rosenmann H, Blum D, Kayed R, Ittner LM. Tau protein: function and pathology. Int J Alzheimers Dis 2012; 2012: 1-2.
[http://dx.doi.org/10.1155/2012/707482] [PMID: 22928147]

[41] Sierra H, Cordova M, Chen CSJ, Rajadhyaksha M. Confocal imaging-guided laser ablation of basal cell carcinomas: an ex vivo study. J Invest Dermatol 2015; 135(2): 612-5.
[http://dx.doi.org/10.1038/jid.2014.371] [PMID: 25178106]

[42] Miao J, Shi R, Li L, *et al.* Pathological tau from alzheimer's brain induces site-specific hyperphosphorylation and SDS- and reducing agent-resistant aggregation of tau *in vivo.* Front Aging Neurosci 2019; 11: 34.
[http://dx.doi.org/10.3389/fnagi.2019.00034] [PMID: 30890929]

[43] DeTure MA, Dickson DW. The neuropathological diagnosis of Alzheimer's disease. Mol

Neurodegener 2019; 14(1): 32.
[http://dx.doi.org/10.1186/s13024-019-0333-5] [PMID: 31375134]

[44] Uddin MS, Ashraf GM, Mamun AA, Mathew B. Toxic tau: structural origins of tau aggregation in Alzheimer's disease. Neural Regen Res 2020; 15(8): 1417-20.
[http://dx.doi.org/10.4103/1673-5374.274329] [PMID: 31997800]

[45] Xia Y, Sorrentino ZA, Kim JD, Strang KH, Riffe CJ, Giasson BI. Impaired tau–microtubule interactions are prevalent among pathogenic tau variants arising from missense mutations. J Biol Chem 2019; 294(48): 18488-503.
[http://dx.doi.org/10.1074/jbc.RA119.010178] [PMID: 31653695]

[46] Arnsten AFT, Datta D, Del Tredici K, Braak H. Hypothesis: Tau pathology is an initiating factor in sporadic Alzheimer's disease. Alzheimers Dement 2021; 17(1): 115-24.
[http://dx.doi.org/10.1002/alz.12192] [PMID: 33075193]

[47] Dietrich K, Bouter Y, Müller M, Bayer T. Synaptic alterations in mouse models for alzheimer disease—a special focus on N-truncated abeta 4-42. Molecules 2018; 23(4): 718.
[http://dx.doi.org/10.3390/molecules23040718] [PMID: 29561816]

[48] Derisbourg M, Leghay C, Chiappetta G, *et al.* Role of the Tau N-terminal region in microtubule stabilization revealed by newendogenous truncated forms. Sci Rep 2015; 5(1): 9659.
[http://dx.doi.org/10.1038/srep09659] [PMID: 25974414]

[49] van Ameijde J, Crespo R, Janson R, *et al.* Enhancement of therapeutic potential of a naturally occurring human antibody targeting a phosphorylated Ser^{422} containing epitope on pathological tau. Acta Neuropathol Commun 2018; 6(1): 59.
[http://dx.doi.org/10.1186/s40478-018-0562-9] [PMID: 30001207]

[50] Chong FP, Ng KY, Koh RY, Chye SM. Tau proteins and tauopathies in alzheimer's disease. Cell Mol Neurobiol 2018; 38(5): 965-80.
[http://dx.doi.org/10.1007/s10571-017-0574-1] [PMID: 29299792]

[51] Haukedal H, Freude KK. Implications of glycosylation in alzheimer's disease. Front Neurosci 2021; 14: 625348.
[http://dx.doi.org/10.3389/fnins.2020.625348] [PMID: 33519371]

[52] Zhao J, Lang M. New insight into protein glycosylation in the development of Alzheimer's disease. Cell Death Discov 2023; 9(1): 314.
[http://dx.doi.org/10.1038/s41420-023-01617-5] [PMID: 37626031]

[53] Diniz Pereira J, Gomes Fraga V, Morais Santos AL, Carvalho MG, Caramelli P, Braga Gomes K. Alzheimer's disease and type 2 diabetes mellitus: A systematic review of proteomic studies. J Neurochem 2021; 156(6): 753-76.
[http://dx.doi.org/10.1111/jnc.15166] [PMID: 32909269]

[54] Chou PS, Wu MN, Yang CC, Shen CT, Yang YH. Effect of advanced glycation end products on the progression of alzheimer's disease. J Alzheimers Dis 2019; 72(1): 191-7.
[http://dx.doi.org/10.3233/JAD-190639] [PMID: 31561370]

[55] Li WY, Lee CY, Lee KM, Zhang G, Lyu A, Yue KKM. Advanced glycation end-product precursor methylglyoxal may lead to development of alzheimer's disease. Diabetes Metab Syndr Obes 2022; 15: 3153-66.
[http://dx.doi.org/10.2147/DMSO.S382927] [PMID: 36262805]

[56] Zhang YJ, Xu YF, Chen XQ, Wang XC, Wang JZ. Nitration and oligomerization of tau induced by peroxynitrite inhibit its microtubule-binding activity. FEBS Lett 2005; 579(11): 2421-7.
[http://dx.doi.org/10.1016/j.febslet.2005.03.041] [PMID: 15848182]

[57] Mylvaganam S, Earnshaw R, Heymann G, Kalia SK, Kalia LV. C-terminus of Hsp70 Interacting Protein (CHIP) and Neurodegeneration: Lessons from the Bench and Bedside. Curr Neuropharmacol 2021; 19(7): 1038-68.

[http://dx.doi.org/10.2174/1570159X18666201116145507] [PMID: 33200713]

[58] Pohanka M. Oxidative stress in Alzheimer disease as a target for therapy. Bratisl Med J 2018; 119(9): 535-43.
[http://dx.doi.org/10.4149/BLL_2018_097] [PMID: 30226062]

[59] Tamagno E, Guglielmotto M, Vasciaveo V, Tabaton M. Oxidative stress and beta amyloid in alzheimer's disease. which comes first: The chicken or the egg? Antioxidants 2021; 10(9): 1479.
[http://dx.doi.org/10.3390/antiox10091479] [PMID: 34573112]

[60] Mustafa AG, Alfaqih MA, Al-Shboul O. The 4-hydroxynonenal mediated oxidative damage of blood proteins and lipids involves secondary lipid peroxidation reactions. Experimental and therapeutic medicine.20158; 16(3): 2132–2137.

[61] Sensi SL, Granzotto A, Siotto M, Squitti R. Copper and zinc dysregulation in alzheimer's disease. Trends Pharmacol Sci 2018; 39(12): 1049-63.
[http://dx.doi.org/10.1016/j.tips.2018.10.001] [PMID: 30352697]

[62] Liu Y, Nguyen M, Robert A, Meunier B. Metal ions in alzheimer's disease: A key role or not? Acc Chem Res 2019; 52(7): 2026-35.
[http://dx.doi.org/10.1021/acs.accounts.9b00248] [PMID: 31274278]

[63] Bhatt S, Puli L, Patil CR. Role of reactive oxygen species in the progression of Alzheimer's disease. Drug Discov Today 2021; 26(3): 794-803.
[http://dx.doi.org/10.1016/j.drudis.2020.12.004] [PMID: 33306995]

[64] Perez Ortiz JM, Swerdlow RH. Mitochondrial dysfunction in Alzheimer's disease: Role in pathogenesis and novel therapeutic opportunities. Br J Pharmacol 2019; 176(18): 3489-507.
[http://dx.doi.org/10.1111/bph.14585] [PMID: 30675901]

[65] Uddin MS, Kabir MT, Mamun AA, *et al.* Pharmacological approaches to mitigate neuroinflammation in Alzheimer's disease. Int Immunopharmacol 2020; 84: 106479.
[http://dx.doi.org/10.1016/j.intimp.2020.106479] [PMID: 32353686]

[66] Marttinen M, Takalo M, Natunen T, *et al.* Molecular Mechanisms of Synaptotoxicity and Neuroinflammation in Alzheimer's Disease. Front Neurosci 2018; 12: 963.
[http://dx.doi.org/10.3389/fnins.2018.00963] [PMID: 30618585]

[67] Merighi S, Nigro M, Travagli A, Gessi S. Microglia and Alzheimer's Disease. Int J Mol Sci 2022; 23(21): 12990.
[http://dx.doi.org/10.3390/ijms232112990] [PMID: 36361780]

[68] Navarro V, Sanchez-Mejias E, Jimenez S, *et al.* Microglia in alzheimer's disease: activated, dysfunctional or degenerative. Front Aging Neurosci 2018; 10: 140.
[http://dx.doi.org/10.3389/fnagi.2018.00140] [PMID: 29867449]

[69] Zhou J, Yu W, Zhang M, Tian X, Li Y, Lü Y. Imbalance of microglial TLR4/TREM2 in LPS-Treated APP/PS1 transgenic mice: A potential link between alzheimer's disease and systemic inflammation. Neurochem Res 2019; 44(5): 1138-51.
[http://dx.doi.org/10.1007/s11064-019-02748-x] [PMID: 30756214]

[70] Liu Y, Dai Y, Li Q, *et al.* Beta-amyloid activates NLRP3 inflammasome *via* TLR4 in mouse microglia. Neurosci Lett 2020; 736: 135279.
[http://dx.doi.org/10.1016/j.neulet.2020.135279] [PMID: 32726591]

[71] Preman P, Alfonso-Triguero M, Alberdi E, Verkhratsky A, Arranz AM. Astrocytes in alzheimer's disease: Pathological significance and molecular pathways. Cells 2021; 10(3): 540.
[http://dx.doi.org/10.3390/cells10030540] [PMID: 33806259]

[72] Chun H, Lee CJ. Reactive astrocytes in Alzheimer's disease: A double-edged sword. Neurosci Res 2018; 126: 44-52.
[http://dx.doi.org/10.1016/j.neures.2017.11.012] [PMID: 29225140]

[73] Javonillo DI, Tran KM, Phan J, *et al.* Systematic phenotyping and characterization of the 3xTg-AD mouse model of alzheimer's disease. Front Neurosci 2022; 15: 785276. [http://dx.doi.org/10.3389/fnins.2021.785276] [PMID: 35140584]

[74] Mitew S, Kirkcaldie MTK, Halliday GM, Shepherd CE, Vickers JC, Dickson TC. Focal demyelination in Alzheimer's disease and transgenic mouse models. Acta Neuropathol 2010; 119(5): 567-77. [http://dx.doi.org/10.1007/s00401-010-0657-2] [PMID: 20198482]

[75] Eid A, Mhatre I, Richardson JR. Gene-environment interactions in Alzheimer's disease: A potential path to precision medicine. Pharmacol Ther 2019; 199: 173-87. [http://dx.doi.org/10.1016/j.pharmthera.2019.03.005] [PMID: 30877021]

[76] Jackson RJ, Hyman BT, Serrano-Pozo A. Multifaceted roles of APOE in Alzheimer disease. Nat Rev Neurol 2024; 20(8): 457-74. [http://dx.doi.org/10.1038/s41582-024-00988-2] [PMID: 38906999]

[77] Uddin MS, Kabir MT, Al Mamun A, Abdel-Daim MM, Barreto GE, Ashraf GM. APOE and alzheimer's disease: evidence mounts that targeting APOE4 may combat alzheimer's pathogenesis. Mol Neurobiol 2019; 56(4): 2450-65. [http://dx.doi.org/10.1007/s12035-018-1237-z] [PMID: 30032423]

[78] Medehouenou TCM, AyotteP, Carmichael PH,*et al.*, Exposure to polychlorinated biphenyls and organochlorine pesticides and risk of dementia, Alzheimer's disease and cognitive decline in an older population: a prospective analysis from the Canadian Study of Health and Aging. Environmental health: a global access science source.2019;18(1):57.

[79] O'Piela DR, Durisek GR III, Escobar YNH, Mackos AR, Wold LE. Particulate matter and Alzheimer's disease: an intimate connection. Trends Mol Med 2022; 28(9): 770-80. [http://dx.doi.org/10.1016/j.molmed.2022.06.004] [PMID: 35840480]

[80] Carmona S, Zahs K, Wu E, Dakin K, Bras J, Guerreiro R. The role of TREM2 in Alzheimer's disease and other neurodegenerative disorders. Lancet Neurol 2018; 17(8): 721-30. [http://dx.doi.org/10.1016/S1474-4422(18)30232-1] [PMID: 30033062]

[81] Cummings J, Lee G, Ritter A, Zhong K. Alzheimer's disease drug development pipeline: 2018. Alzheimers Dement (N Y) 2018; 4(1): 195-214. [http://dx.doi.org/10.1016/j.trci.2018.03.009] [PMID: 29955663]

[82] McDade E, Voytyuk I, Aisen P, *et al.* The case for low-level BACE1 inhibition for the prevention of Alzheimer disease. Nat Rev Neurol 2021; 17(11): 703-14. [http://dx.doi.org/10.1038/s41582-021-00545-1] [PMID: 34548654]

[83] Li X, Wang H, Long J, *et al.* Systematic analysis and biomarker study for alzheimer's disease. Sci Rep 2018; 8(1): 17394. [http://dx.doi.org/10.1038/s41598-018-35789-3] [PMID: 30478411]

[84] Lee SJC, Nam E, Lee HJ, Savelieff MG, Lim MH. Towards an understanding of amyloid-β oligomers: characterization, toxicity mechanisms, and inhibitors. Chem Soc Rev 2017; 46(2): 310-23. [http://dx.doi.org/10.1039/C6CS00731G] [PMID: 27878186]

[85] Chen G, Xu T, Yan Y, *et al.* Amyloid beta: structure, biology and structure-based therapeutic development. Acta Pharmacol Sin 2017; 38(9): 1205-35. [http://dx.doi.org/10.1038/aps.2017.28] [PMID: 28713158]

[86] Utsuki T, Yu Q, Davidson D, *et al.* Identification of novel small molecule inhibitors of amyloid precursor protein synthesis as a route to lower Alzheimer's disease amyloid-beta peptide. J Pharmacol Exp Ther 2006; 318(2): 855-62. [http://dx.doi.org/10.1124/jpet.106.103309] [PMID: 16690718]

[87] Atluri VSR, Tiwari S, Rodriguez M, *et al.* Inhibition of amyloid-beta production, associated neuroinflammation, and histone deacetylase 2-mediated epigenetic modifications prevent neuropathology in alzheimer's disease *in vitro* model. Front Aging Neurosci 2020; 11: 342.

[http://dx.doi.org/10.3389/fnagi.2019.00342] [PMID: 32009938]

[88] Vassar R, Bennett BD, Babu-Khan S, *et al.* Beta-secretase cleavage of Alzheimer's amyloid precursor protein by the transmembrane aspartic protease BACE. Science 1999; 286(5440): 735-41. [http://dx.doi.org/10.1126/science.286.5440.735] [PMID: 10531052]

[89] May PC, Willis BA, Lowe SL, *et al.* The potent BACE1 inhibitor LY2886721 elicits robust central Aβ pharmacodynamic responses in mice, dogs, and humans. J Neurosci 2015; 35(3): 1199-210. [http://dx.doi.org/10.1523/JNEUROSCI.4129-14.2015] [PMID: 25609634]

[90] Zhang Y, Chen H, Li R, Sterling K, Song W. Amyloid β-based therapy for Alzheimer's disease: Challenges, successes and future. Signal Transduct Target Ther 2023; 8(1): 248. [http://dx.doi.org/10.1038/s41392-023-01484-7] [PMID: 37386015]

[91] Sperling R, Henley D, Aisen PS, *et al.* Findings of efficacy, safety, and biomarker outcomes of atabecestat in preclinical alzheimer disease. JAMA Neurol 2021; 78(3): 293-301. [http://dx.doi.org/10.1001/jamaneurol.2020.4857] [PMID: 33464300]

[92] Madrasi K, Das R, Mohmmadabdul H, *et al.* Systematic *in silico* analysis of clinically tested drugs for reducing amyloid-beta plaque accumulation in Alzheimer's disease. Alzheimers Dement 2021; 17(9): 1487-98. [http://dx.doi.org/10.1002/alz.12312] [PMID: 33938131]

[93] Sakamoto K, Matsuki S, Matsuguma K, *et al.* BACE1 inhibitor lanabecestat (AZD3293) in a phase 1 study of healthy japanese subjects: pharmacokinetics and effects on plasma and cerebrospinal fluid Aβ peptides. J Clin Pharmacol 2017; 57(11): 1460-71. [http://dx.doi.org/10.1002/jcph.950] [PMID: 28618005]

[94] Neumann U, Ufer M, Jacobson LH, *et al.* The BACE-1 inhibitor CNP 520 for prevention trials in Alzheimer's disease. EMBO Mol Med 2018; 10(11): e9316. [http://dx.doi.org/10.15252/emmm.201809316] [PMID: 30224383]

[95] de Felice FG, Vieira MNN, Saraiva LM, *et al.* Targeting the neurotoxic species in Alzheimer's disease: inhibitors of Aβ oligomerization. FASEB J 2004; 18(12): 1366-72. [http://dx.doi.org/10.1096/fj.04-1764com] [PMID: 15333579]

[96] Zhao W, Wang J, Ho L, Ono K, Teplow DB, Pasinetti GM. Identification of antihypertensive drugs which inhibit amyloid-beta protein oligomerization. J Alzheimers Dis 2009; 16(1): 49-57. [http://dx.doi.org/10.3233/JAD-2009-0925] [PMID: 19158421]

[97] McKoy AF, Chen J, Schupbach T, Hecht MH. A novel inhibitor of amyloid β (Aβ) peptide aggregation: from high throughput screening to efficacy in an animal model of Alzheimer disease. J Biol Chem 2012; 287(46): 38992-9000. [http://dx.doi.org/10.1074/jbc.M112.348037] [PMID: 22992731]

[98] Xiao XQ, Zhang HY, Tang XC. Huperzine A attenuates amyloid β-peptide fragment 25-35-induced apoptosis in rat cortical neurons *via* inhibiting reactive oxygen species formation and caspase-3 activation. J Neurosci Res 2002; 67(1): 30-6. [http://dx.doi.org/10.1002/jnr.10075] [PMID: 11754078]

[99] Huang M, Jiang X, Liang Y, Liu Q, Chen S, Guo Y. Berberine improves cognitive impairment by promoting autophagic clearance and inhibiting production of β-amyloid in APP/tau/PS1 mouse model of Alzheimer's disease. Exp Gerontol 2017; 91: 25-33. [http://dx.doi.org/10.1016/j.exger.2017.02.004] [PMID: 28223223]

[100] Yin Y, Huang L, Liu Y, *et al.* Effect of tanshinone on the levels of nitric oxide synthase and acetylcholinesterase in the brain of Alzheimer's disease rat model. Clin Invest Med 2008; 31(5): E248-57. [http://dx.doi.org/10.25011/cim.v31i5.4871] [PMID: 18980714]

[101] Hirai K, Hayako H, Kato K, Miyamoto M. Idebenone protects hippocampal neurons against amyloid β-peptide-induced neurotoxicity in rat primary cultures. Naunyn Schmiedebergs Arch Pharmacol

1998; 358(5): 582-5.
[http://dx.doi.org/10.1007/PL00005296] [PMID: 9840428]

[102] Rosales Jubal E, Schwalm M, dos Santos Guilherme M, *et al.* Acitretin reverses early functional network degradation in a mouse model of familial Alzheimer's disease. Sci Rep 2021; 11(1): 6649.
[http://dx.doi.org/10.1038/s41598-021-85912-0] [PMID: 33758244]

[103] Hardy JA, Higgins GA. Alzheimer's disease: the amyloid cascade hypothesis. Science 1992; 256(5054): 184-5.
[http://dx.doi.org/10.1126/science.1566067] [PMID: 1566067]

[104] Ehrnhoefer DE, Bieschke J, Boeddrich A, *et al.* EGCG redirects amyloidogenic polypeptides into unstructured, off-pathway oligomers. Nat Struct Mol Biol 2008; 15(6): 558-66.
[http://dx.doi.org/10.1038/nsmb.1437] [PMID: 18511942]

[105] Ono K, Li L, Takamura Y, *et al.* Phenolic compounds prevent amyloid β-protein oligomerization and synaptic dysfunction by site-specific binding. J Biol Chem 2012; 287(18): 14631-43.
[http://dx.doi.org/10.1074/jbc.M111.325456] [PMID: 22393064]

[106] Bengoa-Vergniory N, Faggiani E, Ramos-Gonzalez P, *et al.*, CLR01 protects dopaminergic neurons *in vitro* and in mouse models of Parkinson's disease. Nat Commun 2020; 11: 4885.
[http://dx.doi.org/10.1038/s41467-020-18689-x]

[107] Monroy A, Lithgow GJ, Alavez S. Curcumin and neurodegenerative diseases. Biofactors 2013; 39(1): 122-32.
[http://dx.doi.org/10.1002/biof.1063] [PMID: 23303664]

[108] Endo H, Nikaido Y, Nakadate M, Ise S, Konno H. Structure activity relationship study of curcumin analogues toward the amyloid-beta aggregation inhibitor. Bioorg Med Chem Lett 2014; 24(24): 5621-6.
[http://dx.doi.org/10.1016/j.bmcl.2014.10.076] [PMID: 25467149]

[109] Rigacci S, Guidotti V, Bucciantini M, *et al.* Aβ(1-42) aggregates into non-toxic amyloid assemblies in the presence of the natural polyphenol oleuropein aglycon. Curr Alzheimer Res 2011; 8(8): 841-52.
[http://dx.doi.org/10.2174/156720511798192682] [PMID: 21592051]

[110] Cao Y, Yu F, Lyu Y, Lu X. Promising candidates from drug clinical trials: Implications for clinical treatment of Alzheimer's disease in China. Front Neurol 2022; 13: 1034243.
[http://dx.doi.org/10.3389/fneur.2022.1034243] [PMID: 36457865]

[111] Wang T, Kuang W, Chen W, *et al.* A phase II randomized trial of sodium oligomannate in Alzheimer's dementia. Alzheimers Res Ther 2020; 12(1): 110.
[http://dx.doi.org/10.1186/s13195-020-00678-3] [PMID: 32928279]

[112] Cantillon M, Andreasen N, Prins N. Phase 1/2a intravenous and subcutaneous oligomer-specific antibody KHK6640 in mild to moderate alzheimer's disease. J Prev Alzheimers Dis 2024; 11(1): 65-70.
[http://dx.doi.org/10.14283/jpad.2024.2] [PMID: 38230718]

[113] Salloway S, Sperling R, Keren R, *et al.* A phase 2 randomized trial of ELND005, scyllo-inositol, in mild to moderate Alzheimer disease. Neurology 2011; 77(13): 1253-62.
[http://dx.doi.org/10.1212/WNL.0b013e3182309fa5] [PMID: 21917766]

[114] Maccecchini ML, Chang MY, Pan C, John V, Zetterberg H, Greig NH. Posiphen as a candidate drug to lower CSF amyloid precursor protein, amyloid-β peptide and τ levels: target engagement, tolerability and pharmacokinetics in humans. J Neurol Neurosurg Psychiatry 2012; 83(9): 894-902.
[http://dx.doi.org/10.1136/jnnp-2012-302589] [PMID: 22791904]

[115] Cebers G, Alexander RC, Haeberlein SB, *et al.* AZD3293: Pharmacokinetic and pharmacodynamic effects in healthy subjects and patients with alzheimer's disease. J Alzheimers Dis 2016; 55(3): 1039-53.
[http://dx.doi.org/10.3233/JAD-160701] [PMID: 27767991]

[116] Bachurin SO, Bovina EV, Ustyugov AA. Current trends in thedevelopment of drugs for the treatment of Alzheimer's diseaseand their clinical trials. Biomedical Chemistry: Research and Methods 2018; 1(3): e00015.
[http://dx.doi.org/10.18097/BMCRM00015]

[117] Aisen PS, Gauthier S, Ferris SH, *et al.* Tramiprosate in mild-to-moderate Alzheimer's disease – a randomized, double-blind, placebo-controlled, multi-centre study (the Alphase Study). Arch Med Sci 2011; 1(1): 102-11.
[http://dx.doi.org/10.5114/aoms.2011.20612] [PMID: 22291741]

[118] Kutzsche J, Jürgens D, Willuweit A, *et al.* Safety and pharmacokinetics of the orally available antiprionic compound PRI-002: A single and multiple ascending dose phase I study. Alzheimers Dement (N Y) 2020; 6(1): e12001.
[http://dx.doi.org/10.1002/trc2.12001] [PMID: 32211506]

[119] Decourt B, Wilson J, Ritter A, *et al.* MCLENA-1: A phase ii clinical trial for the assessment of safety, tolerability, and efficacy of lenalidomide in patients with mild cognitive impairment due to alzheimer's disease. Open Access J Clin Trials 2020; 12: 1-13.
[http://dx.doi.org/10.2147/OAJCT.S221914] [PMID: 32123490]

[120] Yoon SS, AhnJo S-M. Mechanisms of amyloid-β peptide clearance: Potential therapeutic targets for alzheimer's disease. Biomol Ther (Seoul) 2012; 20(3): 245-55.
[http://dx.doi.org/10.4062/biomolther.2012.20.3.245] [PMID: 24130920]

[121] Turner AJ, Nalivaeva NN. New insights into the roles of metalloproteinases in neurodegeneration and neuroprotection. Int Rev Neurobiol 2007; 82: 113-35.
[http://dx.doi.org/10.1016/S0074-7742(07)82006-X] [PMID: 17678958]

[122] Qian C, Yang C, Lu M, *et al.* Activating AhR alleviates cognitive deficits of Alzheimer's disease model mice by upregulating endogenous Aβ catabolic enzyme Neprilysin. Theranostics 2021; 11(18): 8797-812.
[http://dx.doi.org/10.7150/thno.61601] [PMID: 34522212]

[123] Ullah R, Lee EJ. Advances in amyloid-β clearance in the brain and periphery: Implications for neurodegenerative diseases. Exp Neurobiol 2023; 32(4): 216-46.
[http://dx.doi.org/10.5607/en23014] [PMID: 37749925]

[124] Weller RO, Subash M, Preston SD, Mazanti I, Carare RO. Perivascular drainage of amyloid-beta peptides from the brain and its failure in cerebral amyloid angiopathy and Alzheimer's disease. Brain Pathol 2008; 18(2): 253-66.
[http://dx.doi.org/10.1111/j.1750-3639.2008.00133.x] [PMID: 18363936]

[125] Hemming ML, Selkoe DJ, Farris W. Effects of prolonged angiotensin-converting enzyme inhibitor treatment on amyloid β-protein metabolism in mouse models of Alzheimer disease. Neurobiol Dis 2007; 26(1): 273-81.
[http://dx.doi.org/10.1016/j.nbd.2007.01.004] [PMID: 17321748]

[126] Oba R, Igarashi A, Kamata M, Nagata K, Takano S, Nakagawa H. The N-terminal active centre of human angiotensin-converting enzyme degrades Alzheimer amyloid β-peptide. Eur J Neurosci. 2005; 21(3): 733-740.
[http://dx.doi.org/10.1111/j.1460-9568.2005.03912.x]

[127] Xu C, Garcia D, Lu Y, Ozuna K, Adjeroh DA, Wang K. Levels of angiotensin-converting enzyme and apolipoproteins are associated with alzheimer's disease and cardiovascular diseases. Cells 2021; 11(1): 29.
[http://dx.doi.org/10.3390/cells11010029] [PMID: 35011591]

[128] Qiu WQ, Walsh DM, Ye Z, *et al.* Insulin-degrading enzyme regulates extracellular levels of amyloid beta-protein by degradation. J Biol Chem 1998; 273(49): 32730-8.
[http://dx.doi.org/10.1074/jbc.273.49.32730] [PMID: 9830016]

[129] Pérez A, Morelli L, Cresto JC, Castaño EM. Degradation of soluble amyloid beta-peptides 1-40, 1-42, and the Dutch variant 1-40Q by insulin degrading enzyme from Alzheimer disease and control brains. Neurochem Res 2000; 25(2): 247-55.
[http://dx.doi.org/10.1023/A:1007527721160] [PMID: 10786709]

[130] Sahoo BR, Panda PK, Liang W, Tang WJ, Ahuja R, Ramamoorthy A. Degradation of alzheimer's amyloid-β by a catalytically inactive insulin-degrading enzyme. J Mol Biol 2021; 433(13): 166993.
[http://dx.doi.org/10.1016/j.jmb.2021.166993] [PMID: 33865867]

[131] Yan P, Hu X, Song H, *et al.* Matrix metalloproteinase-9 degrades amyloid-beta fibrils *in vitro* and compact plaques in situ. J Biol Chem 2006; 281(34): 24566-74.
[http://dx.doi.org/10.1074/jbc.M602440200] [PMID: 16787929]

[132] Deb S, Gottschall PE. Increased production of matrix metalloproteinases in enriched astrocyte and mixed hippocampal cultures treated with beta-amyloid peptides. J Neurochem 1996; 66(4): 1641-7.
[http://dx.doi.org/10.1046/j.1471-4159.1996.66041641.x] [PMID: 8627321]

[133] Hoogmartens J, Hens E, Engelborghs S, *et al.* Investigation of the role of matrix metalloproteinases in the genetic etiology of Alzheimer's disease. Neurobiol Aging 2021; 104: 105.e1-6.
[http://dx.doi.org/10.1016/j.neurobiolaging.2021.03.011] [PMID: 33892965]

[134] Taniguchi M, Matsuura K, Nakamura R, Kojima A, Konishi M, Akizawa T. MMP-7 cleaves amyloid β fragment peptides and copper ion inhibits the degradation. Biometals 2017; 30(5): 797-807.
[http://dx.doi.org/10.1007/s10534-017-0048-4] [PMID: 28871443]

[135] Porter KN, Sarkar SN, Dakhlallah DA, Vannoy ME, Quintana DD, Simpkins JW. Medroxyprogesterone acetate impairs amyloid beta degradation in a matrix metalloproteinase-9 dependent manner. Front Aging Neurosci 2020; 12: 92.
[http://dx.doi.org/10.3389/fnagi.2020.00092] [PMID: 32317959]

[136] Liao MC, Ahmed M, Smith SO, Van Nostrand WE. Degradation of amyloid beta protein by purified myelin basic protein. J Biol Chem 2009; 284(42): 28917-25.
[http://dx.doi.org/10.1074/jbc.M109.050856] [PMID: 19692707]

[137] Jacobsen JS, Comery TA, Martone RL, *et al.* Enhanced clearance of Aβ in brain by sustaining the plasmin proteolysis cascade. Proc Natl Acad Sci USA 2008; 105(25): 8754-9.
[http://dx.doi.org/10.1073/pnas.0710823105] [PMID: 18559859]

[138] Yamin R, Bagchi S, Hildebrant R, Scaloni A, Widom RL, Abraham CR. Acyl peptide hydrolase, a serine proteinase isolated from conditioned medium of neuroblastoma cells, degrades the amyloid-β peptide. J Neurochem 2007; 100(2): 458-67.
[http://dx.doi.org/10.1111/j.1471-4159.2006.04251.x] [PMID: 17241160]

[139] Sun B, Zhou Y, Halabisky B, *et al.* Cystatin C-cathepsin B axis regulates amyloid beta levels and associated neuronal deficits in an animal model of Alzheimer's disease. Neuron 2008; 60(2): 247-57.
[http://dx.doi.org/10.1016/j.neuron.2008.10.001] [PMID: 18957217]

[140] Yang CN, Shiao YJ, Shie FS, *et al.* Mechanism mediating oligomeric Aβ clearance by naïve primary microglia. Neurobiol Dis 2011; 42(3): 221-30.
[http://dx.doi.org/10.1016/j.nbd.2011.01.005] [PMID: 21220023]

[141] Sakamoto T, Saito H, Ishii K, Takahashi H, Tanabe S, Ogasawara Y. Aluminum inhibits proteolytic degradation of amyloid β peptide by cathepsin D: A potential link between aluminum accumulation and neuritic plaque deposition. FEBS Lett 2006; 580(28-29): 6543-9.
[http://dx.doi.org/10.1016/j.febslet.2006.10.075] [PMID: 17112520]

[142] Suire CN, Leissring MA. Cathepsin D: A candidate link between amyloid β-protein and tauopathy in Alzheimer disease. J Exp Neurol. 2021; 2(1): 10-15.
[PMID: 33665647]

[143] Oberstein TJ, Utz J, Spitzer P, *et al.* The role of cathepsin b in the degradation of Aβ and in the production of Aβ peptides starting with Ala2 in cultured astrocytes. Front Mol Neurosci 2021; 13:

615740.
[http://dx.doi.org/10.3389/fnmol.2020.615740] [PMID: 33510618]

[144] Zhang X, Wang J, Zhang Z, Ye K. Tau in neurodegenerative diseases: molecular mechanisms, biomarkers, and therapeutic strategies. Transl Neurodegener 2024; 13(1): 40.
[http://dx.doi.org/10.1186/s40035-024-00429-6] [PMID: 39107835]

[145] Parra Bravo C, Naguib SA, Gan L. Cellular and pathological functions of tau. Nat Rev Mol Cell Biol 2024; 25(11): 845-64.
[http://dx.doi.org/10.1038/s41580-024-00753-9] [PMID: 39014245]

[146] Rawat P, Sehar U, Bisht J, *et al.*, Phosphorylated tau in alzheimer's disease and other tauopathies. Int J Mol Sci 2022; 23(21): 12841.
[http://dx.doi.org/10.3390/ijms232112841] [PMID: 36361631]

[147] Hong X, Huang L, Lei F, *et al.*, The role and pathogenesis of tau protein in alzheimer's disease. Biomolecules 2025; 15(6): 824.
[http://dx.doi.org/10.3390/biom15060824]

[148] Goedert M, Spillantini MG, Davies SW. Filamentous nerve cell inclusions in neurodegenerative diseases. Curr Opin Neurobiol 1998; 8(5): 619-32.
[http://dx.doi.org/10.1016/S0959-4388(98)80090-1] [PMID: 9811617]

[149] Brunden KR, Trojanowski JQ, Lee VMY. Advances in tau-focused drug discovery for Alzheimer's disease and related tauopathies. Nat Rev Drug Discov 2009; 8(10): 783-93.
[http://dx.doi.org/10.1038/nrd2959] [PMID: 19794442]

[150] Jadhav S, Avila J, Schöll M, *et al.* A walk through tau therapeutic strategies. Acta Neuropathol Commun. 2019; 7(1): 22.
[http://dx.doi.org/10.1186/s40478-019-0664-z]

[151] Aillaud I, Funke SA. Tau aggregation inhibiting peptides as potential therapeutics for alzheimer disease. Cell Mol Neurobiol 2023; 43(3): 951-61.
[http://dx.doi.org/10.1007/s10571-022-01230-7] [PMID: 35596819]

[152] Cummings JL, Gonzalez MI, Pritchard MC, May PC, Toledo-Sherman LM, Harris GA. The therapeutic landscape of tauopathies: challenges and prospects. Alzheimers Res Ther 2023; 15(1): 168.
[http://dx.doi.org/10.1186/s13195-023-01321-7] [PMID: 37803386]

[153] Xia Y, Prokop S, Giasson BI. "Don't Phos Over Tau": recent developments in clinical biomarkers and therapies targeting tau phosphorylation in Alzheimer's disease and other tauopathies. Mol Neurodegener 2021; 16(1): 37.
[http://dx.doi.org/10.1186/s13024-021-00460-5] [PMID: 34090488]

[154] Medeiros R, Baglietto-Vargas D, LaFerla FM. The role of tau in Alzheimer's disease and related disorders. CNS Neurosci Ther 2011; 17(5): 514-24.
[http://dx.doi.org/10.1111/j.1755-5949.2010.00177.x] [PMID: 20553310]

[155] Pooler AM, Polydoro M, Wegmann S, Nicholls SB, Spires-Jones TL, Hyman BT. Propagation of tau pathology in Alzheimer's disease: identification of novel therapeutic targets. Alzheimers Res Ther 2013; 5(5): 49.
[http://dx.doi.org/10.1186/alzrt214] [PMID: 24152385]

[156] Samudra N, Lane-Donovan C, VandeVrede L, Boxer AL. Tau pathology in neurodegenerative disease: disease mechanisms and therapeutic avenues. J Clin Invest 2023; 133(12): e168553.
[http://dx.doi.org/10.1172/JCI168553] [PMID: 37317972]

[157] Yang J, Zhi W, Wang L. Role of tau protein in neurodegenerative diseases and development of its targeted drugs: A literature review. Molecules 2024; 29(12): 2812.
[http://dx.doi.org/10.3390/molecules29122812] [PMID: 38930877]

[158] Davidowitz EJ, Lopez P, Jimenez H, Adrien L, Davies P, Moe JG. Small molecule inhibitor of tau self-association in a mouse model of tauopathy: A preventive study in P301L tau JNPL3 mice. PLoS

One 2023; 18(8): e0286523.
[http://dx.doi.org/10.1371/journal.pone.0286523] [PMID: 37556474]

[159] Wang D, Huang X, Yan L, *et al.* The structure biology of tau and clue for aggregation inhibitor design. Protein J 2021; 40(5): 656-68.
[http://dx.doi.org/10.1007/s10930-021-10017-6] [PMID: 34401998]

[160] Martic S. Inhibition of tau protein aggregation using small molecule inhibitors and immunotherapies. Alzheimers Dement. 2022; 18(Suppl 1): e065627.
[http://dx.doi.org/10.1002/alz.065627]

[161] Gerson JE, Kayed R. Formation and propagation of tau oligomeric seeds. Front Neurol 2013; 4: 93.
[http://dx.doi.org/10.3389/fneur.2013.00093] [PMID: 23882255]

[162] Yang J, Shen N, Shen J, Yang Y, Li HL. Complicated role of post-translational modification and protease-cleaved fragments of tau in alzheimer's disease and other tauopathies. Mol Neurobiol 2024; 61(7): 4712-31.
[http://dx.doi.org/10.1007/s12035-023-03867-x] [PMID: 38114762]

[163] Pir GJ, Choudhary B, Kaniyappan S, *et al.* Suppressing tau aggregation and toxicity by an anti-aggregant tau fragment. Mol Neurobiol 2019; 56(5): 3751-67.
[http://dx.doi.org/10.1007/s12035-018-1326-z] [PMID: 30196394]

[164] Benn J, Cheng S, Keeling S, *et al.* Aggregate-selective removal of pathological tau by clustering-activated degraders. Science 2024; 385(6712): 1009-16.
[http://dx.doi.org/10.1126/science.adp5186] [PMID: 39208111]

[165] Gauthier S, Feldman HH, Schneider LS, *et al.* Efficacy and safety of tau-aggregation inhibitor therapy in patients with mild or moderate Alzheimer's disease: a randomised, controlled, double-blind, parallel-arm, phase 3 trial. Lancet 2016; 388(10062): 2873-84.
[http://dx.doi.org/10.1016/S0140-6736(16)31275-2] [PMID: 27863809]

[166] Wischik CM, Staff RT, Wischik DJ, *et al.* Tau aggregation inhibitor therapy: an exploratory phase 2 study in mild or moderate Alzheimer's disease. J Alzheimers Dis 2024; 41(4): 1145-58.
[PMID: 38995790]

[167] Wagner J, Ryazanov S, Leonov A, *et al.* Anle138b: a novel oligomer modulator for disease-modifying therapy of neurodegenerative diseases such as prion and Parkinson's disease. Acta Neuropathol 2013; 125(6): 795-813.
[http://dx.doi.org/10.1007/s00401-013-1114-9] [PMID: 23604588]

[168] Zhang CC, Xing A, Tan MS, Tan L, Yu JT. The role of MAPT in neurodegenerative diseases: Genetics, mechanisms and therapy. Mol Neurobiol 2016; 53(7): 4893-904.
[http://dx.doi.org/10.1007/s12035-015-9415-8] [PMID: 26363795]

[169] Haji S, Fujita K, Oki R, *et al.* An exploratory trial of EPI-589 in amyotrophic lateral sclerosis (EPIC-ALS): Protocol for a multicenter, open-labeled, 24-week, single-group study. JMIR Res Protoc 2023; 12: e42032.
[http://dx.doi.org/10.2196/42032] [PMID: 36716091]

[170] Willis BA, Lo AC, Dage JL, *et al.* Safety, tolerability, and pharmacokinetics of zagotenemab in participants with symptomatic alzheimer's disease: A phase I clinical trial. J Alzheimers Dis Rep 2023; 7(1): 1015-24.
[http://dx.doi.org/10.3233/ADR-230012] [PMID: 37849628]

[171] Mummery CJ, Börjesson-Hanson A, Blackburn DJ, *et al.* Tau-targeting antisense oligonucleotide $MAPT_{Rx}$ in mild Alzheimer's disease: a phase 1b, randomized, placebo-controlled trial. Nat Med 2023; 29(6): 1437-47.
[http://dx.doi.org/10.1038/s41591-023-02326-3] [PMID: 37095250]

[172] Novak P, Kovacech B, Katina S, *et al.* ADAMANT: a placebo-controlled randomized phase 2 study of AADvac1, an active immunotherapy against pathological tau in Alzheimer's disease. Nature Aging

2021; 1(6): 521-34.
[http://dx.doi.org/10.1038/s43587-021-00070-2] [PMID: 37117834]

[173] Wang X, Li W, Marcus J, *et al.* MK-8719, a novel and selective *O*-GlcNAcase inhibitor that reduces the formation of pathological tau and ameliorates neurodegeneration in a mouse model of tauopathy. J Pharmacol Exp Ther 2020; 374(2): 252-63.
[http://dx.doi.org/10.1124/jpet.120.266122] [PMID: 32493725]

[174] Cowan CM, Bossing T, Page A, Shepherd D, Mudher A. Soluble hyper-phosphorylated tau causes microtubule breakdown and functionally compromises normal tau *in vivo.* Acta Neuropathol 2010; 120(5): 593-604.
[http://dx.doi.org/10.1007/s00401-010-0716-8] [PMID: 20617325]

[175] Alavi Naini SM, Soussi-Yanicostas N. Tau hyperphosphorylation and oxidative stress, a critical vicious circle in neurodegenerative tauopathies? Oxid Med Cell Longev 2015; 2015: 1-17.
[http://dx.doi.org/10.1155/2015/151979] [PMID: 26576216]

[176] Basheer N, Smolek T, Hassan I, *et al.* Does modulation of tau hyperphosphorylation represent a reasonable therapeutic strategy for Alzheimer's disease? From preclinical studies to the clinical trials. Mol Psychiatry 2023; 28(6): 2197-214.
[http://dx.doi.org/10.1038/s41380-023-02113-z] [PMID: 37264120]

[177] Trushina NI, Bakota L, Mulkidjanian AY, Brandt R. The evolution of tau phosphorylation and interactions. Front Aging Neurosci 2019; 11: 256.
[http://dx.doi.org/10.3389/fnagi.2019.00256] [PMID: 31619983]

[178] Do Carmo S, Kautzmann MAI, Bhattacharjee S, *et al.* Differential effect of an evolving amyloid and tau pathology on brain phospholipids and bioactive lipid mediators in rat models of Alzheimer-like pathology. J Neuroinflammation 2024; 21(1): 185.
[http://dx.doi.org/10.1186/s12974-024-03184-7] [PMID: 39080670]

[179] Martínez-González L, Gonzalo-Consuegra C, Gómez-Almería M, *et al.* Tideglusib, a non-ATP competitive inhibitor of GSK-3β as a drug candidate for the treatment of amyotrophic lateral sclerosis. Int J Mol Sci 2021; 22(16): 8975.
[http://dx.doi.org/10.3390/ijms22168975] [PMID: 34445680]

[180] Forlenza OV, Diniz BS, Radanovic M, Santos FS, Talib LL, Gattaz WF. Disease-modifying properties of long-term lithium treatment for amnestic mild cognitive impairment: randomised controlled trial. Br J Psychiatry 2011; 198(5): 351-6.
[http://dx.doi.org/10.1192/bjp.bp.110.080044] [PMID: 21525519]

[181] Hirokawa T, Horie T, Fukiyama Y, *et al.* Roscovitine, a cyclin-dependent kinase-5 inhibitor, decreases phosphorylated tau formation and death of retinal ganglion cells of rats after optic nerve crush. Int J Mol Sci 2021; 22(15): 8096.
[http://dx.doi.org/10.3390/ijms22158096] [PMID: 34360858]

[182] van Eersel J, Ke YD, Liu X, *et al.* Sodium selenate mitigates tau pathology, neurodegeneration, and functional deficits in Alzheimer's disease models. Proc Natl Acad Sci USA 2010; 107(31): 13888-93.
[http://dx.doi.org/10.1073/pnas.1009038107] [PMID: 20643941]

[183] Luo W, Dou F, Rodina A, *et al.* Roles of heat-shock protein 90 in maintaining and facilitating the neurodegenerative phenotype in tauopathies. Proc Natl Acad Sci USA 2007; 104(22): 9511-6.
[http://dx.doi.org/10.1073/pnas.0701055104] [PMID: 17517623]

[184] Dickey CA, Kamal A, Lundgren K, *et al.* The high-affinity HSP90-CHIP complex recognizes and selectively degrades phosphorylated tau client proteins. J Clin Invest 2007; 117(3): 648-58.
[http://dx.doi.org/10.1172/JCI29715] [PMID: 17304350]

[185] Younas, N., Saleem, T., Younas, A. *et al.*, Nuclear face of Tau: an inside player in neurodegeneration. acta neuropatholcommun 11.2023; 196.

[186] Ballatore C, Lee VMY, Trojanowski JQ. Tau-mediated neurodegeneration in Alzheimer's disease and

related disorders. Nat Rev Neurosci 2007; 8(9): 663-72.
[http://dx.doi.org/10.1038/nrn2194] [PMID: 17684513]

[187] Barbier P, Zejneli O, Martinho M, *et al.*, Role of tau as a microtubule-associated protein: Structural and functional aspects. Front Aging Neurosci 2019; 11: 204.
[http://dx.doi.org/10.3389/fnagi.2019.00204] [PMID: 31447664]

[188] Varidaki A, Hong Y, Coffey ET. Repositioning microtubule stabilizing drugs for brain disorders. Front Cell Neurosci 2018; 12: 226.
[http://dx.doi.org/10.3389/fncel.2018.00226] [PMID: 30135644]

[189] Cross DJ, Huber BR, Silverman MA, *et al.* Intranasal paclitaxel alters alzheimer's disease phenotypic features in 3xTg-AD mice. J Alzheimers Dis 2021; 83(1): 379-94.
[http://dx.doi.org/10.3233/JAD-210109] [PMID: 34308901]

[190] Brunden KR, Zhang B, Carroll J, *et al.* Epothilone D improves microtubule density, axonal integrity, and cognition in a transgenic mouse model of tauopathy. J Neurosci 2010; 30(41): 13861-6.
[http://dx.doi.org/10.1523/JNEUROSCI.3059-10.2010] [PMID: 20943926]

[191] Tsai RM, Miller Z, Koestler M, *et al.* Reactions to multiple ascending doses of the microtubule stabilizer TPI-287 in patients with alzheimer disease, progressive supranuclear palsy, and corticobasal syndrome. JAMA Neurol 2020; 77(2): 215-24.
[http://dx.doi.org/10.1001/jamaneurol.2019.3812] [PMID: 31710340]

[192] Kabir MT, Uddin MS, Jeandet P, *et al.* Anti-alzheimer's molecules derived from marine life: Understanding molecular mechanisms and therapeutic potential. Mar Drugs 2021; 19(5): 251.
[http://dx.doi.org/10.3390/md19050251] [PMID: 33925063]

[193] Altinoz MA, Guloksuz S, Ozpinar A. Immunomodifying and neuroprotective effects of noscapine: Implications for multiple sclerosis, neurodegenerative, and psychiatric disorders. Chem Biol Interact 2022; 352: 109794.
[http://dx.doi.org/10.1016/j.cbi.2021.109794] [PMID: 34963564]

[194] Alanazi FK, Radwan AA, Aou-Auda H. Molecular scaffold and biological activities of anti-Alzheimer agents. Trop J Pharm Res 2022; 21(2): 439-51.
[http://dx.doi.org/10.4314/tjpr.v21i2.30]

[195] Ringman JM, Frautschy SA, Teng E, *et al.* Oral curcumin for Alzheimer's disease: tolerability and efficacy in a 24-week randomized, double blind, placebo-controlled study. Alzheimers Res Ther 2012; 4(5): 43.
[http://dx.doi.org/10.1186/alzrt146] [PMID: 23107780]

[196] Azargoonjahromi A, Abutalebian F. Unraveling the therapeutic efficacy of resveratrol in Alzheimer's disease: an umbrella review of systematic evidence. Nutr Metab (Lond) 2024; 21(1): 15.
[http://dx.doi.org/10.1186/s12986-024-00792-1] [PMID: 38504306]

[197] Bahn G, Jo DG. Therapeutic approaches to alzheimer's disease through modulation of NRF2. Neuromolecular Med 2019; 21(1): 1-11.
[http://dx.doi.org/10.1007/s12017-018-08523-5] [PMID: 30617737]

[198] Howard R, Zubko O, Bradley R, *et al.* Minocycline at 2 different dosages *vs* placebo for patients with mild alzheimer disease. JAMA Neurol 2020; 77(2): 164-74.
[http://dx.doi.org/10.1001/jamaneurol.2019.3762] [PMID: 31738372]

[199] Li X, Sun Y, Zhou Z, *et al.* Deep learning-driven exploration of pyrroloquinoline quinone neuroprotective activity in alzheimer's disease. Adv Sci (Weinh) 2024; 11(18): 2308970.
[http://dx.doi.org/10.1002/advs.202308970] [PMID: 38454653]

[200] Bargagna B, Ciccone L, Nencetti S, *et al.* Multifunctional small molecules as potential anti-alzheimer's disease agents. Molecules 2021; 26(19): 6015.
[http://dx.doi.org/10.3390/molecules26196015] [PMID: 34641559]

[201] Kassab AE, Gedawy EM, Sayed AS. Fused thiophene as a privileged scaffold: A review on anti-

Alzheimer's disease potentials *via* targeting cholinesterases, monoamine oxidases, glycogen synthase kinase-3, and Aβ aggregation. Int J Biol Macromol 2024; 265(Pt 2): 131018. [http://dx.doi.org/10.1016/j.ijbiomac.2024.131018] [PMID: 38518928]

[202] Tumiatti V, Minarini A, Bolognesi ML, Milelli A, Rosini M, Melchiorre C. Tacrine derivatives and Alzheimer's disease. Curr Med Chem 2010; 17(17): 1825-38. [http://dx.doi.org/10.2174/092986710791111206] [PMID: 20345341]

[203] Remya C, Dileep KV, Koti Reddy E, *et al.* Neuroprotective derivatives of tacrine that target NMDA receptor and acetyl cholinesterase – Design, synthesis and biological evaluation. Comput Struct Biotechnol J 2021; 19: 4517-37. [http://dx.doi.org/10.1016/j.csbj.2021.07.041] [PMID: 34471497]

[204] Eghtedari M, Sarrafi Y, Nadri H, *et al.* New tacrine-derived AChE/BuChE inhibitors: Synthesis and biological evaluation of 5-amino-2-phenyl-4H-pyrano[2,3-b]quinoline-3-carboxylates. Eur J Med Chem 2017; 128: 237-46. [http://dx.doi.org/10.1016/j.ejmech.2017.01.042] [PMID: 28189905]

[205] Szymański P, Skibiński R, Inglot T, *et al.* New tacrine analogs as acetylcholinesterase inhibitors - theoretical study with chemometric analysis. Molecules 2013; 18(3): 2878-94. [http://dx.doi.org/10.3390/molecules18032878] [PMID: 23459299]

[206] Milelli A, De Simone A, Ticchi N, *et al.* Tacrine-based multifunctional agents in Alzheimer's disease: an old story in continuous development§. Curr Med Chem 2017; 24(32): 3522-46. [PMID: 28294041]

[207] Sabolová D, Kristian P, Kožurková M. Multifunctional properties of novel tacrine congeners: cholinesterase inhibition and cytotoxic activity. J Appl Toxicol 2018; 38(11): 1377-87. [http://dx.doi.org/10.1002/jat.3622] [PMID: 29624715]

[208] Mitra S, Muni M, Shawon NJ, *et al.* Tacrine derivatives in neurological disorders: Focus on molecular mechanisms and neurotherapeutic potential. Oxid Med Cell Longev 2022; 2022(1): 7252882. [http://dx.doi.org/10.1155/2022/7252882] [PMID: 36035218]

[209] Cacabelos R. Donepezil in Alzheimer's disease: From conventional trials to pharmacogenetics. Neuropsychiatr Dis Treat 2007; 3(3): 303-33. [PMID: 19300564]

[210] Silva MA, Kiametis AS, Treptow W. Donepezil inhibits acetylcholinesterase *via* multiple binding modes at room temperature. J Chem Inf Model 2020; 60(7): 3463-71. [http://dx.doi.org/10.1021/acs.jcim.9b01073] [PMID: 32096991]

[211] Brewster JT II, Dell'Acqua S, Thach DQ, Sessler JL. Classics in chemical neuroscience: Donepezil. ACS Chem Neurosci 2019; 10(1): 155-67. [http://dx.doi.org/10.1021/acschemneuro.8b00517] [PMID: 30372021]

[212] Moreira NCS, Lima JEBF, Marchiori MF, Carvalho I, Sakamoto-Hojo ET. Neuroprotective effects of cholinesterase inhibitors: current scenario in therapies for Alzheimer's disease and future perspectives. J Alzheimers Dis Rep 2022; 6(1): 177-93. [http://dx.doi.org/10.3233/ADR-210061] [PMID: 35591949]

[213] Kandiah N, Pai MC, Senanarong V, *et al.* Rivastigmine: the advantages of dual inhibition of acetylcholinesterase and butyrylcholinesterase and its role in subcortical vascular dementia and Parkinson's disease dementia. Clin Interv Aging 2017; 12: 697-707. [http://dx.doi.org/10.2147/CIA.S129145] [PMID: 28458525]

[214] Onor ML, Trevisiol M, Aguglia E. Rivastigmine in the treatment of Alzheimer's disease: an update. Clin Interv Aging 2007; 2(1): 17-32. [http://dx.doi.org/10.2147/ciia.2007.2.1.17] [PMID: 18044073]

[215] Szeto JY, Lewis SJ. JG Lewis S. Current treatment options for Alzheimer's disease and Parkinson's disease dementia. Curr Neuropharmacol 2016; 14(4): 326-38.

[http://dx.doi.org/10.2174/1570159X14666151208112754] [PMID: 26644155]

[216] Marucci G, Buccioni M, Ben DD, Lambertucci C, Volpini R, Amenta F. Efficacy of acetylcholinesterase inhibitors in Alzheimer's disease. Neuropharmacology 2021; 190: 108352. [http://dx.doi.org/10.1016/j.neuropharm.2020.108352] [PMID: 33035532]

[217] Colović MB, Krstić DZ, Lazarević-Pašti TD, Bondžić AM, Vasić VM. Acetylcholinesterase inhibitors: pharmacology and toxicology. Curr Neuropharmacol 2013; 11(3): 315-35. [http://dx.doi.org/10.2174/1570159X11311030006] [PMID: 24179466]

[218] Seltzer B. Galantamine-ER for the treatment of mild-to-moderate Alzheimer's disease. Clin Interv Aging 2010; 5: 1-6.
[PMID: 20169037]

[219] Falvey A, Palandira SP, Chaudhry S, *et al.*, The cholinergic drug galantamine ameliorates acute and subacute peripheral and brain manifestations of acute respiratory distress syndrome in mice. Sci Rep 2025; 15: 33217.
[http://dx.doi.org/10.1038/s41598-025-18542-5]

[220] Zhou B, Hu B. Anti-inflammatory effect of curcumin on neurological disorders: a narrative review. Front Pharmacol 2025; 16: 1658115.
[http://dx.doi.org/10.3389/fphar.2025.1658115] [PMID: 41132526]

[221] dos Santos MG, da Luz DB, de Miranda FB, *et al.*, Resveratrol and neuroinflammation: total-scale analysis of the scientific literature. Nutraceuticals 2024; 4(2): 165-180.
[http://dx.doi.org/10.3390/nutraceuticals4020011]

[222] Birks JS, Harvey RJ. Donepezil for dementia due to Alzheimer's disease. Cochrane Libr 2018; 2018(6): CD001190.
[http://dx.doi.org/10.1002/14651858.CD001190.pub3] [PMID: 29923184]

[223] Athar T, Al Balushi K, Khan SA. Recent advances on drug development and emerging therapeutic agents for Alzheimer's disease. Mol Biol Rep 2021; 48(7): 5629-45.
[http://dx.doi.org/10.1007/s11033-021-06512-9] [PMID: 34181171]

[224] Li T, Martin E, Abada Y, *et al.* Effects of chronic masitinib treatment in APPswe/PSEN1dE9 transgenic mice modeling alzheimer's disease. J Alzheimers Dis 2020; 76(4): 1339-45.
[http://dx.doi.org/10.3233/JAD-200466] [PMID: 32623401]

[225] Piette F, Belmin J, Vincent H, *et al.* Masitinib as an adjunct therapy for mild-to-moderate Alzheimer's disease: a randomised, placebo-controlled phase 2 trial. Alzheimers Res Ther 2011; 3(2): 16.
[http://dx.doi.org/10.1186/alzrt75] [PMID: 21504563]

[226] Geldmacher DS, Fritsch T, McClendon MJ, Landreth G. A randomized pilot clinical trial of the safety of pioglitazone in treatment of patients with Alzheimer disease. Arch Neurol 2011; 68(1): 45-50.
[http://dx.doi.org/10.1001/archneurol.2010.229] [PMID: 20837824]

[227] Saunders AM, Burns DK, Gottschalk WK. Reassessment of pioglitazone for alzheimer's disease. Front Neurosci 2021; 15: 666958.
[http://dx.doi.org/10.3389/fnins.2021.666958] [PMID: 34220427]

[228] Burns DK, Alexander RC, Welsh-Bohmer KA, *et al.* Safety and efficacy of pioglitazone for the delay of cognitive impairment in people at risk of Alzheimer's disease (TOMMORROW): a prognostic biomarker study and a phase 3, randomised, double-blind, placebo-controlled trial. Lancet Neurol 2021; 20(7): 537-47.
[http://dx.doi.org/10.1016/S1474-4422(21)00043-0] [PMID: 34146512]

[229] Dailah HG. Potential of therapeutic small molecules in apoptosis regulation in the treatment of neurodegenerative diseases: An updated review. Molecules 2022; 27(21): 7207.
[http://dx.doi.org/10.3390/molecules27217207] [PMID: 36364033]

[230] Mattei D, Djodari-Irani A, Hadar R, et al. Minocycline rescues decrease in neurogenesis, increase in microglia cytokines and deficits in sensorimotor gating in an animal model of schizophrenia. Brain,

Behavior, and Immunity 2014; 38: 175-184.
[http://dx.doi.org/10.1016/j.bbi.2014.01.019]

[231] Yao W, Yang H, Yang J. Small-molecule drugs development for Alzheimer's disease. Front Aging Neurosci 2022; 14: 1019412.
[http://dx.doi.org/10.3389/fnagi.2022.1019412] [PMID: 36389082]

[232] Akhtar A, Gupta SM, Dwivedi S, Kumar D, Shaikh MF, Negi A. Preclinical models for alzheimer's disease: Past, present, and future approaches. ACS Omega 2022; 7(51): 47504-17.
[http://dx.doi.org/10.1021/acsomega.2c05609] [PMID: 36591205]

CHAPTER 11

New Insights into Drug Development and Immunotherapy for Alzheimer's Disease

Sakuntala Gayen[1], **Souvik Roy**[1,*], **Md Alfaj Uddin**[2] and **Dishani Sukul**[2]

[1] *Department of Pharmacy, NSHM Knowledge Campus Kolkata – Group of Institutions, Kolkata, West Bengal, India*

[2] *Department of Pharmaceutical Technology, Maulana Abul Kalam Azad University of Technology, Haringhata, West Bengal, India*

Abstract: Alzheimer's disease, the most prevalent form of dementia and a chronic neurodegenerative disorder, accounts for 60-80% of all cases, which poses a significant challenge to healthcare systems worldwide. According to the Global Burden of Disease Study, approximately 57.4 million people were living with dementia in 2019, a number projected to rise to 152.8 million in 2050. The underlying pathophysiology of AD includes the buildup of β-amyloid plaques outside cells and the formation of neurofibrillary tangles due to tau protein accumulation within cells. Acetylcholinesterase inhibitors and N-methyl-D-aspartate (NMDA) receptor antagonists are the main drugs used for diagnosis and treatment right now. Moreover, these treatments can temporarily mitigate dementia symptoms but do not halt disease progression or prevent symptom emergence. In this period, there is an urgent need for newer strategies to address AD effectively. Recently, immunotherapies have gained attention as a promising therapeutic avenue for treating AD by leveraging the immune system to downregulate several pathological protein expressions in the brain. In this review, we discuss the pathophysiological mechanisms of AD, newer strategies for drug development, and the potential of immunotherapies to prevent or manage AD.

Keywords: Alzheimer's disease, Current treatment strategies, Immunotherapy, Neurodegenerative disorder, Pathophysiology.

INTRODUCTION

Alzheimer's disease, a neurodegenerative disorder characterized by a progressive decline in cognitive function that mainly affects the elderly population globally, was expected to be the predominant form of dementia, and in 2025, it will affect more than 100 million people worldwide [1]. Therefore, the WHO classifies AD

* **Corresponding author Souvik Roy:** Department of Pharmacy, NSHM Knowledge Campus Kolkata – Group of Institutions, Kolkata, West Bengal, India E-mail: souvikroy35@gmail.com; souvik.roy@nshm.com

as a public health priority. The global burden of Alzheimer's disease is underscored by its escalating prevalence, incidence, and mortality rates that remain estimated due to the widespread underdiagnosis of AD [2]. Clinically, AD is characterized by progressive loss of memory and development of cognitive impairments. The mild cognitive impairment caused by AD can subsequently promote AD dementia, which estimates the etiology among patients at 40% to 75%, depending on the population studied and whether the diagnosis has been made clinically or in combination with biomarkers [3]. The epidemiological study of dementia and AD in Portugal stated that both occurrence and prevalence rates are dramatically increased with age, replicating tentatively every 5 years [4]. The risk of AD dementia is significantly escalated as cognitive function declines, commencing with normal cognition and no amyloid-beta accumulation, advancing to early neurodegenerative alterations, and eventually progressing to mild cognitive impairment (MCI). The pathogenesis of AD is typically characterized by the aberrant accumulation of toxic protein fragments in the nervous system, including β-amyloid deposition within senile plaques and outside neurons, intracellular accumulation of hyperphosphorylated tau protein associated with microtubules, oxidative stress, inflammation, and depletion of central cholinergic neurotransmitters [5, 6].

Numerous researchers have developed effective drug molecules that cure this fatal disease, but these investigations remain stopped due to their numerous adverse effects. Recently, there are five marketed drugs, including acetylcholinesterase (AChEIs) inhibitors—Donepezil, Tacrine, Rivastigmine, and Galantamine—and N-methyl-D-aspartate (NMDA) receptor antagonist Memantine, that have been approved by the Food and Drug Administration (FDA) for AD treatment. Moreover, these marketed drugs could substantially inhibit the progression of AD and alleviate symptoms, while they may not eventually cure the disease [7, 8]. Hence, there is an urgent need for the advancement of AD treatment, which can significantly prevent and downregulate AD progression. New drug development in AD is remarkable due to the growing global burden of the disease and the limited efficacy of existing therapies. As AD progresses, it leads to the deterioration of cognitive ability, memory loss, and subsequently death. Despite extensive research, most existing therapies exclusively manage symptoms without reversing the underlying neurodegeneration. The complexity of AD pathophysiology, including β-amyloid plaques, tau protein tangles, neuroinflammation, and synaptic dysfunction, requires the development of innovative therapeutic strategies for AD treatment [5]. Developing new drugs could address AD etiology and pathogenesis, which are comprehensive and multidimensional, essential to slowing disease progression, improving quality of life, and potentially offering a cure. Recent advances in precision medicine, biomarker identification, and neuroprotective strategies open new avenues for drug discovery. However, drug development in AD faces several challenges, including the high failure rate in clinical investigations due to the heterogeneity of the disease [9, 10]. Nonetheless, continued efforts in exploring novel targets, such as neuroinflammation, synaptic plasticity, and autophagy pathways, hold promise for transformative therapies that could address the unmet needs of AD patients.

Recently, immunotherapies have been at the forefront of controlling AD pathogenesis by immunological modification. Immunotherapy refers to the immunological arena, which primarily aims to identify target sites by activating, suppressing, and inducing immune responses [11]. Intriguingly, immunotherapy in AD management is a relatively novel strategy for non-infectious diseases. Currently, antibody-mediated passive immunotherapy that targets β-amyloid and tau proteins, aimed at obstructing β-amyloid peptide fibrillization and tau protein phosphorylation, and disrupting pre-existing fibrils, has become a dominant one in AD immunotherapy due to the repeated failures of active immunotherapy for AD [12, 13]. The most rational and safest strategies will focus on targeting toxic molecules without provoking an excessive immune response, thereby facilitating therapeutic benefits and improving the efficiency of clinical trial design. This review provides a concise overview of novel insights in drug development and encompasses immunotherapeutic strategies, including active and passive immunotherapy in AD management.

PATHOPHYSIOLOGY OF ALZHEIMER'S DISEASE

Despite the cumulative knowledge about the molecular, biochemical, and cellular mechanisms of the disease, the accurate etiology and pathogenesis of AD remain unclear. Therefore, the development of innovative, effective, disease-modifying drugs faces significant challenges. The pivotal pathological hallmarks are a significant accumulation of β-amyloid to form plaques, neurofibrillary tangles, and loss of neuronal function. Despite a genetic predisposition, several lines of evidence indicate that AD pathogenesis involves inflammation, gliosis, an imbalance in the production and clearance of reactive oxygen species (ROS), excessive metal ion accumulation, and mitochondrial dysfunction (Fig. **1**) [6, 14, 15]. The following discussion highlights the most relevant pathophysiology of AD and putative drug targets for the AD therapeutic arsenal.

β-amyloid Plaques

The proteolytic fragment of amyloid precursor protein (APP) cleavage produces -amyloid, a key factor of AD pathogenesis, and localizes it in the somatodendritic and axonal compartments of neurons, as highlighted by the -amyloid cascade [16]. APP is a single-pass type-I membrane protein, which consists of a single transmembrane domain with a large extracellular domain and a small cytoplasmic tail. The cleavage of APP in the extracellular domain can occur through two distinctive mechanisms, including amyloidogenic and non-amyloidogenic signaling pathways [17]. Primarily, α/β secretase has the credibility to cleave APP in the extracellular domain, producing soluble, membrane-tethered C-terminal fragments and ectodomains. Subsequently, γ-secretases are essential for the transmembrane cleavage of membrane-tethered C-terminal fragments and generating undistinguishable cytosolic polypeptides called APP intracellular domains. In a non-amyloidogenic signaling pathway, APP activities are involved with α-secretase enzyme, followed by γ-secretase action [18]. Initially, α-secretase breakdown encourages the production of soluble ectodomain APPα and C-terminal fragment α. Subsequently, the C-terminal fragment α can be cleaved by γ-secretase, which yields an APP fragment called p3, designated as a non-amyloidogenic protein deficient in pathological activities. Furthermore, the amyloidogenic pathway encompasses thc β-site APP cleaving enzyme 1 (BACE-1), β-secretase, followed by γ-secretase processing. Firstly, the APP cleaved by β-secretase forms the soluble ectodomain APPβ and the C-terminal fragment β. Then, the C-terminal fragment β is cleaved by γ-secretase at multiple sites, producing β-amyloid peptides [19, 20]. The β-amyloid peptides can often self-aggregate and significantly initiate neurotoxicity. Certainly, β-amyloid monomers are susceptible to oligomerization, aggregation into protofibrils and fibrils, whose toxicity is demonstrated by their ability to induce oxidative stress, modification of membrane permeability, mitochondrial dysfunction, synaptic dysfunction, and inflammation [21]. Additionally, β-amyloid proteins are also involved with channels, membrane proteins, and receptors, leading to impaired cellular signaling [22, 23].

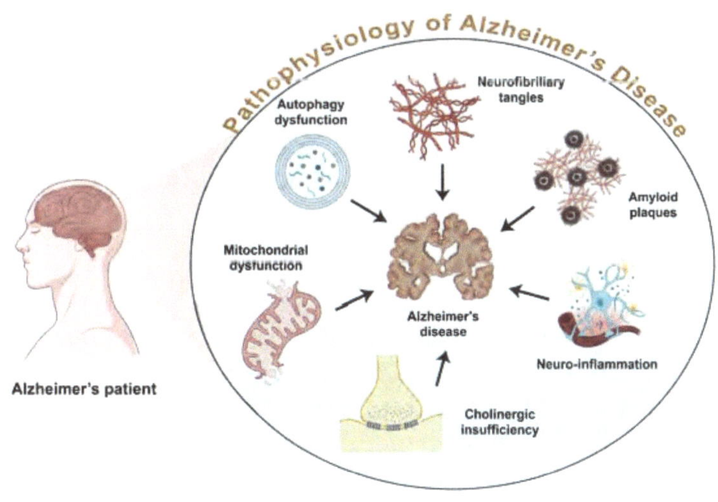

Fig. (1). Pathophysiology of Alzheimer's disease.

Hyperphosphorylation of Tau Proteins

The second most important histopathological feature of AD is the buildup of neurofibrillary tangles, which are made up of tau proteins clumped together inside neurons. The tau is a phosphoprotein, belonging to the microtubule-associated protein family, which is primarily found in axons and, to a lesser extent, in somatodendritic regions and glial cells [24, 25]. Tau protein is crucial for maintaining the stability and assembly of microtubules, thereby promoting axonal transport and dendritic structure [26, 27]. Moreover, its biological activities are directly associated with post-translational modifications, such as phosphorylation at multiple sites. The uncharacteristic phosphorylation of tau protein can reduce its affinity for microtubules, increasing the protein's tendency to form aggregates within the neurons. Thus, tau hyperphosphorylation damages its inherent effector functions, promoting downstream processes such as microtubule assembly, axonal trafficking, immature dendritic cells, loss of synapses, neuronal death, and ultimately contributing to dementia [28]. Likely, β-amyloid and prefibrillar accumulation are accountable for the tau-associated neurotoxicity. The phosphorylated tau accumulates to form oligomers, which further mature into paired helical and straight filaments [29, 30]. Multiple factors, including oxidative stress and disruption of calcium balance, contribute to the development of tau-associated toxicity [31]. Additionally, two chief influencers remain causes of the hyperphosphorylation of tau proteins: (i) conformational modifications of tau in AD-affected brains and an imbalance between the protein kinases and protein phosphorylation 1 (PP1) and 2A (PP2A) activities, whose joint balance actions maintain the normal phosphorylation state of tau proteins. Tau phosphorylation involves more than 30 serine/threonine residues in AD and associates with different kinases, including cyclin-dependent protein kinase 5 (cdk5), glycogen synthase kinase 3 (GSK-3), calcium- and calmodulin-dependent protein kinase II (CaMKII), and protein kinase A (PKA) [32, 33]. In AD, the serine-threonine kinase GSK-3 isoform β (GSK-3β) plays an essential intermediary role to enhance tau hyperphosphorylation. The dephosphorylation of tau, facilitated by PP1 and PP2A, restores abnormal tau to its normal state [34].

Oxidative Stress

Oxidative stress is caused by an imbalance between the production and elimination of oxidants, followed by an ineffective action of the antioxidants. Therefore, the increased levels of accretion of reactive species originated from the nitrogen and oxygen. On the other hand, oxidative stress has been generated due to the oxidative modification of proteins, nucleic acids, and lipids (lipid peroxidation). Reactive species are produced both endogenously, through molecular oxygen metabolism and cellular signaling, and in response to exogenous stimuli, and play a pivotal role in maintaining biological functions [35]. They are responsible for adjusting cellular homeostasis to regulate apoptosis, particularly through their involvement in receptor-associated signaling pathways. Reactive oxygen species include hydroxyl radical, hydrogen peroxide, superoxide anion radical, singlet oxygen, peroxide, hydroxide ion, and hydroperoxyl radical, while nitrogen-containing oxidants include nitric oxide, nitrogen dioxide, and peroxynitrite [36, 37]. In addition, nicotinamide adenine dinucleotide phosphate (NADPH) oxidase, transferring electrons to oxygen from NADPH, enhances the generation of superoxide anion radicals, an essential origin for intracellular ROS formation [38, 39]. Moreover, oxidants can significantly contribute to disease progression and exacerbation of its symptoms through direct and indirect transduction mechanisms. Indeed, reactive species can directly divert cellular functions, which augments cell death. Circuitously, this species acts as a second messenger; for example, H2O2 can disrupt redox mechanisms and affect typical biological functions by altering protein expression and mitochondrial function, thereby triggering inflammatory responses, apoptosis, and autophagy [40, 41]. Oxidative stress is closely associated with inducing neurodegeneration in AD *via* addressing four major features: (i) β-amyloid generation and accumulation; (ii) microglia stimulation; (iii) redox-active metal ion deregulation; and (iv) mitochondrial deregulation [42, 43].

Several studies have demonstrated that reactive species are involved in the development of senile plaques due to the inhibition of α-secretase activity while increasing β- and γ-secretase activities [44]. In addition, oligomeric accumulation also raises oxidant levels, as it has been anticipated that β-amyloid is able to initiate a concentration-dependent accumulation of reactive species and activate NADPH oxidase [45]. Moreover, oxidant species may stimulate the transcription of pro-inflammatory genes in both astrocytes and microglia. The stimulated microglial cells can encourage the production of both oxidants and pro-inflammatory cytokines, including interleukin-1β (IL-1β), IL-6, and tumor necrosis factor-α (TNF-α), which favor β-amyloid production and accumulation, thus facilitating inflammatory responses in AD brains [46, 47]. The production of inflammatory mediators, followed by microglia activation, could also promote reactive astrocytosis, facilitating a secondary inflammatory response. Astrocytes communicate with neurons to support neurotransmitter function, regulate blood flow, and facilitate the formation and maturation of synapses [48]. Nevertheless, in AD, reactive astrocytes play a crucial role in neuroinflammation and the production of ROS and RNS, which can accelerate the development of neurodegeneration and neuropathological disorders [49]. Numerous studies have enlightened the role of reactive astrocytes in the formation of β-amyloid plaques for AD pathology. Due to the activation of both microglia and astrocytes by oxidative stress, as a result of significant loss of synaptic function, enhanced tau pathology by the upsurge of kinase-mediated hyperphosphorylation of tau contributes to the formation and accumulation of β-amyloid and releases pro-inflammatory cytokines, thus augmenting neuronal death through apoptosis [50, 51]. Hence, the accumulated evidence suggests that astrocytes are emerging as a putative therapeutic target for developing new treatment strategies to alleviate neurodegenerative diseases.

Ferroptosis

As the most abundantly produced redox-active metal in the human body, Fe generation and accumulation in the brain are hallmarks for the development of neurodegenerative disorders. In AD, Fe accumulation facilitates ROS generation, increasing β-amyloid aggregation and oligomerization, and hyperphosphorylation and aggregation of tau protein, thus inducing cellular damage. All these mechanistic reactions are mainly promoted by Fenton chemistry [6, 52]. Lately, Fe activity has been attributed to a new form of programmed cell death named ferroptosis. Ferroptosis is a form of iron-dependent cell death induced through oxidative stress that can be frequently promoted by the deactivation of the antioxidant GSH-dependent pathway, thus enhancing the accumulation of toxic lipid-ROS. Indeed, the cells became more prone to inducing ferroptotic cell death *via* an increment of lipid-ROS production [53, 54]. The morphological and biochemical characteristics of ferroptosis diverge from those of apoptosis, necrosis, and autophagy. The three important hallmarks are attributed to ferroptotic cell death, such as (i) iron-dependent peroxidation enzymes like CYP450 and lipoxygenases, and labile redox-active Fe contributes to catalyze the peroxidation of polyunsaturated fatty acids, producing lipid peroxyl radicals; (ii) ferroptosis is driven through peroxidation of phospholipids with polyunsaturated fatty acids; and (iii) decrease lipid-ROS clearance, promoting lipid oxidative stress by the inactivation of GSH-glutathione peroxidase 4 (GPX4) enzyme activity. GPX4 utilizes GSH to regulate downstream lipid peroxidation in the cell membranes [55, 56]. Furthermore, a significant level of labile Fe(II) promotes non-enzymatic lipid peroxidation by the Fenton reaction, which enhances excessive ROS generation and augments ferroptosis. The synthesis of the tripeptide GSH plays a vital role in regulating GPX4 activity, which is essential for providing a safeguard for cells from this programmed cell death. This antiporter system, Xc-, encourages glutamate and cysteine exchange, participating in the biosynthesis of GSH by providing increased levels of cysteine, an amino acid utilized for GSH biosynthesis. Conversely, dysregulation of this antiporter system leads to GSH depletion, thereby suppressing GPX4-dependent ferroptotic cell death [57 - 59]. Ferroptosis-mediated cell death can be abrogated through the activation of iron chelation and antioxidant levels, facilitating the downregulation of ferroptosis *via* iron as well as lipid-ROS-dependent cell death. Several studies have identified cellular mechanisms underlying the storage and uptake of iron, a fundamental regulator of ferroptosis [60, 61]. The higher level of iron uptake caused the reduction of storage, or even deregulation of its regulatory pathways, which could mitigate ferroptotic cell death. Indeed, lipid peroxidation, decreased levels of GSH, and iron overload have been substantially observed in the brains of AD patients [62]. Therefore, the inhibition of ferroptosis has emerged as a potential therapeutic approach for managing AD pathogenesis.

Apolipoprotein E-epsilon 4 (APOE-ε4)

APOE-ε4 genotype has been identified as another reason for the development of late-onset AD, which demonstrates the synergistic action of APOE-ε4 with inflammation and vascular factors, suggesting a possible mechanistic pathway for AD progression [63]. The APOE gene in humans consists of three isoforms, including APOE2, APOE3, and APOE4, with corresponding proteins. The expression of the APOE4 allele is the primary genetic risk factor for AD, and higher polygenic scores for cognitive impairment in older people [64, 65].

Triggering Receptor Expressed on Myeloid Cells 2 (TREM2)

TREM2, a biomarker of microglial inflammatory cells, is a crucial factor for AD progression. The soluble TREM2 (sTREM2) secretion is dependent upon the microglial stimulation; consequently, the elevated level of sTREM2 found in the CSF of AD patients is facilitating APOE4-mediated downstream stimulation of microglia [66]. TREM2 can also activate microglia and promote clustering surrounding β-amyloid and neurofibrillary tangles (NFTs), thus enhancing amyloid uptake, plaque compaction, and phagocytic activity in the primary stage of AD [67, 68].

ROLE OF THE IMMUNE SYSTEM IN ALZHEIMER'S DISEASE

The adaptive immune system is the fundamental regulator for the manifestation and progression of AD pathophysiology. Notably, T-lymphocytes and glial cells are key influencers for neuroinflammation and neuronal destruction [69]. Astroglia and microglia are the brain-resident immune cells that regulate neuroinflammatory responses in AD. Microglia are the chief immune regulator in the CNS, functioning both as antigen-presenting cells (APCs) and phagocytes [70]; however, their role in the clearance of β-amyloid after activation remains unclear. Recently, the advancements in neuroinflammation studies have led to the discovery of numerous inflammatory signaling pathways controlling several cerebral diseases, like the 5-lipoxygenase (ALOX5) pathway [71].

The brain lymphatic system transports immune cells from CSF and connects to the deep cervical lymph nodes, allowing peripheral T-lymphocytes to generate responses in response to brain antigens. The accumulation of both CD8+ effector T-lymphocytes and CD4+ helperT-lymphocytes in the brains of AD patients plays a vital role in the occurrence and progression of the disease. Unlike peripheral mechanisms, the primary APCs in AD are microglial cells, which exhibit elevated expression of genes and markers linked to the T-lymphocyte interactions [72, 73]. There seems to be a reduction of natural immunosuppressive mechanisms linked to AD, with temporary depletion of Foxp3+ regulatory T-cells affecting the choroid plexus. This depletion is followed by the recruitment of immunoregulatory cells, including monocyte-derived macrophages and regulatory T-cells, to the cerebral regions of the brain where plaque pathology is present [74]. In aging, these regulatory and effector functions of lymphocytes have been modified, and other immune manifestations encourage the AD progression [75]. Neurodegeneration, along with concurrent association of the peripheral immune systems in AD patients, has been demonstrated to stimulate leukocyte proliferation and telomere shortening [76].

In neuroinflammation, microglia and astrocytes elicit multiple roles in brain tissues *via* cytokine activity, an important aspect for AD pathophysiology that requires substantial management. When microglia are activated, and astrocytes detect cell death, they release pro-inflammatory cytokines into the extracellular environment and trigger various biological responses [77, 78]. TNF-α is an extremely prolific cytokine in the pathogenesis of AD. For instance, the increased levels of TNF-α with excessive cognitive decline have been identified in the brain tissues of the transgenic AD mice model [79]. Additionally, the downstream tumor necrosis factor receptor 1 (TNFR1) gene expression in transgenic AD mice displayed a depletion of β-amyloid accumulation, BACE1 expression, plaque load, and cognitive impairments [80]. A lot of research has shown that TNF-α is directly linked to the removal of β-amyloid deposits by microglia. Other cytokines, such as interleukin (IL)-1α, IL-6, IL-12, and IL-23, play a substantial role in neuroinflammation [81]. IL-1α causes amyloid precursor protein (APP) overexpression in the AD brain as compared with the healthy brain, which may make a loop of IL-1 secretion and APP synthesis [82, 83]. IL-6 contributes a pivotal role in AD. Although its exact effects are not yet fully understood, it is recognized for the enhancement of TNF-α expression and microglial stimulation. However, the inhibition of IL-6 activation can significantly improve hippocampal and long-term memory function [84]. Additionally, IL-12/IL-23-mediated signaling pathways could deplete AD pathogenesis and cognitive impairment. It is not yet evidenced, but the exclusion of p40 subunit from IL-12/IL-23 pathways has been demonstrated to reduce the proportion of soluble β-amyloid and improve cognitive functionality in the AD mice model [85, 86].

CURRENT TREATMENT STRATEGIES

ACE Inhibitors' Effects on Alzheimer's Disease Pathogenesis

There is a lot of preclinical and clinical evidence supporting that ACE-mediated hypertension can cause cognitive impairment. Disruptions to the blood-brain barrier and certain neurovascular structures lead to increased oxidative stress and neuroinflammation [87]. These conditions exacerbate cognitive impairment. The fact that stroke and hypertension both have significant impacts on cerebral circulation adds credence to the risk of dementia [88, 89]. ACEIs, especially captopril and perindopril, seem to play a role in decreasing Ang II production in both the brain and the rest of the body. This phenomenon has also been observed in clinical trials, where male patients treated with captopril for 24 weeks showed improvements in cognitive function and reduced blood pressure [89]. However, propranolol did not have the same effect on patients. By stopping brain RAS, ACEI treatment has been shown to slow down the cognitive decline that comes with Alzheimer's disease (AD) and other neurodegenerative diseases [90, 91]. Based on preclinical data showing that ACEIs protected against neuronal damage in animal models of AD, researchers have examined ACEIs in Japanese people with AD and high blood pressure at the same time. When ACEIs crossed the blood-brain barrier (BBB), it was found that the correlation between brain RAS and neurodegenerative disorders had a beneficial effect on memory and learning processes. The inhibition of Ang II formation and cholinergic neurotransmission likely caused this improvement in cognitive functions [92, 93].

The degree of lipophilicity of these inhibitors determines whether or not they can cross the blood-brain barrier, and this affects their effectiveness. Captopril, for example, does not seem to dissolve well in lipids according to some research, but it does dissolve in cerebrospinal fluid (CSF) when given to mice and people, respectively. Other inhibitors that have affinity for the central nervous system (CNS) include enalapril, perindopril, and lisinopril. These inhibitors block the effects of brain RAS at this level, and in animal models of AD, enalapril and perindopril have been shown to have antioxidant activity by reducing ischemic brain oedema and preventing oxidative stress-induced cognitive impairment [94 - 96].

In a mouse model of AD dementia caused by intracerebroventricular streptozotocin, lisinopril reduces inflammation, reverses oxidative stress, boosts learning and memory, and raises cholinergic activity in the brain. Peroxisome proliferator-activated receptor-γ (PPAR-γ) regulation was linked to its beneficial effects [97]. According to a study by Thomas *et al.*, lisinopril improved learning and memory deficits and reduced climbing deficits in a Drosophila melanogaster model of AD. The fact that lisinopril significantly lowers reactive oxygen species (ROS) in the thoraces of AD flies after they were given the drug [98] could explain why it improves physical performance. Additionally, preclinical experiments in a mouse model of AD found that perindopril improved cognitive performance [99]. Table **1** compiles the preventive mechanisms of ACEIs during AD progression.

Table 1. Mechanisms of protection of ACEIs in AD prevention.

Mechanisms of ACEI Protection in the Prevention of AD	Defence Mechanism	Impact	Refs.
Cognitive decline	Suppression of brain RAS.	A reduction in ACE activity lessening of cognitive aging.	[90, 91]
Hypothesis Cholinergic	Inhibition of the production of Ang II MDA suppression leads to a reduction in oxidative stress at the brain level.	Enhancement of mental abilities → Avoidance of scopolamine-induced amnesia	[92, 93]
Aggregation of β-amyloid peptides	Neprilysin activity is increased.	A preference toward amplifying the degradation of Aβ.	[89]

In middle age, hypertension has been linked to mild cognitive impairment leading to dementia. Numerous preclinical research studies have examined the relationship between neurodegenerative susceptibility and hypertension. Neuroprotection was enhanced by ACEIs through Ang I/II inhibition. The favorable modulation of cognitive functioning by ACEIs has confirmed the relationship between RAS and dementia, as well as cognitive improvement. Furthermore, a rat model of the lipopolysaccharide (LPS)-induced neuroinflammation paradigm showed neurodegeneration. Also, taking perindopril by mouth for 15 days at a dose of 0.1 mg/kg body weight proved that Ang plays a part in LPS-induced neuroinflammation. This treatment worked, as shown by the noticeable improvement in cognitive skills (Table **2**) [91].

Table 2. ACEIs' influence on biological pathways for possible therapeutic insights in AD.

Compound	Impact on the Biological Channel	The Species and The Disease Model	Refs.
Captopril/ Perindopril	Reduced NO synthesis-induced prevention of neuroinflammation and neurodegeneration.	*In vitro* studies	[94]
Perindopril	Interfering with microglia and astrocytes.	*In vitro* studies	[94]
Enalapril	Suppression of the synthesis of neurotoxic Aβ linked to zinc (1-16).	*In vitro* studies	[94]

(Table 2) cont.....

Compound	Impact on the Biological Channel	The Species and The Disease Model	Refs.
Enalapril/ Perindopril	Activity of antioxidants → Reduction of ischemic brain swelling, preventing oxidative stress-induced cognitive impairment.	*In vivo* studies	[94-96]
Enalapril	Cortical cholinergic deficiency did not improve because of its poor BBB penetration.	*In vivo* studies	[94, 101]
Perindopril	Enhancement of mental abilities.	*In vivo* study	[99]
Perindopril	Remarkable enhancement of cognitive abilities.	Model of LPS-induced neuroinflammation in vivo	[91]
Ramipril Captopril	Preventing the decrease in cognitive abilities.	Scapolamine-induced dementia *in vivo* model	[100]
Lisinopril	Positive benefits on improving memory and learning, reducing oxidative stress, reducing inflammation, and modulating PPAR-γ.	An *in vivo* model of intracerebroventricular streptozotocin-induced AD dementia in mice.	[97]
Lisinopril	Improvement in the treatment of learning and memory deficiencies and climbing impairment → significant drop in ROS levels in AD flies' thoraces.	The Drosophila melanogaster model of AD was studied *in vivo.*	[98]
Captopril	Reduction in Ang II production in the brain as well as in the periphery enhancement of cognitive function.	Clinical trials: 24-week treatment for male patients	[89]

Patients with AD have been shown to have increased ACE activity, and the treatment of ACEIs that pass the blood-brain barrier can control the decrease in ACE activity levels, reducing the rate at which cognitive function declines [90]. *In-vitro* studies have demonstrated that perindopril can significantly interfere with astrocytes and microglia, thus reducing neuroinflammation and neurodegeneration caused by lesser NO production. There are concerns about how well enalapril works in *in-vivo* studies because it is hard for it to cross the blood-brain barrier. Not only that, but lab tests have shown that it stops the growth of zinc-bound A^2(1-16), which could lead to AD because it is neurotoxic [89]. Several preclinical studies have shown that ACEIs can stop amnesia caused by scopolamine by blocking angiotensin-converting enzyme. This lowers MDA levels and reduces oxidative stress in the brain [90]. Cholinergic neurotransmission plays a crucial role in cognition. Studies have shown that the administration of ramipril and captopril, due to their anticholinergic activities, can halt cognitive impairment in a mouse dementia model [100]. However, enalapril administration, due to its poor ability to cross the blood-brain barrier, did not restore the cortical cholinergic deficit [94, 101]. Still, clinical trials have shown that ACEIs only have limited benefits. For example, cognitive function only gets better during the first nine months of treatment and not after that [102].

Aβ: Amyloid beta; ACE: Angiotensin-converting enzyme; Ang I/II: Angiotensin I/II; MDA: Malondialdehyde; RAS: Renin-angiotensin system.

Clinical Evidence: ACE Inhibitors for Alzheimer's Disease

There has been conflicting evidence about the relationship between angiotensin-converting enzyme inhibitors (ACEIs) and cognitive impairment. It was found that ACEI exposure may decrease cognitive impairment and substantially lower the risk of dementia [103]. For instance, perindopril and captopril are two examples of ACEIs that can pass the blood-brain barrier (BBB), but imidapril and enalapril cannot [104 - 106]. But there was no discernible difference in cognitive results between centrally and non-centrally active ACEIs. One more thing that the Italian Longitudinal Study [107] found was that enalapril (alone or with lisinopril) lowered the risk of moderate cognitive impairment (MCI) compared to other blood pressure drugs. Ramipril did not improve the cognitive abilities of AD patients in a pilot study, but it did lower the activity of ACEI in the cerebrospinal fluid (CSF), which suggests that brain activity may be changed [108, 109]. Researchers have also created retrospective studies of patients using ACEIs to evaluate their effects on AD patients (Table **3**).

Table 3. Clinical data on the impact of ACEIs on the Alzheimer's disease model.

Study Design	Study Sample	Objectives	Results	Refs.
Retrospective Cohort Study	117 019 individuals with a single ACEI; - >66 years old	Analyze the usage of ACEIs that penetrate the BBB against those that do not penetrate the BBB in AD.	When compared to non-BBB-penetrating ACEIs, BBB-penetrating ACEIs did not show any correlation with cognitive deterioration within three years after index medication.	[108]
Case-control Study	Individuals aged 60 years or older who have been diagnosed with AD, VaD, or unspecified/other dementia.	Compare the AD risk for those on non-RAS antihypertensive medications.	Patients utilizing ACEIs 24% decreased chance of acquiring AD, respectively.	[110]
Post hoc analysis of the randomized controlled Ginkgo Evaluation of Memory Study (GEMS) trial	3069 individuals who were either 70 years of age or older and had normal cognitive function.	To determine the prevalence of AD among various users of antihypertensive medications.	ACEIs were linked to 50% decreased risk, respectively.	[111]

(Table 3) cont.....

Study Design	Study Sample	Objectives	Results	Refs.
Prospective cohort analysis	819 491 individuals who had cardiovascular disease; - older than 65 years	The risk of getting AD while using ARBs with lisinopril and other AHT	When combined with ACEIs, ARBs not only had additive effects but also a dose-response.	[112]
Four-year prospective multicentre cohort study with a biannual assessment	616 individuals with mild to moderate AD; -78 years old on average.	Find out if treating older persons with ADs with ACEIs results in less mental decline than treating them with other AHT or not at all.	Separating the lowering effect on blood pressure, ACEIs facilitated a slower pace of cognitive impairment in people with AD	[103]
Longitudinal data from a prospective multi-center, population-based cohort study	1054 individuals with a mean age of 75 years who were taking at least one AHT.	Determine if chronic exposure to ACEIs was linked to a decreased incidence of incident dementia or cognitive impairment in comparison to other AHT.	A 6-year exposure to ACEIs did not appear to be linked to a lower risk of dementia development; -ACEIs that penetrate the blood-brain barrier were linked to a 65% reduction in cognitive decline each year of exposure.	[106]
Longitudinal Study	1445 patients receiving hypertension treatment; ages ranged from 65 to 84	Determine if ACEIs lower the risk of MCI in people with cognitive normalcy.	There was no significant effect of ACEIs as a class on the incidence of MCI in hypertensive older adults; -Enalapril was linked to an 83% decreased chance of getting MCI and a 73% decreased risk when used in conjunction with Lisinopril.	[107]
Randomized, prospective, parallel group trial	162 subjects, aged 65 years or older, with mild to severe AD and hypertension	Determine if BBB-piercing ACEIs can reduce the rate of cognitive deterioration in people with mild-t--moderate AD who also have hypertension.	Patients with mild to severe AD may see a slower pace of deterioration while using BBB-penetrating ACEIs;	[105]
Observational study	406 individuals over 50 years old with mild to moderate AD	Compare the decrease rates between individuals with moderate AD using BBB-penetrating ACEIs and those who are not on BBB-penetrating ACEI treatment at this time;	Perindopril, in particular, and other BBB-penetrating ACEIs are linked to a lower rate of cognitive deterioration in persons with mild to moderate AD;	[104]

Antagonists of the N-methyl-d-aspartate Receptor (NMDAR)

NMDAR-mediated excitatory glutamatergic neurotransmission is essential for neuron survival and synaptic plasticity. But when NMDARs are highly activated, they cause excitotoxicity and cell death, which starts the pathophysiology of AD that is linked to neurodegeneration. The neurotransmitter glutamate controls the cationic channels known as NMDARs, which are crucial for learning, memory, synaptic integration, and excitatory transmission [113]. It has been said that Aβ initiates an NMDAR-mediated chain of events that prevent microglial recruitment of glutamates, alter glutamatergic neurotransmission, raise intracellular calcium as a neurotoxic mechanism, and alter the internalization of both NMDA and AMPA/kainate receptors [114, 115]. Therefore, NMDA receptor deactivation can lessen Aβ neurotoxicity. In 2003, researchers used memantine, a non-competitive, low-to-moderate potency NMDA receptor antagonist, to treat moderate to severe AD. A 24-week study in people with moderate to severe Alzheimer's disease found that memantine therapy had a significant effect on functional, global, and cognitive domains [116]. However, its effectiveness is still up for debate.

Targeting individual NMDAR subunits offers a potentially effective treatment for AD. By changing how active the GluN2A and GluN2B subunits are, it might be possible to lessen the negative effects of β-amyloid and get synapses working again. Researchers have shown that memantine and other drugs that stop too much NMDAR activity can help people with AD slow down the rate of cognitive loss. Still, the fact that NMDAR subunits play different roles in synaptic and extra-synaptic transmission and are involved in the production of β-amyloid makes it clear that we need more targeted treatments [117]. In order to treat AD and other neurodegenerative illnesses more effectively, future research will probably concentrate on creating medications that can specifically alter the activity of NMDAR subunits.

Several studies have implicated excitotoxicity as a key factor in the pathogenesis of most neurodegenerative disorders. This shows how important it may be to investigate NMDA receptor antagonists as a potential treatment for these conditions [118]. Researchers have investigated numerous NMDA antagonists as neuroprotective agents, but developing them into effective therapies remains challenging. A major hurdle is that blocking NMDA receptors can lead to side effects, such as cognitive impairment, hallucinations, and psychosis, due to the disruption of normal physiological function. Even with these problems, focusing on specific receptor subunits, especially the GluN2 subunit, offers hope for developing antagonists with fewer side effects [119]. Based on their binding sites, NMDA antagonists fall into three categories: competitive, non-competitive, and negative allosteric antagonists. Research into the molecular causes of neurodegenerative diseases led to the development of competitive NMDA receptor antagonists like D-CPP, D-AP5, and DCKA. These medicines change the structure of GluN1 or GluN2 subunits by focusing on their glycine or glutamate parts. This stops the ion channel pore from opening. Clinical studies have failed due to adverse effects such as drowsiness, disorientation, and hallucinations, despite their potential as neuroprotective and anticonvulsant drugs. No competitive antagonist has proven safe or effective in humans, and most struggle to cross the blood-brain barrier. While GluN1 antagonists show promise, additional research is necessary, especially to tackle conditions like Alzheimer's. Non-competitive NMDA receptor antagonists, such as PCP, MK-801, and ketamine, were developed to treat Alzheimer's disease (AD) by blocking calcium-mediated responses at the NMDA receptor's PCP site. Even though these drugs helped protect neurons, their strong binding affinity meant that their effects lasted for a long time, which led to side effects like psychosis and dopaminergic activation. These side effects have limited their clinical use in treating AD, despite their initial promise in targeting excitotoxicity associated with the disease. The discovery of memantine and amantadine as clinically tolerated non-competitive NMDA receptor antagonists offered new hope, particularly for treating neurodegenerative disorders like Alzheimer's. These drugs bind to NMDA receptors more quickly than MK-801, which means they have fewer side effects while still working when NMDA receptors are overactive [118, 120].

Current NMDA Receptor Antagonist: Memantine

El Lilly was the first to develop memantine, an amino-alkyl cyclohexane derivative (1-amino-3,5-dimethyladamantane). The FDA now approves and recommends memantine as a medication for treating average to severe AD symptoms. Its effectiveness has been demonstrated in numerous clinical trials, with small but statistically significant benefits [121 - 124]. Memantine has moderate efficacy but beneficial effects on behaviour, mood, cognition, and the ability to carry out everyday tasks in AD patients, according to several systematic reviews of randomized controlled trials [125 - 127]. However, the drug's mechanism of action in mild to moderate AD is still explicitly unknown. Notably, memantine does not exhibit the side effects typically associated with high-affinity NMDA blockers and appears to achieve its pharmacological effects in a clinically well-tolerated manner. The main side effects associated with memantine were rare and similar to placebo in trials that reported them. These included dizziness, sporadic restlessness/agitation, diarrhoea, ocular effects (cataracts, conjunctive inflammation), feeling dizzy, dyspnoea, confusion, fatigue, migraine, irritation, diarrhoea, and incontinence of urine [128, 129]. Based on the outcomes of fruitful clinical studies, memantine may potentially represent a valuable therapeutic approach for AD when used to modulate glutamatergic activity [130, 131].

Memantine has been shown to be safe and effective in placebo-controlled trials for people with mild to severe AD. It seems that memantine and other cholinesterase inhibitors work in different ways and are well tolerated together [132, 133]. Currently, the second-generation memantine derivatives are under development, which may even possess more neuroprotective qualities than memantine [134, 135].

THE CHALLENGES IN DRUG DEVELOPMENT STRATEGIES ALZHEIMER'S DISEASE

There have been numerous challenges in translating the preclinical success of NMDA receptor antagonists into clinical therapy for AD and other neurodegenerative illnesses. The brain's NMDA receptor activities are complicated, making it challenging to strike a balance between therapeutic benefits and preserving essential brain functioning. Their therapeutic usage has also been restricted by side effects, including psychosis, symptoms similar to schizophrenia, and disruption of dopaminergic transmission. Despite their success, medications like amantadine and memantine still have negative effects. Although there are few side effects and new allosteric modulators, such as ifenprodil, show promise with their low bioavailability and cross-reactivity with other receptors, such as serotonin and histamine [136, 137]. Due to the development of multiple serious side effects, there is a necessity to establish newer approaches for AD treatment.

Immunotherapies for AD

Currently, most drugs used to treat AD, like NMDA antagonists and cholinesterase inhibitors, only help with symptoms. They don't halt the disease progression from getting worse. Much more effort is required to establish newer therapeutic approaches for AD. To overcome such limitations, immunotherapies have emerged as one of the most promising approaches to halt or slow down the AD progression [138, 139]. Fortunately, several preclinical and clinical studies are ongoing that will open new avenues for unraveling disease mechanisms and developing treatment strategies for AD diagnosis and drug development. For example, immunotherapeutic approaches targeting β-amyloid and tau expression were initially thought to be very promising for treating people with Alzheimer's disease because they showed promising results in animal studies [140, 141]. Significant efforts have focused on developing multitarget immunotherapies for AD, optimizing antibody titers and epitopes, validating the immunization process using pharmacogenetic and pharmacogenomic methods, offering preventive treatment for genetically stratified patients in the pre-symptomatic phase, and establishing primary endpoints for prevention using objective, multifunctional biomarkers [142]. Researchers suggest that active immunization through vaccination and/or passive immunization with specific antibodies, which aims to enhance β-amyloid clearance, is promising, whereas focusing on targets beyond β-amyloid, such as tau proteins, is essential [143, 144]. Furthermore, microglia-based immunotherapeutic strategies targeting different immune cells, including CD38, toll-like receptors (TLRs), and triggering receptors expressed on myeloid cells 2 (TREM2), are being investigated as well [145]. Both active and passive immunotherapy for AD treatment have advantages. Active immunization by vaccination depends upon humoral and cellular immunity and the accumulation of endogenous antibodies. On the other hand, passive immunization with antibodies is thought to be a better and more effective way to treat older AD patients whose bodies no longer respond well to vaccines [146].

Active Vaccination for AD

Active vaccination strategies for AD aim to stimulate the immune system to recognize and target pathological proteins, such as β-amyloid and tau, that accumulate in the brain. This approach involves administering a vaccine containing a specific antigen, which prompts the body to develop antibodies to prevent the accumulation of these proteins (Fig. **2**) [147]. Consequently, one of the most studied antigens in AD vaccines is β-amyloid, as its deposition forms amyloid plaques, a hallmark of AD pathology. Early clinical trials have demonstrated that these vaccines can successfully activate immune responses and lower amyloid levels. However, challenges remain, including ensuring long-term safety, avoiding excessive inflammation, and achieving efficacy across diverse AD patient populations [148, 149]. Another strategy is tau-targeted vaccines, which aim to prevent the formation of neurofibrillary tangles [150, 151]. It has been reported that about 85% immunization against β-amyloid deposition and 15% against tau have been documented, while the FDA has not approved any AD vaccines to date [152]. A DNA vaccine targeting $A\beta_{42}$ trimers could pave the way for new options in preventing AD pathogenesis. AV-1959D is another DNA vaccine that targets N-terminal epitopes of β-amyloid antigen. It has been tested on mice, rabbits, and nonhuman primates, and it works in the AD mice model. Petrushina and colleagues conducted a study that revealed no short- or long-term adverse effects of repeated-dose safety assessments in mice. Consequently, researchers have observed an increase in anti-amyloid antibody levels over time [153]. Early studies using a conjugated $A\beta_{3\text{-}10}$ keyhole limpet hemocyanin vaccine showed a notable reduction in tau hyperphosphorylation, but this immunotherapy is not clinically effective when administered too late [154]. Other research groups have investigated the impact of combining systemic immunomodulators with influenza vaccines to enhance immune responses against amyloid plaques. Particularly, the blocking of PD-1/PD-L1 checkpoint interaction prevents T-cell apoptosis and exhaustion and leads to decreased AD pathology. When combined with an influenza vaccine, this therapy may activate two immune-boosting pathways, potentially benefiting patients. Using monocyte-derived macrophages to bring these cells to the CNS of the APP/PS1 mouse model has been shown to significantly reduce cognitive impairment and β-amyloid deposition [155, 156]. Recently, Y-5A15, a vaccine produced by genetically altering yeast cells to express $A\beta_{1-15}$ on their cell surface, has been shown to improve cognitive function, reduce β-amyloid plaque formation, and attenuate neuronal damage in animal models [157]. Accumulating evidence suggests that active vaccination holds promise as a potential therapeutic to obstruct AD progression; however, additional clinical studies are needed to optimize the efficacy and safety of these treatments.

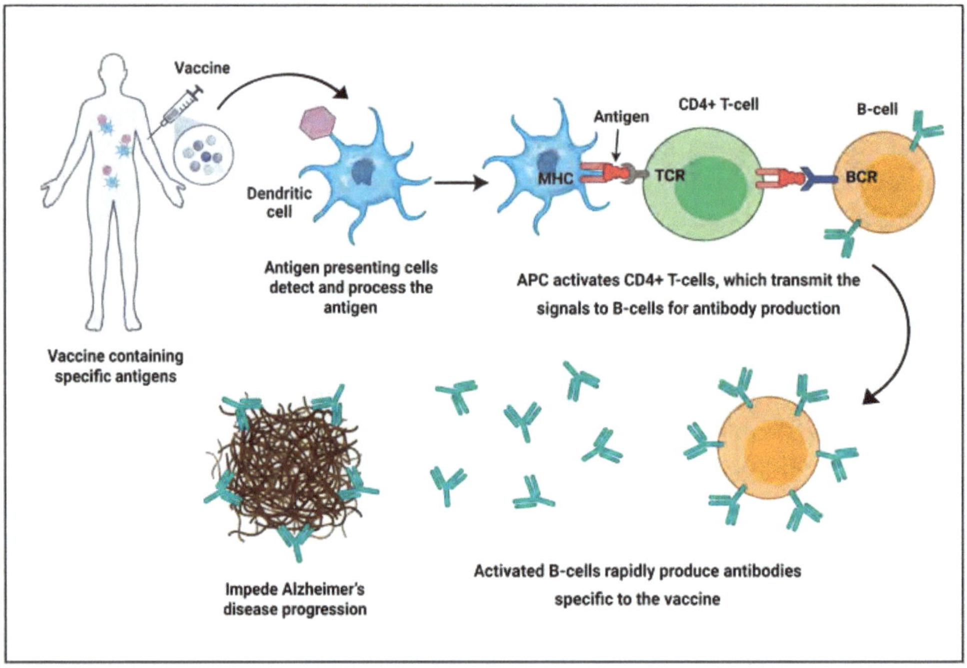

Fig. (2). Active immunization against Alzheimer's disease.

Antibodies for AD

In early clinical studies of AD patients, treatment with anti-amyloid antibodies reduced the buildup of plaques. This suggests that passive immunotherapy warrants significant attention as a means to change the course of the disease [158 - 160]. The FDA recently approved aducanumab, a monoclonal antibody (mAb) targeting β-amyloid for AD. This drug shows promise for reducing β-amyloid levels in AD patients [161]. Single-chain fragment variables (scFvs), which are composed of antibody light- and heavy-chain variable regions, have shown great promise for treating AD [162]. Passive immunotherapy involves monoclonal antibodies (mAbs) targeting β-amyloid and is currently in the advanced stages of clinical development (Fig. **3**). Solanezumab and bapineuzumab potentially target the N-terminal and mid-domain of β-amyloid, but these mAbs are unsuccessful in providing therapeutic effects in cognition and daily living activities in phase III clinical studies. Notably, solanezumab, bapineuzumab, gantenerumab, and crenezumab were discontinued following phase-III clinical trials due to their failure to improve cognitive function [163, 164]. Additionally, BAN2401, which is also known as Lecanemab, went through a phase-III clinical study in July 2020. The results showed that it prevented β-amyloid from clumping and provided patients with AD greater clinical benefits [165]. The post-translational modification of the β-amyloid peptide involves a pyroglutamate at the N-terminus (pGlu3), which is a crucial antibody target due to its neo-epitope characteristics and propensity to form neurotoxic oligomer aggregates [166]. The antibody targeting p-Glu-Aβ, PBD-C06, effectively addresses inflammatory concerns by inactivating immune responses, potentially clearing the most toxic β-amyloid aggregates, and improving cognition in AD patients at therapeutic doses [167].

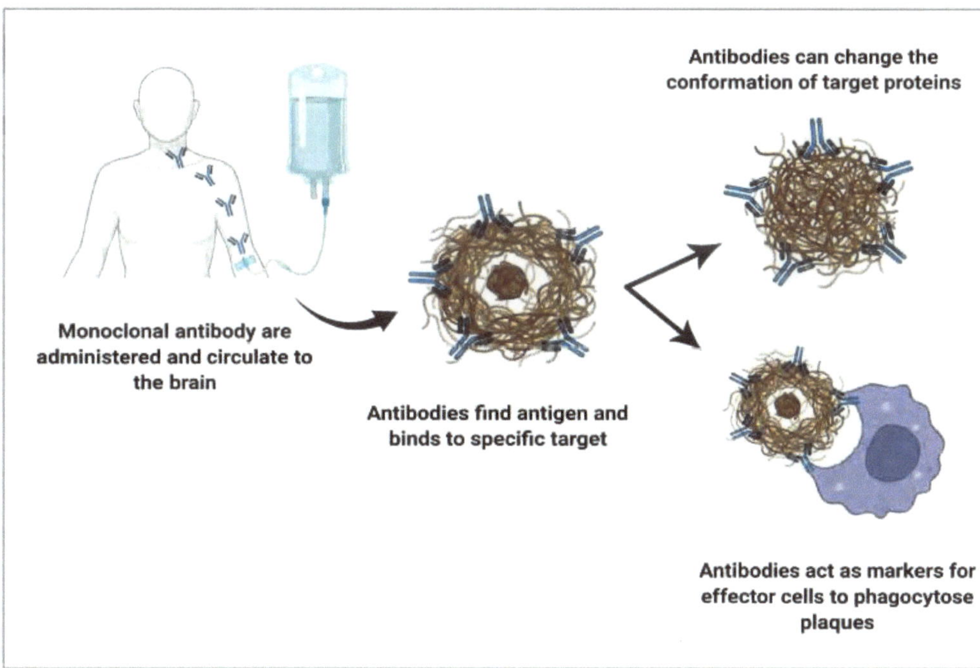

Fig. (3). Antibody therapies in Alzheimer's disease.

RECENT ADVANCEMENT IN IMMUNOTHERAPY FOR ALZHEIMER'S DISEASE

Immunotherapy Targeting β-amyloid

β-amyloid is considered central to the pathogenesis of AD, which is characterized by synaptic impairment, neurodegeneration, and cognitive dysfunction. Hence, several therapeutic approaches targeting β-amyloid may be efficient in curbing AD progression. Mechanistically, β-amyloid inhibitors could significantly prevent β-amyloid production and aggregation and simultaneously enhance β-amyloid clearance. Earlier, numerous drugs have been examined for their capability to reduce β-amyloid production and agglomeration [168, 169]. Nevertheless, all attempts have been unsuccessful, prompting a reevaluation of whether β-amyloid remains an essential therapeutic target and merits continued research. Considering that β-amyloid accumulation is the primary driver of the neurodegenerative disorder in AD, enhancing its clearance could be a promising approach. So, immunotherapy for AD has become very important to help get rid of β-amyloid and speed up research on anti-β-amyloid therapy [170].

Vaccines and antibodies, which are called active and passive immunotherapy, are now part of the most advanced anti-β-amyloid immunotherapy [171, 172]. Active immunotherapy meticulously encourages the immune system through administering β-amyloid, thus stimulating immune responses to the production of endogenous antibodies to counter β-amyloid progression. Active immunization was first reported in 1999, demonstrating that it curbs β-amyloid deposition in the brains of the PDAPP transgenic mouse model [173]. Lately, AN1792, a vaccine to target full-length β-amyloid, has been established and undertaken in clinical studies. Nonetheless, this investigation has been stopped as the manifestation of T-cells induced meningoencephalitis in 6% of recruited AD patients [174]. The reduction of overactive immune responses has led to the establishment of second-generation vaccines, such as CAD106, that lack T-lymphocyte epitopes. The advantage of active immunization is the ability to administer a short course of drug while producing more efficient, long-lasting antibodies at a limited cost. However, at the same time, the overactive immune responses and side effects have been predicted, especially in elderly patients [175, 176].

Due to the low immunogenicity of vaccines and the development of T-cel--dependent adverse effects, significant effort has shifted toward passive immunotherapy, in which, humanized monoclonal antibodies have been utilized to facilitate the clearance of β-amyloid [177]. Passive immunization promises relatively consistent antibody titers, but this is mostly achieved at the cost of cerebral amyloid angiopathy with microhemorrhages, vasogenic oedema, and other side effects. Mechanistically, passive immunotherapy causes antibody opsonization of antigens that facilitate macrophage phagocytosis, antibody-dependent peripheral reduction in β-amyloid production by β-amyloid efflux from the CNS, antibody-catalyzed alteration in the secondary structure of β-amyloid monomers to curb oligomer formation, and increases the outflow of antigen-antibody complexes through Fc receptors across the BBB [178]. In 2000, Brad and his colleagues first executed the *in-vivo* experiment of a β-amyloid antibody on a mouse model, suggesting that administering an antibody targeting the N-terminus of β-amyloid peripherally could stimulate microglia to phagocytize β-amyloid, hence this intervention successfully alleviates β-amyloid-mediated AD pathogenesis. Subsequently, β-amyloid antibodies targeting the N-terminus, as well as other regions such as the C-terminus and mid-region, have been evaluated for their potential to enhance β-amyloid clearance and improve cognitive dysfunction in a mouse model [179]. Recently, antibody targeting to a single small peptide sequence of β-amyloid has achieved some therapeutic efficacy. Additionally, Aducanumab has gained market approval and entered into clinical trials for AD [180].

Immunotherapy Targeting Tau Aggregation

Tau is a soluble protein that promotes tubulin assembly, cytoskeletal integrity, and microtubule stability, thus tau pathology facilitates the dysregulation of neuronal cell functions. Indeed, the development of neurofibrillary tangles leads to a significant loss of axonal integrity, which in turn reduces connectivity with synapses and contributes to dementia in AD patients. This intracellular tangle was later obtained extracellularly, after neuronal death and subsequently composed of hyperphosphorylated tau proteins. The definitive role of tau pathology in neurodegeneration has been explicitly established through the discovery of tau mutations associated with frontotemporal dementia and Parkinsonism linked to chromosome 17 (FTDP-17) [181, 182]. The aim of immunotherapy targeting tau pathology is to develop antibodies that specifically identify the abnormal hyperphosphorylated tau proteins. These antibodies effectively lead to the clearance of tau protein aggregates, which may substantially improve neuronal functional abilities [183]. A potential side effect of targeting tau pathology is the risk of interfering with its normal cellular functions. However, the prototype immunogen was specifically designed to stimulate the production of antibodies that primarily recognize the pathological tau proteins. Likewise, tau knockout animals demonstrate the typical phenotype, suggesting that other microtubule-associated proteins can perform similar functions, and eliminating endogenous tau aggregation alleviates β-amyloid-induced dysfunction in a transgenic mouse model [184]. The new study, on the other hand, showed that β-amyloid immunotherapy was indirectly linked to the removal of early tau pathology.

However, hyperphosphorylated tau aggregation still existed, just like in clinical studies. Intriguingly, immunotherapy targeting β-amyloid significantly reduces both soluble β-amyloid and tau protein, thereby improving cognition in mice with neurofibrillary tangles and plaques [185].

LIMITATIONS OF IMMUNOTHERAPY IN ALZHEIMER'S DISEASE

Immunotherapy, while showing promise in cancer treatment, faces significant limitations in Alzheimer's disease (AD) due to the unique challenges of targeting the brain. One major issue is the blood-brain barrier (BBB), which restricts many therapeutic agents from entering thebrain and limits the effectiveness of immune-based treatments. Additionally, the brain regulates immune response differently than other organs, and excessive immune activation can lead to neuroinflammation, potentially worsening AD symptoms rather than alleviating them [163]. Another challenge is the specificity of immunotherapy in targeting β-amyloid plaques and tau proteins, the key pathological markers in AD. Though some antibodies have been developed to clear these proteins, they often have limited efficacy and can cause adverse side effects, such as brain swelling or bleeding, as seen in some clinical trials [186]. Furthermore, AD is a highly complex and multifactorial disease, influenced by genetic, environmental, and lifestyle factors, which complicates the design of a one-size-fits-all immunotherapeutic approach [187]. Lastly, the aging immune system itself presents limitations, as older adults are the primary affected population with reduced immune responses, which may affect the potential efficacy of immunotherapy in AD [188]. Therefore, while immunotherapy holds potential, overcoming these limitations is essential for it to become a viable treatment option for Alzheimer's disease.

CONCLUSION AND FUTURE PERSPECTIVE

Immunotherapy for AD has shown promising yet complex potential in recent years. Traditionally, symptomatic treatments have managed AD, but immunotherapy introduces a targeted approach that targets key pathological drivers, particularly β-amyloid plaques and tau tangles. Active and passive immunization strategies targeting these proteins have demonstrated some success in reducing plaque burden and regressing cognitive impairment in early studies. Monoclonal antibodies, in particular, have been at the forefront, with some gaining regulatory approval based on their effects on β-amyloid and modest clinical benefits. Yet, challenges remain; adverse effects, such as β-amyloi--related imaging abnormalities (ARIA) and limited efficacy in later stages of the disease, highlight the need for optimized treatment protocols and patient selection.

Future perspectives in immunotherapy for AD are shifting towards multi-targeted approaches that combine β-amyloid and tau immunotherapy, as well as integrate anti-inflammatory and neuroprotective strategies to address the disease's multifaceted nature. Innovations in targeted delivery mechanisms by utilizing nanoparticles may further enhance therapeutic precision, while biomarker-driven personalized treatments are likely to improve efficacy and safety. In AD progression, immunotherapy holds considerable promise as part of a more comprehensive strategy, potentially transforming the clinical landscape of AD management.

REFERENCES

[1] DeTure MA, Dickson DW. The neuropathological diagnosis of Alzheimer's disease. Mol Neurodegener 2019; 14(1): 32.
[http://dx.doi.org/10.1186/s13024-019-0333-5] [PMID: 31375134]

[2] Lanctôt KL, Hahn-Pedersen JH, Eichinger CS, *et al.* Burden of illness in people with alzheimer's disease: A systematic review of epidemiology, comorbidities and mortality. J Prev Alzheimers Dis 2024; 11(1): 97-107.
[http://dx.doi.org/10.14283/jpad.2023.61] [PMID: 38230722]

[3] Lee J. Mild cognitive impairment in relation to alzheimer's disease: An investigation of principles, classifications, ethics, and problems. Neuroethics 2023; 16: 16.
[http://dx.doi.org/10.1007/s12152-023-09522-5]

[4] Gonçalves-Pereira M, Cardoso A, Verdelho A, *et al.* The prevalence of dementia in a Portuguese community sample: a 10/66 Dementia Research Group study. BMC Geriatr 2017; 17(1): 261.
[http://dx.doi.org/10.1186/s12877-017-0647-5] [PMID: 29115922]

[5] Jeremic D, Jiménez-Díaz L, Navarro-López JD. Past, present and future of therapeutic strategies against amyloid-β peptides in Alzheimer's disease: a systematic review. Ageing Res Rev 2021; 72: 101496.
[http://dx.doi.org/10.1016/j.arr.2021.101496] [PMID: 34687956]

[6] Rajmohan R, Reddy PH. Amyloid-beta and phosphorylated tau accumulations cause abnormalities at synapses of alzheimer's disease neurons. J Alzheimers Dis 2017; 57(4): 975-99.
[http://dx.doi.org/10.3233/JAD-160612] [PMID: 27567878]

[7] Yao W, Yang H, Yang J. Small-molecule drugs development for Alzheimer's disease. Front Aging Neurosci 2022; 14: 1019412.
[http://dx.doi.org/10.3389/fnagi.2022.1019412] [PMID: 36389082]

[8] Oliver DMA, Reddy PH. Small molecules as therapeutic drugs for Alzheimer's disease. Mol Cell Neurosci 2019; 96: 47-62.
[http://dx.doi.org/10.1016/j.mcn.2019.03.001] [PMID: 30877034]

[9] Langbaum JB, Zissimopoulos J, Au R, *et al.* Recommendations to address key recruitment challenges of Alzheimer's disease clinical trials. Alzheimers Dement 2023; 19(2): 696-707.
[http://dx.doi.org/10.1002/alz.12737] [PMID: 35946590]

[10] Marques L, Costa B, Pereira M, *et al.* Advancing precision medicine: A review of innovative in silico approaches for drug development, clinical pharmacology and personalized healthcare. Pharmaceutics 2024; 16(3): 332.
[http://dx.doi.org/10.3390/pharmaceutics16030332] [PMID: 38543226]

[11] Aljassabi A, Zieneldien T, Kim J, Regmi D, Cao C. Alzheimer's disease immunotherapy: Current strategies and future prospects. J Alzheimers Dis 2024; 98(3): 755-72.
[http://dx.doi.org/10.3233/JAD-231163] [PMID: 38489183]

[12] Valiukas Z, Ephraim R, Tangalakis K, Davidson M, Apostolopoulos V, Feehan J. Immunotherapies for Alzheimer's Disease—A Review. Vaccines (Basel) 2022; 10(9): 1527. [http://dx.doi.org/10.3390/vaccines10091527] [PMID: 36146605]

[13] Barrera-Ocampo A, Lopera F. Amyloid-beta immunotherapy: the hope for Alzheimer disease? Colomb Med (Cali) 2016; 47(4): 203-12. [http://dx.doi.org/10.25100/cm.v47i4.2640] [PMID: 28293044]

[14] Rather MA, Khan A, Alshahrani S, *et al.* Inflammation and alzheimer's disease: Mechanisms and therapeutic implications by natural products. Mediators Inflamm 2021; 2021(1): 9982954. [http://dx.doi.org/10.1155/2021/9982954] [PMID: 34381308]

[15] Karran E, De Strooper B. The amyloid hypothesis in Alzheimer disease: new insights from new therapeutics. Nat Rev Drug Discov 2022; 21(4): 306-18. [http://dx.doi.org/10.1038/s41573-022-00391-w] [PMID: 35177833]

[16] Zhang Y, Chen H, Li R, Sterling K, Song W. Amyloid β-based therapy for Alzheimer's disease: challenges, successes and future. Signal Transduct Target Ther 2023; 8(1): 248. [http://dx.doi.org/10.1038/s41392-023-01484-7] [PMID: 37386015]

[17] Pfundstein G, Nikonenko AG, Sytnyk V. Amyloid precursor protein (APP) and amyloid β (Aβ) interact with cell adhesion molecules: Implications in Alzheimer's disease and normal physiology. Front Cell Dev Biol 2022; 10: 969547. [http://dx.doi.org/10.3389/fcell.2022.969547] [PMID: 35959488]

[18] Steiner H, Fukumori A, Tagami S, Okochi M. Making the final cut: pathogenic amyloid-β peptide generation by γ-secretase. Cell Stress 2018; 2(11): 292-310. [http://dx.doi.org/10.15698/cst2018.11.162] [PMID: 31225454]

[19] Liu X, Liu Y, Ji S. Secretases related to amyloid precursor protein processing. Membranes (Basel) 2021; 11(12): 983. [http://dx.doi.org/10.3390/membranes11120983] [PMID: 34940484]

[20] Zhao J, Liu X, Xia W, Zhang Y, Wang C. Targeting amyloidogenic processing of APP in alzheimer's disease. Front Mol Neurosci 2020; 13: 137. [http://dx.doi.org/10.3389/fnmol.2020.00137] [PMID: 32848600]

[21] Ono K, Tsuji M. Protofibrils of amyloid-β are important targets of a disease-modifying approach for alzheimer's disease. Int J Mol Sci 2020; 21(3): 952. [http://dx.doi.org/10.3390/ijms21030952] [PMID: 32023927]

[22] Wiatrak B, Piasny J, Kuźniarski A, Gąsiorowski K. Interactions of amyloid-β with membrane proteins. Int J Mol Sci 2021; 22(11): 6075. [http://dx.doi.org/10.3390/ijms22116075] [PMID: 34199915]

[23] Mroczko B, Groblewska M, Litman-Zawadzka A, Kornhuber J, Lewczuk P. Cellular receptors of amyloid β oligomers (AβOs) in alzheimer's disease. Int J Mol Sci 2018; 19(7): 1884. [http://dx.doi.org/10.3390/ijms19071884] [PMID: 29954063]

[24] Barbier P, Zejneli O, Martinho M, *et al.* Role of tau as a microtubule-associated protein: structural and functional aspects. Front Aging Neurosci 2019; 11: 204. [http://dx.doi.org/10.3389/fnagi.2019.00204] [PMID: 31447664]

[25] Alavi Naini SM, Soussi-Yanicostas N. Tau hyperphosphorylation and oxidative stress, a critical vicious circle in neurodegenerative tauopathies? Oxid Med Cell Longev 2015; 2015: 1-17. [http://dx.doi.org/10.1155/2015/151979] [PMID: 26576216]

[26] Mueller RL, Combs B, Alhadidy MM, Brady ST, Morfini GA, Kanaan NM. Tau: A signaling hub protein. Front Mol Neurosci 2021; 14: 647054. [http://dx.doi.org/10.3389/fnmol.2021.647054] [PMID: 33815057]

[27] Hervy J, Bicout DJ. Dynamical decoration of stabilized-microtubules by Tau-proteins. Sci Rep 2019;

9(1): 12473.
[http://dx.doi.org/10.1038/s41598-019-48790-1] [PMID: 31462746]

[28] Cario A, Berger CL. Tau, microtubule dynamics, and axonal transport: New paradigms for neurodegenerative disease. 2023; 45(8).

[29] Holper S, Watson R, Yassi N. Tau as a Biomarker of Neurodegeneration. Int J Mol Sci 2022; 23(13): 7307.
[http://dx.doi.org/10.3390/ijms23137307] [PMID: 35806324]

[30] Rawat P, Sehar U, Bisht J, Selman A, Culberson J, Reddy PH. Phosphorylated Tau in Alzheimer's Disease and Other Tauopathies. Int J Mol Sci 2022; 23(21): 12841.
[http://dx.doi.org/10.3390/ijms232112841] [PMID: 36361631]

[31] Baracaldo-Santamaría D, Avendaño-Lopez SS, Ariza-Salamanca DF, *et al.* Role of Calcium Modulation in the Pathophysiology and Treatment of Alzheimer's Disease. Int J Mol Sci 2023; 24(10): 9067.
[http://dx.doi.org/10.3390/ijms24109067] [PMID: 37240413]

[32] Guo T, Zhang D, Zeng Y, Huang TY, Xu H, Zhao Y. Molecular and cellular mechanisms underlying the pathogenesis of Alzheimer's disease. Mol Neurodegener 2020; 15(1): 40.
[http://dx.doi.org/10.1186/s13024-020-00391-7] [PMID: 32677986]

[33] Bartolome F, Carro E, Alquezar C. Oxidative stress in tauopathies: From cause to therapy. Antioxidants 2022; 11(8): 1421.
[http://dx.doi.org/10.3390/antiox11081421] [PMID: 35892623]

[34] Basheer N, Smolek T, Hassan I, *et al.* Does modulation of tau hyperphosphorylation represent a reasonable therapeutic strategy for Alzheimer's disease? From preclinical studies to the clinical trials. Mol Psychiatry 2023; 28(6): 2197-214.
[http://dx.doi.org/10.1038/s41380-023-02113-z] [PMID: 37264120]

[35] Hong Y, Boiti A, Vallone D, Foulkes NS. Reactive oxygen species signaling and oxidative stress: Transcriptional regulation and evolution. Antioxidants 2024; 13(3): 312.
[http://dx.doi.org/10.3390/antiox13030312] [PMID: 38539845]

[36] Phaniendra A, Jestadi DB, Periyasamy L. Free radicals: properties, sources, targets, and their implication in various diseases. Indian J Clin Biochem 2015; 30(1): 11-26.
[http://dx.doi.org/10.1007/s12291-014-0446-0] [PMID: 25646037]

[37] Collin F. Chemical basis of reactive oxygen species reactivity and involvement in neurodegenerative diseases. Int J Mol Sci 2019; 20(10): 2407.
[http://dx.doi.org/10.3390/ijms20102407] [PMID: 31096608]

[38] Vermot A, Petit-Härtlein I, Smith SME, Fieschi F. NADPH oxidases (NOX): An overview from discovery, molecular mechanisms to physiology and pathology. Antioxidants 2021; 10(6): 890.
[http://dx.doi.org/10.3390/antiox10060890] [PMID: 34205998]

[39] Cipriano A, Viviano M, Feoli A, *et al.* NADPH oxidases: From molecular mechanisms to current inhibitors. J Med Chem 2023; 66(17): 11632-55.
[http://dx.doi.org/10.1021/acs.jmedchem.3c00770] [PMID: 37650225]

[40] Sies H. Hydrogen peroxide as a central redox signaling molecule in physiological oxidative stress: Oxidative eustress. Redox Biol 2017; 11: 613-9.
[http://dx.doi.org/10.1016/j.redox.2016.12.035] [PMID: 28110218]

[41] Lennicke C, Cochemé HM. Redox metabolism: ROS as specific molecular regulators of cell signaling and function. Mol Cell 2021; 81(18): 3691-707.
[http://dx.doi.org/10.1016/j.molcel.2021.08.018] [PMID: 34547234]

[42] Houldsworth A. Role of oxidative stress in neurodegenerative disorders: a review of reactive oxygen species and prevention by antioxidants. Brain Commun 2023; 6(1): fcad356.
[http://dx.doi.org/10.1093/braincomms/fcad356] [PMID: 38214013]

[43] Singh A, Kukreti R, Saso L, Kukreti S. Oxidative stress: A key modulator in neurodegenerative diseases. Molecules 2019; 24(8): 1583.
[http://dx.doi.org/10.3390/molecules24081583] [PMID: 31013638]

[44] MacLeod R, Hillert EK, Cameron RT, Baillie GS. The role and therapeutic targeting of α-, β- and γ-secretase in Alzheimer's disease. Future Sci OA 2015; 1(3): FSO11.
[http://dx.doi.org/10.4155/fso.15.9] [PMID: 28031886]

[45] Tamagno E, Guglielmotto M, Vasciaveo V, Tabaton M. Oxidative stress and beta amyloid in alzheimer's disease. which comes first: The chicken or the egg? Antioxidants 2021; 10(9): 1479.
[http://dx.doi.org/10.3390/antiox10091479] [PMID: 34573112]

[46] Simpson DSA, Oliver PL. ROS generation in microglia: Understanding oxidative stress and inflammation in neurodegenerative disease. Antioxidants 2020; 9(8): 743.
[http://dx.doi.org/10.3390/antiox9080743] [PMID: 32823544]

[47] García-Revilla J, Alonso-Bellido IM, Burguillos MA, *et al.* Reformulating Pro-Oxidant Microglia in Neurodegeneration. J Clin Med 2019; 8(10): 1719.
[http://dx.doi.org/10.3390/jcm8101719] [PMID: 31627485]

[48] Gąssowska-Dobrowolska M, Chlubek M, Kolasa A, *et al.* Microglia and astroglia—the potential role in neuroinflammation induced by pre- and neonatal exposure to lead (Pb). Int J Mol Sci 2023; 24(12): 9903.
[http://dx.doi.org/10.3390/ijms24129903] [PMID: 37373050]

[49] Lawrence JM, Schardien K, Wigdahl B, Nonnemacher MR. Roles of neuropathology-associated reactive astrocytes: a systematic review. Acta Neuropathol Commun 2023; 11(1): 42.
[http://dx.doi.org/10.1186/s40478-023-01526-9] [PMID: 36915214]

[50] Pal A, Rani I, Pawar A, Picozza M, Rongioletti M, Squitti R. Microglia and Astrocytes in Alzheimer's Disease in the Context of the Aberrant Copper Homeostasis Hypothesis. Biomolecules 2021; 11(11): 1598.
[http://dx.doi.org/10.3390/biom11111598] [PMID: 34827595]

[51] Price BR, Johnson LA, Norris CM. Reactive astrocytes: The nexus of pathological and clinical hallmarks of Alzheimer's disease. Ageing Res Rev 2021; 68: 101335.
[http://dx.doi.org/10.1016/j.arr.2021.101335] [PMID: 33812051]

[52] Wang J, Fu J, Zhao Y, Liu Q, Yan X, Su J. Iron and targeted iron therapy in alzheimer's disease. Int J Mol Sci 2023; 24(22): 16353.
[http://dx.doi.org/10.3390/ijms242216353] [PMID: 38003544]

[53] Feng S, Tang D, Wang Y, *et al.* The mechanism of ferroptosis and its related diseases. Mol Biomed 2023; 4(1): 33.
[http://dx.doi.org/10.1186/s43556-023-00142-2] [PMID: 37840106]

[54] Yan H, Zou T, Tuo Q, *et al.* Ferroptosis: mechanisms and links with diseases. Signal Transduct Target Ther 2021; 6(1): 49.
[http://dx.doi.org/10.1038/s41392-020-00428-9] [PMID: 33536413]

[55] Chen F, Kang R, Tang D, Liu J. Ferroptosis: principles and significance in health and disease. J Hematol Oncol 2024; 17(1): 41.
[http://dx.doi.org/10.1186/s13045-024-01564-3] [PMID: 38844964]

[56] Zhou Q, Meng Y, Li D, *et al.* Ferroptosis in cancer: from molecular mechanisms to therapeutic strategies. Signal Transduct Target Ther 2024; 9(1): 55.
[http://dx.doi.org/10.1038/s41392-024-01769-5] [PMID: 38453898]

[57] Xie Y, Kang R, Klionsky DJ, Tang D. GPX4 in cell death, autophagy, and disease. Autophagy 2023; 19(10): 2621-38.
[http://dx.doi.org/10.1080/15548627.2023.2218764] [PMID: 37272058]

[58] Jiang Y, Glandorff C, Sun M. GSH and Ferroptosis: Side-by-Side Partners in the Fight against Tumors. Antioxidants 2024; 13(6): 697.
[http://dx.doi.org/10.3390/antiox13060697] [PMID: 38929136]

[59] Ma H, Dong Y, Chu Y, Guo Y, Li L. The mechanisms of ferroptosis and its role in alzheimer's disease. Front Mol Biosci 2022; 9: 965064.
[http://dx.doi.org/10.3389/fmolb.2022.965064] [PMID: 36090039]

[60] Yu Y, Yan Y, Niu F, *et al.* Ferroptosis: a cell death connecting oxidative stress, inflammation and cardiovascular diseases. Cell Death Discov 2021; 7(1): 193.
[http://dx.doi.org/10.1038/s41420-021-00579-w] [PMID: 34312370]

[61] Rochette L, Dogon G, Rigal E, Zeller M, Cottin Y, Vergely C. Lipid peroxidation and iron metabolism: Two corner stones in the homeostasis control of ferroptosis. Int J Mol Sci 2022; 24(1): 449.
[http://dx.doi.org/10.3390/ijms24010449] [PMID: 36613888]

[62] Chen K, Jiang X, Wu M, Cao X, Bao W, Zhu LQ. Ferroptosis, a potential therapeutic target in alzheimer's disease. Front Cell Dev Biol 2021; 9: 704298.
[http://dx.doi.org/10.3389/fcell.2021.704298] [PMID: 34422824]

[63] Troutwine BR, Hamid L, Lysaker CR, Strope TA, Wilkins HM. Apolipoprotein E and Alzheimer's disease. Acta Pharm Sin B 2022; 12(2): 496-510.
[http://dx.doi.org/10.1016/j.apsb.2021.10.002] [PMID: 35256931]

[64] Raulin AC, Doss SV, Trottier ZA, Ikezu TC, Bu G, Liu CC. ApoE in Alzheimer's disease: pathophysiology and therapeutic strategies. Mol Neurodegener 2022; 17(1): 72.
[http://dx.doi.org/10.1186/s13024-022-00574-4] [PMID: 36348357]

[65] Huq AJ, Fransquet P, Laws SM, *et al.* Genetic resilience to Alzheimer's disease in *APOE* ε4 homozygotes: A systematic review. Alzheimers Dement 2019; 15(12): 1612-23.
[http://dx.doi.org/10.1016/j.jalz.2019.05.011] [PMID: 31506248]

[66] Yang J, Fu Z, Zhang X, Xiong M, Meng L, Zhang Z. TREM2 ectodomain and its soluble form in Alzheimer's disease. J Neuroinflammation 2020; 17(1): 204.
[http://dx.doi.org/10.1186/s12974-020-01878-2] [PMID: 32635934]

[67] Li Y, Xu H, Wang H, Yang K, Luan J, Wang S. TREM2: Potential therapeutic targeting of microglia for Alzheimer's disease. Biomed Pharmacother 2023; 165: 115218.
[http://dx.doi.org/10.1016/j.biopha.2023.115218] [PMID: 37517293]

[68] Nabizadeh F, Seyedmirzaei H, Karami S. Neuroimaging biomarkers and CSF sTREM2 levels in Alzheimer's disease: a longitudinal study. Sci Rep 2024; 14(1): 15318.
[http://dx.doi.org/10.1038/s41598-024-66211-w] [PMID: 38961148]

[69] Wu KM, Zhang YR, Huang YY, Dong Q, Tan L, Yu JT. The role of the immune system in Alzheimer's disease. Ageing Res Rev 2021; 70: 101409.
[http://dx.doi.org/10.1016/j.arr.2021.101409] [PMID: 34273589]

[70] Wu Y, Eisel ULM. Microglia-Astrocyte Communication in Alzheimer's Disease. J Alzheimers Dis 2023; 95(3): 785-803.
[http://dx.doi.org/10.3233/JAD-230199] [PMID: 37638434]

[71] Chen F, Ghosh A, Lin J, *et al.* 5-lipoxygenase pathway and its downstream cysteinyl leukotrienes as potential therapeutic targets for Alzheimer's disease. Brain Behav Immun 2020; 88: 844-55.
[http://dx.doi.org/10.1016/j.bbi.2020.03.022] [PMID: 32222525]

[72] Afsar A, Chen M, Xuan Z, Zhang L. A glance through the effects of $CD4^+$ T cells, $CD8^+$ T cells, and cytokines on Alzheimer's disease. Comput Struct Biotechnol J 2023; 21: 5662-75.
[http://dx.doi.org/10.1016/j.csbj.2023.10.058] [PMID: 38053545]

[73] Zeng J, Liao Z, Yang H, *et al.* T cell infiltration mediates neurodegeneration and cognitive decline in

Alzheimer's disease. Neurobiol Dis 2024; 193: 106461.
[http://dx.doi.org/10.1016/j.nbd.2024.106461] [PMID: 38437992]

[74] Dai L, Shen Y. Insights into T-cell dysfunction in Alzheimer's disease. Aging Cell 2021; 20(12): e13511.
[http://dx.doi.org/10.1111/acel.13511] [PMID: 34725916]

[75] Rajendiran A, Tenbrock K. Regulatory T cell function in autoimmune disease. J Transl Autoimmun 2021; 4: 100130.
[http://dx.doi.org/10.1016/j.jtauto.2021.100130] [PMID: 35005594]

[76] Zhang Q, Yang G, Luo. Neuroinflammation in Alzheimer's disease: insights from peripheral immune cells. Immun Ageing. 2024; 21: 38 (2024).

[77] Tjalkens RB, Popichak KA, Kirkley KA. Inflammatory Activation of Microglia and Astrocytes in Manganese Neurotoxicity. Adv Neurobiol 2017; 18: 159-81.
[http://dx.doi.org/10.1007/978-3-319-60189-2_8] [PMID: 28889267]

[78] Gao C, Jiang J, Tan Y, Chen S. Microglia in neurodegenerative diseases: mechanism and potential therapeutic targets. Signal Transduct Target Ther 2023; 8(1): 359.
[http://dx.doi.org/10.1038/s41392-023-01588-0] [PMID: 37735487]

[79] Plantone D, Pardini M, Righi D, Manco C, Colombo BM, De Stefano N. The Role of TNF-α in Alzheimer's Disease: A Narrative Review. Cells 2023; 13(1): 54.
[http://dx.doi.org/10.3390/cells13010054] [PMID: 38201258]

[80] Steeland S, Gorlé N, Vandendriessche C, *et al.* Counteracting the effects of TNF receptor-1 has therapeutic potential in Alzheimer's disease. EMBO Mol Med 2018; 10(4): e8300.
[http://dx.doi.org/10.15252/emmm.201708300] [PMID: 29472246]

[81] Yadav V, C M, Kumarasamy M. Natural products as potential modulators of pro-inflammatory cytokines signalling in Alzheimer's disease. Brain Behavior and Immunity Integrative 2024; 5: 100048.
[http://dx.doi.org/10.1016/j.bbii.2024.100048]

[82] Kinney JW, Bemiller SM, Murtishaw AS, et al. Inflammation as a central mechanism in Alzheimer's disease. Alzheimers Dement (N Y) 2018; 4: 575-590.
[http://dx.doi.org/10.1016/j.trci.2018.06.014] [PMID: 30406177]

[83] van der Kant R, Goldstein LSB. Cellular functions of the amyloid precursor protein from development to dementia. Dev Cell 2015; 32(4): 502-15.
[http://dx.doi.org/10.1016/j.devcel.2015.01.022] [PMID: 25710536]

[84] Barreto Chang OL, Maze M. Defining the role of Interleukin-6 for the development of perioperative neurocognitive disorders: Evidence from clinical and preclinical studies. Front Aging Neurosci 2023; 14: 1097606.
[http://dx.doi.org/10.3389/fnagi.2022.1097606] [PMID: 36778590]

[85] vom Berg J, Prokop S, Miller KR, *et al.* Inhibition of IL-12/IL-23 signaling reduces Alzheimer's disease–like pathology and cognitive decline. Nat Med 2012; 18(12): 1812-9.
[http://dx.doi.org/10.1038/nm.2965] [PMID: 23178247]

[86] Nitsch L, Schneider L, Zimmermann J, Müller M. Microglia-Derived Interleukin 23: A Crucial Cytokine in Alzheimer's Disease? Front Neurol 2021; 12: 639353.
[http://dx.doi.org/10.3389/fneur.2021.639353] [PMID: 33897596]

[87] Kim S, Jung UJ, Kim SR. Role of Oxidative Stress in Blood–Brain Barrier Disruption and Neurodegenerative Diseases. Antioxidants 2024; 13(12): 1462.
[http://dx.doi.org/10.3390/antiox13121462] [PMID: 39765790]

[88] Faraco G, Iadecola C. Hypertension. Hypertension 2013; 62(5): 810-7.
[http://dx.doi.org/10.1161/HYPERTENSIONAHA.113.01063] [PMID: 23980072]

[89] Wright JW, Harding JW. The brain RAS and Alzheimer's disease. Exp Neurol 2010; 223(2): 326-33. [http://dx.doi.org/10.1016/j.expneurol.2009.09.012] [PMID: 19782074]

[90] Wzgarda A, Kleszcz R, Prokop M, *et al.* Unknown face of known drugs – what else can we expect from angiotensin converting enzyme inhibitors? Eur J Pharmacol 2017; 797: 9-19. [http://dx.doi.org/10.1016/j.ejphar.2016.12.031] [PMID: 28087255]

[91] Goel R, Bhat SA, Rajasekar N, Hanif K, Nath C, Shukla R. Hypertension exacerbates predisposition to neurodegeneration and memory impairment in the presence of a neuroinflammatory stimulus: Protection by angiotensin converting enzyme inhibition. Pharmacol Biochem Behav 2015; 133: 132-45. [http://dx.doi.org/10.1016/j.pbb.2015.04.002] [PMID: 25869103]

[92] Kehoe PG, Miners S, Love S. Angiotensins in Alzheimer's disease – friend or foe? Trends Neurosci 2009; 32(12): 619-28. [http://dx.doi.org/10.1016/j.tins.2009.07.006] [PMID: 19796831]

[93] Ohrui T, Matsui T, Yamaya M, *et al.* Angiotensin-converting enzyme inhibitors and incidence of Alzheimer's disease in Japan. J Am Geriatr Soc 2004; 52(4): 649-50. [http://dx.doi.org/10.1111/j.1532-5415.2004.52178_7.x] [PMID: 15066094]

[94] Gouveia F, Camins A, Ettcheto M, *et al.* Targeting brain Renin-Angiotensin System for the prevention and treatment of Alzheimer's disease: Past, present and future. Ageing Res Rev 2022; 77: 101612. [http://dx.doi.org/10.1016/j.arr.2022.101612] [PMID: 35346852]

[95] Panahpour H, Dehghani GA, Bohlooli S. Enalapril attenuates ischaemic brain oedema and protects the blood–brain barrier in rats *via* an anti-oxidant action. Clin Exp Pharmacol Physiol 2014; 41(3): 220-6. [http://dx.doi.org/10.1111/1440-1681.12210] [PMID: 24471927]

[96] Szczepanska-Sadowska E, Zera T, Kowara M, *et al.* The contribution of angiotensin peptides to cardiovascular neuroregulation in health and disease. Angiotesin. Academic Press 2023; pp. 21-75. [http://dx.doi.org/10.1016/B978-0-323-99618-1.00009-X]

[97] Singh B, Sharma B, Jaggi AS, Singh N. Attenuating effect of lisinopril and telmisartan in intracerebroventricular streptozotocin induced experimental dementia of Alzheimer's disease type: possible involvement of PPAR-γ agonistic property. J Renin Angiotensin Aldosterone Syst 2013; 14(2): 124-36. [http://dx.doi.org/10.1177/1470320312459977] [PMID: 23060470]

[98] Thomas J, Smith H, Smith CA, *et al.* The angiotensin-converting enzyme inhibitor lisinopril mitigates memory and motor deficits in a drosophila model of alzheimer's disease. Pathophysiology 2021; 28(2): 307-19. [http://dx.doi.org/10.3390/pathophysiology28020020] [PMID: 35366264]

[99] Yamada K, Horita T, Takayama M, *et al.* Effect of a centrally active angiotensin converting enzyme inhibitor, perindopril, on cognitive performance in chronic cerebral hypo-perfusion rats. Brain Res 2011; 1421: 110-20. [http://dx.doi.org/10.1016/j.brainres.2011.09.016] [PMID: 21981801]

[100] Ababei DC, Bild V, Ciobică A, Lefter RM, Rusu RN, Bild W. A Comparative study on the memory-enhancing actions of oral renin-angiotensin system altering drugs in scopolamine-treated mice. Am J Alzheimers Dis Other Demen 2019; 34(5): 329-36. [http://dx.doi.org/10.1177/1533317519847042] [PMID: 31106575]

[101] Ongali B, Nicolakakis N, Tong XK, Aboulkassim T, Imboden H, Hamel E. Enalapril alone or co-administered with losartan rescues cerebrovascular dysfunction, but not mnemonic deficits or amyloidosis in a mouse model of Alzheimer's disease. J Alzheimers Dis 2016; 51(4): 1183-95. [http://dx.doi.org/10.3233/JAD-150868] [PMID: 26923013]

[102] Wong Zhang DE, Sobey CG, De Silva TM. The role of angiotensin peptides in the brain during health and disease. In: Angiotensin: From the Kidney to Coronavirus. In: Molecular Mediators in Health and

Disease: How Cells Communicate. 2023: 749-773.
[http://dx.doi.org/10.1016/B978-0-323-99618-1.00026-X]

[103] Soto ME, Abellan van Kan G, Nourhashemi F, *et al.* Angiotensin-converting enzyme inhibitors and Alzheimer's disease progression in older adults: results from the Réseau sur la Maladie d'Alzheimer Français cohort. J Am Geriatr Soc 2013; 61(9): 1482-8.
[http://dx.doi.org/10.1111/jgs.12415] [PMID: 24000874]

[104] O'Caoimh R, Healy L, Gao Y, *et al.* Effects of centrally acting angiotensin converting enzyme inhibitors on functional decline in patients with Alzheimer's disease. J Alzheimers Dis 2014; 40(3): 595-603.
[http://dx.doi.org/10.3233/JAD-131694] [PMID: 24496072]

[105] Ohrui T, Tomita N, Sato-Nakagawa T, *et al.* Effects of brain-penetrating ACE inhibitors on Alzheimer disease progression. Neurology 2004; 63(7): 1324-5.
[http://dx.doi.org/10.1212/01.WNL.0000140705.23869.E9] [PMID: 15477567]

[106] Sink KM, Leng X, Williamson J, *et al.* Angiotensin-converting enzyme inhibitors and cognitive decline in older adults with hypertension: results from the Cardiovascular Health Study. Arch Intern Med 2009; 169(13): 1195-202.
[http://dx.doi.org/10.1001/archinternmed.2009.175] [PMID: 19597068]

[107] Solfrizzi V, Scafato E, Frisardi V, *et al.* Angiotensin-converting enzyme inhibitors and incidence of mild cognitive impairment. Age (Omaha) 2013; 35(2): 441-53.
[http://dx.doi.org/10.1007/s11357-011-9360-z] [PMID: 22203459]

[108] Hebert PL, McBean AM, O'Connor H, Frank B, Good C, Maciejewski ML. Time until incident dementia among Medicare beneficiaries using centrally acting or non-centrally acting ACE inhibitors. Pharmacoepidemiol Drug Saf 2013; 22(6): 641-8.
[http://dx.doi.org/10.1002/pds.3449] [PMID: 23620414]

[109] Wharton W, Stein JH, Korcarz C, *et al.* The effects of ramipril in individuals at risk for Alzheimer's disease: results of a pilot clinical trial. J Alzheimers Dis 2012; 32(1): 147-56.
[http://dx.doi.org/10.3233/JAD-2012-120763] [PMID: 22776970]

[110] Davies NM, Kehoe PG, Ben-Shlomo Y, Martin RM. Associations of anti-hypertensive treatments with Alzheimer's disease, vascular dementia, and other dementias. J Alzheimers Dis 2011; 26(4): 699-708.
[http://dx.doi.org/10.3233/JAD-2011-110347] [PMID: 21709373]

[111] Yasar S, Xia J, Yao W, *et al.* Antihypertensive drugs decrease risk of Alzheimer disease. Neurology 2013; 81(10): 896-903.
[http://dx.doi.org/10.1212/WNL.0b013e3182a35228] [PMID: 23911756]

[112] Li NC, Lee A, Whitmer RA, *et al.* Use of angiotensin receptor blockers and risk of dementia in a predominantly male population: prospective cohort analysis. BMJ 2010; 340(jan12 1): b5465.
[http://dx.doi.org/10.1136/bmj.b5465] [PMID: 20068258]

[113] Zhang Y, Li P, Feng J, Wu M. Dysfunction of NMDA receptors in Alzheimer's disease. Neurol Sci 2016; 37(7): 1039-47.
[http://dx.doi.org/10.1007/s10072-016-2546-5] [PMID: 26971324]

[114] Bezprozvanny I, Mattson MP. Neuronal calcium mishandling and the pathogenesis of Alzheimer's disease. Trends Neurosci 2008; 31(9): 454-63.
[http://dx.doi.org/10.1016/j.tins.2008.06.005] [PMID: 18675468]

[115] Hynd M, Scott HL, Dodd PR. Glutamate-mediated excitotoxicity and neurodegeneration in Alzheimer?s disease. Neurochem Int 2004; 45(5): 583-95.
[http://dx.doi.org/10.1016/j.neuint.2004.03.007] [PMID: 15234100]

[116] Herrmann N, Li A, Lanctôt K. Memantine in dementia: a review of the current evidence. Expert Opin Pharmacother 2011; 12(5): 787-800.
[http://dx.doi.org/10.1517/14656566.2011.558006] [PMID: 21385152]

[117] Wang R, Reddy PH. Role of glutamate and NMDA receptors in Alzheimer's disease. J Alzheimers Dis 2017; 57(4): 1041-8.
[http://dx.doi.org/10.3233/JAD-160763] [PMID: 27662322]

[118] Chen HSV, Lipton SA. The chemical biology of clinically tolerated NMDA receptor antagonists. J Neurochem 2006; 97(6): 1611-26.
[http://dx.doi.org/10.1111/j.1471-4159.2006.03991.x] [PMID: 16805772]

[119] Lipton SA. Failures and successes of NMDA receptor antagonists: Molecular basis for the use of open-channel blockers like memantine in the treatment of acute and chronic neurologic insults. NeuroRx 2004; 1(1): 101-10.
[http://dx.doi.org/10.1602/neurorx.1.1.101] [PMID: 15717010]

[120] Parsons CG, Danysz W, Quack G. Memantine is a clinically well tolerated N-methyl-d-aspartate (NMDA) receptor antagonist—a review of preclinical data. Neuropharmacology 1999; 38(6): 735-67.
[http://dx.doi.org/10.1016/S0028-3908(99)00019-2] [PMID: 10465680]

[121] Agüera-Ortiz LF. [Memantine in the pharmacologic treatment of moderately severe to severe Alzheimer's disease in Spain (MEMORY study)]. Rev Neurol 2010; 51(9): 525-34.
[PMID: 20979032]

[122] Grossberg GT, Pejović V, Miller ML, Graham SM. Memantine therapy of behavioral symptoms in community-dwelling patients with moderate to severe Alzheimer's disease. Dement Geriatr Cogn Disord 2009; 27(2): 164-72.
[http://dx.doi.org/10.1159/000200013] [PMID: 19194105]

[123] Peskind ER, Potkin SG, Pomara N, *et al.* Memantine treatment in mild to moderate Alzheimer disease: a 24-week randomized, controlled trial. Am J Geriatr Psychiatry 2006; 14(8): 704-15.
[http://dx.doi.org/10.1097/01.JGP.0000224350.82719.83] [PMID: 16861375]

[124] van Dyck CH, Tariot PN, Meyers B, Malca Resnick E. A 24-week randomized, controlled trial of memantine in patients with moderate-to-severe Alzheimer disease. Alzheimer Dis Assoc Disord 2007; 21(2): 136-43.
[http://dx.doi.org/10.1097/WAD.0b013e318065c495] [PMID: 17545739]

[125] Areosa SA, Sherriff F, McShane R. Memantine for dementia. Cochrane Database Syst Rev. 2005; (3): CD003154.
[http://dx.doi.org/10.1002/14651858.CD003154.pub4]

[126] Emre M, Mecocci P, Stender K. Pooled analyses on cognitive effects of memantine in patients with moderate to severe Alzheimer's disease. J Alzheimers Dis 2008; 14(2): 193-9.
[http://dx.doi.org/10.3233/JAD-2008-14207] [PMID: 18560130]

[127] Wilcock GK, Ballard CG, Cooper JA, Loft H. Memantine for agitation/aggression and psychosis in moderately severe to severe Alzheimer's disease: a pooled analysis of 3 studies. J Clin Psychiatry 2008; 69(3): 341-8.
[http://dx.doi.org/10.4088/JCP.v69n0302] [PMID: 18294023]

[128] Farlow MR, Graham SM, Alva G. Memantine for the treatment of Alzheimer's disease: tolerability and safety data from clinical trials. Drug Saf 2008; 31(7): 577-85.
[http://dx.doi.org/10.2165/00002018-200831070-00003] [PMID: 18558791]

[129] Rossom R, Adityanjee , Dysken M. Efficacy and tolerability of memantine in the treatment of dementia. Am J Geriatr Pharmacother 2004; 2(4): 303-12.
[http://dx.doi.org/10.1016/j.amjopharm.2004.12.006] [PMID: 15903287]

[130] Periclou AP, Ventura D, Sherman T, Rao N, Abramowitz WT. Lack of pharmacokinetic or pharmacodynamic interaction between memantine and donepezil. Ann Pharmacother 2004; 38(9): 1389-94.
[http://dx.doi.org/10.1345/aph.1D638] [PMID: 15266045]

[131] Wenk GL, Quack G, Moebius HJ, Danysz W. No interaction of memantine with acetylcholinesterase

inhibitors approved for clinical use. Life Sci 2000; 66(12): 1079-83.
[http://dx.doi.org/10.1016/S0024-3205(00)00411-2] [PMID: 10737358]

[132] Grossberg GT. Rationalizing therapeutic approaches in Alzheimer's disease. CNS Spectr 2005; 10(S18) (Suppl. 18): 17-21.
[http://dx.doi.org/10.1017/S109285290001419X] [PMID: 16273026]

[133] Rountree SD, Chan W, Pavlik VN, Darby EJ, Siddiqui S, Doody RS. Persistent treatment with cholinesterase inhibitors and/or memantine slows clinical progression of Alzheimer disease. Alzheimers Res Ther 2009; 1(2): 7.
[http://dx.doi.org/10.1186/alzrt7] [PMID: 19845950]

[134] Albensi BC, Ilkanich E. Open-channel blockers of the NMDA receptor complex. Drug News Perspect 2004; 17(9): 557-62.
[http://dx.doi.org/10.1358/dnp.2004.17.9.872569] [PMID: 15645013]

[135] Lipton S. The molecular basis of memantine action in Alzheimer's disease and other neurologic disorders: low-affinity, uncompetitive antagonism. Curr Alzheimer Res 2005; 2(2): 155-65.
[http://dx.doi.org/10.2174/1567205053585846] [PMID: 15974913]

[136] Tatulian SA. Challenges and hopes for Alzheimer's disease. Drug Discov Today 2022; 27(4): 1027-43.
[http://dx.doi.org/10.1016/j.drudis.2022.01.016] [PMID: 35121174]

[137] Zhang J, Zhang Y, Wang J, Xia Y, Zhang J, Chen L. Recent advances in Alzheimer's disease: mechanisms, clinical trials and new drug development strategies. Signal Transduct Target Ther 2024; 9(1): 211.
[http://dx.doi.org/10.1038/s41392-024-01911-3] [PMID: 39174535]

[138] Golde TE, Levey AI. Immunotherapies for Alzheimer's disease. Science 2023; 382(6676): 1242-4.
[http://dx.doi.org/10.1126/science.adj9255] [PMID: 38096276]

[139] Yiannopoulou KG, Papageorgiou SG. Current and Future Treatments in Alzheimer Disease: An Update. J Cent Nerv Syst Dis 2020; 12: 1179573520907397.
[http://dx.doi.org/10.1177/1179573520907397] [PMID: 32165850]

[140] Valera E, Spencer B, Masliah E. Immunotherapeutic Approaches Targeting Amyloid-β, α-Synuclein, and Tau for the Treatment of Neurodegenerative Disorders. Neurotherapeutics 2016; 13(1): 179-89.
[http://dx.doi.org/10.1007/s13311-015-0397-z] [PMID: 26494242]

[141] Jadhav S, Avila J, Schöll M, et al. A walk-through tau therapeutic strategies. acta neuropathol commun. 2019; 7(1): 1-31.

[142] Gong CX, Dai CL, Liu F, Iqbal K. Multi-Targets: An Unconventional Drug Development Strategy for Alzheimer's Disease. Front Aging Neurosci 2022; 14: 837649.
[http://dx.doi.org/10.3389/fnagi.2022.837649] [PMID: 35222001]

[143] Alshamrani M. Recent Trends in Active and Passive Immunotherapies of Alzheimer's Disease. Antibodies (Basel) 2023; 12(2): 41.
[http://dx.doi.org/10.3390/antib12020041] [PMID: 37366656]

[144] Winblad B, Graf A, Riviere ME, Andreasen N, Ryan JM. Active immunotherapy options for Alzheimer's disease. Alzheimers Res Ther 2014; 6(1): 7.
[http://dx.doi.org/10.1186/alzrt237] [PMID: 24476230]

[145] Di Benedetto G, Burgaletto C, Bellanca CM, Munafò A, Bernardini R, Cantarella G. Role of Microglia and Astrocytes in Alzheimer's Disease: From Neuroinflammation to Ca^{2+} Homeostasis Dysregulation. Cells 2022; 11(17): 2728.
[http://dx.doi.org/10.3390/cells11172728] [PMID: 36078138]

[146] Bhadane P, Roul K, Belemkar S, Kumar D. Immunotherapeutic approaches for Alzheimer's disease: Exploring active and passive vaccine progress. Brain Res 2024; 1840: 149018.
[http://dx.doi.org/10.1016/j.brainres.2024.149018] [PMID: 38782231]

[147] Galasko D. Active immunization in Alzheimer's disease. Nat Aging 2021; 1(6): 493-5. [http://dx.doi.org/10.1038/s43587-021-00076-w] [PMID: 37117835]

[148] Mantile F, Prisco A. Vaccination against β-Amyloid as a Strategy for the Prevention of Alzheimer's Disease. Biology (Basel) 2020; 9(12): 425. [http://dx.doi.org/10.3390/biology9120425] [PMID: 33260956]

[149] Wang W, Fan L, Xu D, et al. Immunotherapy for Alzheimer's disease. Acta Biochimica et Biophysica Sinica 2012; 44(10): 807-814.. [http://dx.doi.org/10.1093/abbs/gms065]

[150] Tan W, Thiruppathi J, Hong SH, *et al.* Development of an anti-tauopathy mucosal vaccine specifically targeting pathologic conformers. NPJ Vaccines 2024; 9(1): 108. [http://dx.doi.org/10.1038/s41541-024-00904-1] [PMID: 38879560]

[151] Soeda Y, Takashima A. New Insights Into Drug Discovery Targeting Tau Protein. Front Mol Neurosci 2020; 13: 590896. [http://dx.doi.org/10.3389/fnmol.2020.590896] [PMID: 33343298]

[152] Cacabelos R. How plausible is an Alzheimer's disease vaccine? Expert Opin Drug Discov 2020; 15(1): 1-6. [http://dx.doi.org/10.1080/17460441.2019.1667329] [PMID: 31526140]

[153] Petrushina I, Hovakimyan A, Harahap-Carrillo IS, *et al.* Characterization and preclinical evaluation of the cGMP grade DNA based vaccine, AV-1959D to enter the first-in-human clinical trials. Neurobiol Dis 2020; 139: 104823. [http://dx.doi.org/10.1016/j.nbd.2020.104823] [PMID: 32119976]

[154] Cao Y-P, Wang J-C, Zhu K, Zhang H-Y, Wang G-Q, Liu H-Y. Early active immunization with Aβ $_{3\text{-}10}$ -KLH vaccine reduces tau phosphorylation in the hippocampus and protects cognition of mice. Neural Regen Res 2020; 15(3): 519-27. [http://dx.doi.org/10.4103/1673-5374.266061] [PMID: 31571664]

[155] Xing Z, Zuo Z, Hu D, *et al.* Influenza vaccine combined with moderate-dose PD1 blockade reduces amyloid-β accumulation and improves cognition in APP/PS1 mice. Brain Behav Immun 2021; 91: 128-41. [http://dx.doi.org/10.1016/j.bbi.2020.09.015] [PMID: 32956831]

[156] Saresella M, Calabrese E, Marventano I, *et al.* A potential role for the PD1/PD-L1 pathway in the neuroinflammation of Alzheimer's disease. Neurobiol Aging 2012; 33(3): 624.e11-22. [http://dx.doi.org/10.1016/j.neurobiolaging.2011.03.004] [PMID: 21514692]

[157] Liu D, Lu S, Zhang L, *et al.* Yeast-Based Aβ1-15 Vaccine Elicits Strong Immunogenicity and Attenuates Neuropathology and Cognitive Deficits in Alzheimer's Disease Transgenic Mice. Vaccines (Basel) 2020; 8(3): 351. [http://dx.doi.org/10.3390/vaccines8030351] [PMID: 32630299]

[158] Fedele E. Anti-Amyloid Therapies for Alzheimer's Disease and the Amyloid Cascade Hypothesis. Int J Mol Sci 2023; 24(19): 14499. [http://dx.doi.org/10.3390/ijms241914499] [PMID: 37833948]

[159] Song C, Shi J, Zhang P, *et al.* Immunotherapy for Alzheimer's disease: targeting β-amyloid and beyond. Transl Neurodegener 2022; 11(1): 18. [http://dx.doi.org/10.1186/s40035-022-00292-3] [PMID: 35300725]

[160] Guo X, Yan L, Zhang D, Zhao Y. Passive immunotherapy for Alzheimer's disease. Ageing Res Rev 2024; 94: 102192. [http://dx.doi.org/10.1016/j.arr.2024.102192] [PMID: 38219962]

[161] Vaz M, Silva V, Monteiro C, Silvestre S. Role of Aducanumab in the Treatment of Alzheimer's Disease: Challenges and Opportunities. Clin Interv Aging 2022; 17: 797-810. [http://dx.doi.org/10.2147/CIA.S325026] [PMID: 35611326]

[162] Fu L, Zhang Y, Zhang X, *et al.* Preparation and *in vitro* activity of single chain antibodies against Alzheimer's disease. Immunol Lett 2020; 227: 1-7.
[http://dx.doi.org/10.1016/j.imlet.2020.07.009] [PMID: 32781005]

[163] Yi LX, Tan EK, Zhou ZD. Passive immunotherapy for Alzheimer's disease: challenges & future directions. J Transl Med 2024; 22(1): 430.
[http://dx.doi.org/10.1186/s12967-024-05248-x] [PMID: 38715084]

[164] van Dyck CH. Anti-Amyloid-β Monoclonal Antibodies for Alzheimer's Disease: Pitfalls and Promise. Biol Psychiatry 2018; 83(4): 311-9.
[http://dx.doi.org/10.1016/j.biopsych.2017.08.010] [PMID: 28967385]

[165] Vitek GE, Decourt B, Sabbagh MN. Lecanemab (BAN2401): an anti–beta-amyloid monoclonal antibody for the treatment of Alzheimer disease. Expert Opin Investig Drugs 2023; 32(2): 89-94.
[http://dx.doi.org/10.1080/13543784.2023.2178414] [PMID: 36749830]

[166] Crehan H, Liu B, Kleinschmidt M, *et al.* Effector function of anti-pyroglutamate-3 Aβ antibodies affects cognitive benefit, glial activation and amyloid clearance in Alzheimer's-like mice. Alzheimers Res Ther 2020; 12(1): 12.
[http://dx.doi.org/10.1186/s13195-019-0579-8] [PMID: 31931873]

[167] Hettmann T, Gillies SD, Kleinschmidt M, *et al.* Development of the clinical candidate PBD-C06, a humanized pGlu3-Aβ-specific antibody against Alzheimer's disease with reduced complement activation. Sci Rep 2020; 10(1): 3294.
[http://dx.doi.org/10.1038/s41598-020-60319-5] [PMID: 32094456]

[168] Selkoe DJ, Hardy J. The amyloid hypothesis of Alzheimer's disease at 25 years. EMBO Mol Med 2016; 8(6): 595-608.
[http://dx.doi.org/10.15252/emmm.201606210] [PMID: 27025652]

[169] Benilova I, Karran E, De Strooper B. The toxic Aβ oligomer and Alzheimer's disease: an emperor in need of clothes. Nat Neurosci 2012; 15(3): 349-57.
[http://dx.doi.org/10.1038/nn.3028] [PMID: 22286176]

[170] Panza F, Lozupone M, Seripa D, Imbimbo BP. Amyloid-β immunotherapy for alzheimer disease: Is it now a long shot? Ann Neurol 2019; 85(3): 303-15.
[http://dx.doi.org/10.1002/ana.25410] [PMID: 30635926]

[171] Yadollahikhales G, Rojas JC. Anti-Amyloid Immunotherapies for Alzheimer's Disease: A 2023 Clinical Update. Neurotherapeutics 2023; 20(4): 914-31.
[http://dx.doi.org/10.1007/s13311-023-01405-0] [PMID: 37490245]

[172] Mo JJ, Li J, Yang Z, Liu Z, Feng JS. Efficacy and safety of anti-amyloid- *β* immunotherapy for Alzheimer's disease: a systematic review and network meta-analysis. Ann Clin Transl Neurol 2017; 4(12): 931-42.
[http://dx.doi.org/10.1002/acn3.469] [PMID: 29296624]

[173] Schenk D, Barbour R, Dunn W, *et al.* Immunization with amyloid-β attenuates Alzheimer-disease-like pathology in the PDAPP mouse. Nature 1999; 400(6740): 173-7.
[http://dx.doi.org/10.1038/22124] [PMID: 10408445]

[174] Vukicevic M, Fiorini E, Siegert S, *et al.* An amyloid beta vaccine that safely drives immunity to a key pathological species in Alzheimer's disease: pyroglutamate amyloid beta. Brain Commun 2022; 4(1): fcac022.
[http://dx.doi.org/10.1093/braincomms/fcac022] [PMID: 35479516]

[175] Panza F, Solfrizzi V, Imbimbo BP, Tortelli R, Santamato A, Logroscino G. Amyloid-based immunotherapy for Alzheimer's disease in the time of prevention trials: the way forward. Expert Rev Clin Immunol 2014; 10(3): 405-19.
[http://dx.doi.org/10.1586/1744666X.2014.883921] [PMID: 24490853]

[176] Winblad B, Andreasen N, Minthon L, *et al.* Safety, tolerability, and antibody response of active Aβ

immunotherapy with CAD106 in patients with Alzheimer's disease: randomised, double-blind, placebo-controlled, first-in-human study. Lancet Neurol 2012; 11(7): 597-604.
[http://dx.doi.org/10.1016/S1474-4422(12)70140-0] [PMID: 22677258]

[177] Wang A, Das P, Switzer RC III, Golde TE, Jankowsky JL. Robust amyloid clearance in a mouse model of Alzheimer's disease provides novel insights into the mechanism of amyloid-beta immunotherapy. J Neurosci 2011; 31(11): 4124-36.
[http://dx.doi.org/10.1523/JNEUROSCI.5077-10.2011] [PMID: 21411653]

[178] Plotkin SS, Cashman NR. Passive immunotherapies targeting Aβ and tau in Alzheimer's disease. Neurobiol Dis 2020; 144: 105010.
[http://dx.doi.org/10.1016/j.nbd.2020.105010] [PMID: 32682954]

[179] Bard F, Cannon C, Barbour R, *et al.* Peripherally administered antibodies against amyloid β-peptide enter the central nervous system and reduce pathology in a mouse model of Alzheimer disease. Nat Med 2000; 6(8): 916-9.
[http://dx.doi.org/10.1038/78682] [PMID: 10932230]

[180] Tampi RR, Forester BP, Agronin M. Aducanumab: evidence from clinical trial data and controversies. Drugs Context 2021; 10: 1-9.
[http://dx.doi.org/10.7573/dic.2021-7-3] [PMID: 34650610]

[181] Kempf SJ, Metaxas A. Neurofibrillary tangles in Alzheimer's disease: elucidation of the molecular mechanism by immunohistochemistry and tau protein phospho-proteomics. Neural Regen Res 2016; 11(10): 1579-81.
[http://dx.doi.org/10.4103/1673-5374.193234] [PMID: 27904486]

[182] Salvadores N, Gerónimo-Olvera C, Court FA. Axonal degeneration in AD: The contribution of Aβ and tau. Front Aging Neurosci 2020; 12: 581767.
[http://dx.doi.org/10.3389/fnagi.2020.581767] [PMID: 33192476]

[183] Kadmiri NE. Tau-targeted immunotherapy for alzheimer's disease: insight into clinical trials. OBM Neurobiol 2024; 8(3): 1-7.
[http://dx.doi.org/10.21926/obm.neurobiol.2403238]

[184] Zhou L, McInnes J, Wierda K, *et al.* Tau association with synaptic vesicles causes presynaptic dysfunction. Nat Commun 2017; 8(1): 15295.
[http://dx.doi.org/10.1038/ncomms15295] [PMID: 28492240]

[185] Feng X, Hou Y, Liu J, *et al.* A multi-targeting immunotherapy ameliorates multiple facets of Alzheimer's disease in 3xTg mice. NPJ Vaccines 2024; 9(1): 153.
[http://dx.doi.org/10.1038/s41541-024-00942-9] [PMID: 39164276]

[186] Vander Zanden CM, Chi EY. Passive immunotherapies targeting amyloid beta and tau oligomers in alzheimer's disease. J Pharm Sci 2020; 109(1): 68-73.
[http://dx.doi.org/10.1016/j.xphs.2019.10.024] [PMID: 31647950]

[187] Arafah A, Khatoon S, Rasool I, *et al.* The future of precision medicine in the cure of alzheimer's disease. Biomedicines 2023; 11(2): 335.
[http://dx.doi.org/10.3390/biomedicines11020335] [PMID: 36830872]

[188] Cao W, Zheng H. Peripheral immune system in aging and Alzheimer's disease. Mol Neurodegener 2018; 13(1): 51.
[http://dx.doi.org/10.1186/s13024-018-0284-2] [PMID: 30285785]

CHAPTER 12

Natural Products as Effective Treatment Approach for Alzheimer's Disease: *In silico* Justification

Piyali Khamkat[1,*], **Bramhajit Chatterjee**[1], **Vivek Barik**[1], **Suman Sahu**[2] and **Swarupananda Mukherjee**[3]

[1] *Department of Pharmaceutical Technology, Brainware University, Kolkata, West Bengal, India*

[2] *Department of Pharmacognosy, Bharat Technology, Uluberia, West Bengal, India*

[3] *Department of Pharmaceutical Technology, NSHM Knowledge Campus, Kolkata-Group of Institutions, Kolkata, West Bangal, India*

Abstract: Despite its complicated pathology and the lack of predefined curative treatments, Alzheimer's disease (AD) is still a challenge to this day. This chapter has focused on modern medical drug design for the use of natural products as therapeutic tools by providing a range of bioactive compounds in their spectra against which more than one pathological pathway in AD could be targeted. *In silico* approaches have provided powerful tools in evaluating the efficacy of these compounds in a cost-effective and time-efficient manner. This chapter discusses the current utility of *in silico* approaches like molecular docking, molecular dynamics simulations, and absorption, distribution, metabolism, elimination, and toxicity (ADMET) predictions towards confirming the application of naturalproducts as potential therapeutic alternatives for AD treatment. Some of the bioactive compounds originate from natural sources and encompass polyphenols, alkaloids, and terpenoids that display strong potential to inhibit fundamental pathological pathways such as Aβ aggregation, AChE inhibition, oxidative stress, and neuroinflammation. The computational assessment of such compounds predicts favourable pharmacokinetic profiles and drug-likeness. Such will pave the way for further investigations of these new chemical entities through *in vitro* and *in vivo* studies. Thus, *in silico* methodologies are a solid justification for developing natural products as effective therapeutic agents in AD.

Keywords: Alzheimer's disease, Amyloid-β aggregation, Acetylcholinesterase inhibition, Admet, *In silico*, Molecular docking, Natural products, Neuroinflammation, Oxidative stress.

* **Corresponding author Piyali Khamkat:** Department of Pharmaceutical Technology, Brainware University, Kolkata, West Bengal, India; E-mail: piyalikhamkat95@gmail.com

Swarupananda Mukherjee, Souvik Roy & Dipanjan Karati (Eds.)

INTRODUCTION

Alzheimer's disease (AD) is a worsening neurodegenerative illness affecting mental activity, function, and personality, with 25 million cases globally. It progresses from preclinical to dementia, and a rise in dementia cases is expected over the next 30 years. Understanding the illness process is crucial for improved patient treatment and preparedness [1, 2]. Symptoms include difficulty recalling events, uncertainty about time and location, and problem-solving challenges. The National Institute of Neurological and Communicative Disorders and Stroke and Alzheimer's Disease and Related Disorders Association established the criteria in 1984 for AD, stating that dementia develops gradually and no other brain disorders can explain memory loss and cognitive impairments [3]. Histological confirmation of clinical diagnosis is the only way to diagnose AD definitively. Advances in understanding pathogenic variants and presymptomatic individual clinical investigations have led to advancements in monogenic AD. An estimated 6.7 million Americans 65 and older are thought to be affected by Alzheimer's disease, and by 2060, that figure is predicted to rise to 13.8 million [4, 5]. With COVID-19 exacerbating the trend, the disease is now the sixth most common cause of death in the United States. More than 11 million relatives and unpaid carers gave 18 billion hours of care in 2022, worth $339.5 billion. Family carers now face higher expenses due to the lack of paid healthcare professionals [6]. Medicare and Medicaid pay three times as much per person on average for services provided to people with dementia as they do to people without the condition. In 2023, the total amount paid for hospice services, health care, and long-term care is expected to reach $345 billion [7, 8].

The amyloid cascade theory states that an accumulation of amyloid-beta peptides in the brain sets off degenerative processes that ultimately result in neurodegeneration. The cost of more recent monoclonal antibody treatments makes them less accessible, and patient noncompliance can reduce the effectiveness and tolerability of the treatment [9, 10]. Limited therapeutic methods exist for AD, but physical activity improves cognitive performance, reduces inflammation, boosts brain health, and encourages neurogenesis while addressing lifestyle, reducing symptoms, and managing cardiovascular risk factors. Acetylcholinesterase inhibitors (AChEIs) and N-methyl-D-aspartate antagonists (NMDA) are approved therapies for AD [11, 12]. These drugs reduce the overactivation of the NMDAR glutamate receptor, restoring regular activity. However, they only treat AD symptoms. AChEIs increase ACH levels in the synaptic cleft but are often ineffective due to poor solubility and bioavailability [13]. However, due to poor solubility, limited bioavailability, and inability to penetrate the blood-brain barrier (BBB), acetylcholinesterase inhibitors are often ineffective as a therapeutic approach. The BBB is crucial for treating disorders and AD pathophysiology, but few drugs can cross it, necessitating effective BBB techniques, understanding of BBB transportation, and therapeutic agent transfer [14, 15].

AD has no effective treatment. By blocking the synthesis of Aβ-peptides, encouraging Aβ breakdown, blocking AChE, lowering oxidative stress, and lowering neuroinflammation, these substances can combat AD in many ways [16, 17]. Additionally, several beneficial herbs can be utilized to treat AD and lessen dementia. Natural substances like curcumin, resveratrol, and Ginkgo biloba extract have antioxidant properties, which can lower oxidative stress, reduce brain inflammation, and maintain neuron health and cognitive capacity. However, further clinical research is needed to assess the effectiveness, ideal doses, and long-term safety of these compounds [18, 19]. The use of natural components in treating AD is examined in this chapter, highlighting their effectiveness and potential benefits. It emphasizes the need to understand their pharmacokinetics, bioavailability, and safety characteristics, as including natural ingredients could enhance patient outcomes and advance neurodegenerative treatments. Physical activity improves cognitive performance in the elderly, reduces inflammation, and promotes neurogenesis. Advances in understanding pathogenic variants and presymptomatic clinical investigations have led to advancements in monogenic AD. *In-silico* justification of natural products offers a new therapeutic approach without side effects, inhibiting Aβ-peptide production and reducing oxidative stress.

COMPREHENSION OF ALZHEIMER'S DISEASE

Pathogenesis of Alzheimer's Disease

AD is a worsening neurological condition causing dementia in senior populations, leading to behavioral abnormalities, loss of functional independence, and cognitive deterioration, primarily in memory. This chapter explores the disease's pathophysiology (Fig. **1**), molecular processes, and potential treatment options [20 - 22].

Core Histopathological Features of Alzheimer's Disease

AD is characterized by some hallmark traits that exacerbate the neurodegenerative process:

- AD is a condition distinguished by the accumulation of two key proteins, tau and amyloid-beta (Aβ), which form the pathological lesions that define the disease.

- **Amyloid-beta plaques,** found in Alzheimer's patients' brains, are extracellular deposits primarily composed of Aβ peptides, which aggregate to form fibrils, disrupt neuronal function, and trigger neurotoxic events [23, 24].
- **Neurofibrillary Tangles (NFTs):** Neurofibrillary tangles, a form of AD, are a result of the accumulation of hyperphosphorylated tau protein, which disrupts transport and synaptic function and ultimately leads to neuronal death.
- **Neuronal Loss and Brain Atrophy:** AD, distinguished by the accumulation of neurofibrillary tangles and amyloid plaques, leads to extensive neuronal loss, particularly in the hippocampus and cortex, causing significant brain atrophy [25, 26].

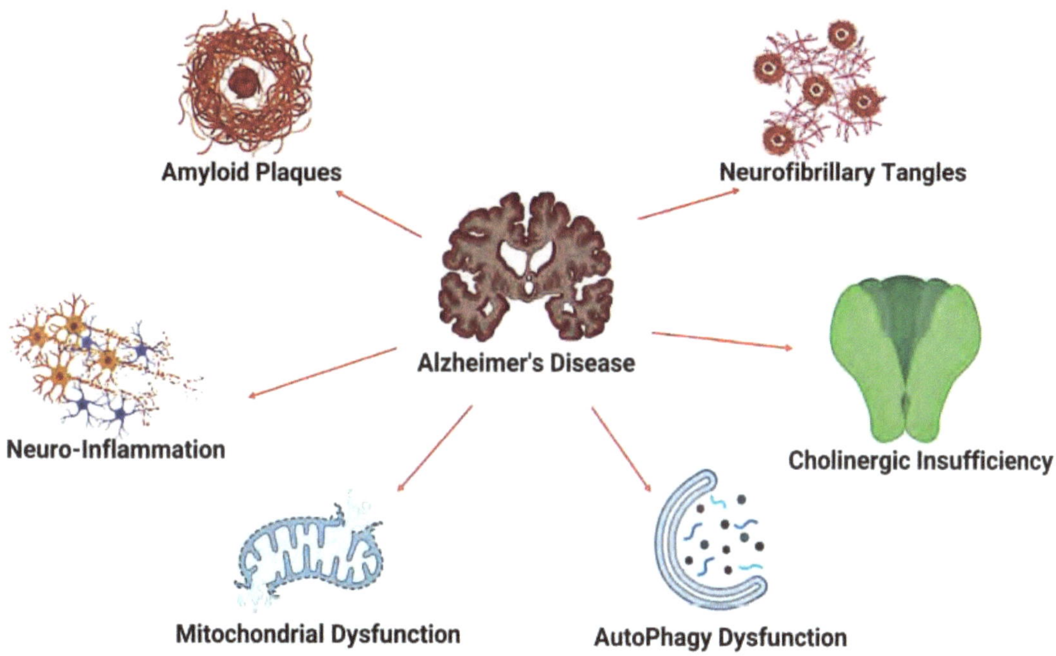

Fig. (1). Pathophysiological diagram of AD.

Molecular Mechanisms of Alzheimer's Disease

- A complex interaction of molecular pathways results in neurofibrillary tangles and amyloid-beta plaques, which in turn cause neurodegeneration and Alzheimer's disease.
- **Amyloidogenic Pathway:** The amyloidogenic pathway is essential for the formation of amyloid-beta peptides, which are cleaved by BACE1 and Aβ, forming amyloid plaques that cause synaptic dysfunction.
- **Tau Pathology and Hyperphosphorylation:** In Alzheimer's disease, tau protein undergoes hyperphosphorylation, reducing its affinity for microtubules and causing neurofibrillary tangles. This pathology correlates with cognitive

decline severity, making it a crucial target for therapeutic intervention.

- **Synaptic Dysfunction and Neuronal Death:** Synaptic dysfunction in Alzheimer's disease leads to cognitive decline, as toxic Aβ oligomers impair synaptic plasticity, causing neuronal death and contributing to the disease's clinical manifestations [27 - 29].

Mitochondrial Dysfunction and Oxidative Stress

Mitochondrial dysfunction and oxidative stress are closely intertwined processes that play a crucial role in the pathogenesis of AD.

- **Oxidative Stress:** One of the main causes of AD is oxidative stress, which is brought on by an imbalance between the generation of reactive oxygen species and brain detoxification. Damage to lipids, DNA, and proteins results in cellular malfunction and death.
- **Mitochondrial Dysfunction:** Mitochondria, the primary energy source in neurons, are a significant cause of AD, leading to synaptic failure, neurodegeneration, and cognitive decline [30 - 32].

Current Treatment Approaches and Limitations

In-depth research is still being done on disease-modifying therapeutic applications for AD.

- **Cholinesterase Inhibitors**

Cholinesterase inhibitors are a primary treatment for AD, especially in early to moderate stages. By preventing acetylcholinesterase from functioning, they raise the amount of acetylcholine, a neurotransmitter that is required for learning and memory. This increases acetylcholine concentration at synaptic junctions and improves nerve cell communication, temporarily alleviating some symptoms but not halting or reversing the progression of neurodegeneration [33].

- **NMDA Receptor Antagonists**

NMDA receptor antagonists are drugsused to treat AD, targeting the NMDA receptor, which regulates learning, brainactivity, and memory. Excessive glutamate release in Alzheimer's leads to excitotoxicity, causingneurons to be damaged or killed due to excessive calcium influx. NMDA receptor antagonists partially block the NMDA receptor, preventing excessive calcium influx and allowing normal neurotransmission for memory and cognition. This helps reduce excitotoxicity and improve cognitive function.

- **Anti-amyloid Therapies**

The goal of Aβ therapy for AD is to lessen or stop the development of Aβ plaques in the brain, which are a crucial aspect of the disease's pathophysiology. According to the amyloid cascade theory, the build-up of Aβ peptides increases the risk of AD by starting a chain reaction of pathological processes that include inflammation, tau tangles, and neurodegeneration [34 - 36].

Need for Novel Therapeutic Strategies

- **Targeting Tau and Amyloid-β Pathology**

Recent advancements in anti-amyloid therapies, including monoclonal antibodies like aducanumab and lecanemab, aim to reduce Aβ plaques, a key characteristic of AD.

Anti-Tau Therapies: Another pathogenic feature of AD is tangled tau proteins. Anti-tau antibodies, microtubule stabilizers, and tau aggregation inhibitors are among the treatments being researched.

- **Boosting Synaptic Plasticity and Neuroprotection**

Neuroprotective Agents: By lowering the synthesis of harmful amyloid-β peptides, substances like BACE inhibitors (β-secretase inhibitors) seek to prevent neuronal damage.

Synaptic Plasticity Enhancers: Using neurotrophic factors such as BDNF (Brain-derived Neurotrophic Factor) and small molecules that alter synaptic receptors are two ways to improve synaptic function and plasticity [37 - 39].

- **Targeting Metabolic and Mitochondrial Dysfunction**

Mitochondrial Protection: Research is underway to improve mitochondrial health in AD, using treatments like coenzyme Q10, antioxidants, and mitochondrial stabilizers.

Metabolic Interventions: To address metabolic dysregulation in AD, therapies such as insulin sensitizers, glucose metabolism enhancers, and ketogenic diets are being investigated.

• **Precision Medicine and Gene Therapy**

Gene Editing: Genetic mutations linked to AD, such as those in the APP or PSEN1/2 genes, may be corrected with the use of CRISPR/Cas9 and other gene-editing techniques.

Precision Medicine: By customizing therapy according to a patient's genetic composition, illness stage, and biomarkers, treatment results may be enhanced. For instance, focusing on particular APOE genetic variations, which are a significant risk factor for AD [40].

• **Cell-based Therapies**

Stem Cell Therapy: Research on using stem cells to supply neuroprotective substances or replace damaged neurons is very promising. Among the cell types under investigation are induced pluripotent stem cells (iPSCs) and mesenchymal stem cells [41].

NATURAL PRODUCTS: POTENTIAL THERAPEUTIC AGENTS

Overview of Natural Products

Research has indicated that medicinal plants can mitigate the progression and signs of several illnesses, such as AD. Several medicinal plant extracts have been studied for their impact on AD, and the active chemicals involved have been discovered. Natural products have been shown to exhibit neuroprotective effects *via* a variety of molecular mechanisms, such as increasing cholinergic signaling, inhibiting Aβ and tau protein aggregation, and having anti-oxidative and anti-inflammatory properties [42, 43]. These benefits are usually seen in combinations and extracts, indicating that by targeting several pathogenic sites, natural compounds may be capable of delaying or stopping the progression and onset of AD. Many substances have demonstrated advantageous pharmacological effects, such as anti-amyloidogenic, anticholinesterase, antioxidant, and anti-inflammatory qualities (Fig. **2**) [44]. These substances include alkaloids, lignans, polyphenols, flavonoids, sterols, tannins, and triterpenes. Certain substances, such as garlic extract, green tea extract, melatonin, vitamins E and C, resveratrol, curcumin, and Ginkgo biloba extract, have been utilized in AD patients [45, 46]. Research has demonstrated that the plant Bacopa monnieri, which is used in traditional therapy, improves memory and cognitive function. Saponins and triterpenoids are among its main ingredients. Because of its active components, Convolvulus pluricaulis possesses nootropic and memory-improving effects. It has been demonstrated that Centella asiatica enhances intellect, memory, longevity, and brain cell renewal. Ginkgo biloba leaves have been utilized for their memory-enhancing and anti-aging properties.

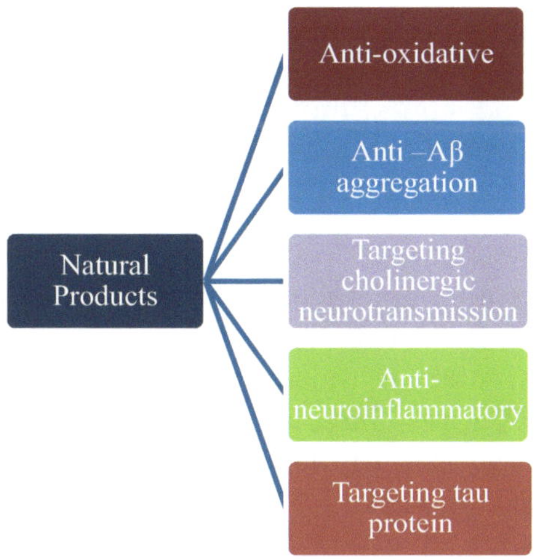

2A

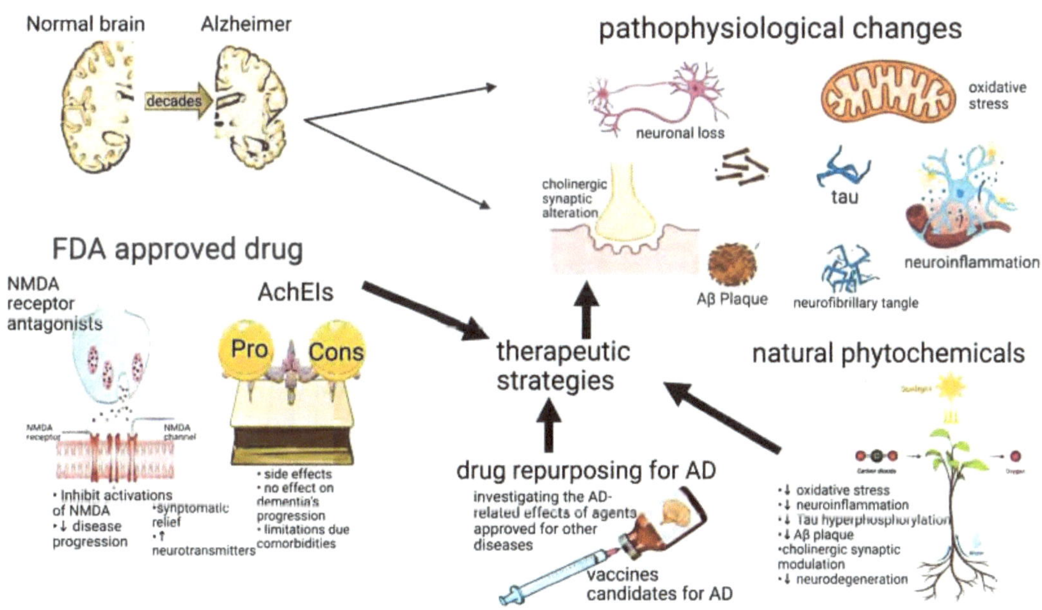

Fig. (2). Functions of natural products in AD (2A) and Mechanism of action of Phytoconstituents for AD treatment (2B).

Bioactive Compounds for Alzheimer's Disease

Natural products have demonstrated anti-neuroinflammatory efficacy by inhibiting the activation of microglia, minimizing the production of pro-inflammatory cytokines, and preventing the activation of NF-κB and p38 MAPK. In addition, certain products stimulate Nrf2, which enhances their anti-neuroinflammatory properties.

Alkaloids

Alkaloids are secondary compounds with pharmacological activity that frequently have nitrogen as a constituent of the ring. They have been connected to several pharmacological actions, such as those that reduce inflammation. COX-2 and iNOS protein and mRNA levels have been observed to decrease in the central nervous system (CNS) as a result of the alkaloid cryptolepine, which is present in Cryptolepis sanguinolenta. It works by preventing NF-κB and p38 MAPK from becoming activated in microglia [47]. It is not known how cryptolepine affects animal models of neuroinflammation or AD. Animal models of peripheral inflammation nevertheless demonstrated anti-inflammatory action. Due to its cytotoxicity and potential to harm DNA, this alkaloid has faced significant obstacles in its development as a therapy for AD.

Tetrandrine, an alkaloid derived from Radix Stephania tetrandra and synthesized from bisbenzylisoquinoline, has demonstrated promising anti-inflammatory activity *via* NF-κB in BV-2 microglia stimulated by fibrillar Aβ. Furthermore, *via* inhibiting NF-κB activation, it reduced hippocampus neuroinflammation in a rat model of AD caused by amyloid beta. Although tetrandrine's clinical effectiveness in AD has not been studied, its lipophilic nature has led to suggestions that it may penetrate the blood-brain barrier and aid stroke patients [48 - 50].

Berberine is a well-known isoquinoline alkaloid and quaternary ammonium salt with cholesterol-lowering properties, AChE, and butyrylcholinesterase inhibition with antioxidant qualities. It has been demonstrated to lessen β-amyloid-induced expressions in BV2 microglia cells and to improve learning and spatial memory in Tg mice. Additionally, berberine significantly suppresses the MAPK and PI3K/protein kinase B pathways, which lowers NF-κB production. Traditional medicine has utilized Huperzine A, a sesquiterpene alkaloid group present in Huperzia serrata, as a remedy for fever and edema and as a dietary supplement to enhance memory. A powerful AChE inhibitor, the novel tacrine-Huperzine A combination (Huprines), can considerably lessen Aβ-induced memory damage. Based on clinical investigations, Huperzine A has extremely low minimal side effects, including headaches, nausea, dizziness, and decreased heart rate. It may block many apoptotic processes, control nerve growth factor expression and release, improve memory and learning in Tg mice, and decrease the quantity of oligomeric A and β-amyloid plaques in the cortex and hippocampus. To completely understand the effectiveness of Huperzine A against Alzheimer's disease, more research is necessary [51].

Flavonoids

Numerous plant components, including vegetables, flowers, fruits, bark, roots, and stems, naturally contain flavonoids and phenolic compounds. Their ability to reduce inflammation has been proven, and research has shown that the flavonoid kaempferol suppresses neuroinflammation by reducing the production of pro-inflammatory mediators in BV2 microglial cells, which are activated by LPS and mediated *via* p38 MAPK and NF-κB pathways. Tiroside, a glycosidic flavonoid, is similar to kaempferol in that it has been demonstrated to inhibit p38 MAPK, activate Nrf2, and attenuate NF-κB, among other pathways, therefore preventing neuroinflammation in BV-2 microglia [48, 49].

Flavones such as apigenin (4′,7-trihydroxyflavone) that are present in celery, parsley, and chamomile have been demonstrated to inhibit activated microglia's generation of TNFα and pro-inflammatory IL-6. In models of AD, apigenin has been confirmed to have neuroprotective effects, which may be related to its anti-inflammatory properties, according to animal studies. Quercetin is a common natural anti-inflammatory and antioxidant flavonoid that can be found in a wide variety of fruits, vegetables, and seeds, similar to kaempferol [52]. BV-2 microglia activated with LPS produced less NO through iNOS-mediated synthesis when quercetin was added, possibly due to mechanisms that blocked NF-κB activation. Quercetin's anti-inflammatory properties depend on the antioxidant transcription factor Nrf2. Quercetin's impact on cognitive performance in the APP/PS1 mice model of AD has been connected to its anti-inflammatory activities. According to studies by Lv *et al.*, (2018), treating APP/PS1 mice with quercetin dramatically decreased neuroinflammation, p-Tau, and Aβ plaques. Furthermore, apigenin enhanced memory and spatial learning after inducing amnesia with Aβ25–35 (Fig. **3**) [53].

Green tea contains a flavone called quercetin, which has been demonstrated to exhibit strong antioxidant and anti-inflammatory properties in microglia. These properties are important for neuroprotection and potential treatment advantages in AD. However, because AD medication does not penetrate the BBB, it is not clinically effective. Related flavones such as luteolin have been discovered to have similar anti-inflammatory and neuroprotective properties [54]. Because of its capacity to suppress neuroinflammation, the flavanol epigallocatechin-3-gallate (EGCG), which is present in green tea, has been proposed to possess anti-amyloidogenic and neuroprotective properties. *In vitro* studies have demonstrated that EGCG can reduce Aβ-stimulated EOC13.31 microglia's levels of TNFα, IL-1β, IL-6, and iNOS *via* processes involving NF-κB. When lipopolysaccharide (LPS) was injected systemically into mice, EGCG decreased Aβ production and neurotoxicity and avoided memory impairment in animals. Additionally, *in vivo* research showed that EGCG enhanced neuroprotection in animal models of AD. Although EGCG has been studied *in vitro* and in animal models of AD, human studies have not assessed how well it enhances cognitive performance. For instance, giving healthy individuals 300 mg of EGCG enhanced their brain activity without having a corresponding impact on task performance. Additionally, a double-blind, placebo-controlled crossover investigation of the effects of a single oral dosage of 135 mg of EGCG on cerebral blood flow (CBF), mood, and cognitive performance in healthy adult humans was conducted. The results did not reveal any appreciable differences between the EGCG and placebo groups in terms of mood and cognitive function. The translational gap between the compound's bioactivity *in vitro* and animal studies and its effects in human trials may be caused by the poor oral bioavailability of EGCG and the variations in metabolism between humans and animals [55].

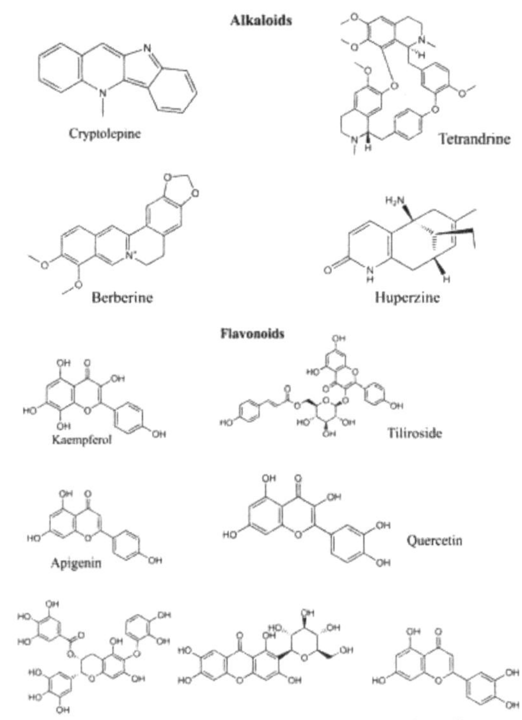

Fig. (3). Structure of bioactive components of alkaloids and flavonoids.

Further investigations involving humans are invaluable to ascertain the impact of EGCG on cognitive performance. Mangiferin, a glucosylxanthone that is naturally found in the leaves, stem, and bark of mango trees, has been shown to decrease the production of prostaglandin E2 and COX-2 expression when triggered by lipopolysaccharide (LPS) [56]. *In vivo* research indicated that mangiferin improved cognitive deficits and decreased neuroinflammation in APP/PS1 mice. However, no human study has confirmed the efficacy of mangiferin in treating AD outcomes. Flavonoids remain a significant class of natural substances for decreasing neuroinflammation in AD due to their basic inhibitory actions on pro-inflammatory transcription factors and activation of anti-inflammatory and antioxidant transcription factors. However, because of their high polarity, parent flavonoids typically have limited overall bioavailability and have difficulty crossing the blood-brain barrier. Moreover, luteolin can prevent apoptosis by enhancing endogenous antioxidant systems, reducing intracellular ROS production, and stimulating the NRF2 pathway. It has been demonstrated to reduce lipid peroxide formation, enhance antioxidant systems, alleviate cognitive impairment, and prevent inflammatory responses in brain tissue brought on by long-term cerebral hypoperfusion. In a study, luteolin enhanced memory and cognitive function in a streptozotocin-induced rat model of AD. Nevertheless, additional evidence from clinical trials is required to validate luteolin's preventive benefits against AD. The rhizomatous perennial plant Curcuma longa contains the water-insoluble curcuminoids curcumin, demethoxycurcumin, and bis-demethoxycurcumin. Curcumin is a recognized medication for the treatment of AD because of its antibacterial, anticancer, anti-inflammatory, and antioxidant qualities [57].

Polyphenols

Berries and grapes contain a polyphenol called resveratrol, which has been researched extensively as a possible therapy for several illnesses. Resveratrol has been shown in numerous pharmacological investigations to have anti-neuroinflammatory and neuroprotective properties in both *in vitro* and animal models. In 2007, Candelario-Jalil *et al*., found the first proof that resveratrol can stop neuroinflammation. They found that resveratrol reduced the production of molecules that caused free radicals and PGE2 to be made in primary rat microglia that were activated by LPS. This study also demonstrated that resveratrol is the only known inhibitor that selectively inhibits the synthesis of microsomal prostaglandin E synthase-1 (mPGES-1) without influencing COX-2 [58]. Later, Abraham and Johnson (2009) found that resveratrol consumption decreased LPS-induced IL-1β levels in plasma and IL-1β mRNA in aged mouse hippocampal tissues and cultured BV-2 microglia cells [59]. Recent research by Sun *et al*., (2019) provided fresh evidence linking resveratrol's ability to control neuroinflammation to its capability to repair tau-induced neuropathology and cognitive deficits in a mouse model of AD. In mice, resveratrol treatment avoided neuroinflammation and synapse loss, decreased phosphorylated tau levels, and improved cognitive impairments. These preclinical resveratrol studies are encouraging and call for additional clinical research [60].

Perhaps the most studied naturally occurring neuroprotective polyphenol for the treatment of AD is curcumin, which is found in *Curcuma longa*, or turmeric. Numerous pharmacological actions and therapeutic advantages, such as anti-inflammatory, anticancer, antibacterial, antioxidant, and wound-healing properties, have been associated with it. Studies conducted on BV-2 microglia demonstrated that curcumin suppressed neuroinflammation in LTA-stimulated microglial cells by lowering TNFα, PGE2, and nitric oxide (NO) production and blocking NF-κB and MAPK activation. However, a 24-week placebo-controlled clinical experiment using curcumin failed to show any benefit in AD. The lack of efficacy might be caused by differences in the biology between rat models of AD and human AD, as well as the product's bioavailability, according to the researchers' hypothesis. Following a 4-week treatment, a subsequent randomized, double-blind, placebo-controlled study in older, healthy individuals found a significant increase in working memory and mood [61, 62].

Rosmarinic acid, a polyphenol-type carboxylic acid with a variety of pharmacological characteristics such as neuroprotective, antiviral, antibacterial, anti-inflammatory, and antioxidant qualities, is found in several Lamiaceae species. It can prevent β-amyloid-induced memory loss by inhibiting NF-κB and TNF-α production, protecting neuronal PC12 cells from beta-amyloid-induced cytotoxicity, and lowering tau protein hyperphosphorylation. Moreover, it blocks the production of ROS, the activation of caspase-3, and DNA fragmentation to obstruct apoptotic pathways.

Lutein is a flavonoid compound found in medicinal plants, including Magnoliophyta, Pteridophyta, Bryophyta, and Pinophyta. It has a range of biological actions, including anti-inflammatory, antioxidant, anticancer, antibacterial, and neuroprotective qualities. It can reduce the number of β-amyloids produced, the amount of amyloid precursor protein expressed, and the extent of tau protein hyperphosphorylation caused by zinc [45, 51].

Terpenes

Terpenoids are a class of molecules derived from the union of two or more isoprene units. They have been shown to reduce neuroinflammation both *in vitro* and in animal models. *Tanacetum parthenium* contains parthenolide, a physiologically active sesquiterpene lactone that has been shown to enhance cognitive performance and lower IL-6 and TNF-α levels in the cortex and hippocampus regions of rats (Fig. **4**). Additionally, it has been documented to suppress neuroinflammation in rats with intracerebral hemorrhage-induced brain damage by lowering TLR4/NF-κB-mediated TNF-α, IL-17, and IL-6 levels in the ipsilateral hemispheres of the brain. In AD clinical studies, parthenolide's neuroprotection needs to be further verified.

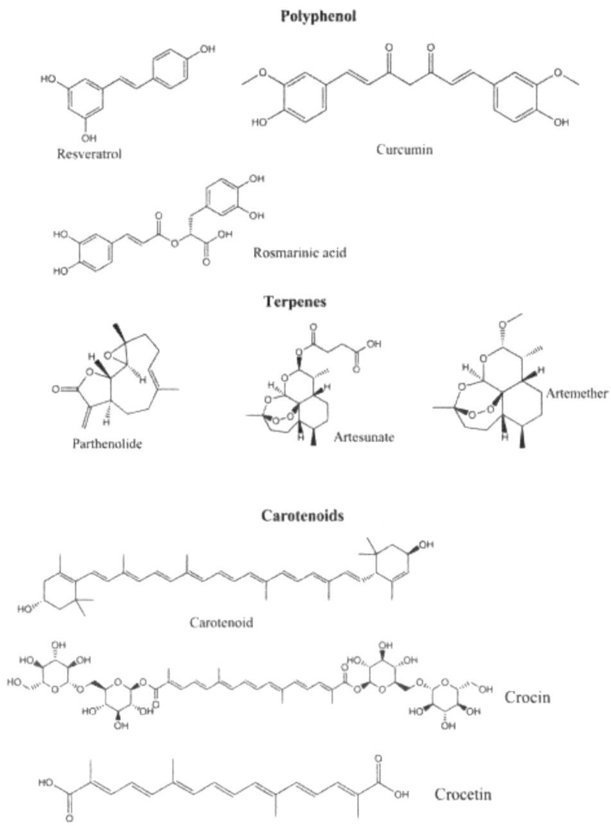

Fig. (4). Structure of bioactive components of Polyphenols, Terpenes, Carotenoids.

Artemisinin, a sesquiterpene lactone found in *Artemisia annua*, may have neuroprotective effects on AD patients, in part because of its anti-inflammatory properties [51]. Research has shown that in BV-2 microglia exposed to LPS, artemisinin inhibited the release of TNFα, IL-6, MCP-1, and NO. Furthermore, it has been observed to have modulatory effects on the microglial NF-κB signaling pathway. Artemisinin analogs, including artesunate and artemether, diminish neuroinflammation by concentrating on NF-κB signaling in BV-2 microglia [63].

Carotenoids

The spice saffron, or *Crocus sativus*, has many therapeutic applications, such as the treatment of cancer, diabetes, atherosclerosis, depression, and neurological illnesses. Various studies, including *in vitro* experiments, AD model organisms, and clinical investigations, have shown that saffron flowers contain carotenoids, crocin, and crocetin, which are natural compounds with neuroprotective qualities and potential therapeutic uses. Crocin and crocetin were found to inhibit the production of IL-1β, reactive oxygen species (ROS), NO/iNOS, and TNF-α in BV-2 microglial cells following LPS stimulation through pathways associated with NF-κB, as demonstrated in BV-2 microglia research. The brain function of animals with Alzheimer's disease was improved by these anti-inflammatory carotenoids [51]. According to research conducted by Mazumder *et al.*, (2017), crocin can improve mice's cognitive function in addition to having anti-inflammatory and antioxidant properties. Currently, no clinical research has been done to demonstrate the effects of crocin and crocetin in AD [61].

Marine Products

Many marine species contain astaxanthin, a xanthophyll carotenoid that has been studied for its potential as a neuroprotective natural product. Astaxanthin reduces the synthesis of IL-6 generated by LPS in BV-2 microglia by blocking NO/iNOS and COX-2, which is achieved through the activation of NF-κB, ERK1/2, and MSK-1. It has been demonstrated that astaxanthin inhibits neuroinflammation in animal models of neurodegeneration, improving cognitive impairments in diabetic mice and preventing NF-κB-mediated neuroinflammation. Studies have shown encouraging outcomes in enhancing cognitive function, and the results suggest that astaxanthin has significant potential for developing novel therapeutics for neurodegenerative illnesses like AD. Overall, astaxanthin is a promising candidate for novel therapy development due to its neuroprotective properties [63, 64].

Problems with Delivering Natural Compounds into the Brain

It is difficult to treat AD because of physical barriers such as the brain's blood-brain barrier (BBB). Due to their poor pharmacokinetic profiles and limited bioavailability, the BBB significantly affects the activity of neuroprotective natural substances, as the passage of endogenous chemicals from blood to brain depends on this critical mechanism. Some anti-inflammatory natural products, such as resveratrol and curcumin, have poor bioavailability because of extensive metabolism.

Lipid-based nanocarrier delivery methods have been explored to enhance BBB penetration and the bioavailability of these compounds. Liposomes, for instance, are vesicles composed of lipid bilayers that self-assemble when amphiphilic compounds like phospholipids are present. A newer class of submicron-sized lipid emulsions, called solid lipid nanoparticles (SLNs), can penetrate the BBB and exert pharmacological effects on the central nervous system. Lipid nanoparticles have gained attention as protective carriers for active compounds. Several natural anti-inflammatory agents have demonstrated improved brain permeability through these novel delivery strategies [44, 51]. Table **1** describes natural products and their mode of action against AD.

Table 1. Drugs and antibodies derived from natural products targeting Alzheimer's disease and their mechanisms of action.

Drugs	Source Organism / TherapeuticAntibodies	Action Mechanism	Refs.
Physostigmine	*Physostigmavenensosum Balf.* (Leguminosae)	Reversibly inhibits AChE, leading to improved cognitive abilities *in vivo*.	[50]
Galantamine	*LycorisradiataHerb., Galanthusnivalis L., Narcissus*spp. (Amaryllidaceae)	Reversibly blocks AChE and potentiates nicotinicacetyl cholinereceptors through allosteric mechanisms.	[65]
Huperzine A	*HuperziaserrataTrevis.* (Lycopodiaceae)	Exhibits selective and reversible inhibition of the AChE enzyme	[66]
ZT-1	Prodrug of huperzine	SuppressesAChE action and re-establishes proper acetylcholine levels	[67]
Curcumin	*Curcuma longa L.* (Zingiberaceae)	Inhibits the formation of Aβ aggregates, prevents Aβ-induced inflammation, and interferes with β-secretase and AChE activities	[68]
Resveratrol	*Vitis vinifera L.* (Vitaceae)	Promotes the decomposition and clearance of intracellular Aβ aggregates	[69]
Bryostatin-1	*Bugulaneritina L.* (Bugulidae)	Promotes α-secretase activity in human fibroblast cells, reduces Aβ 42 levels, and minimizes mortality in transgenic models of Alzheimer's disease	[70]
Rifampicin	*Amycolatopsisrifamycinica* (Pseudonocardiaceae)	Blocks the formation of Aβ aggregates *in vitro*	[71]
Scyllocyclohexanehexol (ELND005, AZD-103)	*Cornusflorida L.* (Cornaceae) and *Cocos nucifera L.* (Arecaceae)	Disassembles neurotoxic fibrils, promoting the elimination of amyloid peptides ratherthan plaque formation	[72]

(Table 1) cont.....

Drugs	Source Organism / TherapeuticAntibodies	Action Mechanism	Refs.
Bapineuzumab (AN-1792)	Humanized monoclonal antibody	Aβ plaque-specific antibody	[73]
Ponezumab (PF04360365)	Humanized monoclonal antibody	Aβ plaque-specific antibody	[74]
Solanezumab, Crenezumab	Monoclonal antibody	Neutralizes Aβ plaques with a specific antibody	[75]
Gantenerumab	Humanized monoclonal antibody	Strong ability to bind and eliminate Aβ plaques from the brain.	[76]
BAN2401	Humanized immunoglobulin-1 monoclonal antibody	Specifically binds to large, soluble Aβ oligomers, neutralizing their harmful effects on brain cells.	[77]
Cyclosporin A	*Tolypocladium inflatum* (fungus)	The strongest neuroprotectant for stroke and traumatic brain injury.	[77]

COMPUTATIONAL APPROACHES AND RATIONALE FOR NATURAL PRODUCTS IN DRUG DISCOVERY

The Importance of Computational Methods in the Drug Development Pipeline

A computer-based approach to the identification and development of potential drug candidates, *in-silico* drug discovery involves the refinement of structures through computer-aided drug design (CADD) methodologies, such as *in-silico* structure prediction and virtual ligand screening, and optimization. It is an indispensable element of modern drug research, as it minimises the need for time and money to identify and develop therapeutic candidates. The combination of *in-silico* strategies and physical screening techniques is often employed to maximize the discovery of promising drug candidates. *In-silico* research helps with drug development in many ways. It makes it easier to screen, create, and predict the therapeutic potential of new medicines. It also helps find new and interesting molecules that help figure out how toxic they are because *in-silico* research uses current knowledge to inform future operations, it also improves flexibility and morality in early drug development [24, 78].

An $8.3 billion industry was founded in 2022 by *in-silico* drug development, which produced a large number of potential medicinal candidates. Examples include cancer drug vemurafenib, the HIV therapy drug raltegravir, and COVID-19 therapeutic options such as molnupiravir. Because it helps identify potential drugs, *in-silico* drug discovery is an essential part of the drug development process, including the prediction of binding modes and process optimization.

Although frequently employed alongside traditional experimental methodologies, *in vivo* and *in vitro* procedures cannot be entirely replaced by *in-silico* techniques.

Methods such as databases, homology models, pharmacophores, and quantitative structure-activity relationships (QSAR) are increasingly used in drug development to screen and evaluate candidates (Fig. **5**). These techniques also support the generation of structure-based drugs by analyzing large datasets and predicting potential therapeutic targets. For example, virtual screening predicts each molecule's binding score using a virtual library of compounds.

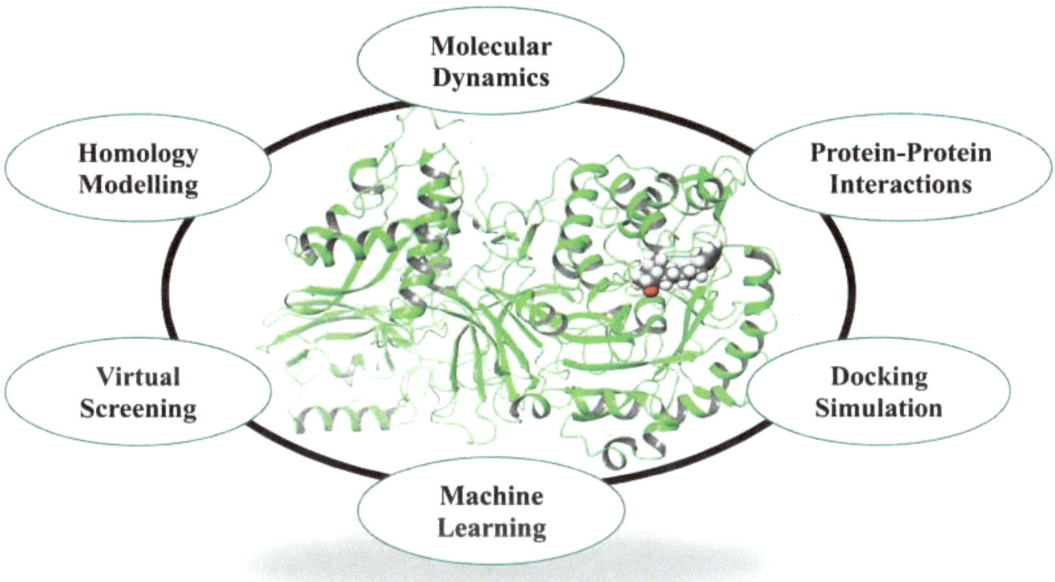

Fig. (5). Different applications of *in-silico* methods.

Advantages of *in-silico* research in drug discovery include reducing time and resource requirements, utilizing existing information, integrating with other methodologies, predictive capabilities, and cost-effectiveness. However, implementing *in-silico* research presents several challenges, including validation and accuracy, the complexity of biological systems, regulatory approval, data availability and quality, and interdisciplinary expertise. Ensuring the accuracy and precision of *in-silico* predictions depends on proper validation. Accurately modeling biological systems *in-silico* is challenging due to their inherent complexity. Another difficulty is obtaining regulatory acceptance, as authorities require strong evidence of reliability and applicability. Successful *in-silico* research also depends on high-quality data and multidisciplinary knowledge [67, 79].

In silico Techniques

Both academic and commercial institutions have made substantial investments in NP research due to the resurgence of interest in these compounds. These investments include NP searches, isolation, characterization, and biological evaluation. *In silico*-based techniques have made it much cheaper to bring new medicines to market, which has been very helpful for both the pharmaceutical business and academics.To find NP-based hit molecules, virtual screening (VS) methods and machine learning approaches have been applied extensively. Many compounds fail to reach the market due to inadequate pharmacokinetic properties, which are usually detected late in the discovery process. Early computational predictions of ADMET profiles (absorption, distribution, metabolism, elimination, and toxicity) for natural product drugs have become an essential part of the drug development process. This has reduced the time and cost associated with ADMET profiling using conventional experimental methods. Therefore, to generate NP analogs with acceptable ADMET qualities, rational drug design-based procedures need to rely on *in silico*-based approaches. The scientific community faces difficulties in identifying less expensive treatment options for illnesses and medications with few adverse effects. Natural products have the potential to transform drug discovery. Major pharmaceutical corporations continue to focus less on NPs, yet NPs still make up half of FDA-approved medications, especially antibiotics and anticancer compounds [51, 63]. "Drug-likeness" means how similar biochemical properties are, like polarity, hydrophobicity, lipophilicity, molecular mass, and hydrogen bond donors/acceptors. Drug-likeness can be predicted from molecular structure through *in silico* approaches before synthesis and evaluation. The medicinal chemistry community uses the rule of five (Ro5) to estimate the "drug-likeness" of important compounds. It often serves as an initial filter in VS of chemical libraries. QED (Quantitative Estimate of Drug-likeness) is a refined measure that focuses on the appeal of a drug candidate. It scores a molecule between zero and one depending on its characteristics. In QED, an unfavourable feature is tolerated if other features are almost ideal, providing a rich view of drug-likeness. Molecular docking is the most widely used technique in structure-based drug design (Fig. **6**). Pharmacophore use was initiated in the late 1970s for maximizing the separation of the partners with particular orientations for better structural modelling. Such a model does permit rigid docking as well as changes in relative orientation. Advances in computational capacity [51, 80] now make it possible to predict hypothetical changes in interior geometry during complex development, commonly referred to as flexible docking. The technique of Molecular Dynamics Simulations connects with the time-dependent motion of atoms and molecules. As a matter of fact, it lets them picture how the proteins associated with Alzheimer's change.

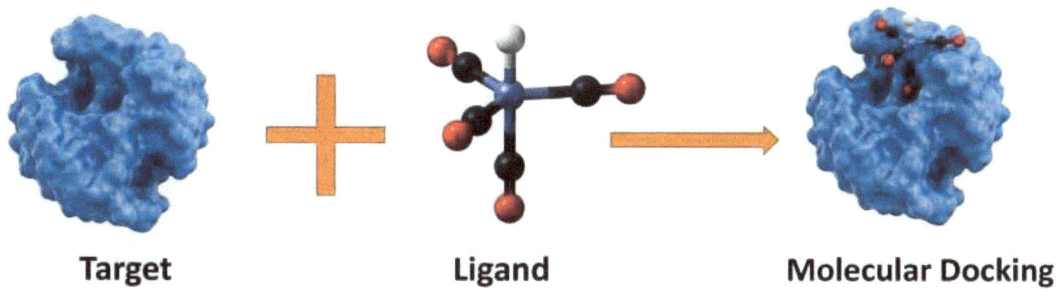

Fig. (6). Diagram of molecular docking.

Development of Natural Product Databases (NPD)

NPD comprises an all-inclusive database of all information related to natural products, including structures, biological activities, and source information. Poor hit rates from synthetic combinatorial screenings have led researchers to either boost the diversity of combinatorial databases by improving synthetic reactions or revisit NPs, which have historically been instrumental in drug discovery, notably in therapies targeting cancer and microbial infections. Because of their great structural diversity and complexity, NPs have produced novel lead compounds with distinctive scaffolds.

PubChem is a complementary database provided by the National Institutes of Health (NIH). This database encompasses data regarding the biological roles of smaller molecules and several other small molecules derived from natural sources. NPD plays a vital role in sharing, recording, and protecting collections.

Tropical Plant Database: This database catalogs tropical plants for their use and certain compounds, which can have any neuroprotective/anti-inflammatory properties applicable in Alzheimer's research.

NCI Database: The National Cancer Institute's database contains information on natural products and their tested biological activities, such as neuroprotective effects.

ChEMBL: It is a database of bioactive drug-like small molecules, some of which are natural products with known pharmacological effects. This database, named KNApSAcK, is specifically dedicated to natural products from plants and their biological activities; it can prove quite helpful in finding new treatments for Alzheimer's [62, 80].

To identify new drugs, the chemical space of tiny compounds has been investigated using *in-silico*-based drug design techniques. However, there are issues with focusing on synthetic, natural, or pseudo-natural items in the chemical realm, as well as which areas should be studied. NPs possess distinctive qualities such as structural complexity and diversity of scaffolds, which can be investigated for novel medicinal treatments. Expanding the searchable drug-like chemical space, going back to ignored or unconventional chemical regions, and the time-consuming procedure of isolating a single chemical constituent are some of the challenges.

CURRENT SCENARIO AND FUTURE ASPECTS OF *IN-SILICO* TECHNIQUES IN AD USING NPS

In 2013, Ntie-Kang assessed 2400 NPs from the Gram-positive bacterium database StreptomeDB 2.0 for drug-likeness. The study found 52.5% of compounds had at least one Ro5 violation, according to the research, and 22.7% had more than two. Among microbial NPs, polyketides constituted the bulk of compounds possessing multiple Ro5 violations. Pilkington classified the 179 marine NPs in three kingdoms into three categories: known drug space, lead-like space, and drug-like space. According to the PCA study, various descriptors contributed to the observed variability, with TPSA, logP, and logS having the greatest impact on the second principal component. For marine NPs in these categories, the chemical space distribution is 0.5%, 39.7%, and 64.8%, in that order [80].

Mexican NPs from the BIOFACQUIM were subjected to a computational ADMET review in 2020 by Medina-Franco *et al.*, who also compared the results with datasets from AfroDB, NuBBEDB, TCM, and FDA-approved medicines. They discovered that the profiles of toxicity, hepatotoxicity, excretion, metabolism, and absorption of BIOFACQUIM were comparable to those of other NPs [81].

The calculated ADMET profile of datasets containing protein-protein interface inhibitors (iPPIs) and non-iPPIs was published by Lagorce *et al.*, in 2017. They discovered that usual binding sites on proteins that molecularly recognize other proteins are only accessible by beyond-Ro5 molecules rather than by conventional small-molecule ligands. Several very effective iPPIs are NP (macrocyclic) polyketides.

Many studies have been conducted in response to the COVID-19 pandemic to recommend novel antivirals and treatment plans that will lower morbidity and mortality. One such research proposed paclitaxel (Taxol) and other medication candidates as possible antivirals. It is difficult to get significant amounts of Taxol for commercial supply and biological screening, nevertheless.

In another study, the inhibitory actions of histone deacetylase (HDAC) isoforms in natural products (NPs) from an African NP database collection were evaluated. The study discovered that NPs from African source species are comparable to HDAC inhibitors and occupy chemical regions not previously documented in published databases. Unfortunately, since it was hard to get actual samples of the seventeen proposed compounds, or because some of them were very expensive, only three of them were tested experimentally.

Using the pan-African Natural Products Library (pANAPL), Karaman *et al.*, performed a virtual screening (VS) to determine that bichalcones were sirtuin inhibitors. Only five of the 22 suggested hits have enough amounts for additional research. Two of these substances, rhuschalcone IV and rhuschalcone I counterpart, showed action *in vitro*, indicating that they may be further refined to enhance their biological effects as inhibitors of sirtuins. In addition, the writers offered recommendations for additional development [82].

The study focuses on the neuroprotective properties of a furanoflavonoid that was isolated from Pongamia pinnata in Alzheimer's disease. Although several health advantages of furanoflavonoids have been documented, their impact on certain conditions has not been well studied. According to the study, Karanjin has appropriate ADMET profiles for therapeutic usage and complies with Lipinski's drug-likeness guidelines. Compared to typical medications, the docking scores demonstrated greater potency against AD targets. Fig. (**7**) shows a strong correlation between the results and previous studies on karanjin in an Alzheimer's disease animal model. But further *in vivo* studies, clinical trials, bioavailability, permeability, and safe dose administration are needed before Karanjin may be utilised to treat AD [83].

In 2023, Vasanth Kanth TL, with his team, worked on bioactive compounds and demonstrated that the Tau protein plays an important part in the increasingly difficult-to-treat neurodegenerative illnesses, such as Alzheimer's. The side effects of many modern medications are intolerable to the body and are quite costly. To solve this, scientists used *in silico* techniques to repurpose already-existing molecules. They took substances from the Selleckchem natural product library, looked at their ADMET characteristics and blood-brain barrier-crossing capability, and evaluated the Tau protein's structure. Ligustroflavone has the best binding affinity among the 92 compounds that met the ADMET screening requirements [84].

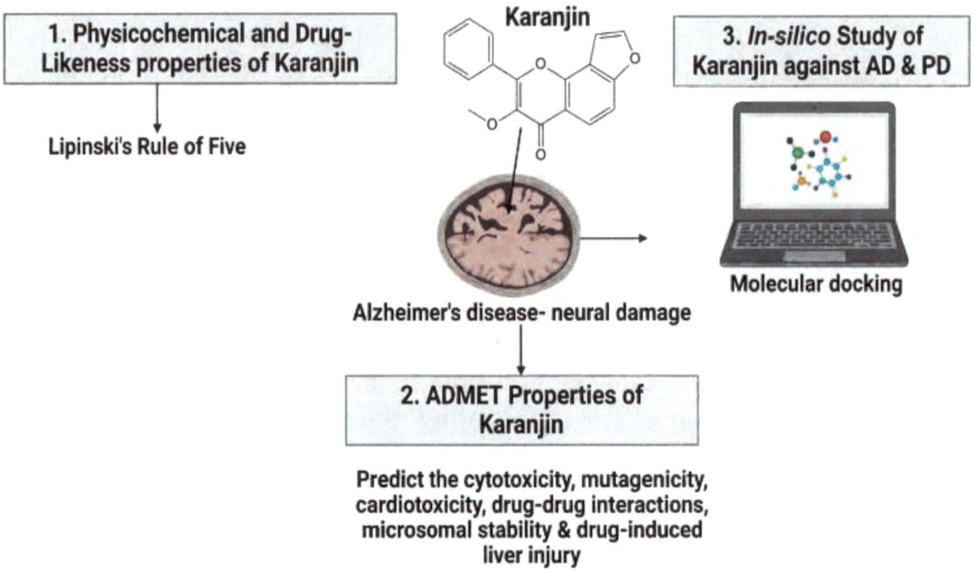

Fig. (7). *In silico* molecular docking analysis of Karanjin.

CONCLUSION

The diverse bioactive compounds and NPs' neuroprotective properties make them a potential candidate for drugs with beneficial effects in AD. *In-silico* approaches involving the evaluation of such compounds provide a powerful tool in the exploration of their potential mechanisms of action, thus rendering screening large numbers of compounds both inexpensive and time-effective. Alongside supporting the potential of natural products, *in-silico* screening and modeling also aid the prediction of drug-likeness, bioavailability, and safety profiles. This way, the computational approach optimizes the choice of candidates for further *in vitro* and *in vivo* testing. Moreover, those candidates that show positive pharmacokinetic and pharmacodynamic profiles can be rationally modified through structure-based drug design to have enhanced efficacy.

In conclusion, the *in-silico* studies provide sufficient justification to continue with further studies on natural products as therapeutic agents for AD. These computational tools boost the pipeline for developing such compounds by predetermining key interactions with disease-related proteins and their drug-like properties, all of which together qualify natural products as an effective and attractive treatment approach for AD.

REFERENCES

[1] Hippius H, Neundörfer G. The discovery of Alzheimer's disease. Dialogues Clin Neurosci 2003; 5(1): 101-8. [http://dx.doi.org/10.31887/DCNS.2003.5.1/hhippius] [PMID: 22034141]

[2] Congdon EE, Sigurdsson EM. Tau-targeting therapies for Alzheimer disease. Nat Rev Neurol 2018; 14(7): 399-415. [http://dx.doi.org/10.1038/s41582-018-0013-z] [PMID: 29895964]

[3] Oliveira BCL, Bellozi PMQ, Reis HJ, de Oliveira ACP. QuaglioBellozi PM, Reis HJ, Pinheiro de Oliveia AC. Inflammation as a possible link between dyslipidemia and alzheimer's disease. Neuroscience 2018; 376: 127-41. [http://dx.doi.org/10.1016/j.neuroscience.2018.02.012]

[4] Porsteinsson AP, Isaacson RS, Knox S, Sabbagh MN, Rubino I. Diagnosis of early alzheimer's disease: Clinical practice in 2021. J Prev Alzheimers Dis 2021; 8(3): 371-86. [http://dx.doi.org/10.14283/jpad.2021.23] [PMID: 34101796]

[5] Chen G, Xu T, Yan Y, *et al.* Amyloid beta: structure, biology and structure-based therapeutic development. Acta Pharmacol Sin 2017; 38(9): 1205-35. [http://dx.doi.org/10.1038/aps.2017.28] [PMID: 28713158]

[6] Huang SY, Yang YX, Kuo K, *et al.* Herpesvirus infections and Alzheimer's disease: a Mendelian randomization study. Alzheimers Res Ther 2021; 13(1): 158. [http://dx.doi.org/10.1186/s13195-021-00905-5] [PMID: 34560893]

[7] Hebert LE, Weuve J, Scherr PA, Evans DA. Alzheimer disease in the United States (2010–2050) estimated using the 2010 census. Neurology 2013; 80(19): 1778-83. [http://dx.doi.org/10.1212/WNL.0b013e31828726f5] [PMID: 23390181]

[8] Asiful Islam M, Saif Khandker S, Alam F, Ibrahim Khalil M, Amjad Kamal M, Hua Gan S. Alzheimer';s disease and natural products: Future regimens emerging from nature. Curr Top Med Chem 2017; 17(12): 1408-28. [http://dx.doi.org/10.2174/1568026617666170103163054] [PMID: 28049401]

[9] Kirova AM, Bays RB, Lagalwar S. Working memory and executive function decline across normal aging, mild cognitive impairment, and Alzheimer's disease. BioMed Res Int 2015; 2015: 1-9. [http://dx.doi.org/10.1155/2015/748212] [PMID: 26550575]

[10] Gu Y, Scarmeas N. Dietary patterns in Alzheimer's disease and cognitive aging. Curr Alzheimer Res 2011; 8(5): 510-9. [http://dx.doi.org/10.2174/156720511796391836] [PMID: 21605048]

[11] Morris MC, Tangney CC, Wang Y, *et al.* MIND diet slows cognitive decline with aging. Alzheimers Dement 2015; 11(9): 1015-22. [http://dx.doi.org/10.1016/j.jalz.2015.04.011] [PMID: 26086182]

[12] Scarmeas N, Anastasiou CA, Yannakoulia M. Nutrition and prevention of cognitive impairment. Lancet Neurol 2018; 17(11): 1006-15. [http://dx.doi.org/10.1016/S1474-4422(18)30338-7] [PMID: 30244829]

[13] Kumar K, Kumar A, Keegan RM, Deshmukh R. Recent advances in the neurobiology and neuropharmacology of Alzheimer's disease. Biomed Pharmacother 2018; 98: 297-307. [http://dx.doi.org/10.1016/j.biopha.2017.12.053] [PMID: 29274586]

[14] Yin RH, Yu JT, Tan L. The Role of SORL1 in Alzheimer's Disease. Mol Neurobiol 2015; 51(3): 909-18. [http://dx.doi.org/10.1007/s12035-014-8742-5] [PMID: 24833601]

[15] Sharma P, Srivastava P, Seth A, Tripathi PN, Banerjee AG, Shrivastava SK. Comprehensive review of mechanisms of pathogenesis involved in Alzheimer's disease and potential therapeutic strategies. Prog Neurobiol 2019; 174: 53-89.

[http://dx.doi.org/10.1016/j.pneurobio.2018.12.006] [PMID: 30599179]

[16] Klose J, Griehl C, Roßner S, Schilling S. Natural products from plants and algae for treatment of alzheimer's disease: A review. Biomolecules 2022; 12(5): 694.
[http://dx.doi.org/10.3390/biom12050694] [PMID: 35625622]

[17] Chen X, Drew J, Berney W, Lei W. Neuroprotective natural products for alzheimer's disease. Cells 2021; 10(6): 1309.
[http://dx.doi.org/10.3390/cells10061309] [PMID: 34070275]

[18] Essa MM, Vijayan RK, Castellano-Gonzalez G, Memon MA, Braidy N, Guillemin GJ. Neuroprotective effect of natural products against Alzheimer's disease. Neurochem Res 2012; 37(9): 1829-42.
[http://dx.doi.org/10.1007/s11064-012-0799-9] [PMID: 22614926]

[19] Dey A, Bhattacharya R, Mukherjee A, Pandey DK. Natural products against Alzheimer's disease: Pharmaco-therapeutics and biotechnological interventions. Biotechnol Adv 2017; 35(2): 178-216.
[http://dx.doi.org/10.1016/j.biotechadv.2016.12.005] [PMID: 28043897]

[20] Desai SK, Pandey CH, Mulgaonkar SS. Memory-strengthening activity of aqueous liquorice extract and glabridin extract in behavioral models. Int J Pharm Sci Rev Res 2012; 16: 120-4.

[21] Folch J, Petrov D, Ettcheto M, *et al.* Current research therapeutic strategies for alzheimer's disease treatment. Neural Plast 2016; 2016: 1-15.
[http://dx.doi.org/10.1155/2016/8501693] [PMID: 26881137]

[22] Albuquerque EX, Santos MD, Alkondon M, Pereira EFR, Maelicke A. Modulation of nicotinic receptor activity in the central nervous system: a novel approach to the treatment of Alzheimer disease. Alzheimer Dis Assoc Disord 2001; 15 (Suppl. 1): S19-25.
[http://dx.doi.org/10.1097/00002093-200108001-00004] [PMID: 11669505]

[23] Long JM, Holtzman DM. Alzheimer disease: An update on pathobiology and treatment strategies. Cell 2019; 179(2): 312-39.
[http://dx.doi.org/10.1016/j.cell.2019.09.001] [PMID: 31564456]

[24] Bojić T, Sencanski M, Perovic V, Milicevic J, Glisic S. *In silico* screening of natural compounds for candidates 5HT6 receptor antagonists against alzheimer's disease. Molecules 2022; 27(9): 2626.
[http://dx.doi.org/10.3390/molecules27092626] [PMID: 35565976]

[25] Huang LK, Chao SP, Hu CJ. Clinical trials of new drugs for Alzheimer disease. J Biomed Sci 2020; 27(1): 18.
[http://dx.doi.org/10.1186/s12929-019-0609-7] [PMID: 31906949]

[26] Kucwaj-Brysz K, Baltrukevich H, Czarnota K, Handzlik J. Chemical update on the potential for serotonin 5-HT_6 and 5-HT_7 receptor agents in the treatment of Alzheimer's disease. Bioorg Med Chem Lett 2021; 49: 128275.
[http://dx.doi.org/10.1016/j.bmcl.2021.128275] [PMID: 34311086]

[27] Lang FM, Mo Y, Sabbagh M, *et al.* Intepirdine as adjunctive therapy to donepezil for mild-t--moderate Alzheimer's disease: A randomized, placebo-controlled, phase 3 clinical trial (MINDSET). Alzheimers Dement (N Y) 2021; 7(1): e12136.
[http://dx.doi.org/10.1002/trc2.12136] [PMID: 34095437]

[28] Ivachtchenko AV, Lavrovsky Y, Okun I. AVN-101: A multi-target drug candidate for the treatment of CNS disorders. J Alzheimers Dis 2016; 53(2): 583-620.
[http://dx.doi.org/10.3233/JAD-151146] [PMID: 27232215]

[29] Ivachtchenko AV, Lavrovsky Y, Ivanenkov YA. AVN-211, novel and highly selective 5-HT $_6$ receptor small molecule antagonist, for the treatment of alzheimer's disease. Mol Pharm 2016; 13(3): 945-63.
[http://dx.doi.org/10.1021/acs.molpharmaceut.5b00830] [PMID: 26886442]

[30] Nirogi R, Shinde A, Jayarajan P, *et al.* Potential benefits of Masupirdine (SUVN-502) on Behavioral and Psychological symptoms in patients with moderate Alzheimer's Disease (5090). Neurology 2020;

94(15_supplement): 5090.
[http://dx.doi.org/10.1212/WNL.94.15_supplement.5090]

[31] Nirogi R, Abraham R, Benade V, *et al.* SUVN-502, a novel, potent, pure, and orally active 5-HT6 receptor antagonist: pharmacological, behavioral, and neurochemical characterization. Behav Pharmacol 2019; 30(1): 16-35.
[http://dx.doi.org/10.1097/FBP.0000000000000414] [PMID: 29847336]

[32] Khoury R, Grysman N, Gold J, Patel K, Grossberg GT. The role of 5 HT6-receptor antagonists in Alzheimer's disease: an update. Expert Opin Investig Drugs 2018; 27(6): 523-33.
[http://dx.doi.org/10.1080/13543784.2018.1483334] [PMID: 29848076]

[33] Ramírez MJ. 5-HT6 receptors and Alzheimer's disease. Alzheimers Res Ther 2013; 5(2): 15.
[http://dx.doi.org/10.1186/alzrt169] [PMID: 23607787]

[34] Codony X, Vela JM, Ramírez MJ. 5-HT6 receptor and cognition. Curr Opin Pharmacol 2011; 11(1): 94-100.
[http://dx.doi.org/10.1016/j.coph.2011.01.004] [PMID: 21330210]

[35] Grimaldi B, Bonnin A, Fillion MP, Ruat M, Traiffort E, Fillion G. Characterization of 5-ht6 receptor and expression of 5-ht6 mRNA in the rat brain during ontogenetic development. Naunyn Schmiedebergs Arch Pharmacol 1998; 357(4): 393-400.
[http://dx.doi.org/10.1007/PL00005184] [PMID: 9606024]

[36] Ferrero H, Solas M, Francis PT, Ramirez MJ. Serotonin 5-HT_6 Receptor Antagonists in Alzheimer's Disease: Therapeutic Rationale and Current Development Status. CNS Drugs 2017; 31(1): 19-32.
[http://dx.doi.org/10.1007/s40263-016-0399-3] [PMID: 27914038]

[37] Kanagaratnam L, Dramé M, Trenque T, *et al.* Adverse drug reactions in elderly patients with cognitive disorders: A systematic review. Maturitas 2016; 85: 56-63.
[http://dx.doi.org/10.1016/j.maturitas.2015.12.013] [PMID: 26857880]

[38] Azam S, Haque ME, Jakaria M, Jo SH, Kim IS, Choi DK. G-Protein-Coupled Receptors in CNS: A Potential Therapeutic Target for Intervention in Neurodegenerative Disorders and Associated Cognitive Deficits. Cells 2020; 9(2): 506.
[http://dx.doi.org/10.3390/cells9020506] [PMID: 32102186]

[39] Sudoł S, Cios A, Jastrzębska-Więsek M, *et al.* The Phenoxyalkyltriazine Antagonists for 5-HT_6 Receptor with Promising Procognitive and Pharmacokinetic Properties *In Vivo* in Search for a Novel Therapeutic Approach to Dementia Diseases. Int J Mol Sci 2021; 22(19): 10773.
[http://dx.doi.org/10.3390/ijms221910773] [PMID: 34639113]

[40] Li X, Gao L, Liu J, *et al.* Safety, tolerability and pharmacokinetics of the serotonin 5-HT6 receptor antagonist, HEC30654, in healthy chinese subjects. Front Pharmacol 2021; 12: 726536.
[http://dx.doi.org/10.3389/fphar.2021.726536] [PMID: 34489712]

[41] Di Giovanni G, De Deurwaerdère P. Serotonin research: Crossing scales and boundaries. Neuropharmacology 2020; 181: 108340.
[http://dx.doi.org/10.1016/j.neuropharm.2020.108340] [PMID: 33007358]

[42] Noori T, Dehpour AR, Sureda A, Sobarzo-Sanchez E, Shirooie S. Role of natural products for the treatment of Alzheimer's disease. Eur J Pharmacol 2021; 898: 173974.
[http://dx.doi.org/10.1016/j.ejphar.2021.173974] [PMID: 33652057]

[43] Paroni G, Bisceglia P, Seripa D. Understanding the amyloid hypothesis in Alzheimer's disease. J Alzheimers Dis 2019; 68(2): 493-510.
[http://dx.doi.org/10.3233/JAD-180802] [PMID: 30883346]

[44] Duara R, Barker W. Heterogeneity in alzheimer's disease diagnosis and progression rates: Implications for therapeutic trials. Neurotherapeutics 2022; 19(1): 8-25.
[http://dx.doi.org/10.1007/s13311-022-01185-z] [PMID: 35084721]

[45] Breijyeh Z, Karaman R. Comprehensive review on Alzheimer's disease: causes and treatment.

Molecules 2020; 25(24): 5789.
[http://dx.doi.org/10.3390/molecules25245789] [PMID: 33302541]

[46] Kamat PK, Kalani A, Rai S, *et al.* Mechanism of Oxidative stress and synapse dysfunction in the pathogenesis of Alzheimer's Disease: understanding the therapeutics strategies. Mol Neurobiol 2016; 53(1): 648-61.
[http://dx.doi.org/10.1007/s12035-014-9053-6] [PMID: 25511446]

[47] Resende R, Moreira PI, Proença T, *et al.* Brain oxidative stress in a triple-transgenic mouse model of Alzheimer disease. Free Radic Biol Med 2008; 44(12): 2051-7.
[http://dx.doi.org/10.1016/j.freeradbiomed.2008.03.012] [PMID: 18423383]

[48] Power R, Prado-Cabrero A, Mulcahy R, Howard A, Nolan JM. The role of nutrition for the aging population: implications for cognition and Alzheimer's disease. Annu Rev Food Sci Technol 2019; 10(1): 619-39.
[http://dx.doi.org/10.1146/annurev-food-030216-030125] [PMID: 30908950]

[49] Serra JA, Domínguez RO, de Lustig ES, *et al.* Parkinson's disease is associated with oxidative stress: comparison of peripheral antioxidant profiles in living Parkinson's, Alzheimer's and vascular dementia patients. J Neural Transm (Vienna) 2001; 108(10): 1135-48.
[http://dx.doi.org/10.1007/s007020170003] [PMID: 11725816]

[50] Khamkat P, Chatterjee B, Barık V, Patra D, Chakraborty A. Extraction, characterization and antibacterial potential assessment of polar phytoconstituents of Caesalpinia bonducella seeds extract. YYU J Agric Sci 2024; 34(1): 115-27.
[http://dx.doi.org/10.29133/yyutbd.1362736]

[51] Olajide OA, Sarker SD. Alzheimer's disease: natural products as inhibitors of neuroinflammation. Inflammopharmacology 2020; 28(6): 1439-55.
[http://dx.doi.org/10.1007/s10787-020-00751-1] [PMID: 32930914]

[52] Kheiri G, Dolatshahi M, Rahmani F, Rezaei N. Role of p38/MAPKs in Alzheimer's disease: implications for amyloid beta toxicity targeted therapy. Rev Neurosci 2018; 30(1): 9-30.
[http://dx.doi.org/10.1515/revneuro-2018-0008] [PMID: 29804103]

[53] Lv M, Yang S, Cai L, Qin L, Li B, Wan Z. Effects of querce tin intervention on cognition function in app/ps1 mice was affected by vitamin D status. Mol Nutr Food Res 2018; 62(24): 1800621.
[http://dx.doi.org/10.1002/mnfr.201800621] [PMID: 30328681]

[54] Hu J, Webster D, Cao J, Shao A. The safety of green tea and green tea extract consumption in adults – Results of a systematic review. Regul Toxicol Pharmacol 2018; 95: 412-33.
[http://dx.doi.org/10.1016/j.yrtph.2018.03.019] [PMID: 29580974]

[55] Seong KJ, Lee HG, Kook MS, Ko HM, Jung JY, Kim WJ. Epigallocatechin-3-gallate rescues LPS-impaired adult hippocampal neurogenesis through suppressing the TLR4-NF-κB signaling pathway in mice. Korean J Physiol Pharmacol 2016; 20(1): 41-51.
[http://dx.doi.org/10.4196/kjpp.2016.20.1.41] [PMID: 26807022]

[56] Lee YJ, Choi DY, Yun YP, Han SB, Oh KW, Hong JT. Epigallocatechin-3-gallate prevents systemic inflammation-induced memory deficiency and amyloidogenesis *via* its anti-neuroinflammatory properties. J Nutr Biochem 2013; 24(1): 298-310.
[http://dx.doi.org/10.1016/j.jnutbio.2012.06.011] [PMID: 22959056]

[57] Infante-Garcia C, Ramos-Rodriguez JJ, Delgado-Olmos I, *et al.* Long-term mangiferin extract treatment improves central pathology and cognitive deficits in APP/PS1 Mice. Mol Neurobiol 2017; 54(6): 4696-704.
[http://dx.doi.org/10.1007/s12035-016-0015-z] [PMID: 27443159]

[58] Candelario-Jalil E, de Oliveira ACP, Gräf S, *et al.* Resveratrol potently reduces prostaglandin E2production and free radical formation in lipopolysaccharide-activated primary rat microglia. J Neuroinflammation 2007; 4(1): 25.
[http://dx.doi.org/10.1186/1742-2094-4-25] [PMID: 17927823]

[59] Abraham J, Johnson RW. Consuming a diet supplemented with resveratrol reduced infection-related neuroinflammation and deficits in working memory in aged mice. Rejuvenation Res 2009; 12(6): 445-53.
[http://dx.doi.org/10.1089/rej.2009.0888] [PMID: 20041738]

[60] Sun GY, Chen Z, Jasmer KJ, *et al.* Quercetin attenuates inflammatory responses in BV-2 microglial cells: role of MAPKs on the Nrf2 pathway and induction of heme oxygenase-1. PLoS One 2015; 10(10): e0141509.
[http://dx.doi.org/10.1371/journal.pone.0141509] [PMID: 26505893]

[61] Mazumder AG, Sharma P, Patial V, Singh D. Crocin attenuates kindling development and associated cognitive impairments in mice *via* inhibiting reactive oxygen species-mediated NF-κB activation. Basic Clin Pharmacol Toxicol 2017; 120(5): 426-33.
[http://dx.doi.org/10.1111/bcpt.12694] [PMID: 27800651]

[62] Zhang J, Zheng Y, Luo Y, Du Y, Zhang X, Fu J. Curcumin inhibits LPS-induced neuroinflammation by promoting microglial M2 polarization *via* TREM2/ TLR4/ NF-κB pathways in BV2 cells. Mol Immunol 2019; 116: 29-37.
[http://dx.doi.org/10.1016/j.molimm.2019.09.020] [PMID: 31590042]

[63] Soares TB, Loureiro L, Carvalho A, *et al.* Lipid nanocarriers loaded with natural compounds: Potential new therapies for age related neurodegenerative diseases? Prog Neurobiol 2018; 168: 21-41.
[http://dx.doi.org/10.1016/j.pneurobio.2018.04.004] [PMID: 29641983]

[64] Cuello AC. Early and late CNS inflammation in Alzheimer's disease: two extremes of a continuum? Trends Pharmacol Sci 2017; 38(11): 956-66.
[http://dx.doi.org/10.1016/j.tips.2017.07.005] [PMID: 28867259]

[65] Furukawa S, Yang L, Sameshima H. Galantamine, an acetylcholinesterase inhibitor, reduces brain damage induced by hypoxia-ischemia in newborn rats. Int J Dev Neurosci 2014; 37(1): 52-7.
[http://dx.doi.org/10.1016/j.ijdevneu.2014.06.011] [PMID: 24972037]

[66] Qian ZM, Ke Y. Huperzine A: is it an effective disease-modifying drug for Alzheimer's disease? Front Aging Neurosci 2014; 6: 216.
[http://dx.doi.org/10.3389/fnagi.2014.00216] [PMID: 25191267]

[67] Jia J, Zhao Q, Liu Y, *et al.* Phase I study on the pharmacokinetics and tolerance of ZT-1, a prodrug of huperzine A, for the treatment of Alzheimer's disease. Acta Pharmacol Sin 2013; 34(7): 976-82.
[http://dx.doi.org/10.1038/aps.2013.7] [PMID: 23624756]

[68] Yang F, Lim GP, Begum AN, *et al.* Curcumin inhibits formation of amyloid β oligomers and fibrils, binds plaques, and reduces amyloid *in vivo*. J Biol Chem 2005; 280(7): 5892-901.
[http://dx.doi.org/10.1074/jbc.M404751200] [PMID: 15590663]

[69] Marambaud P, Zhao H, Davies P. Resveratrol promotes clearance of Alzheimer's disease amyloid-β peptides. J Biol Chem 2005; 280(45): 37377-82.
[http://dx.doi.org/10.1074/jbc.M508246200] [PMID: 16162502]

[70] Sun MK, Alkon DL. Dual effects of bryostatin-1 on spatial memory and depression. Eur J Pharmacol 2005; 512(1): 43-51.
[http://dx.doi.org/10.1016/j.ejphar.2005.02.028] [PMID: 15814089]

[71] Tomiyama T, Kaneko H, Kataoka K, Asano S, Endo N. Rifampicin inhibits the toxicity of pre-aggregated amyloid peptides by binding to peptide fibrils and preventing amyloid-cell interaction. Biochem J 1997; 322(3): 859-65.
[http://dx.doi.org/10.1042/bj3220859] [PMID: 9148761]

[72] Schenk D, Barbour R, Dunn W, *et al.* Immunization with amyloid-β attenuates Alzheimer-disease-like pathology in the PDAPP mouse. Nature 1999; 400(6740): 173-7.
[http://dx.doi.org/10.1038/22124] [PMID: 10408445]

[73] Rinne JO, Brooks DJ, Rossor MN, *et al.* 11C-PiB PET assessment of change in fibrillar amyloid-β

load in patients with Alzheimer's disease treated with bapineuzumab: a phase 2, double-blind, placebo-controlled, ascending-dose study. Lancet Neurol 2010; 9(4): 363-72. [http://dx.doi.org/10.1016/S1474-4422(10)70043-0] [PMID: 20189881]

[74] Burstein AH, Zhao Q, Ross J, *et al.* Safety and pharmacology of ponezumab (PF-04360365) after a single 10-minute intravenous infusion in subjects with mild to moderate Alzheimer disease. Clin Neuropharmacol 2013; 36(1): 8-13. [http://dx.doi.org/10.1097/WNF.0b013e318279bcfa] [PMID: 23334069]

[75] Zampar S, Wirths O. Immunotherapy targeting Amyloid-β peptides in Alzheimer's disease. Exon Publications. 2020 Dec 19: 23-49.

[76] Ostrowitzki S, Deptula D, Thurfjell L, *et al.* Mechanism of amyloid removal in patients with Alzheimer disease treated with gantenerumab. Arch Neurol 2012; 69(2): 198-207. [http://dx.doi.org/10.1001/archneurol.2011.1538] [PMID: 21987394]

[77] Babitha K, Vazhayil R, Shanmuga SVM. Natural products and its derived drugs for the treatment of neurodegenerative disorders: Alzheimer's disease-a review. Br Biomed Bull 2014; 2: 359-70.

[78] Ancajas CMF, Oyedele AS, Butt CM, Walker AS. Advances, opportunities, and challenges in methods for interrogating the structure activity relationships of natural products. Nat Prod Rep 2024; 41(10): 1543-78. [http://dx.doi.org/10.1039/D4NP00009A] [PMID: 38912779]

[79] Barik V, Samsuddin MD, Khamkat P, Barik BB. Mental health and well-being in sustainable practices. In: Prabhakar PK, Leal Filho W, editors. Preserving Health, Preserving Earth: The Path to Sustainable Healthcare. World Sustainability Series. Cham: Springer; 2024: 169-179. [http://dx.doi.org/10.1007/978-3-031-60545-1_10]

[80] Simoben CV, Babiaka SB, Moumbock AFA, *et al.* Challenges in natural product-based drug discovery assisted with *in silico* -based methods. RSC Advances 2023; 13(45): 31578-94. [http://dx.doi.org/10.1039/D3RA06831E] [PMID: 37908659]

[81] Brogi S, Ramalho TC, Kuca K, Medina-Franco JL, Valko M. Editorial: *In silico* Methods for Drug Design and Discovery. Front Chem 2020; 8: 612. [http://dx.doi.org/10.3389/fchem.2020.00612] [PMID: 32850641]

[82] Lagorce D, Douguet D, Miteva MA, Villoutreix BO. Computational analysis of calculated physicochemical and ADMET properties of protein-protein interaction inhibitors. Sci Rep 2017; 7(1): 46277. [http://dx.doi.org/10.1038/srep46277] [PMID: 28397808]

[83] Gnanaraj C, Sekar M, Fuloria S, *et al. In silico* molecular docking analysis of karanjin against alzheimer's and parkinson's diseases as a potential natural lead molecule for new drug design, development and therapy. Molecules 2022; 27(9): 2834. [http://dx.doi.org/10.3390/molecules27092834] [PMID: 35566187]

[84] Vasanth Kanth TLB, Raha A, Vijay Murali RM, *et al.* Repurposing of clinically proven bioactive compounds for targeted treatment of Alzheimer's disease using molecular docking approach. *In Silico* Pharmacol 2023; 11(1): 33. [http://dx.doi.org/10.1007/s40203-023-00173-1] [PMID: 37920821]

CHAPTER 13

Biopolymer-based Therapeutic Approaches as Effective Treatment Methods for Alzheimer's Disease

Dipanjan Karati[1,*] and **Shreyasi Meur**[2]

[1] *Department of Pharmaceutical Technology, School of Pharmacy, Techno India University, Kolkata, West Bengal, India*

[2] *Department of Pharmaceutical Technology, NSHM Knowledge Campus Kolkata – Group of Institutions, Kolkata, West Bengal, India*

Abstract: Alzheimer's disease (AD) is a complex neurodegenerative disorder marked by progressive cognitive decline, memory impairment, and neuroinflammation, with no curative therapies currently available. The complexity of its pathogenesis, which involves amyloid-beta (Aβ) plaques and tau protein aggregation, presents significant challenges to effective therapeutic development. Despite advances in pharmacological interventions, the lack of curative therapies highlights the need for innovative approaches. Biopolymers, owing to their unique properties such as biocompatibility, biodegradability, and the ability to cross the blood-brain barrier (BBB), have emerged as promising candidates for therapeutic applications in AD. These materials enable targeted delivery of therapeutic agents, sustained release, and enhanced bioavailability, minimizing off-target effects. This chapter delves into the potential of biopolymers as innovative tools for addressing AD's therapeutic challenges. It categorizes biopolymer systems into polysaccharides, proteins, peptides, and nucleic acids, exploring their ability to encapsulate drugs, ensure sustained release, and achieve targeted delivery across the blood-brain barrier (BBB). Emphasis is placed on their capacity to modulate critical AD mechanisms, including Aβ aggregation, tau pathology, oxidative damage, and neuroinflammation. Strategies such as nanoparticle engineering, targeted delivery, and phytochemical-based therapies are discussed, emphasizing their potential to overcome existing challenges in drug delivery and therapeutic efficacy. Novel nanocarrier-based drug delivery systems highlight the transformative potential of these approaches, though challenges related to biodegradation, stability, and regulatory compliance remain. By synthesizing cutting-edge research, this chapter highlights biopolymer-based therapies as transformative strategies poised to address the unmet clinical needs of AD, paving the way for novel, targeted, and patient-centric treatment paradigms.

[*] **Corresponding author Dipanjan Karati:** Department of Pharmaceutical Technology, School of Pharmacy, Techno India University, Kolkata, West Bengal, India E-mail: karatibabai@gmail.com

Swarupananda Mukherjee, Souvik Roy & Dipanjan Karati (Eds.)

Keywords: Alzheimer's disease, Biopolymer, Blood-brain barrier, Nanoparticles, Tau protein.

INTRODUCTION

Alzheimer's disease (AD) is one of the most devastating neurodegenerative disorders, characterized by progressive memory loss, cognitive decline, and behavioral impairments [1]. Despite extensive research efforts, the complexity of AD pathogenesis—which encompasses amyloid-beta (Aβ) plaques, tau protein aggregation, oxidative stress, and chronic neuroinflammation—continues to pose significant challenges to effective treatment development [2]. Current pharmacological approaches provide only symptomatic relief, leaving an unmet need for innovative and holistic therapeutic strategies that target the disease's multifactorial nature. Biopolymers have garnered increasing attention in recent years for their potential to revolutionize the therapeutic landscape of AD [3]. These natural polymeric materials, such as polysaccharides, proteins, peptides, and nucleic acid-based systems, offer remarkable versatility in addressing key challenges in drug delivery and therapeutic targeting [4]. Biopolymers are not only biocompatible and biodegradable but also capable of encapsulating, protecting, and delivering therapeutic agents directly to the brain. Their tunable properties allow for advanced functionalities, including sustained drug release, precision targeting, and the ability to cross the blood-brain barrier (BBB) [3].

This chapter delves into the transformative potential of biopolymers in Alzheimer's disease therapy. It highlights their unique ability to overcome critical barriers, such as crossing the blood-brain barrier (BBB), delivering therapeutics with precision, and enabling sustained release of bioactive agents. The focus shifts to innovative biopolymer-based systems, classified by their origin and function. Polysaccharide-based systems like chitosan and hyaluronic acid offer solutions for drug encapsulation, while protein-based formulations, including collagen and silk fibroin, enable targeted delivery to brain cells. Peptide-based polymers and nucleic acid delivery platforms further expand the toolkit for combating amyloid-beta aggregation, tau pathology, and other neurodegenerative mechanisms with unprecedented specificity and efficacy. These systems, optimized for size, surface characteristics, and ligand targeting, exemplify the strides made in enhancing bioavailability and therapeutic precision. Moreover, innovative nanocarrier-based combination therapies are discussed, showcasing how biopolymer systems can synergize with other modalities to enhance therapeutic efficacy. A comprehensive exploration of biopolymer-based strategies in AD treatment is presented here, emphasizing their promise in overcoming current therapeutic barriers. By addressing challenges such as stability, biodegradation, and regulatory concerns, it sets the stage for advancing these systems toward personalized and precision medicine approaches for Alzheimer's disease.

BIOPOLYMERS IN DRUG DELIVERY

Biopolymers are an extensive and highly adaptable class of compounds originating from biological systems or synthesized using biological precursors. Similar to other polymers, biopolymers are constructed from repeating structural units, or monomers, linked in sequence [5]. Their unique features, including biodegradability, accessibility, and customizable physicochemical properties, make them attractive for advanced formulations. As the global emphasis shifts toward sustainability, biopolymers have become pivotal in designing systems aligned with environmental preservation. Recently, their utility in drug delivery systems (DDS) has garnered significant interest [6]. DDS refers to strategies for incorporating therapeutic agents, ensuring their precise delivery to specific diseased locations while minimizing systemic side effects. The ideal DDS enables both targeted delivery and controlled drug release, safeguarding drugs from premature degradation within the body before they reach their intended target. Moreover, these systems leverage biocompatibility and biodegradability to reduce adverse effects while optimizing therapeutic outcomes [7].

Both natural and synthetic polymers have shown potential in DDS development. While natural polymers excel in biocompatibility and biodegradability, their limited mechanical strength, thermal stability, and solubility often restrict their broader applications [8]. To address these challenges, functionalization and blending techniques are employed, creating advanced materials that exhibit enhanced properties derived from the parent polymers [7, 8]. Such hybrid systems combine complementary attributes, minimizing drawbacks and enhancing the efficiency of DDS [9]. The development of polymeric nanobiocomposites often involves combining polymers with fillers like metal nanoparticles, hydroxyapatite, or organic and inorganic clays. This approach enables high drug-loading efficiency while minimizing the quantity of carrier material used. Drug incorporation into nanocomposites is achieved through two main methods: impregnation, which involves incubating nanocomposites in a drug solution, and integration, where drugs are encapsulated during the material's synthesis (Fig. **1**) [10].

Polymer–drug complexes typically form through interactions such as hydrogen bonding, hydrophobic forces, electrostatic attractions, or van der Waals forces. To improve mechanical strength and system stability, cross-linking agents are often introduced, providing robust structural integrity. In certain applications, supramolecular aggregates with cavity-like structures are required to host guest molecules during inclusion complexation. Various preparation methods are employed based on the properties of thc biopolymers and active compounds, as well as the desired DDS characteristics. For instance, nanoprecipitation is a commonly used technique for hydrophobic polymers. Alternatively, the supercritical fluid method involves dissolving polymers and drugs in a liquid or gaseous medium above their critical points to create nanoparticles. Numerous factors, including the stability of bioactive components, the potential toxicity of residual solvents, the particle size of the resulting DDS, and the desired drug release profile influence the selection of a preparative method. Drying techniques such as freeze-drying and spray-drying are frequently utilized. Freeze-drying is preferred for thermally sensitive materials, while spray-drying involves evaporating solvents rapidly with hot air, leading to particle aggregation. These versatile methodologies allow the tailoring of DDS to meet specific therapeutic needs while preserving the stability of sensitive bioactive compounds [11, 12].

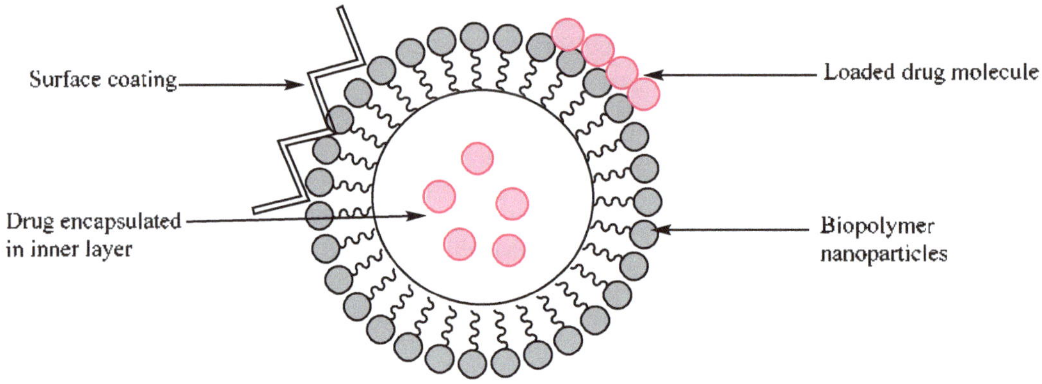

Fig. (1). The fundamental architecture of a biopolymer-based nanoparticle (NP) consists of a drug encapsulated within a nanocapsule or dispersed throughout a nanosphere. Additionally, surface modifications can be applied to improve the nanoparticle's stability, targeting efficiency, or overall performance.

MECHANISMS OF ALZHEIMER'S DISEASE

Central to the pathophysiology of Alzheimer's disease are amyloid beta (Aβ) plaques and tau protein neurofibrillary tangles, which disrupt neuronal function and structure. These hallmark pathologies are exacerbated by oxidative stress and chronic neuroinflammation [13]. Aβ deposition activates microglia and astrocytes, leading to inflammation and oxidative stress, which in turn exacerbate Aβ and tau pathologies, creating a vicious self-reinforcing cycle of neurodegeneration [14]. Together, these mechanisms underline the complexity of AD and provide a framework for exploring therapeutic targets to mitigate its progression.

Amyloid Beta (Aβ) Pathway

The amyloid beta (Aβ) pathway is a cornerstone in Alzheimer's disease (AD) pathogenesis, driven by the abnormal cleavage of amyloid precursor protein (APP) [15]. APP, a transmembrane protein, is processed through two major pathways: the non-amyloidogenic pathway, mediated by α-secretase, and the amyloidogenic pathway, involving β-secretase and γ-secretase [16]. In the amyloidogenic pathway, APP is cleaved to produce Aβ peptides, primarily $A\beta_{40}$ and $A\beta_{42}$. $A\beta_{42}$ is more aggregation-prone and is implicated in the formation of soluble oligomers, fibrils, and extracellular plaques. These plaques disrupt neuronal signaling and lead to synaptic dysfunction, triggering a cascade of events that exacerbate neuronal damage [17]. Aβ accumulation also interacts with neuronal and non-neuronal cells, stimulating microglial activation and the release of pro-inflammatory cytokines [18]. Furthermore, genetic mutations in APP and presenilin genes (PSEN1 and PSEN2), which are involved in γ-secretase activity, increase the production of pathogenic Aβ species, reinforcing their central role in familial AD [19].

Tau Protein Pathway

Tau protein pathology is another hallmark of AD, characterized by the hyperphosphorylation of tau, a microtubule-associated protein critical for maintaining neuronal structure and intracellular transport [20]. Hyperphosphorylation of tau, mediated by kinases such as GSK-3β and CDK-5, reduces its affinity for microtubules, causing tau to aggregate into paired helical filaments and neurofibrillary tangles (NFTs) [21]. NFTs disrupt the cytoskeletal framework, impairing axonal transport and leading to synaptic and neuronal loss. The propagation of misfolded tau between neurons amplifies the disease process [22]. Evidence suggests a bidirectional relationship between Aβ and tau pathologies; Aβ oligomers can activate kinases involved in tau phosphorylation, while tau pathology exacerbates Aβ toxicity, creating a synergistic cycle of neurodegeneration [22].

Oxidative Stress

Oxidative stress, characterized by excessive production of reactive oxygen species (ROS), is a key contributor to neuronal injury in AD [23]. Neurons are particularly vulnerable due to their high metabolic demand and limited antioxidant capacity [24]. Aβ peptides exacerbate oxidative stress by disrupting mitochondrial function, leading to electron transport chain inefficiencies and heightened ROS production. This mitochondrial dysfunction is observed in post-mortem AD brains, where Aβ aggregates are often found associated with mitochondrial membranes. ROS damage cellular components, including lipids, proteins, and nucleic acids, compromising neuronal integrity [25]. Lipid peroxidation disrupts membrane function, while protein oxidation impairs enzymatic activity and receptor signaling. Oxidative damage to nucleic acids can lead to mitochondrial DNA mutations, further amplifying mitochondrial dysfunction [26]. Additionally, trace metals such as iron and copper, which are dysregulated in AD, catalyze ROS formation, exacerbating oxidative damage [27].

Neuroinflammation

Neuroinflammation is characterized by chronic activation of microglia and astrocytes in response to Aβ deposits and neuronal injury [28]. Microglia, the brain's resident immune cells, are initially protective, attempting to phagocytose Aβ and clear debris. However, prolonged activation leads to a sustained inflammatory state, marked by the release of pro-

inflammatory cytokines such as IL-1β, TNF-α, and IL-6 [29]. These cytokines exacerbate neuronal damage, impair Aβ clearance mechanisms, and promote tau hyperphosphorylation [30]. Astrocytes also play a dual role in AD. While they support neuronal metabolism and neurotransmitter recycling [31], chronic astrocytic activation contributes to excitotoxicity by failing to regulate extracellular glutamate levels. This glutamate accumulation overstimulates NMDA receptors, causing calcium influx and neuronal injury [32]. Furthermore, astrocytes release neurotoxic substances, including reactive nitrogen species, which augment oxidative damage [33].

BIOPOLYMER-BASED THERAPEUTIC APPROACHES FOR ALZHEIMER'S DISEASE

Polysaccharide-based Systems

Various designs have been created by combining the polysaccharide with other inorganic or naturally occurring components to create hybrid or core-shell systems, or by employing it as a special component of nanosized carriers [34], some of which are summarized in Table **1**.

Table 1. Polysaccharide-based systems developed for the treatment of Alzheimer's disease

Targeting Strategy	Polysaccharide-Based Systems	Type of System/Preparation	Target	Route of Administration	Encapsulated Drug	Preclinical Performance			Refs.
						In vivo	*In vitro*	Outcome	
Passive targeting	Chitosan	Nanoparticle (γ-ray)	Permeation enhancement	Oral	Memantine	Albino rats	-	Neurological amelioration	[35]

(Table 1) cont.....

Targeting Strategy	Polysaccharide-Based Systems	Type of System/Preparation	Target	Route of Administration	Encapsulated Drug	Preclinical Performance			Refs.
						In vivo	*In vitro*	Outcome	
	Chitosan	Nanoparticle (ion gelation)	Magnevist®/ IgG4.1	Systemic	Curcumin/ Dexamethasone	B6/SJL mice; Tg2576 transgenic mice	hCMEC/D3 BBB cell line	Improved pharmacokinetics	[36]
Active targeting	Chitosan	Nanoparticle (ion gelation)	Magnevist®/ $F(ab')_2$	Systemic	Cyclophosphamide	B6SJLF1/J mice	hCMEC/D3 BBB cell line	Improved pharmacokinetics	[37]
	Chitosan	Nanoparticle (ion gelation)	L-Valine	Systemic	Saxagliptin	Wistar rats	-	Improved pharmacokinetics	[38]
	Chitosan	Nanosuspension (ion gelation)		Nose-to-brain	Donepezil	SD rats	-	Improved pharmacokinetics	[39]
	Chitosan	NE (emulsion)		Nose-to-brain	Curcumin	-	SNM	Enhanced permeation	[40]
	Hyaluronic acid	Microparticles (ion interaction)		Nose-to-brain	-	App^{NL-G-F} knock-in mouse	CHO	Improved pharmacokinetics and enhanced uptake	[41]
Administration route targeting	Gellan gum/ Xanthan gum	Gel (melt emulsion-probe sonication)	BBB permeation enhancement, cerebral drug concentration enhancement	Nose-to-brain	Resveratrol	SD rats	SNM	Improved pharmacokinetics and enhanced uptake.	[42]
	Gellan gum	Nano emulsion (spontaneous emulsion)		Nose-to-brain	Resveratrol; Curcumin	Albino rats	SNM	Improved pharmacokinetics and enhanced uptake	[43]
	Chitosan	Microemulsion (water titration)		Nose-to-brain	Rivastigmine	SD rats	SNM	Improved pharmacokinetics and enhanced uptake	[44]

Protein-based Systems

Silk Fibroin-based Formulations

Silk Fibroin (SF) hydrolysis byproducts have neuroprotective properties because they inhibit inflammation and delay the apoptotic process brought on by reactive oxygen species and β-amyloid [45, 46]. In both human and animal experiments, they have been linked to an increase in acetylcholinesterase, which results in a sharp rise in cognitive function as well as mnemonic activity [47]. Furthermore, it has been observed that a number of the effects of silkworm extracts are antagonists of N-methyl-4-phenyl1,2,3,6-tetrahydropyridine effects, which are precursors of the neurotoxin 1-methyl-4-phenylpyridinium, which is generally implicated in the dopaminergic receptors in the substantia nigra [48, 49]. Sha *et al.*, recently discussed the use of a hydrogel coated with hyaluronic acid, silk fibroin, and poly-dopamine that can prolong the release rate of neurotrophin-3 to improve spinal cord regeneration, suggesting that it has a lot of potential for drug delivery to gain CNS regeneration [50]. Combining SF with polypyrrole (PPy) allowed Zao *et al.*, to create conductive composite nanofibers with sufficient biological and mechanical properties. After being electrically stimulated, Schwann cells grown on the scaffold displayed increased motility, proliferation, and production of neurotrophic factors. Additionally, *in vivo* experiments showed that the scaffold, which was created by electrical stimulation, effectively promoted axonal regeneration and remyelination [51]. Also, it is now evident that electrically conductive frameworks are required in order to restore the brain tissues' physiological functions. In a different study, SF scaffolds with regulated pore diameters and porosities were infused with carbon nanofibers (CNFs). It has been demonstrated that adding CNFs enhances mechanical characteristics, electrical conductivity, fibroblast metabolic activity, and cell proliferation. This produced a composite porous structure that can sustain biological stability and structure at physiologically significant stress levels [52].

Gelatin-based Formulations

Nanocomposites based on gelatin-polyvinyl alcohol (Ge/PVA) efficiently shield the properties of pharmaceuticals from the surrounding environment and their extracellular route of action, which led to extended release of drugs at the site of action and longer drug retention [53, 54]. A work by Rajkumar *et al.*, used alkali co-precipitation to create a nanocomposite (Ge/PVA/$Mg(OH)_2$) by tying gelatin (Ge) as well as polyvinyl alcohol (PVA) to magnesium hydroxide ($Mg(OH)_2$) [55]. The influence of the Ge/PVA/$Mg(OH)_2$ nanocomposite upon biocompatibility, cellular absorption, decreased expression of the Aβ protein, and protection against neuronal cell death was also clearly shown in an *in vitro* investigation. The decreased levels of Aβ expression were further validated by the confocal analysis. In rats treated with intracerebroventricular streptozotocin (ICV-STZ), the subsequent *in vivo* analysis demonstrated the protective effects of Ge/PVA/$Mg(OH)_2$ nanocomposites against the cognitive and synaptic deficits of AD.

Another novel avenue is the development of Ge/PLA/AuNCs utilizing the medicinally significant plant extract from *Syzygium cumini,* which defines it as a prospective candidate for a variety of biological activities and offers a unique approach with possible therapeutic uses. Using the green synthesis approach, Rajkumar *et al.*, created a new Ge/PLA-loaded Gold nanocomposite (Ge/PLA/AuNCs) from *S. cumini* plant fruit extract [56]. Ge/PLA/AuNCs' anti-Alzheimer effect was verified by inhibiting the enzymes AChE (76.37±1.18%) and BChE (85.94±1.38%). Studies conducted on zebrafish embryos *in vivo* demonstrated the exceptional biocompatibility and nontoxicity of Ge/PLA/AuNCs. After being treated with Ge/PLA/AuNCs, the SH-SY5Y cell line investigation showed increased neuronal cell proliferation and greater cell viability (95.27±1.62%).

Collagen-based Formulations

In order to provide neuroprotection in neurodegenerative illnesses, collagen-based injectable hydrogels are being considered for facilitating the release of neurotrophic factors [57 - 59]. Mesenchymal Stromal Cell (MSC)-based neurotrophic factor delivery to the brain is a potential neuroprotective technique, but its application is constrained by the poor survival of cells following implantation. Although the intra-cerebral application of collagen-based hydrogels has not been well studied, research indicates that these hydrogels may be able to give transplanted cells a supporting matrix, hence increasing cell survival following implantation. In particular, rats were used to test the feasibility of delivering glial-derived neurotrophic factor (GDNF) overexpressing MSCs (GDNF-MSCs) *via* intracerebral transplantation matrices made of collagen hydrogel cross-linked with four-arm Star-poly(ethylene glycol) [57]. The study demonstrated that the application of the collagen hydrogel permitted the release of GDNF inside the striatum parenchyma and had no effect on the survival of cells. Additionally, GDNF-MSC transplantation in a collagen hydrogel dramatically decreased the host brain's responsiveness to cells, reflected by a decline in the recruitment of astrocytes and microglia around the delivery spot [57].

Albumin-based Formulations

Albumin is the most prevalent protein in cerebrospinal fluid (CSF) and blood plasma (about 40 g/L) [60]. Within the CSF, albumin adheres to amyloid-β and contributes to the prevention of fibril formation, particularly in peripheral organs where plasma albumin concentration is high [61, 62]. According to Prajapati *et al.*, [63], albumin accounts for 60% of the overall inhibitory efficacy against amyloid accumulation in plasma and CSF. Albumin-plasma exchange therapy slowed cognitive decline in a phase II/III clinical trial of patients with mild to moderate Alzheimer's disease (AD) when compared to the placebo group. This suggests that removing peripheral albumin-bound amyloid-β may lower the amount of amyloid-β in CSF [64, 65]. According to this research, albumin has the inherent ability to preserve the brain, which makes it a valuable biomaterial for the central nervous system. Additionally, albumin nanoparticles have persistent drug absorption and good mucoadhesion, making them a perfect option for drug administration from the nose to the brain [66, 67]. According to Wong and Ho [68], the albumin nanoparticle method increased the availability of the Alzheimer's disease drug R-flurbiprofen inside the brain as compared to when the drug was administered orally or intranasally.

Peptide-based Systems

The development of short peptides to act as protein inhibitors is justified by their promise for fewer adverse effects and their specificity [69]. This selectivity raises the therapeutic index and lowers the possibility of off-target consequences. Short peptides created by Miksusanti *et al.*, [70], showed strong binding affinity as well as specificity for tau and amyloid-beta proteins, lowering aggregation by approximately 70% *in vitro*. Studies conducted *in vivo* revealed a notable decrease in tau tangles and amyloid plaques, along with enhanced cognitive function in treated mice. The blood-brain barrier was successfully penetrated by these peptides, which then gathered in the desired brain areas.

A G0 ApoE-derived peptide (AEP) delivery system was engineered in a research study by Al-Azzawi *et al.*, [71], and two molecules of Flurbiprofen (FP) were attached to it at both lysine amino terminals to increase the drug's bioavailability in brain tissue. This study demonstrated that this drug delivery method is cytotoxicity-free and can reduce γ-secretase activity in neuroglial cells by FP. In contrast to both the free drug and another adsorptive-mediated transcytosis (AMT)-driven FP peptidic nanocarrier, the transcytosis of FP across a cerebral endothelium model was notably improved [72, 73]. Collagen-mimicking peptide nanofibers were used by Gülseren*et al.*, as a bioactive template to create bimetallic nanoparticles [74]. Blocking amyloid β (Aβ) aggregate development, these green NPs displayed extraordinary activity with over 74% inhibition, outperforming the effects

of Au and Ag NPs alone, which showed inhibition of 66% and 43%, respectively. The bimetallic Au/Ag-NPs transformed into multifunctional therapeutic agents for Alzheimer's disease by exhibiting strong suppression of Aβ as well as inhibitory activities against esterase (about 50%) and reactive oxygen species (approximately 75%). Studies investigating tissue penetration, 3-D uptake, and endosomal escape have demonstrated the great benefits of Au/Ag-NPs in overcoming cellular barriers; these characteristics also offer promise for future therapeutic approaches.

Nucleic Acid-based Systems

Since microglia are crucial to neuroinflammation, controlling target gene transcription along with post-transcriptional translation can either alter microglial activity or regulate the release of inflammatory mediators, which would mitigate neuroinflammation [75]. For synergistic effects on microglia normalization, Aljohani *et al.*, created a material called CMC-Fi-siRNA@$ZnO_{a\text{–}d}$, which is built on carboxymethylcellulose (CMC) encapsulating Fingolimod (Fi), siRNA, along with zinc oxide (ZnO) with variable loading [76]. The CMC-Fi-siRNA@ZnOd significantly reduced microglia priming by raising Brain-derived neurotrophic factor (BDNF) production and decreasing proinflammatory mediator levels. This significantly improved Aβ phagocytosis. After 48 hours of incubation, the hybrid nanocomposite (NP) had no discernible impact on cell survival in the immortalized microglia cells (IMG) cell viability test. Additionally, the NP reduced the cytotoxicity that Aβ produced. In one approach by Samaridou *et al.*, [41], a hydrophobic analogue of octaarginine (r8) that was chemically coupled with lauric acid (C12) and the RNA of interest generated electrostatically driven nanocomplexes for their use as a novel 'nose-to-brain' RNAi delivery strategy. To improve their stability as well as mucodiffusion traversing the olfactory nasal mucosa, such cationic nanocomplexes were then encased (ENCPs) with several protective polymers, such as hyaluronic acid (HA) or polyethyleneglycol-polyglutamic acid (PEG-PGA). Following intranasal delivery, *in vivo* investigations in a murine model of Alzheimer's disease demonstrated a statistically significant increase in a potentially therapeutic miRNA mimic inside the hippocampal area and its subsequent effect on two mRNA targets.

To enhance the bioavailability of Tarenflurbil (R-flurbiprofen), Mu and colleagues developed a nanosystem incorporating the drug into PEGylated poly(lactic acid) (PEG-PLA) nanoparticles [77]. To further optimize its targeting efficiency, these nanoparticles were conjugated with an RNA-based aptamer, FB4 (5′-NH2-spacer-CGCGGAUUGCGGCCGUUGU CUGUGGCGUCCGUUC-3′), which selectively binds to the extracellular domain of the mouse transferrin receptor. The functionalized NPs exhibited a mean size of approximately 25 nm and displayed negative Z-potential values. This formulation significantly increased the solubility of tarenflurbil in aqueous environments and improved its controlled release profile *in vitro*. Moreover, FB4-conjugated nanoparticles markedly enhanced tarenflurbil uptake in Brain-derived Endothelial 5 (bEND.5) cells, confirming the aptamer's specificity in facilitating targeted drug delivery [78]. In a separate study, Mathew *et al.*, investigated the efficacy of the RNA-based aptamer NN2 (5′-UGCCACUCUCCUGGGACCCCCGCCGGAUG-GCCACAUCC-3′), previously identified through SELEX screening for its binding affinity to amyloid-beta (Aβ) peptides [79]. The NN2 aptamer was covalently linked to curcumin-loaded PLGA nanoparticles (Cur-PLGA NPs), resulting in a nanosystem with an average particle diameter of approximately 170 nm [80]. *In vitro* studies demonstrated that these nanoparticles exhibited no cytotoxic effects on LAG cells (mouse fibroblast-like connective tissue), confirming their biocompatibility. Additionally, NN2-functionalized curumin-PLGA NPs effectively reduced the size of amyloid aggregates, supporting their potential as a targeted therapeutic approach for AD [80].

BIOPOLYMER NANOPARTICLES FOR CROSSING THE BLOOD-BRAIN BARRIER (BBB)

Challenges and Strategies of Delivering Therapeutics to the Brain

Developing drugs for central nervous system (CNS) disorders, including certain cancers, dementia, neurodegenerative conditions such as Alzheimer's and Parkinson's diseases, and lysosomal storage disorders (LSDs) that impact the brain, is highly challenging. This complexity arises primarily due to the blood-brain barrier (BBB), a significant hurdle for targeted drug delivery. Current approaches for drug delivery into the CNS include temporary disruption of tight junctions (TJs) within the BBB, chemical modification of therapeutic agents, and direct intracranial administration through surgical interventions. Among these strategies, the use of nanoparticles (NPs) is particularly noteworthy as a cutting-edge technique [81 - 85]. Nanoparticles serve as optimal carriers for drugs, which can be encapsulated within their core or attached to their surface through adsorption or covalent bonding with the polymer structure [86, 87]. Biodegradable NPs, in particular, are considered highly promising for controlled release systems (CRSs). Their fundamental prerequisite is biocompatibility, ensuring safe metabolism without adverse effects. Biodegradable polymers degrade *in vivo* under physiological conditions, forming nanoscale assemblies (ranging from 1 to 1000 nm), commonly referred to as nano-biopolymers [88].

Biopolymer NPs have been extensively utilized as drug carriers due to their numerous benefits. These include enabling the administration of hydrophobic drugs and protecting labile molecules from degradation [11, 89 - 91]. Furthermore, NPs facilitate the delivery of not only pharmaceuticals but also nucleic acids and therapeutic proteins [81, 92 - 96]. Natural polymers such as chitosan, sodium alginate, and gelatin, as well as synthetic polymers like polylactic acid (PLA), polyglycolic acid (PGA), poly(lactic-co-glycolic acid) (PLGA), polybutyl cyanoacrylates (PBCA), and polycaprolactone (PCL), are frequently employed to fabricate biopolymer NPs [11, 96 - 100]. Although synthetic, these polymers degrade into oligomers and monomers, which are subsequently eliminated *via* natural metabolic pathways, such as the Krebs cycle [11, 101, 102]. Additionally, biopolymer NPs must meet critical requirements to function effectively. These include (i) the capacity to traverse physiological barriers such as the BBB or ophthalmic barrier, (ii) the ability to regulate drug concentrations over time, and (iii) the capability to release active agents precisely at the desired site of action. Due to their nanoscale dimensions and the potential for tailored modification for targeted delivery and controlled release, biopolymer NPs stand out as a leading technology in drug delivery systems [103].

BBB Penetration Mechanisms of Biopolymer NPs

The mechanisms by which nanoparticles (NPs) traverse the blood-brain barrier (BBB) align with those used by other molecules and can be broadly classified into two categories: passive transport, which relies on simple diffusion, and active transport, which requires ATP consumption for energy [82, 104, 105]. Similar to small lipophilic molecules that diffuse across the BBB *via* endothelial cells, NPs can leverage this passive diffusion mechanism due to their nanoscale dimensions. Additionally, the ability of NPs to permeate passively can be enhanced by incorporating cationic charges or lipid-based modifications on their surface [81, 104, 106]. Surface functionalization with polyethylene glycol (PEG) is often employed for cationic NPs to extend their systemic circulation time, prevent protein adsorption, evade immune recognition, reduce haemolysis or erythrocyte aggregation, improve colloidal stability, and protect the encapsulated therapeutic molecules from enzymatic degradation [107].

Active transport, by contrast, includes mechanisms such as adsorption-mediated endocytosis and receptor-mediated endocytosis [82, 108 - 110]. In adsorption-mediated endocytosis, positively charged NPs interact electrostatically with negatively charged domains on the cell membrane. To facilitate these interactions, NPs can be modified with molecules like albumin or transactivating transcriptional activator (TAT) peptides, enabling binding to the membrane through electrostatic forces [111 - 114]. Receptor-mediated endocytosis, one of the most widely utilized mechanisms for NP delivery, involves targeting receptors expressed on the apical surface of BBB endothelial cells. In this method, NPs are engineered to display specific antigens on their surface, which bind to these receptors. This binding event triggers membrane invagination and the formation of vesicles that transport the NPs into the cell interior [112, 115]. Similarly, polymeric formulations have been extensively employed in neurodegenerative disease treatment in both *in vitro* studies and animal experiments. PEG, one of the most extensively utilized ligands, not only stabilizes NPs in biological media such as blood but also confers a "stealth" effect, helping NPs evade macrophage-mediated immune responses [116]. Furthermore, Mittal *et al.*, explored the delivery of estradiol-loaded PLGA NPs in a rat model mimicking post-menopausal Alzheimer's disease (AD), given that reduced estradiol levels are associated with increased AD risk in post-menopausal women. Estradiol-loaded PLGA NPs, prepared using a single-emulsion technique and having an average diameter of ~130 nm, effectively inhibited the expression of $A\beta_{42}$ in the rat model, demonstrating their potential in AD therapy [117].

Biopolymer NP based-drug Delivery in Neurodegenerative Diseases

The development of nanoparticles (NPs) using polymers such as poly (lactic-c-glycolic acid) (PLGA), poly (lactic acid) (PLA), poly (glycolic acid) (PGA), and Chitosan has significantly advanced drug delivery for central nervous system (CNS) disorders by overcoming the formidable blood-brain barrier (BBB). Functionalized NPs have been extensively studied to optimize their ability to traverse the BBB. By tailoring surface properties, these nanosystems can interact with specific components of the BBB, enhancing drug delivery to the brain (Fig. **2**) [11]. For instance, Liu *et al.*, demonstrated that PLA-NPs loaded with breviscapine, a flavonoid, could cross the BBB efficiently, with larger particles (~300 nm) achieving superior drug concentrations in the brain compared to smaller particles (~200 nm) [118]. Furthermore, transactivating transcriptional activator (TAT) peptides conjugated to PLA-NP surfaces increased transport efficiency by bypassing efflux transporters at the BBB [119]. Surface-coating strategies with agents like polysorbate 80 and poloxamer 188 on PLGA-NPs have further improved CNS penetration [120]. Another breakthrough involved paclitaxel-loaded PLGA-NPs functionalized with glutathione, which facilitated better BBB crossing and improved drug delivery to the brain [121]. A glyco-heptapeptide modification of PLGA-NPs has also shown success in transporting therapeutic agents, such as loperamide and rhodamine-123, by mimicking opioid peptides through absorption-mediated endocytosis [122, 123]. Recent applications of NPs in neurodegenerative diseases, particularly Alzheimer's disease (AD) and Parkinson's disease (PD), have gained attention due to their increasing prevalence. Dual-functionalized NPs designed to target the BBB and deliver specific drugs are a key area of research. Zhang *et al.*, developed PEGylated PLA-NPs with dual targeting: one peptide aimed at BBB receptors and another targeting amyloid-beta (Aβ) 1-42 aggregates. This system demonstrated excellent targeting efficiency both *in vitro* and *in vivo*, establishing its potential for AD diagnosis and therapy [124]. PLGA-NPs are especially prominent in AD and PD treatment due to their controlled and sustained drug release, low toxicity, and biocompatibility. For example, Sánchez-López *et al.*, loaded memantine (MEM), an FDA-approved drug for AD, into PEG-PLGA-NPs for oral delivery. These NPs exhibited enhanced BBB permeability and a slower release profile compared to free MEM, leading to a significant reduction in Aβ plaques in both *in vitro* and *in vivo* models [125]. Functionalized PLGA-NPs targeting lysosomes have also been explored to restore cellular function in neurodegenerative conditions [126].

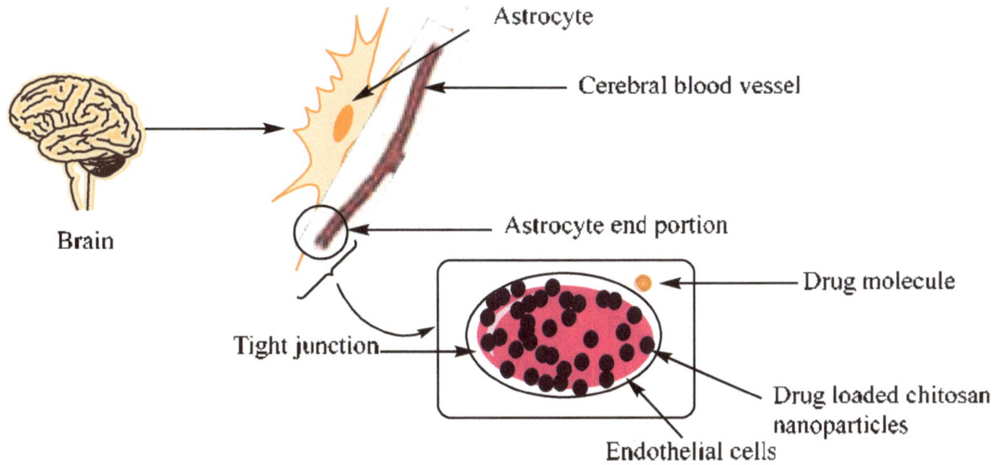

Fig. (2). A schematic illustrates how a chitosan (Cs)-based drug-loaded nanocarrier interacts with the BBB to facilitate controlled drug release into the brain.

THERAPEUTIC TARGETING WITH BIOPOLYMER-BASED SYSTEMS

Targeting Amyloid Plaques

Biopolymer-based nanoparticles (NPs) offer a highly effective strategy for delivering Aβ inhibitors, improving drug stability, prolonging circulation time, and enabling targeted delivery to the brain. Numerous studies have demonstrated that biopolymeric nanoparticles (NPs) can modulate the kinetics of amyloid-beta (Aβ) plaque formation, either by stimulating, inhibiting, or delaying their accumulation. By facilitating the efficient transport of therapeutic agents into neuronal cells, these nanosystems offer a promising avenue for preventing Aβ deposition and mitigating Alzheimer's disease (AD) pathology [4, 127].In preclinical investigations, Cheng *et al.*, developed a curcumin nanoparticle formulation using polyvinylpyrrolidone (PVP) and a polyethylene glycol-polylactic acid (PEG-PLA) co-block polymer [128]. This formulation was tested both in an *in vitro* blood-brain barrier (BBB) model and in an AD mouse model (Tg2576) following oral administration. Compared to control groups, the curcumin-loaded NPs significantly decreased Aβ plaque burden in AD mouse brains and exhibited greater efficacy in improving cue-based and working memory performance than free curcumin, as demonstrated in multiple behavioural assessments. A separate study employed polyethylene glycol-functionalized gold nanoparticles (PEG-AuNPs) to examine their impact on Aβ aggregation [129]. Researchers observed that these NPs effectively reduced the clustering of Aβ peptides *in vitro*. In the AD mouse model, the PEG-AuNPs demonstrated the ability to decrease Aβ toxicity, thereby reducing its neurotoxic effects.

Furthermore, a study employing young mice as a model for the presymptomatic phase of AD evaluated the potential of Aβ-targeting liposomes to prevent the onset of disease symptoms, including cerebral Aβ deposition, structural brain alterations, and cognitive impairment. The liposomal formulation (mApoE-P--LIP) was dual-functionalized with a synthetic peptide (mApoE) containing the receptor-binding domain of apolipoprotein E and phosphatidic acid (PA), which facilitated Aβ binding and BBB penetration [130, 131]. Previously, aged symptomatic transgenic mice (Tg) with advanced AD pathology had been treated with these liposomes in a separate study [103]. In the current investigation, treatment protocols were modified to assess the efficacy of liposomes in delaying the onset of AD symptoms in presymptomatic mice. The findings suggest that mApoE-PA-LIP represents a promising multifunctional approach for early intervention, potentially delaying cognitive decline, structural brain deterioration, and Aβ plaque formation. Additionally, the study highlighted the need for re-evaluating Aβ-targeting therapies at earlier stages of AD progression, as conventional clinical trials have thus far yielded limited success in symptomatic patients [133]. Another investigation described a novel thermosensitive polymeric micelle system designed for amyloid-targeted therapy in AD. This intelligent polymer, composed of two polyethylene glycol (PEG) analogs, PMO37 and POEG38, displayed superior thermoresponsiveness, biocompatibility, and mechanical stability. When subjected to a temperature shift, the polymer transitioned from a hydrophilic to a hydrophobic state, effectively entrapping Aβ fibrils and preventing the formation of neurotoxic Aβ plaques [134]. Clementino *et al.*, investigated the potential of Simvastatin encapsulated within chitosan-lecithin nanoparticles (SVT-LCN) for the treatment of neurodegenerative diseases, particularly Alzheimer's disease (AD) [135]. Simvastatin has been shown to lower cholesterol levels, which in turn reduces Aβ accumulation, a key pathological feature of AD. An *in vitro* release assay, utilizing the dialysis bag diffusion technique, demonstrated a significantly faster release of simvastatin from SVT-LCN compared to its unencapsulated form. Specifically, after eight hours, approximately 40% of the encapsulated drug was released, whereas only 20% was observed in the non-encapsulated suspension. The rapid release profile of Simvastatin was attributed to the enzymatic degradation of the chitosan-lecithin NP shell by lysozymes present in nasal secretions. Within one hour of exposure, the NP's outer structure was disrupted, promoting efficient drug release.

Targeting Tau Pathology

Tau protein undergoes pathological aggregation due to its intrinsic amino acid sequences, specifically VQIVYK and VQIINK, which drive self-association and fibril formation [136]. Developing effective therapeutics capable of preventing tau aggregation is critical for AD treatment. Nadimidla *et al.,* examined the inhibitory effects of the cationic polymer polyethyleneimine (PEI) and the polypeptide arginine (Arg) on tau aggregation, focusing on VQIVYK, GKVQIINKLDL peptides, and the P301L tau mutant commonly associated with tauopathies [137]. Both PEI and Arg significantly impede tau aggregation, highlighting their potential as therapeutic agents. Additionally, these cationic compounds demonstrated efficacy in gene delivery applications [138, 139], suggesting their potential role in Alzheimer's gene therapy. Aggidis *et al.*, developed a potent retro-inverso peptide inhibitor of tau aggregation, RI-AG03 [Ac-rrrrrrrrGpkyk(ac)iqvGr-NH_2], which specifically targets the VQIVYK tau aggregation hotspot [140]. Their findings indicated that RI-AG03 effectively inhibited tau aggregation by over 90% when administered at equimolar concentrations, preventing fibril formation as observed *via* electron microscopy (EM). Additionally, RI-AG03 blocked seeded aggregation when applied during the growth phase of tau fibrils. Fluorescein-labeled RI-AG03 exhibited excellent cellular uptake in HEK-293 cells over a 24-hour period and demonstrated non-toxic behaviour at concentrations up to 30 μM. In transgenic Drosophila models expressing human tau, RI-AG03 significantly improved neurodegenerative symptoms and behavioural impairments, further supporting its therapeutic potential. In a work by Wang *et al.*, functional scaffolds were created by electrospinning a PLGA nanofibrous mat, covering it with graphene oxide (GO), and then physisorbing methylene blue (MB) in mild circumstances [141]. In order to effectively load and release MB from the substrate and control the activities of NPCs, GO was pre-coated on the nanofibrous scaffolds. The autophagy signaling pathway was activated by MB, which kept the NPCs grown on the scaffolds in the quiescent phase. Additionally, tau phosphorylation was diminished, and neural progenitor cells (NPCs) were shielded from apoptosis by the MB-loaded nanofibrous scaffolds. Paul *et al.*, used a range of biophysical, structural, and spectroscopic techniques to assess how native PLGA affected the clustering of tau protein caused by Aβ seed [142]. According to their findings, native PLGA nanoparticles mitigated the effect of $A\beta_{1\text{-}42}$ seeds, which increased tau protein aggregation both with and without heparin. Remarkably, both the 4R and 3R tau isoforms that contribute to the development of neurofibrillary tangles inside AD brains were blocked from aggregating by PLGA. Native PLGA also inhibited tau aggregation generated by Aβ seeds in the presence of arachidonic acid.

Neuroprotective Approaches

One innovative approach involved the intranasal administration of lutein, a carotenoid with potent antioxidant and anti-inflammatory effects, encapsulated in cationic chitosan-modified PLGA core-shell NPs. Intranasal delivery of chitosan-coated lutein NPs proved to be an efficient and non-invasive method for targeting the brain. However, due to its low solubility and poor bioavailability, the therapeutic efficacy of lutein was previously limited. To overcome these challenges, lutein was encapsulated in PLGA NPs, allowing for enhanced solubility and targeted brain delivery. The cationic charge of the chitosan-coated NPs facilitated electrostatic interactions with endothelial cells, promoting internalization of the drug carrier system. As a result, chitosan-coated lutein-PLGA NPs successfully crossed the nasal mucosal barrier and exerted neuroprotective effects on neuronal cells [143]. Another study investigated the nasal-to-brain delivery of Alendronate using chitosan NPs. Alendronate, known for its ability to inhibit cholesterol synthesis and acetylcholinesterase (AChE) activity, was efficiently transported to the brain *via* electrostatic interactions between its amino acid groups and the negatively charged cell membranes. This system demonstrated prolonged drug retention, with less than 39% of the drug being released within the first 30 minutes, ensuring sustained therapeutic action [144]. The development of nanomaterial-based drug delivery systems (DDS) has significantly improved the ability to penetrate the BBB, with starch emerging as a particularly attractive biopolymer due to its biocompatibility, biodegradability, and eco-friendly properties. A study conducted by Prakash *et al.*, explored the neuroprotective effects of starch nanoparticles encapsulating methyl gallate (MG), referred to as starch-encapsulated MG (SEMG). This formulation was designed to combat Aβ-induced neurotoxicity, a key pathological mechanism in AD. The SEMG NPs demonstrated potent acetylcholinesterase inhibition, antioxidant activity, and anti-amyloidogenic effects by preventing Aβ fibrillation and destabilizing preformed fibrils. Furthermore, SEMG was found to mitigate reactive oxygen species (ROS)-mediated cellular damage, restore mitochondrial membrane potential, and reduce apoptosis in Neuro2A cells, with an IC_{50} value of 18.25 ± 0.025 μg/mL [145].

To enhance targeted delivery, antioxidants can be conjugated with small molecules, including viral and non-viral vectors, polyethylene glycol (PEG), or naked oligonucleotides, forming nano-complexes. Lee *et al.*, demonstrated that viral vector-mediated delivery of superoxide dismutase (SOD) and catalase genes significantly upregulated enzymatic activity, thereby improving cellular antioxidant defenses [146]. Similarly, Williams *et al.*, synthesized PEG-glutathione (PEG-GSH) conjugate NPs, which displayed significantly greater protective effects against oxidative stress compared to standard GSH oligomers [147]. Recent research has explored self-assembling nanogels derived from modified hyaluronic acid as carriers for curcumin and epigallocatechin gallate (EGCG). Functional assays demonstrated that these biopolymer-based nanogels exhibit strong antioxidant properties and effectively inhibit Aβ aggregation and cell death *in vitro* [148, 149]. Additionally, Elnaggar *et al.*, developed a chitosan-based hydrogel capable of successfully delivering piperine, a lipophilic antioxidant, to the brain for AD therapy. The effectiveness of chitosan in neutralizing reactive oxygen species (ROS) was found to be dependent on its molecular weight and concentration [150].

Lignin, an inexpensive and abundant biopolymer, has garnered attention due to its biocompatibility, biodegradability, and intrinsic free radical-scavenging properties [151]. Lignin-derived nanogels have been widely studied for drug encapsulation [152] and could serve as viable candidates for neuroprotective therapies in AD. Another emerging approach involves creating biomimetic antioxidant enzymes *via* molecular imprinting on nanogels [153]. Hydrogels possessing antioxidant activity can also serve as dispersants or nanoparticle coatings. Notably, polysaccharides like alginate, derived from brown algae, have demonstrated neuroprotective potential by counteracting H_2O_2-induced oxidative stress and safeguarding neurons [154, 155]. Hybrid alginate-coated chitosan NPs have been utilized to encapsulate the antioxidant Naringenin, further enhancing its therapeutic efficacy [156]. A synergistic antioxidant approach involves the fabrication of biodegradable PLGA microspheres coated with type I collagen(Col) and decorated with manganese dioxide (MnO_2) nanoparticles (PLGA-Col-MnO_2). These hybrid systems effectively mitigate oxidative stress while the collagen coating enhances their biological properties and promotes MnO_2 entrapment [157]. Optimization of microsphere size is necessary to facilitate BBB penetration for *in vivo* applications.

BIOPOLYMERIC NANOCARRIER PLATFORMS FOR ALZHEIMER'S DISEASE TREATMENT

Nanoparticles are widely utilized for site-specific controlled delivery and direct targeting to improve a drug's effectiveness and decrease adverse effects. To mitigate toxicity and boost cellular uptake, polymers are typically employed as nanoparticle carriers since inorganic nanoparticles are potentially toxic. Table **2** shows a handful of biopolymer-coated nanocarriers that have been loaded with potent bioactive agents capable of ameliorating Alzheimer's disease.

Table 2. Bioactive agent-loaded biopolymeric nanocarrier platforms.

Nanocarrier Platform	Nanocarrier Composition	Bioactive Compound	Active Targeting Ligand	Refs.
Polymeric NPs	PS80-coated PLGA NPs	Donepezil	None	[158]
Polymeric NPs	PS80-coated PBCA NPs	Tacrine	None	[159]
Polymeric NPs	PS80-coated PBCA NPs	Rivastigmine	None	[160]
Polymeric NPs	PLGA and PBCA NPs	Rivastigmine	None	[161]

(Table 2) cont.....

Nanocarrier Platform	Nanocarrier Composition	Bioactive Compound	Active Targeting Ligand	Refs.
Polymeric NPs	PEG-PLGA NPs	Memantine	None	[125]
Polymeric NPs	Chitosan	F(ab') fragment of anti-amyloid antibody IgG4.1	None	[162]
Liposomes	PEG-DMPC and PEG-EYPC	Amyloid beta binding llama single-domain antibody fragments (VHH-pa2H)	GSH	[163]
Polymeric NPs	PEG-PLA NPs	TGN and QSH peptides	None	[124]
Polymeric NPs	PLGA NPs with Pluronic F127	iAβ5 peptide, Aβ aggregation inhibitor	Anti-TransferrinRmonoclonal antibody OX26 and anti-Aβ monoclonal antibody DE2B4	[164]
Polymeric NPs	PLGA NPs	Ac-LVFFARK-NH2, Aβ aggregation inhibitor	None	[165]
Dendrimers	KLVFF peptide	Aβ aggregation inhibitor	None	[166]
Gold NPs	LCA10 and VCD10 peptides	Aβ aggregation inhibitors	None	[167]
Polymeric NPs	PLGA NPs	Vitamin D-binding protein	None	[168]
Magnetic NPs	Dextran-coated Fe_3O_4 NPs	Osmotin protein, neuroprotective	None	[169]
Liposomes	DOTAP/DOPE/Chol/DSPE-PEG (4.5:4.5:2:4 molar ratio)	BDNF	Mannose and penetratin or rabies virus glycoprotein	[170]
Polymeric NPs	PS80-coated PBCA NPs	Curcumin	Apolippoprotein E3 peptide	[171]
Polymeric NPs	PLGA NPs	Curcumin	Tet-1 peptide	[172]
Polymeric NPs	PLGA NPs	Curcumin	g7 glycopeptide	[173]
Polymeric NPs	PEG-PLGA NPs	Curcumin	B6 peptide	[174]
Liposomes	DSPC/Chol (2:1 molar ratio) with DPS-PEG2000-Cur (10 or 20 mol %)	Curcumin	Anti-Transferrin R monoclonal antibody OX26	[175]
Polymeric NPs	PAAM-CL-PLGA NPs	Curcumin and rosmarinic acid	83–14 monoclonal antibody	[176]
Liposomes	DSPC/Chol/DSPE-PEG2000/DSPE-PEG2000-COOH (2:1:0.11:0.021 molar ratio)	α-mangostin	Transferrin	[177]
Gold NPs	PEG-coated Au NPs	Anthocyanins	None	[178]
Polymeric NPs	PEG-PLGA NPs	Anthocyanins	None	[179]
Polymeric NPs	PEG-PLGA NPs	EGCG and ascorbic acid	None	[180]

NPs: Nanoparticles; PLGA: Poly(lactic-co-glycolic acid); PBCA: Poly(butyl cyanoacrylate); PS80: Polysorbate 80; PEG: Polyethylene glycol;DMPC: 1,2-Dimyristoyl-sn-glycero-3-phosphocholine; EYPC: Egg yolk phosphatidylcholine; PLA: Polylactic acid; KLVFF: Lys-Leu-Val-Phe-Phe (β-amyloid binding peptide); LCA10 Peptide: Leucine-based amyloid-targeting peptide (specific sequence varies); VCD10 Peptide: Valine-cysteine-aspartate-based peptide (exact composition depends on study); DOTAP: 1,2-Dioleoyl-3-trimethylammonum-propane; DOPE: 1,2-Dioleoyl-sn-glycero-3-phosphoethanolamine; Chol: Cholesterol; DSPE: 1,2-Distearoyl-sn-glycero-3-phosphoethanolamine; DSPC: 1,2-Distearoyl-sn-glycero-3-phosphocholine; DPS: 1,2-Distearoyl-sn-glyceo-3-phosphate; PAAM: Polyacrylamide; Tet-1 peptide: Ten-eleven translocation 1 peptide.

INNOVATIVE BIOPOLYMER NANOPARTICLE-BASED THERAPEUTICS FOR ALZHEIMER'S DISEASE

A diverse range of nanoparticle formulations—ranging from lipid-based, polymeric, and mesoporous silica nanoparticles to hybrid graphene oxide and PEGylated nanocarriers encapsulating potent bioactive compounds such as curcumin, quercetin, coenzyme Q10, and various antioxidants, helping to inhibit Aβ aggregation, reduce oxidative stress, and restore cognitive function (Table **3**).

Table 3. Phytoconstituent-loaded biopolymeric nanocarriers for the treatment of Alzheimer's Disease.

Nanoparticle Type	Size (nm)	Dosage / Concentration	Loaded Phytochemical Agent	Therapeutic Efficacy	Limitations / Challenges	Refs.
Chitosan Nanoparticles	300 - 400 nm	30 μM	Genistein	Improves nasal mucosa permeability, neuroprotection	Poor bioavailability (6.8%)	[181]
Selenium-PLGA Nanospheres	Hybrid / 70.5 ± 6 - 160 ± 5 nm	-	Curcumin	Efficient BBB penetration reduces Aβ accumulation	None reported	[182]
Chitosan-coated Solid Lipid Nanoparticles	182.6 - 184.9 nm	80 mg/kg	Ferulic Acid	Reduces oxidative stress, improves cognitive functions	Low solubility & poor oral bioavailability	[183]
PLGA Nanoparticles	226.6 ± 44.4 nm	2.5 mg/kg	Vitamin D-binding protein	Reduces Aβ accumulation, neuroinflammation & cognitive dysfunction	None reported	[164, 184]

(Table 3) cont.....

Nanoparticle Type	Size (nm)	Dosage / Concentration	Loaded Phytochemical Agent	Therapeutic Efficacy	Limitations / Challenges	Refs.
HPMC-Quercetin Nanoparticles	<1000 nm	30 mg/kg/day	Quercetin	Reduces amyloid plaques & neurofibrillary tangles	Partial inhibition of $AlCl_3$ toxicity	[185]
PLGA Nanoparticles	92 ± 7 nm	2 mg/kg per dose	PAPANONOate (NO donor)	Sustains nitric oxide release, disrupts Aβ fibrils, improves memory & cognition.	Degrades into lactic & glycolic acid, increasing ATP production	[186]
PLGA Nanoparticles	100 nm	5 mg/ml	Ginsenoside Rg3	Reduces Aβ toxicity, improves BBB permeability, and provides neuroprotection	Poor pharmacokinetics & bioavailability	[187]
Surface-Modified PLGA NPs	-	-	Coenzyme Q10	Disrupts amyloid plaques, inhibits Aβ fibrillation.	None reported	[188]
PLGA-Chitosan NPs	136.2 ± 1.09 - 128.8 ± 1.25 nm	4 mg/kg body weight	Lutein	Reduces oxidative stress, enhances pharmacokinetics, and protects against neuronal damage	Poor bioavailability	[143]
PEGylated PLGA NPs	124.8 ± 5.2 nm	40 mg/kg	Quercetin &Rosmarinic acid	Prolonged drug release, increased synaptic protein expression, and reduced Aβ load	Degrades *via* surface erosion, poor bioavailability	[180]
Chitosan Nanoparticles	192.3 nm	0.125 mg/kg body weight	Niruriflavone	Biocompatible, enhances cell viability, increases antioxidant enzyme levels, reduces oxidative damage	None reported	[189]
PLGA Nanoparticles	147.5 ± 20.7 nm	5–10 ng/ml	Triptolide	Sustained drug release, enhances transcellular permeability, and reduces oxidative stress.	Poor solubility & bioavailability	[190]

(Table 3) cont.....

Nanoparticle Type	Size (nm)	Dosage / Concentration	Loaded Phytochemical Agent	Therapeutic Efficacy	Limitations / Challenges	Refs.
PEG-Lys-PCL_2 - Y-Shaped Copolymer NPs	75.4 ± 1.9 - 91.7 ± 3.0 nm	675 mg/kg	Baicalein	Enhances cellular uptake, anti-amyloid and antioxidant effects	Poor bioavailability	[191]
PLGA@QT Nanoparticles	100–150 nm	20 mg/kg	Quercetin	Prevents Zn^{2+}-induced Aβ fibril formation, improves cognition	Limited understanding of pharmacokinetics	[192]
PEGylated NPs	125 nm	40 mg/kg	Anti-$A\beta_{1-42}$	Reduces Aβ oligomer levels, improves memory.	None reported	[193]

NPs: Nanoparticles; PLGA: Poly(lactic-co-glycolicacid); HMPC: Hydroxypropyl methylcellulose; PCL_2:(Poly Caprolactone)$_2$;Aβ: Amyloid-beta; PEG:Poly Ethylene Glycol; Lys: Lysine; QT: Quercetin; BBB: Blood brainbarrier.

Challenges

A significant challenge in utilizing biopolymers for Alzheimer's disease (AD) therapy is their effective delivery across the blood-brain barrier (BBB), which restricts the entry of many therapeutic biomolecules. Strategies such as nanoparticle-based carriers and chemical modifications aim to enhance BBB permeability. However, ensuring that biopolymers do not trigger immune responses remains another obstacle, as some natural biopolymers exhibit immunogenicity that can cause adverse effects. Scientists are modifying biopolymer structures to minimize immunogenicity while maintaining therapeutic efficacy [194]. Another key limitation is the degradation of natural biopolymers over time, which affects their long-term stability and therapeutic impact. Structural modifications are being explored to extend their functional lifespan. Additionally, since AD affects specific brain regions, targeted biopolymer delivery systems are under investigation to enhance treatment precision. Regulatory challenges also pose a barrier, as rigorous preclinical and clinical evaluations are required to establish safety and efficacy, making the approval process costly and time-consuming [195 - 200]. Further challenges arise in the commercialization of biopolymer-based therapies due to limited natural sources, batch-to-batch variability, and high production costs. Variability in biopolymer composition, influenced by source and processing conditions, complicates quality control and reproducibility [201]. Regulatory approval for biopolymer-based therapeutics is another hurdle, requiring extensive safety assessments. Additionally, the absence of standardized nanotechnology guidelines creates disparities in regulatory requirements across different regions, making global clinical trials complex. Compliance with Good Manufacturing Practices (GMP) and stringent quality control measures—covering particle size, drug loading, and release kinetics—is essential for successful commercialization [201 - 204].

A promising research direction is the optimization of nanoparticle-based drug delivery systems for biopolymers, enabling more effective and targeted drug transport to the brain. Since neuroinflammation is a key contributor to AD progression, novel anti-inflammatory biopolymer-based therapies are being explored. Additionally, researchers are investigating mitochondria-targeting nanocarriers to reduce oxidative stress, prevent mitochondrial dysfunction, and enhance energy production in neurons [205]. To accelerate progress, interdisciplinary collaboration between bioengineers, clinicians, and regulatory experts is essential. Organizing international conferences and increasing funding for biopolymer-based AD therapies will foster innovation. Developing specialized educational programs will equip future researchers with expertise in biopolymer engineering for neurodegenerative diseases [206].

FUTURE PERSPECTIVES AND RESEARCH DIRECTION

The application of biopolymers in AD treatment remains an evolving field, with numerous research opportunities yet to be explored. One promising avenue is the advancement of nanoparticle-based drug delivery systems to optimize the therapeutic efficacy of biopolymers. Additionally, novel anti-inflammatory strategies for AD treatment are required, given the crucial role of neuroinflammation in disease progression [207]. Researchers are also investigating a diverse range of natural and synthetic biopolymers to design next-generation systems for targeted drug delivery to the brain, with the ultimate objective of developing a cure for AD [4]. Considering the significant role of mitochondrial dysfunction in AD pathogenesis, future research should focus on designing mitochondria-targeting nanocarriers. These specialized compounds could mitigate mitochondrial reactive oxygen species (ROS) production, prevent mitochondrial permeability transition pore opening, and reduce mitochondrial DNA mutations [205]. Additionally, they may promote mitochondrial biogenesis and enhance mitochondrial bioenergetics in both the brain and peripheral tissues of AD patients [205]. To accelerate progress in biopolymer-based therapies for AD, improved research coordination is necessary. This can be achieved through multidisciplinary collaboration among bioengineers, clinical researchers, healthcare professionals, policymakers, and educators. Hosting international conferences and workshops would foster the exchange of knowledge and encourage innovative research. Additionally, funding agencies should prioritize financial support for biopolymer research in AD, ensuring that researchers have the resources to advance this field. Moreover, developing specialized educational programs would equip the next generation of scientists with the expertise required to innovate in biopolymer-based therapeutics [4, 201, 206,]. Several knowledge gaps must still be addressed to enhance the use of biopolymers in AD management. Key areas include understanding immune responses to biopolymer-based nanomaterials and optimizing immunotherapeutic approaches. Additionally, developing biopolymer-based scaffolds for neuroregeneration remains a priority, with researchers exploring hybrid approaches combining natural biopolymers with synthetic or electroconductive polymers [208]. Identifying the most effective biopolymers for neural tissue engineering is another crucial goal, with particular focus on extracellular matrix-derived proteins and polysaccharides. Lastly, challenges related to sourcing biopolymers, such as collagen, must be overcome by identifying alternative sources or developing synthetic analogs [209].

CONCLUSION

Despite ongoing advancements, biopolymer-based therapies for AD face critical challenges, including immune responses, degradation, regulatory hurdles, and commercialization barriers. However, engineering strategies are being developed to enhance biocompatibility, stability, and BBB penetration, making biopolymers a promising therapeutic avenue. Future research must focus on optimizing immunotherapeutic approaches, developing neuroregenerative scaffolds, and identifying effective biopolymers for neural tissue engineering. Hybrid biopolymer systems combining natural and synthetic materials may offer improved drug delivery precision. Additionally, addressing supply chain challenges through synthetic biopolymer alternatives or alternative natural sources is crucial. Biopolymer-based nanomedicine presents an innovative, targeted approach for AD treatment. The rapid advancement of smart biopolymer technologies is expected to revolutionize patient-centered treatment by enabling precise drug delivery. With continued research and integration into clinical trials, biopolymer-based therapeutics have the potential to provide novel and effective solutions for AD management while overcoming existing limitations.

REFERENCES

[1] Issa AA. Mechanistic insights into the molecular and cellular basis of Alzheimer's disease. In: Essential Guide to Neurodegenerative Disorders. 2025: 211-221. [http://dx.doi.org/10.1016/B978-0-443-15702-8.00013-0]

[2] Anitha K, Singh MK, Kohat K, *et al.* Recent insights into the neurobiology of Alzheimer's disease and advanced treatment strategies. Mol Neurobiol 2025; 62(2): 2314-32. [http://dx.doi.org/10.1007/s12035-024-04384-1]

[3] Singh S, Kumar S, Kumar G, Mukherjee S. Neuro-compatible Biomaterials: Pioneering Solutions for Brain. Biomaterials and Neurodegenerative Disorders.:43.

[4] Zivari-Ghader T, Valioglu F, Eftekhari A, *et al.* Recent progresses in natural based therapeutic

materials for Alzheimer's disease. Heliyon 2024; 10(4): e26351.
[http://dx.doi.org/10.1016/j.heliyon.2024.e26351] [PMID: 38434059]

[5] Wróblewska-Krepsztul J, Rydzkowski T, Michalska-Pożoga I, Thakur VK. Biopolymers for biomedical and pharmaceutical applications: Recent advances and overview of alginate electrospinning. Nanomaterials (Basel) 2019; 9(3): 404.
[http://dx.doi.org/10.3390/nano9030404] [PMID: 30857370]

[6] Talebian S, Foroughi J, Wade SJ, *et al.* Biopolymers for antitumor implantable drug delivery systems: recent advances and future outlook. Adv Mater 2018; 30(31): 1706665.
[http://dx.doi.org/10.1002/adma.201706665] [PMID: 29756237]

[7] Gagliardi A, Paolino D, Iannone M, Palma E, Fresta M, Cosco D. Sodium deoxycholate-decorated zein nanoparticles for a stable colloidal drug delivery system. Int J Nanomedicine 2018; 13: 601-14.
[http://dx.doi.org/10.2147/IJN.S156930] [PMID: 29430179]

[8] Fazal T, Murtaza BN, Shah M, *et al.* Recent developments in natural biopolymer based drug delivery systems. RSC Adv. 2023; 13(33): 23087-23121.
[http://dx.doi.org/10.1039/d3ra03369d] [PMID: 37529365]

[9] Chen X, Fan Y, Wu L, *et al.* Ultra-selective molecular-sieving gas separation membranes enabled by multi-covalent-crosslinking of microporous polymer blends. Nat Commun 2021; 12(1): 6140.
[http://dx.doi.org/10.1038/s41467-021-26379-5] [PMID: 34686671]

[10] Lynch CR, Kondiah PPD, Choonara YE, du Toit LC, Ally N, Pillay V. Hydrogel biomaterials for application in ocular drug delivery. Front Bioeng Biotechnol 2020; 8: 228.
[http://dx.doi.org/10.3389/fbioe.2020.00228] [PMID: 32266248]

[11] Calzoni E, Cesaretti A, Polchi A, Di Michele A, Tancini B, Emiliani C. Biocompatible polymer nanoparticles for drug delivery applications in cancer and neurodegenerative disorder therapies. J Funct Biomater 2019; 10(1): 4.
[http://dx.doi.org/10.3390/jfb10010004] [PMID: 30626094]

[12] Fazal T, Murtaza BN, Shah M, *et al.* Recent developments in natural biopolymer based drug delivery systems. RSC Advances 2023; 13(33): 23087-121.
[http://dx.doi.org/10.1039/D3RA03369D] [PMID: 37529365]

[13] Sighencea MG, Popescu RŞ, Trifu SC. From fundamentals to innovation in alzheimer's disease: Molecular findings and revolutionary therapies. Int J Mol Sci 2024; 25(22): 12311.
[http://dx.doi.org/10.3390/ijms252212311] [PMID: 39596378]

[14] AbuAlrob M. Neuroinflammation in Alzheimer's disease: mechanistic insights, pathological implications, and emerging therapeutic strategies [Internet]. Authorea; 2024.
[http://dx.doi.org/10.22541/au.172838938.84403346/v1]

[15] Zang J. Aβ in alzheimer's disease: significance and potential as a therapeutic target. In: Biological sciences and environmental health. 1st ed. Boca Raton (FL): CRC Press; 2024.

[16] Al-kuraishy HM, Jabir MS, Al-Gareeb AI, *et al.* Evaluation and targeting of amyloid precursor protein (APP)/amyloid beta (Aβ) axis in amyloidogenic and non-amyloidogenic pathways: A time outside the tunnel. Ageing Res Rev 2023; 92: 102119.
[http://dx.doi.org/10.1016/j.arr.2023.102119] [PMID: 37931848]

[17] Azargoonjahromi A. The duality of amyloid-β: its role in normal and Alzheimer's disease states. Mol Brain 2024; 17(1): 44.
[http://dx.doi.org/10.1186/s13041-024-01118-1] [PMID: 39020435]

[18] Merighi S, Nigro M, Travagli A, Gessi S. Microglia and Alzheimer's disease. Int J Mol Sci 2022; 23(21): 12990.
[http://dx.doi.org/10.3390/ijms232112990] [PMID: 36361780]

[19] Hampel H, Hardy J, Blennow K, *et al.* The amyloid-β pathway in Alzheimer's disease. Mol Psychiatry 2021; 26(10): 5481-503.

[http://dx.doi.org/10.1038/s41380-021-01249-0] [PMID: 34456336]

[20] Rawat P, Sehar U, Bisht J, Selman A, Culberson J, Reddy PH. Phosphorylated tau in Alzheimer's disease and other tauopathies. Int J Mol Sci 2022; 23(21): 12841. [http://dx.doi.org/10.3390/ijms232112841] [PMID: 36361631]

[21] Li X, Ba Z, Huang J, *et al.* Comprehensive review on Alzheimer's disease: from the posttranslational modifications of Tau to corresponding treatments. iBrain. 2024; 10(4): 427-438. [http://dx.doi.org/10.1002/ibra.12176] [PMID: 39691421]

[22] Fišar Z. Linking the amyloid, tau, and mitochondrial hypotheses of Alzheimer's disease and identifying promising drug targets. Biomolecules 2022; 12(11): 1676. [http://dx.doi.org/10.3390/biom12111676] [PMID: 36421690]

[23] Buccellato FR, D'Anca M, Fenoglio C, Scarpini E, Galimberti D. Role of oxidative damage in alzheimer's disease and neurodegeneration: From pathogenic mechanisms to biomarker discovery. Antioxidants 2021; 10(9): 1353. [http://dx.doi.org/10.3390/antiox10091353] [PMID: 34572985]

[24] Olufunmilayo EO, Gerke-Duncan MB, Holsinger RMD. Oxidative stress and antioxidants in neurodegenerative disorders. Antioxidants 2023; 12(2): 517. [http://dx.doi.org/10.3390/antiox12020517] [PMID: 36830075]

[25] Jurcău MC, Andronie-Cioara FL, Jurcău A, *et al.* The link between oxidative stress, mitochondrial dysfunction and neuroinflammation in the pathophysiology of Alzheimer's disease: therapeutic implications and future perspectives. Antioxidants 2022; 11(11): 2167. [http://dx.doi.org/10.3390/antiox11112167] [PMID: 36358538]

[26] Dewanjee S, Chakraborty P, Bhattacharya H, *et al.* Altered glucose metabolism in Alzheimer's disease: Role of mitochondrial dysfunction and oxidative stress. Free Radic Biol Med 2022; 193(Pt 1): 134-57. [http://dx.doi.org/10.1016/j.freeradbiomed.2022.09.032] [PMID: 36206930]

[27] Doroszkiewicz J, Farhan JA, Mroczko J, Winkel I, Perkowski M, Mroczko B. Common and trace metals in Alzheimer's and Parkinson's diseases. Int J Mol Sci 2023; 24(21): 15721. [http://dx.doi.org/10.3390/ijms242115721] [PMID: 37958705]

[28] Leng F, Edison P. Neuroinflammation and microglial activation in Alzheimer disease: where do we go from here? Nat Rev Neurol 2021; 17(3): 157-72. [http://dx.doi.org/10.1038/s41582-020-00435-y] [PMID: 33318676]

[29] Cai Y, Liu J, Wang B, Sun M, Yang H. Microglia in the neuroinflammatory pathogenesis of Alzheimer's disease and related therapeutic targets. Front Immunol 2022; 13: 856376. [http://dx.doi.org/10.3389/fimmu.2022.856376] [PMID: 35558075]

[30] Thakur S, Dhapola R, Sarma P, Medhi B, Reddy DH. Neuroinflammation in Alzheimer's disease: current progress in molecular signaling and therapeutics. Inflammation 2023; 46(1): 1-17. [http://dx.doi.org/10.1007/s10753-022-01721-1] [PMID: 35986874]

[31] Preman P, Alfonso-Triguero M, Alberdi E, Verkhratsky A, Arranz AM. Astrocytes in Alzheimer's disease: pathological significance and molecular pathways. Cells 2021; 10(3): 540. [http://dx.doi.org/10.3390/cells10030540] [PMID: 33806259]

[32] Satarker S, Bojja SL, Gurram PC, Mudgal J, Arora D, Nampoothiri M. Astrocytic glutamatergic transmission and its implications in neurodegenerative disorders. Cells 2022; 11(7): 1139. [http://dx.doi.org/10.3390/cells11071139] [PMID: 35406702]

[33] Liu R, Wang J, Chen Y, *et al.* NOX activation in reactive astrocytes regulates astrocytic LCN2 expression and neurodegeneration. Cell Death Dis 2022; 13(4): 371. [http://dx.doi.org/10.1038/s41419-022-04831-8] [PMID: 35440572]

[34] Curcio M, Cirillo G, Rouaen JRC, *et al.* Natural polysaccharide carriers in brain delivery: challenge and perspective. Pharmaceutics 2020; 12(12): 1183.

[http://dx.doi.org/10.3390/pharmaceutics12121183] [PMID: 33291284]

[35] Radwan RR, Abdel Ghaffar AM, Ali HE. Gamma radiation preparation of chitosan nanoparticles for controlled delivery of memantine. J Biomater Appl 2020; 34(8): 1150-62. [http://dx.doi.org/10.1177/0885328219890071] [PMID: 31771402]

[36] Jaruszewski KM, Curran GL, Swaminathan SK, *et al.* Multimodal Nanoprobes to target cerebrovascular amyloid in Alzheimer's disease brain. Biomaterials 2014; 35(6): 1967-76. [http://dx.doi.org/10.1016/j.biomaterials.2013.10.075] [PMID: 24331706]

[37] Agyare EK, Jaruszewski KM, Curran GL, *et al.* Engineering theranostic nanovehicles capable of targeting cerebrovascular amyloid deposits. J Control Release 2014; 185: 121-9. [http://dx.doi.org/10.1016/j.jconrel.2014.04.010] [PMID: 24735640]

[38] Fernandes J, Ghate MV, Basu Mallik S, Lewis SA. Amino acid conjugated chitosan nanoparticles for the brain targeting of a model dipeptidyl peptidase-4 inhibitor. Int J Pharm 2018; 547(1-2): 563-71. [http://dx.doi.org/10.1016/j.ijpharm.2018.06.031] [PMID: 29906562]

[39] Bhavna , Md S, Ali M, *et al.* Donepezil nanosuspension intended for nose to brain targeting: *In vitro* and *in vivo* safety evaluation. Int J Biol Macromol 2014; 67: 418-25. [http://dx.doi.org/10.1016/j.ijbiomac.2014.03.022] [PMID: 24705169]

[40] Sood S, Jain K, Gowthamarajan K. Optimization of curcumin nanoemulsion for intranasal delivery using design of experiment and its toxicity assessment. Colloids Surf B Biointerfaces 2014; 113: 330-7. [http://dx.doi.org/10.1016/j.colsurfb.2013.09.030] [PMID: 24121076]

[41] Samaridou E, Walgrave H, Salta E, *et al.* Nose-to-brain delivery of enveloped RNA - cell permeating peptide nanocomplexes for the treatment of neurodegenerative diseases. Biomaterials 2020; 230: 119657. [http://dx.doi.org/10.1016/j.biomaterials.2019.119657] [PMID: 31837821]

[42] Rajput A, Bariya A, Allam A, Othman S, Butani SB. In situ nanostructured hydrogel of resveratrol for brain targeting: *in vitro-in vivo* characterization. Drug Deliv Transl Res 2018; 8(5): 1460-70. [http://dx.doi.org/10.1007/s13346-018-0540-6] [PMID: 29785574]

[43] Nasr M. Development of an optimized hyaluronic acid-based lipidic nanoemulsion co-encapsulating two polyphenols for nose to brain delivery. Drug Deliv 2016; 23(4): 1444-52. [http://dx.doi.org/10.3109/10717544.2015.1092619] [PMID: 26401600]

[44] Shah B, Khunt D, Misra M, Padh H. Formulation and in-vivo pharmacokinetic consideration of intranasal microemulsion and mucoadhesive microemulsion of rivastigmine for brain targeting. Pharm Res 2018; 35(1): 8. [http://dx.doi.org/10.1007/s11095-017-2279-z] [PMID: 29294189]

[45] Chei S, Oh HJ, Lee K, Jin H, Lee JY, Lee BY. Dietary silk peptide inhibits LPS-induced inflammatory responses by modulating toll-like receptor 4 (TLR4) signaling. Biomolecules 2020; 10(5): 771. [http://dx.doi.org/10.3390/biom10050771] [PMID: 32429220]

[46] Chae HS, Kang YK, Shin YK, *et al.* The role of BF-7 on neuroprotection and enhancement of cognitive function. Korean J Physiol Pharmacol 2004; 8(4): 173-9.

[47] De Giorgio G, Matera B, Vurro D, *et al.* Silk fibroin materials: Biomedical applications and perspectives. Bioengineering (Basel) 2024; 11(2): 167. [http://dx.doi.org/10.3390/bioengineering11020167] [PMID: 38391652]

[48] Kang YK, Nam SH, Sohn HO, Lee DW. Inhibitory effect of silkworm extract on monoamine oxidase activity *in vitro* and *in vivo*. Entomol Res. 2005; 35(3): 189-193. [http://dx.doi.org/10.1111/j.1748-5967.2005.tb00158.x]

[49] Kang YK, Oh HS, Cho YH, Kim YJ, Han YG, Nam SH. Effects of a silkworm extract on dopamine and monoamine oxidase-B activity in an MPTP-induced Parkinsons disease model. Lab Anim Res 2010; 26(3): 287-92.

[http://dx.doi.org/10.5625/lar.2010.26.3.287]

[50] Sha Q, Wang Y, Zhu Z, *et al.* A hyaluronic acid/silk fibroin/poly-dopamine-coated biomimetic hydrogel scaffold with incorporated neurotrophin-3 for spinal cord injury repair. Acta Biomater 2023; 167: 219-33.
[http://dx.doi.org/10.1016/j.actbio.2023.05.044] [PMID: 37257575]

[51] Zhao Y, Liang Y, Ding S, Zhang K, Mao H, Yang Y. Application of conductive PPy/SF composite scaffold and electrical stimulation for neural tissue engineering. Biomaterials 2020; 255: 120164.
[http://dx.doi.org/10.1016/j.biomaterials.2020.120164] [PMID: 32554132]

[52] Tufan Y, Öztatlı H, Garipcan B, Ercan B. Development of electrically conductive porous silk fibroin/carbon nanofiber scaffolds. Biomed Mater 2021; 16(2): 025027.
[http://dx.doi.org/10.1088/1748-605X/abc3db] [PMID: 33091884]

[53] Kim H, Yang GH, Choi CH, Cho YS, Kim G. Gelatin/PVA scaffolds fabricated using a 3D-printing process employed with a low-temperature plate for hard tissue regeneration: Fabrication and characterizations. Int J Biol Macromol 2018; 120(Pt A): 119-27.
[http://dx.doi.org/10.1016/j.ijbiomac.2018.07.159] [PMID: 30056041]

[54] Sun M, Wang Y, Yao L, Li Y, Weng Y, Qiu D. Fabrication and characterization of gelatin/polyvinyl alcohol composite scaffold. Polymers (Basel) 2022; 14(7): 1400.
[http://dx.doi.org/10.3390/polym14071400] [PMID: 35406273]

[55] Rajkumar M, Vimala K, Tamiliniyan DD, *et al.* Gelatin/polyvinyl alcohol loaded magnesium hydroxide nanocomposite attenuates neurotoxicity and oxidative stress in Alzheimer's disease induced rats. Int J Biol Macromol 2022; 222(Pt B): 2122-43.
[http://dx.doi.org/10.1016/j.ijbiomac.2022.10.010] [PMID: 36228820]

[56] Rajkumar M, Davis Presley SI, Thiyagarajulu N, *et al.* Gelatin/PLA-loaded gold nanocomposites synthesis using Syzygium cumini fruit extract and their antioxidant, antibacterial, anti-inflammatory, antidiabetic and anti-Alzheimer's activities. Sci Rep 2025; 15(1): 2110.
[http://dx.doi.org/10.1038/s41598-024-84098-5] [PMID: 39814774]

[57] Hoban DB, Newland B, Moloney TC, Howard L, Pandit A, Dowd E. The reduction in immunogenicity of neurotrophin overexpressing stem cells after intra-striatal transplantation by encapsulation in an in situ gelling collagen hydrogel. Biomaterials 2013; 34(37): 9420-9.
[http://dx.doi.org/10.1016/j.biomaterials.2013.08.073] [PMID: 24054846]

[58] Moriarty N, Pandit A, Dowd E. Encapsulation of primary dopaminergic neurons in a GDNF-loaded collagen hydrogel increases their survival, re-innervation and function after intra-striatal transplantation. Sci Rep 2017; 7(1): 16033.
[http://dx.doi.org/10.1038/s41598-017-15970-w] [PMID: 29167483]

[59] Bellotti E, Schilling AL, Little SR, Decuzzi P. Injectable thermoresponsive hydrogels as drug delivery system for the treatment of central nervous system disorders: A review. J Control Release 2021; 329: 16-35.
[http://dx.doi.org/10.1016/j.jconrel.2020.11.049] [PMID: 33259851]

[60] Ucar B. Natural biomaterials in brain repair: A focus on collagen. Neurochem Int 2021; 146: 105033.
[http://dx.doi.org/10.1016/j.neuint.2021.105033] [PMID: 33785419]

[61] Stanyon HF, Viles JH. Human serum albumin can regulate amyloid-β peptide fiber growth in the brain interstitium: implications for Alzheimer disease. J Biol Chem 2012; 287(33): 28163-8.
[http://dx.doi.org/10.1074/jbc.C112.360800] [PMID: 22718756]

[62] Bohrmann B, Tjernberg L, Kuner P, *et al.* Endogenous proteins controlling amyloid β-peptide polymerization. Possible implications for β-amyloid formation in the central nervous system and in peripheral tissues. J Biol Chem 1999; 274(23): 15990-5.
[http://dx.doi.org/10.1074/jbc.274.23.15990] [PMID: 10347147]

[63] Prajapati KD, Sharma SS, Roy N. Current perspectives on potential role of albumin in

neuroprotection. Reviews in the Neurosciences. 2011; 22(3): 355-363.
[http://dx.doi.org/10.1515/rns.2011.028]

[64] Boada M, Anaya F, Ortiz P, *et al.* Efficacy and safety of plasma exchange with 5% albumin to modify cerebrospinal fluid and plasma amyloid-β concentrations and cognition outcomes in Alzheimer's disease patients: a multicenter, randomized, controlled clinical trial. J Alzheimers Dis 2017; 56(1): 129-43.
[http://dx.doi.org/10.3233/JAD-160565] [PMID: 27911295]

[65] Boada M, López OL, Olazarán J, *et al.* A randomized, controlled clinical trial of plasma exchange with albumin replacement for Alzheimer's disease: Primary results of the AMBAR Study. Alzheimers Dement 2020; 16(10): 1412-25.
[http://dx.doi.org/10.1002/alz.12137] [PMID: 32715623]

[66] Luppi B, Bigucci F, Corace G, *et al.* Albumin nanoparticles carrying cyclodextrins for nasal delivery of the anti-Alzheimer drug tacrine. Eur J Pharm Sci 2011; 44(4): 559-65.
[http://dx.doi.org/10.1016/j.ejps.2011.10.002] [PMID: 22009109]

[67] Piazzini V, Landucci E, D'Ambrosio M, *et al.* Chitosan coated human serum albumin nanoparticles: A promising strategy for nose-to-brain drug delivery. Int J Biol Macromol 2019; 129: 267-80.
[http://dx.doi.org/10.1016/j.ijbiomac.2019.02.005] [PMID: 30726749]

[68] Wong LR, Ho PC. Role of serum albumin as a nanoparticulate carrier for nose-to-brain delivery of R-flurbiprofen: implications for the treatment of Alzheimer's disease. J Pharm Pharmacol 2018; 70(1): 59-69.
[http://dx.doi.org/10.1111/jphp.12836] [PMID: 29034965]

[69] Mehra RR, Basu A, Christman RM, *et al.* Mechanoresponsive, proteolytically stable and biocompatible supergelators from ultra short enantiomeric peptides with sustained drug release propensity. New J Chem 2020; 44(16): 6346-54.
[http://dx.doi.org/10.1039/D0NJ00102C]

[70] Miksusanti M, Razak F, Huda N, Muntasir M. Design of short peptides as targeted protein inhibitors for alzheimer's disease. J Biomed Techno Nanomaterials 2024; 1(3): 106-16.

[71] Al-azzawi S, Masheta D, Guildford A, Phillips G, Santin M. A peptide-based nanocarrier for an enhanced delivery and targeting of flurbiprofen into the brain for the treatment of Alzheimer's disease: An *in vitro* study. Nanomaterials (Basel) 2020; 10(8): 1590.
[http://dx.doi.org/10.3390/nano10081590] [PMID: 32823499]

[72] Al-azzawi S, Masheta D, Guildford AL, Phillips G, Santin M. Dendrimeric poly (epsilon-lysine) delivery systems for the enhanced permeability of flurbiprofen across the blood-brain barrier in Alzheimer's disease. Int J Mol Sci 2018; 19(10): 3224.
[http://dx.doi.org/10.3390/ijms19103224] [PMID: 30340406]

[73] Al-azzawi S, Masheta D, Guildford A, Phillips G, Santin M. Designing and characterization of a novel delivery system for improved cellular uptake by brain using dendronised Apo-E-derived peptide. Front Bioeng Biotechnol 2019; 7: 49.
[http://dx.doi.org/10.3389/fbioe.2019.00049] [PMID: 30972332]

[74] Gülseren G, Demirsoy Z, Şeker M, Büyükünal O. Exploring bimetallic nanoparticles in alzheimer's therapy: A novel bio-assisted synthesis with multitarget potential. Mol Pharm 2024; 21(6): 3006-16.
[http://dx.doi.org/10.1021/acs.molpharmaceut.4c00175] [PMID: 38698500]

[75] Chu J, Zhang W, Liu Y, *et al.* Biomaterials-based anti-inflammatory treatment strategies for Alzheimer's disease. Neural Regen Res 2024; 19(1): 100-15.
[http://dx.doi.org/10.4103/1673-5374.374137] [PMID: 37488851]

[76] Aljohani NB, Qusti SY, Alsiny M, *et al.* Carboxymethylcellulose encapsulated fingolimod, siRNA@ZnO hybrid nanocomposite as a new anti-Alzheimer's material. RSC Advances 2024; 14(30): 22044-55.
[http://dx.doi.org/10.1039/D4RA01965B] [PMID: 39006767]

[77] Chen CB, Dellamaggiore KR, Ouellette CP, *et al.* Aptamer-based endocytosis of a lysosomal enzyme. Proc Natl Acad Sci USA 2008; 105(41): 15908-13. [http://dx.doi.org/10.1073/pnas.0808360105] [PMID: 18838694]

[78] Mu C, Dave N, Hu J, *et al.* Solubilization of flurbiprofen into aptamer-modified PEG–PLA micelles for targeted delivery to brain-derived endothelial cells *in vitro*. J Microencapsul 2013; 30(7): 701-8. [http://dx.doi.org/10.3109/02652048.2013.778907] [PMID: 23517066]

[79] Takahashi T, Tada K, Mihara H. RNA aptamers selected against amyloid β-peptide (Aβ) inhibit the aggregation of Aβ. Mol Biosyst 2009; 5(9): 986-91. [http://dx.doi.org/10.1039/B903391B] [PMID: 19668864]

[80] Mathew A, Aravind A, Brahatheeswaran D, *et al.* Amyloid-binding aptamer conjugated curcumin–PLGA nanoparticle for potential use in Alzheimer's disease. Bionanoscience 2012; 2(2): 83-93. [http://dx.doi.org/10.1007/s12668-012-0040-y]

[81] Zhou Y, Peng Z, Seven ES, Leblanc RM. Crossing the blood-brain barrier with nanoparticles. J Control Release 2018; 270: 290-303. [http://dx.doi.org/10.1016/j.jconrel.2017.12.015] [PMID: 29269142]

[82] Mulvihill JJE, Cunnane EM, Ross AM, Duskey JT, Tosi G, Grabrucker AM. Drug delivery across the blood-brain barrier: recent advances in the use of nanocarriers. Nanomedicine (Lond) 2020; 15(2): 205-14. [http://dx.doi.org/10.2217/nnm-2019-0367] [PMID: 31916480]

[83] Pandit R, Chen L, Götz J. The blood-brain barrier: Physiology and strategies for drug delivery. Adv Drug Deliv Rev 2020; 165-166: 1-14. [http://dx.doi.org/10.1016/j.addr.2019.11.009] [PMID: 31790711]

[84] Lockman PR, Mumper RJ, Khan MA, Allen DD. Nanoparticle technology for drug delivery across the blood-brain barrier. Drug Dev Ind Pharm 2002; 28(1): 1-13. [http://dx.doi.org/10.1081/DDC-120001481] [PMID: 11858519]

[85] Saraiva C, Praça C, Ferreira R, Santos T, Ferreira L, Bernardino L. Nanoparticle-mediated brain drug delivery: Overcoming blood–brain barrier to treat neurodegenerative diseases. J Control Release 2016; 235: 34-47. [http://dx.doi.org/10.1016/j.jconrel.2016.05.044] [PMID: 27208862]

[86] Ezhilarasi PN, Karthik P, Chhanwal N, Anandharamakrishnan C. Nanoencapsulation techniques for food bioactive components: a review. Food Bioprocess Technol 2013; 6(3): 628-47. [http://dx.doi.org/10.1007/s11947-012-0944-0]

[87] Rao JP, Geckeler KE. Polymer nanoparticles: Preparation techniques and size-control parameters. Prog Polym Sci 2011; 36(7): 887-913. [http://dx.doi.org/10.1016/j.progpolymsci.2011.01.001]

[88] Sahoo SK, Labhasetwar V. Nanotech approaches to drug delivery and imaging. Drug Discov Today 2003; 8(24): 1112-20. [http://dx.doi.org/10.1016/S1359-6446(03)02903-9] [PMID: 14678737]

[89] Bhatt P, Lalani R, Mashru R, Misra A. Abstract 2065: Anti-FSHR antibody Fab' fragment conjugated immunoliposomes loaded with cyclodextrin-paclitaxel complex for improved *in vitro* efficacy on ovarian cancer cells. Cancer Res 2016; 76(14_Supplement): 2065. [http://dx.doi.org/10.1158/1538-7445.AM2016-2065]

[90] Vhora I, Patil S, Bhatt P, Misra A. Protein- and Peptide-drug conjugates: an emerging drug delivery technology. Adv Protein Chem Struct Biol 2015; 98: 1-55. [http://dx.doi.org/10.1016/bs.apcsb.2014.11.001] [PMID: 25819275]

[91] Letchford K, Burt H. A review of the formation and classification of amphiphilic block copolymer nanoparticulate structures: micelles, nanospheres, nanocapsules and polymersomes. Eur J Pharm

Biopharm 2007; 65(3): 259-69.
[http://dx.doi.org/10.1016/j.ejpb.2006.11.009] [PMID: 17196803]

[92] Xiao F, Lin L, Chao Z, *et al.* Organic spherical nucleic acids for the transport of a NIR-II-emitting dye across the blood–brain barrier. Angew Chem Int Ed Engl 2020; 59: 9702-10.
[http://dx.doi.org/10.1002/anie.202002312]

[93] Zhu Z, Tian D, Gao P, *et al.* Cell-penetrating peptides transport noncovalently linked thermally activated delayed fluorescence nanoparticles for time-resolved luminescence imaging. J Am Chem Soc 2018; 140(50): 17484-91.
[http://dx.doi.org/10.1021/jacs.8b08438] [PMID: 30525541]

[94] Woodrow KA, Cu Y, Booth CJ, Saucier-Sawyer JK, Wood MJ, Mark Saltzman W. Intravaginal gene silencing using biodegradable polymer nanoparticles densely loaded with small-interfering RNA. Nat Mater 2009; 8(6): 526-33.
[http://dx.doi.org/10.1038/nmat2444] [PMID: 19404239]

[95] Calzoni E, Cesaretti A, Montegiove N, Di Michele A, Emiliani C. Enhanced stability of long-living immobilized recombinant β-d-*N*-acetyl-hexosaminidase a on polylactic acid (PLA) films for potential biomedical applications. J Funct Biomater 2021; 12(2): 32.
[http://dx.doi.org/10.3390/jfb12020032] [PMID: 34064736]

[96] Calzoni E, Cesaretti A, Montegiove N, Di Michele A, Pellegrino RM, Emiliani C. HexA-enzyme coated polymer nanoparticles for the development of a drug-delivery system in the treatment of sandhoff lysosomal storage disease. J Funct Biomater 2022; 13(2): 37.
[http://dx.doi.org/10.3390/jfb13020037] [PMID: 35466219]

[97] Khan AR, Liu M, Khan MW, Zhai G. Progress in brain targeting drug delivery system by nasal route. J Control Release 2017; 268: 364-89.
[http://dx.doi.org/10.1016/j.jconrel.2017.09.001] [PMID: 28887135]

[98] Makadia HK, Siegel SJ. Poly lactic-co-glycolic acid (PLGA) as biodegradable controlled drug delivery carrier. Polymers (Basel) 2011; 3(3): 1377-97.
[http://dx.doi.org/10.3390/polym3031377] [PMID: 22577513]

[99] Claudio P, Reatul K, Brigitte E, Geraldine P. Drug-delivery nanocarriers to cross the blood–brain barrier. InNanobiomaterials in Drug Delivery 2016 Jan 1 (pp. 333-370). William Andrew Publishing.
[http://dx.doi.org/10.1016/B978-0-323-42866-8.00010-1]

[100] Sabbagh F, Kim BS. Recent advances in polymeric transdermal drug delivery systems. J Control Release 2022; 341: 132-46.
[http://dx.doi.org/10.1016/j.jconrel.2021.11.025] [PMID: 34813879]

[101] Lammers T, Subr V, Ulbrich K, Hennink WE, Storm G, Kiessling F. Polymeric nanomedicines for image-guided drug delivery and tumor-targeted combination therapy. Nano Today 2010; 5(3): 197-212.
[http://dx.doi.org/10.1016/j.nantod.2010.05.001]

[102] Grund S, Bauer M, Fischer D. Polymers in drug delivery—state of the art and future trends. Adv Eng Mater 2011; 13(3): B61-87.
[http://dx.doi.org/10.1002/adem.201080088]

[103] Montegiove N, Calzoni E, Emiliani C, Cesaretti A. Biopolymer nanoparticles for nose-to-brain drug delivery: A new promising approach for the treatment of neurological diseases. J Funct Biomater 2022; 13(3): 125.
[http://dx.doi.org/10.3390/jfb13030125] [PMID: 36135560]

[104] Bhaskar S, Tian F, Stoeger T, *et al.* Multifunctional Nanocarriers for diagnostics, drug delivery and targeted treatment across blood-brain barrier: perspectives on tracking and neuroimaging. Part Fibre Toxicol 2010; 7(1): 3.
[http://dx.doi.org/10.1186/1743-8977-7-3] [PMID: 20199661]

[105] Hersh AM, Alomari S, Tyler BM. Crossing the blood-brain barrier: advances in nanoparticle technology for drug delivery in neuro-oncology. Int J Mol Sci 2022; 23(8): 4153. [http://dx.doi.org/10.3390/ijms23084153] [PMID: 35456971]

[106] Mikitsh JL, Chacko AM. Pathways for small molecule delivery to the central nervous system across the blood-brain barrier. Perspectives in medicinal chemistry. 2014 Jan;6:PMC-S13384. [http://dx.doi.org/10.4137/PMC.S13384]

[107] Nelson CE, Kintzing JR, Hanna A, Shannon JM, Gupta MK, Duvall CL. Balancing cationic and hydrophobic content of PEGylated siRNA polyplexes enhances endosome escape, stability, blood circulation time, and bioactivity *in vivo.* ACS Nano 2013; 7(10): 8870-80. [http://dx.doi.org/10.1021/nn403325f] [PMID: 24041122]

[108] Grabrucker AM, Ruozi B, Belletti D, *et al.* Nanoparticle transport across the blood brain barrier. Tissue Barriers 2016; 4(1): e1153568. [http://dx.doi.org/10.1080/21688370.2016.1153568] [PMID: 27141426]

[109] Pulicherla KK, Verma MK. Targeting therapeutics across the blood brain barrier (BBB), prerequisite towards thrombolytic therapy for cerebrovascular disorders-an overview and advancements. AAPS PharmSciTech 2015; 16(2): 223-33. [http://dx.doi.org/10.1208/s12249-015-0287-z] [PMID: 25613561]

[110] Hervé F, Ghinea N, Scherrmann JM. CNS delivery *via* adsorptive transcytosis. AAPS J 2008; 10(3): 455-72. [http://dx.doi.org/10.1208/s12248-008-9055-2] [PMID: 18726697]

[111] Cano A, Sánchez-López E, Ettcheto M, *et al.* Current advances in the development of novel polymeric nanoparticles for the treatment of neurodegenerative diseases. Nanomedicine (Lond) 2020; 15(12): 1239-61. [http://dx.doi.org/10.2217/nnm-2019-0443] [PMID: 32370600]

[112] Ding S, Khan AI, Cai X, *et al.* Overcoming blood–brain barrier transport: Advances in nanoparticle-based drug delivery strategies. Mater Today 2020; 37: 112-25. [http://dx.doi.org/10.1016/j.mattod.2020.02.001] [PMID: 33093794]

[113] Lu W. Adsorptive-mediated brain delivery systems. Curr Pharm Biotechnol 2012; 13(12): 2340-8. [http://dx.doi.org/10.2174/138920112803341851] [PMID: 23016640]

[114] Kristensen M, Kucharz K, Felipe Alves Fernandes E, *et al.* Conjugation of therapeutic psd-95 inhibitors to the cell-penetrating peptide tat affects blood–brain barrier adherence, uptake, and permeation. Pharmaceutics 2020; 12(7): 661. [http://dx.doi.org/10.3390/pharmaceutics12070661] [PMID: 32674358]

[115] Lajoie JM, Shusta EV. Targeting receptor-mediated transport for delivery of biologics across the blood-brain barrier. Annu Rev Pharmacol Toxicol 2015; 55(1): 613-31. [http://dx.doi.org/10.1146/annurev-pharmtox-010814-124852] [PMID: 25340933]

[116] Guerrini L, Alvarez-Puebla RA, Pazos-Perez N. Surface modifications of nanoparticles for stability in biological fluids. Materials (Basel) 2018; 11(7): 1154. [http://dx.doi.org/10.3390/ma11071154] [PMID: 29986436]

[117] Mittal G, Carswell H, Brett R, Currie S, Kumar MNVR. Development and evaluation of polymer nanoparticles for oral delivery of estradiol to rat brain in a model of Alzheimer's pathology. J Control Release 2011; 150(2): 220-8. [http://dx.doi.org/10.1016/j.jconrel.2010.11.013] [PMID: 21111014]

[118] Liu M, Li H, Luo G, Liu Q, Wang Y. Pharmacokinetics and biodistribution of surface modification polymeric nanoparticles. Arch Pharm Res 2008; 31(4): 547-54. [http://dx.doi.org/10.1007/s12272-001-1191-8] [PMID: 18449515]

[119] Rao KS, Reddy MK, Horning JL, Labhasetwar V. TAT-conjugated nanoparticles for the CNS delivery of anti-HIV drugs. Biomaterials 2008; 29(33): 4429-38.

[http://dx.doi.org/10.1016/j.biomaterials.2008.08.004] [PMID: 18760470]

[120] Kulkarni SA, Feng SS. Effects of surface modification on delivery efficiency of biodegradable nanoparticles across the blood-brain barrier. Nanomedicine (Lond) 2011; 6(2): 377-94. [http://dx.doi.org/10.2217/nnm.10.131] [PMID: 21385139]

[121] Geldenhuys W, Mbimba T, Bui T, Harrison K, Sutariya V. Brain-targeted delivery of paclitaxel using glutathione-coated nanoparticles for brain cancers. J Drug Target 2011; 19(9): 837-45. [http://dx.doi.org/10.3109/1061186X.2011.589435] [PMID: 21692650]

[122] Tosi G, Costantino L, Rivasi F, *et al.* Targeting the central nervous system: *In vivo* experiments with peptide-derivatized nanoparticles loaded with Loperamide and Rhodamine-123. J Control Release 2007; 122(1): 1-9. [http://dx.doi.org/10.1016/j.jconrel.2007.05.022] [PMID: 17651855]

[123] Vergoni AV, Tosi G, Tacchi R, Vandelli MA, Bertolini A, Costantino L. Nanoparticles as drug delivery agents specific for CNS: *in vivo* biodistribution. Nanomedicine 2009; 5(4): 369-77. [http://dx.doi.org/10.1016/j.nano.2009.02.005] [PMID: 19341816]

[124] Zhang C, Wan X, Zheng X, *et al.* Dual-functional nanoparticles targeting amyloid plaques in the brains of Alzheimer's disease mice. Biomaterials 2014; 35(1): 456-65. [http://dx.doi.org/10.1016/j.biomaterials.2013.09.063] [PMID: 24099709]

[125] Sánchez-López E, Ettcheto M, Egea MA, *et al.* Memantine loaded PLGA PEGylated nanoparticles for Alzheimer's disease: *in vitro* and *in vivo* characterization. J Nanobiotechnology 2018; 16(1): 32. [http://dx.doi.org/10.1186/s12951-018-0356-z] [PMID: 29587747]

[126] Bourdenx M, Daniel J, Genin E, *et al.* Nanoparticles restore lysosomal acidification defects: Implications for Parkinson and other lysosomal-related diseases. Autophagy 2016; 12(3): 472-83. [http://dx.doi.org/10.1080/15548627.2015.1136769] [PMID: 26761717]

[127] Pradhan N, Jana NR. Nanomodulators that target alzheimer's disease: A review. ACS Appl Nano Mater 2024; 7(4): 3515-45. [http://dx.doi.org/10.1021/acsanm.3c04846]

[128] Cheng KK, Yeung CF, Ho SW, Chow SF, Chow AHL, Baum L. Highly stabilized curcumin nanoparticles tested in an *in vitro* blood-brain barrier model and in Alzheimer's disease Tg2576 mice. AAPS J 2013; 15(2): 324-36. [http://dx.doi.org/10.1208/s12248-012-9444-4] [PMID: 23229335]

[129] Ali T, Kim MJ, Rehman SU, Ahmad A, Kim MO. Anthocyanin-loaded PEG-gold nanoparticles enhanced the neuroprotection of anthocyanins in an Aβ 1–42 mouse model of Alzheimer's disease. Mol Neurobiol 2017; 54(8): 6490-506. [http://dx.doi.org/10.1007/s12035-016-0136-4] [PMID: 27730512]

[130] Re F, Gregori M, Masserini M. Nanotechnology for neurodegenerative disorders. Maturitas 2012; 73(1): 45-51. [http://dx.doi.org/10.1016/j.maturitas.2011.12.015] [PMID: 22261367]

[131] Bana L, Minniti S, Salvati E, *et al.* Liposomes bi-functionalized with phosphatidic acid and an ApoE-derived peptide affect Aβ aggregation features and cross the blood–brain-barrier: Implications for therapy of Alzheimer disease. Nanomedicine 2014; 10(7): 1583-90. [http://dx.doi.org/10.1016/j.nano.2013.12.001] [PMID: 24333591]

[132] Park TE, Singh B, Li H, *et al.* Enhanced BBB permeability of osmotically active poly(mannitol-c--PEI) modified with rabies virus glycoprotein *via* selective stimulation of caveolar endocytosis for RNAi therapeutics in Alzheimer's disease. Biomaterials 2015; 38: 61-71. [http://dx.doi.org/10.1016/j.biomaterials.2014.10.068] [PMID: 25457984]

[133] Mancini S, Balducci C, Micotti E, *et al.* Multifunctional liposomes delay phenotype progression and prevent memory impairment in a presymptomatic stage mouse model of Alzheimer disease. J Control Release 2017; 258: 121-9.

[http://dx.doi.org/10.1016/j.jconrel.2017.05.013] [PMID: 28501671]

[134] Agrawal M, Prathyusha E, Ahmed H, *et al.* Biomaterials in treatment of Alzheimer's disease. Neurochem Int 2021; 145: 105008.
[http://dx.doi.org/10.1016/j.neuint.2021.105008] [PMID: 33684545]

[135] Clementino AR, Marchi C, Pozzoli M, Bernini F, Zimetti F, Sonvico F. Anti-inflammatory properties of statin-loaded biodegradable lecithin/chitosan nanoparticles: a step toward nose-to-brain treatment of neurodegenerative diseases. Front Pharmacol 2021; 12: 716380.
[http://dx.doi.org/10.3389/fphar.2021.716380] [PMID: 34630094]

[136] Montgomery KM, Samelson AJ, Gestwicki JE. The cellular environment guides self-assembly and structural conformations of microtubule-associated protein tau (MAPT). Isr J Chem 2023; 64(12): e202300104.
[http://dx.doi.org/10.1002/ijch.202300104]

[137] Nadimidla K, Ismail T, Kanapathipillai M. Tau peptides and tau mutant protein aggregation inhibition by cationic polyethyleneimine and polyarginine. Biopolymers 2017; 107(9): e23024.
[http://dx.doi.org/10.1002/bip.23024] [PMID: 28456996]

[138] Pandey AP, Sawant KK. Polyethylenimine: A versatile, multifunctional non-viral vector for nucleic acid delivery. Mater Sci Eng C 2016; 68: 904-18.
[http://dx.doi.org/10.1016/j.msec.2016.07.066] [PMID: 27524093]

[139] Wang X, Niu D, Hu C, Li P. Polyethyleneimine-based nanocarriers for gene delivery. Curr Pharm Des 2015; 21(42): 6140-56.
[http://dx.doi.org/10.2174/1381612821666151027152907] [PMID: 26503146]

[140] Aggidis A, Chatterjee S, Townsend D, *et al.* Peptide-based inhibitors of Tau aggregation as a potential therapeutic for Alzheimer's disease and other Tauopathies. bioRxiv 2021.

[141] Wang L, Liu X, Fu J, *et al.* Release of methylene blue from graphene oxide-coated electrospun nanofibrous scaffolds to modulate functions of neural progenitor cells. Acta Biomater 2019; 88: 346-56.
[http://dx.doi.org/10.1016/j.actbio.2019.02.036] [PMID: 30822551]

[142] Paul PS, Patel T, Cho JY, *et al.* Native PLGA nanoparticles attenuate Aβ-seed induced tau aggregation under *in vitro* conditions: potential implication in Alzheimer's disease pathology. Sci Rep 2024; 14(1): 144.
[http://dx.doi.org/10.1038/s41598-023-50465-x] [PMID: 38167993]

[143] Dhas N, Mehta T. Cationic biopolymer functionalized nanoparticles encapsulating lutein to attenuate oxidative stress in effective treatment of Alzheimer's disease: A non-invasive approach. Int J Pharm 2020; 586: 119553.
[http://dx.doi.org/10.1016/j.ijpharm.2020.119553] [PMID: 32561306]

[144] Zameer S, Ali J, Vohora D, Najmi AK, Akhtar M. Development, optimisation and evaluation of chitosan nanoparticles of alendronate against Alzheimer's disease in intracerebroventricular streptozotocin model for brain delivery. J Drug Target 2021; 29(2): 199-216.
[http://dx.doi.org/10.1080/1061186X.2020.1817041] [PMID: 32876502]

[145] Prakashkumar N, Sivamaruthi BS, Chaiyasut C, Suganthy N. Decoding the neuroprotective potential of methyl gallate-loaded starch nanoparticles against beta amyloid-induced oxidative stress-mediated apoptosis: An *in vitro* study. Pharmaceutics 2021; 13(3): 299.
[http://dx.doi.org/10.3390/pharmaceutics13030299] [PMID: 33668877]

[146] Lee WH, Kumar A, Rani A, *et al.* Influence of viral vector-mediated delivery of superoxide dismutase and catalase to the hippocampus on spatial learning and memory during aging. Antioxid Redox Signal 2012; 16(4): 339-50.
[http://dx.doi.org/10.1089/ars.2011.4054] [PMID: 21942371]

[147] Williams SR, Lepene BS, Thatcher CD, Long TE. Synthesis and characterization of poly(ethylene

glycol)-glutathione conjugate self-assembled nanoparticles for antioxidant delivery. Biomacromolecules 2009; 10(1): 155-61.
[http://dx.doi.org/10.1021/bm801058j] [PMID: 19086778]

[148] Jiang Z, Dong X, Liu H, Wang Y, Zhang L, Sun Y. Multifunctionality of self-assembled nanogels of curcumin-hyaluronic acid conjugates on inhibiting amyloid β-protein fibrillation and cytotoxicity. React Funct Polym 2016; 104: 22-9.
[http://dx.doi.org/10.1016/j.reactfunctpolym.2016.04.019]

[149] Jiang Z, Dong X, Yan X, Liu Y, Zhang L, Sun Y. Nanogels of dual inhibitor-modified hyaluronic acid function as a potent inhibitor of amyloid β-protein aggregation and cytotoxicity. Sci Rep 2018; 8(1): 3505.
[http://dx.doi.org/10.1038/s41598-018-21933-6] [PMID: 29472606]

[150] Feng T, Du Y, Li J, Hu Y, Kennedy JF. Enhancement of antioxidant activity of chitosan by irradiation. Carbohydr Polym 2008; 73(1): 126-32.
[http://dx.doi.org/10.1016/j.carbpol.2007.11.003]

[151] Lu Q, Zhu M, Zu Y, *et al.* Comparative antioxidant activity of nanoscale lignin prepared by a supercritical antisolvent (SAS) process with non-nanoscale lignin. Food Chem 2012; 135(1): 63-7.
[http://dx.doi.org/10.1016/j.foodchem.2012.04.070]

[152] Figueiredo P, Lintinen K, Hirvonen JT, Kostiainen MA, Santos HA. Properties and chemical modifications of lignin: Towards lignin-based nanomaterials for biomedical applications. Prog Mater Sci 2018; 93: 233-69.
[http://dx.doi.org/10.1016/j.pmatsci.2017.12.001]

[153] Chen Z, Hua Z, Wang J, Guan Y, Zhao M, Li Y. Molecularly imprinted soluble nanogels as a peroxidase-like catalyst in the oxidation reaction of homovanillic acid under aqueous conditions. Appl Catal A Gen 2007; 328(2): 252-8.
[http://dx.doi.org/10.1016/j.apcata.2007.05.040]

[154] Eftekharzadeh B, Khodagholi F, Abdi A, Maghsoudi N. Alginate protects NT2 neurons against H2O2-induced neurotoxicity. Carbohydr Polym 2010; 79(4): 1063-72.
[http://dx.doi.org/10.1016/j.carbpol.2009.10.040]

[155] Matyash M, Despang F, Mandal R, Fiore D, Gelinsky M, Ikonomidou C. Novel soft alginate hydrogel strongly supports neurite growth and protects neurons against oxidative stress. Tissue Eng Part A 2012; 18(1-2): 55-66.
[http://dx.doi.org/10.1089/ten.tea.2011.0097] [PMID: 21770866]

[156] Maity S, Mukhopadhyay P, Kundu PP, Chakraborti AS. Alginate coated chitosan core-shell nanoparticles for efficient oral delivery of naringenin in diabetic animals—An *in vitro* and *in vivo* approach. Carbohydr Polym 2017; 170: 124-32.
[http://dx.doi.org/10.1016/j.carbpol.2017.04.066] [PMID: 28521977]

[157] Tapeinos C, Larrañaga A, Sarasua JR, Pandit A. Functionalised collagen spheres reduce H_2O_2 mediated apoptosis by scavenging overexpressed ROS. Nanomedicine 2018; 14(7): 2397-405.
[http://dx.doi.org/10.1016/j.nano.2017.03.022] [PMID: 28552642]

[158] Md S, Ali M, Baboota S, Sahni JK, Bhatnagar A, Ali J. Preparation, characterization, *in vivo* biodistribution and pharmacokinetic studies of donepezil-loaded PLGA nanoparticles for brain targeting. Drug Dev Ind Pharm 2014; 40(2): 278-87.
[http://dx.doi.org/10.3109/03639045.2012.758130] [PMID: 23369094]

[159] Wilson B, Samanta M, Santhi K, Kumar K, Paramakrishnan N, Suresh B. Targeted delivery of tacrine into the brain with polysorbate 80-coated poly(n-butylcyanoacrylate) nanoparticles. Eur J Pharm Biopharm 2008; 70(1): 75-84.
[http://dx.doi.org/10.1016/j.ejpb.2008.03.009] [PMID: 18472255]

[160] Wilson B, Samanta MK, Santhi K, Kumar KPS, Paramakrishnan N, Suresh B. Poly(n-butylcyanoacrylate) nanoparticles coated with polysorbate 80 for the targeted delivery of rivastigmine

into the brain to treat Alzheimer's disease. Brain Res 2008; 1200: 159-68. [http://dx.doi.org/10.1016/j.brainres.2008.01.039] [PMID: 18291351]

[161] Joshi SA, Chavhan SS, Sawant KK. Rivastigmine-loaded PLGA and PBCA nanoparticles: Preparation, optimization, characterization, *in vitro* and pharmacodynamic studies. Eur J Pharm Biopharm 2010; 76(2): 189-99. [http://dx.doi.org/10.1016/j.ejpb.2010.07.007] [PMID: 20637869]

[162] Agyare EK, Curran GL, Ramakrishnan M, Yu CC, Poduslo JF, Kandimalla KK. Development of a smart nano-vehicle to target cerebrovascular amyloid deposits and brain parenchymal plaques observed in Alzheimer's disease and cerebral amyloid angiopathy. Pharm Res 2008; 25(11): 2674-84. [http://dx.doi.org/10.1007/s11095-008-9688-y] [PMID: 18712585]

[163] Rotman M, Welling MM, Bunschoten A, *et al.* Enhanced glutathione PEGylated liposomal brain delivery of an anti-amyloid single domain antibody fragment in a mouse model for Alzheimer's disease. J Control Release 2015; 203: 40-50. [http://dx.doi.org/10.1016/j.jconrel.2015.02.012] [PMID: 25668771]

[164] Loureiro JA, Gomes B, Fricker G, Coelho MAN, Rocha S, Pereira MC. Cellular uptake of PLGA nanoparticles targeted with anti-amyloid and anti-transferrin receptor antibodies for Alzheimer's disease treatment. Colloids Surf B Biointerfaces 2016; 145: 8-13. [http://dx.doi.org/10.1016/j.colsurfb.2016.04.041] [PMID: 27131092]

[165] Xiong N, Dong XY, Zheng J, Liu FF, Sun Y. Design of LVFFARK and LVFFARK-functionalized nanoparticles for inhibiting amyloid β-protein fibrillation and cytotoxicity. ACS Appl Mater Interfaces 2015; 7(10): 5650-62. [http://dx.doi.org/10.1021/acsami.5b00915] [PMID: 25700145]

[166] Chafekar SM, Malda H, Merkx M, *et al.* Branched KLVFF tetramers strongly potentiate inhibition of β-amyloid aggregation. ChemBioChem 2007; 8(15): 1857-64. [http://dx.doi.org/10.1002/cbic.200700338] [PMID: 17763487]

[167] Xiong N, Zhao Y, Dong X, Zheng J, Sun Y. Design of a molecular hybrid of dual peptide inhibitors coupled on AuNPs for enhanced inhibition of amyloid β-protein aggregation and cytotoxicity. Small 2017; 13(13): 1601666. [http://dx.doi.org/10.1002/smll.201601666] [PMID: 28112856]

[168] Jeon SG, Cha MY, Kim J, *et al.* Vitamin D-binding protein-loaded PLGA nanoparticles suppress Alzheimer's disease-related pathology in 5XFAD mice. Nanomedicine 2019; 17: 297-307. [http://dx.doi.org/10.1016/j.nano.2019.02.004] [PMID: 30794963]

[169] Amin FU, Hoshiar AK, Do TD, *et al.* Osmotin-loaded magnetic nanoparticles with electromagnetic guidance for the treatment of Alzheimer's disease. Nanoscale 2017; 9(30): 10619-32. [http://dx.doi.org/10.1039/C7NR00772H] [PMID: 28534925]

[170] Arora S, Sharma D, Singh J. GLUT-1: an effective target to deliver brain-derived neurotrophic factor gene across the blood brain barrier. ACS Chem Neurosci 2020; 11(11): 1620-33. [http://dx.doi.org/10.1021/acschemneuro.0c00076] [PMID: 32352752]

[171] Mulik RS, Mönkkönen J, Juvonen RO, Mahadik KR, Paradkar AR. ApoE3 mediated poly(butyl) cyanoacrylate nanoparticles containing curcumin: study of enhanced activity of curcumin against beta amyloid induced cytotoxicity using *in vitro* cell culture model. Mol Pharm 2010; 7(3): 815-25. [http://dx.doi.org/10.1021/mp900306x] [PMID: 20230014]

[172] Mathew A, Fukuda T, Nagaoka Y, *et al.* Curcumin loaded-PLGA nanoparticles conjugated with Tet-1 peptide for potential use in Alzheimer's disease. PLoS One 2012; 7(3): e32616. [http://dx.doi.org/10.1371/journal.pone.0032616] [PMID: 22403681]

[173] Barbara R, Belletti D, Pederzoli F, *et al.* Novel Curcumin loaded nanoparticles engineered for Blood-Brain Barrier crossing and able to disrupt Abeta aggregates. Int J Pharm 2017; 526(1-2): 413-24. [http://dx.doi.org/10.1016/j.ijpharm.2017.05.015] [PMID: 28495580]

[174] Fan S, Zheng Y, Liu X, *et al.* Curcumin-loaded PLGA-PEG nanoparticles conjugated with B6 peptide for potential use in Alzheimer's disease. Drug Deliv 2018; 25(1): 1091-102. [http://dx.doi.org/10.1080/10717544.2018.1461955] [PMID: 30107760]

[175] Mourtas S, Lazar AN, Markoutsa E, Duyckaerts C, Antimisiaris SG. Multifunctional nanoliposomes with curcumin–lipid derivative and brain targeting functionality with potential applications for Alzheimer disease. Eur J Med Chem 2014; 80: 175-83. [http://dx.doi.org/10.1016/j.ejmech.2014.04.050] [PMID: 24780594]

[176] Kuo YC, Tsai HC. Rosmarinic acid- and curcumin-loaded polyacrylamide-cardiolipin-poly(lactide-co-glycolide) nanoparticles with conjugated 83-14 monoclonal antibody to protect β-amyloid-insulted neurons. Mater Sci Eng C 2018; 91: 445-57. [http://dx.doi.org/10.1016/j.msec.2018.05.062] [PMID: 30033276]

[177] Chen ZL, Huang M, Wang XR, *et al.* Transferrin-modified liposome promotes α-mangostin to penetrate the blood–brain barrier. Nanomedicine 2016; 12(2): 421-30. [http://dx.doi.org/10.1016/j.nano.2015.10.021] [PMID: 26711963]

[178] Kim MJ, Rehman SU, Amin FU, Kim MO. Enhanced neuroprotection of anthocyanin-loaded PEG-gold nanoparticles against $A\beta_{1\text{-}42}$-induced neuroinflammation and neurodegeneration *via* the NF-$_{\kappa}$B /JNK/GSK3β signaling pathway. Nanomedicine 2017; 13(8): 2533-44. [http://dx.doi.org/10.1016/j.nano.2017.06.022] [PMID: 28736294]

[179] Amin FU, Shah SA, Badshah H, Khan M, Kim MO. Anthocyanins encapsulated by PLGA@PEG nanoparticles potentially improved its free radical scavenging capabilities *via* p38/JNK pathway against $A\beta_{1\text{-}42}$-induced oxidative stress. J Nanobiotechnology 2017; 15(1): 12. [http://dx.doi.org/10.1186/s12951-016-0227-4] [PMID: 28173812]

[180] Cano A, Ettcheto M, Chang JH, *et al.* Dual-drug loaded nanoparticles of Epigallocatechin-3-gallate (EGCG)/Ascorbic acid enhance therapeutic efficacy of EGCG in a APPswe/PS1dE9 Alzheimer's disease mice model. J Control Release 2019; 301: 62-75. [http://dx.doi.org/10.1016/j.jconrel.2019.03.010] [PMID: 30876953]

[181] Rassu G, Porcu EP, Fancello S, *et al.* Intranasal delivery of genistein-loaded nanoparticles as a potential preventive system against neurodegenerative disorders. Pharmaceutics 2018; 11(1): 8. [http://dx.doi.org/10.3390/pharmaceutics11010008] [PMID: 30597930]

[182] Huo X, Zhang Y, Jin X, Li Y, Zhang L. A novel synthesis of selenium nanoparticles encapsulated PLGA nanospheres with curcumin molecules for the inhibition of amyloid β aggregation in Alzheimer's disease. J Photochem Photobiol B 2019; 190: 98-102. [http://dx.doi.org/10.1016/j.jphotobiol.2018.11.008] [PMID: 30504054]

[183] Saini S, Sharma T, Jain A, Kaur H, Katare OP, Singh B. Systematically designed chitosan-coated solid lipid nanoparticles of ferulic acid for effective management of Alzheimer's disease: A preclinical evidence. Colloids Surf B Biointerfaces 2021; 205: 111838. [http://dx.doi.org/10.1016/j.colsurfb.2021.111838] [PMID: 34022704]

[184] Anand B, Wu Q, Nakhaei-Nejad M, Karthivashan G, Dorosh L, Amidian S, Dahal A, Li X, Stepanova M, Wille H, Giuliani F. Significance of native PLGA nanoparticles in the treatment of Alzheimer's disease pathology. Bioactive materials. 2022 Nov 1;17: 506-25. [http://dx.doi.org/10.1016/j.nano.2019.02.004] [PMID: 30794963]

[185] Rifaai RA, Mokhemer SA, Saber EA, El-Aleem SAA, El-Tahawy NFG. Neuroprotective effect of quercetin nanoparticles: A possible prophylactic and therapeutic role in alzheimer's disease. J Chem Neuroanat 2020; 107: 101795. [http://dx.doi.org/10.1016/j.jchemneu.2020.101795] [PMID: 32464160]

[186] Samir M, Abdelkader RM, Boushehri MS, Mansour S, Lamprecht A, Tammam SN. Enhancement of mitochondrial function using NO releasing nanoparticles; a potential approach for therapy of Alzheimer's disease. Eur J Pharm Biopharm 2023; 184: 16-24. [http://dx.doi.org/10.1016/j.ejpb.2023.01.006] [PMID: 36640916]

[187] Aalinkeel R, Kutscher HL, Singh A, *et al.* Neuroprotective effects of a biodegradable poly(lactic-c--glycolic acid)-ginsenoside Rg3 nanoformulation: a potential nanotherapy for Alzheimer's disease? J Drug Target 2018; 26(2): 182-93.
[http://dx.doi.org/10.1080/1061186X.2017.1354002] [PMID: 28697660]

[188] Chakraborty A, Mohapatra SS, Barik S, Roy I, Gupta B, Biswas A. Impact of nanoparticles on amyloid β-induced Alzheimer's disease, tuberculosis, leprosy and cancer: a systematic review. Biosci Rep 2023; 43(2): BSR20220324.
[http://dx.doi.org/10.1042/BSR20220324] [PMID: 36630532]

[189] Rajamanickam G, Manju SL. Formulation and characterization of chitosan nanoparticles loaded with neuroprotective flavonoid from Phyllanthus niruri Linn. Macromol Res 2023; 31(1): 13-24.
[http://dx.doi.org/10.1007/s13233-023-00114-z]

[190] Jia L, Nie X, Ji H, Yuan Z, Li R. Multiple-coated plga nanoparticles loading triptolide attenuate injury of a cellular model of alzheimer's disease. BioMed Res Int 2021; 2021(1): 8825640.
[http://dx.doi.org/10.1155/2021/8825640] [PMID: 33708996]

[191] Aghajanzadeh M, Andalib S, Danafar H, Rostamizadeh K, Sharafi A. The effect of baicalein-loaded Y-shaped miktoarm copolymer on spatial memory and hippocampal expression of DHCR24, SELADIN and SIRT6 genes in rat model of Alzheimer. Int J Pharm 2020; 586: 119546.
[http://dx.doi.org/10.1016/j.ijpharm.2020.119546] [PMID: 32544519]

[192] Sun D, Li N, Zhang W, *et al.* Design of PLGA-functionalized quercetin nanoparticles for potential use in Alzheimer's disease. Colloids Surf B Biointerfaces 2016; 148: 116-29.
[http://dx.doi.org/10.1016/j.colsurfb.2016.08.052] [PMID: 27591943]

[193] Carradori D, Balducci C, Re F, *et al.* Antibody-functionalized polymer nanoparticle leading to memory recovery in Alzheimer's disease-like transgenic mouse model. Nanomedicine 2018; 14(2): 609-18.
[http://dx.doi.org/10.1016/j.nano.2017.12.006] [PMID: 29248676]

[194] Eswar K, Mukherjee S, Ganesan P, Rengan AK. Immunomodulatory natural polysaccharides: An overview of the mechanisms involved. Eur Polym J 2023; 188: 111935.
[http://dx.doi.org/10.1016/j.eurpolymj.2023.111935]

[195] Jatoi S, Hafeez DRA, Riaz SU, Ali A, Ghauri MI, Zehra M. Low vitamin B12 levels: an underestimated cause of minimal cognitive impairment and dementia. Cureus 2020; 12(2): e6976.
[http://dx.doi.org/10.7759/cureus.6976] [PMID: 32206454]

[196] Cho HS, Huang LK, Lee YT, Chan L, Hong CT. Suboptimal baseline serum vitamin B12 is associated with cognitive decline in people with Alzheimer's disease undergoing cholinesterase inhibitor treatment. Front Neurol 2018; 9: 325.
[http://dx.doi.org/10.3389/fneur.2018.00325] [PMID: 29867734]

[197] Cipriani G, Dolciotti C, Picchi L, Bonuccelli U. Alzheimer and his disease: a brief history. Neurol Sci 2011; 32(2): 275-9.
[http://dx.doi.org/10.1007/s10072-010-0454-7] [PMID: 21153601]

[198] McKhann GM, Knopman DS, Chertkow H, *et al.* The diagnosis of dementia due to Alzheimer's disease: Recommendations from the National Institute on Aging-Alzheimer's Association workgroups on diagnostic guidelines for Alzheimer's disease. Alzheimers Dement 2011; 7(3): 263-9.
[http://dx.doi.org/10.1016/j.jalz.2011.03.005] [PMID: 21514250]

[199] Mayeux R, Stern Y. Epidemiology of Alzheimer disease. Cold Spring Harb Perspect Med 2012; 2(8): a006239.
[http://dx.doi.org/10.1101/cshperspect.a006239] [PMID: 22908189]

[200] Yaari R, Fleisher AS, Tariot PN. Updates to diagnostic guidelines for Alzheimer's disease. Prim Care Companion CNS Disord 2011; 13(5): 26971.
[http://dx.doi.org/10.4088/PCC.11f01262] [PMID: 22295259]

[201] Joye IJ, McClements DJ. Julian McClements D. Biopolymer-based delivery systems: challenges and opportunities. Curr Top Med Chem 2016; 16(9): 1026-39.
[http://dx.doi.org/10.2174/1568026615666150825143130] [PMID: 26303423]

[202] Papadimitriou L, Manganas P, Ranella A, Stratakis E. Biofabrication for neural tissue engineering applications. Mater Today Bio 2020; 6: 100043.
[http://dx.doi.org/10.1016/j.mtbio.2020.100043] [PMID: 32190832]

[203] Montazersaheb S, Ahmadian E, Dizaj SM, *et al.* Emerging nanotherapeutic strategies in alzheimer's disease. Frontiers in Clinical Drug Research-Dementia 2021; 2: 173-203.
[http://dx.doi.org/10.2174/9789815039474121020006]

[204] Srivastava GK, Martinez-Rodriguez S, Md Fadilah NI, *et al.* Progress in Wound-Healing Products Based on Natural Compounds, Stem Cells, and MicroRNA-Based Biopolymers in the European, USA, and Asian Markets: Opportunities, Barriers, and Regulatory Issues. Polymers (Basel) 2024; 16(9): 1280.
[http://dx.doi.org/10.3390/polym16091280] [PMID: 38732749]

[205] Blagov AV, Grechko AV, Nikiforov NG, Borisov EE, Sadykhov NK, Orekhov AN. Role of impaired mitochondrial dynamics processes in the pathogenesis of Alzheimer's disease. Int J Mol Sci 2022; 23(13): 6954.
[http://dx.doi.org/10.3390/ijms23136954] [PMID: 35805958]

[206] Weerarathna IN, Kumar P, Luharia A, Mishra G. Engineering with biomedical sciences changing the horizon of healthcare-a review. Bioengineered 2024; 15(1): 2401269.
[http://dx.doi.org/10.1080/21655979.2024.2401269] [PMID: 39285709]

[207] Fu WY, Wang X, Ip NY. Targeting neuroinflammation as a therapeutic strategy for Alzheimer's disease: mechanisms, drug candidates, and new opportunities. ACS Chem Neurosci 2019; 10(2): 872-9.
[http://dx.doi.org/10.1021/acschemneuro.8b00402] [PMID: 30221933]

[208] Sarker MD, Naghieh S, McInnes AD, Schreyer DJ, Chen X. Regeneration of peripheral nerves by nerve guidance conduits: Influence of design, biopolymers, cells, growth factors, and physical stimuli. Prog Neurobiol 2018; 171: 125-50.
[http://dx.doi.org/10.1016/j.pneurobio.2018.07.002] [PMID: 30077776]

[209] Veeman D, Sai MS, Sureshkumar P, *et al.* Additive manufacturing of biopolymers for tissue engineering and regenerative medicine: an overview, potential applications, advancements, and trends. Int J Polym Sci 2021; 2021(1): 1-20.
[http://dx.doi.org/10.1155/2021/4907027]

CHAPTER 14

Integrative Molecular Approaches in Targeted Therapy for AD: Bridging Complex Mechanisms and Future Innovations

Tiyas Pal[1], **Swarupananda Mukherjee**[1,*], **Dipanjan Karati**[2], **Nilanjan Pahari**[3], **Chowdhury Mobaswar Hossain**[4] and **Saheli Naskar**[1]

[1] *Department of Pharmaceutical Technology, NSHM Knowledge Campus, Kolkata-Group of Institutions, Kolkata, West Bengal, India*

[2] *Department of Pharmaceutical Technology, School of Pharmacy, Techno India University, Kolkata, West Bengal, India*

[3] *Department of Pharmaceutical Technology, Calcutta Institute of Pharmaceutical Technology and Allied Health Sciences, Uluberia, West Bengal, India*

[4] *Department of Pharmaceutical Technology, Maulana Abul Kalam Azad University of Technology, Haringhata, West Bengal, India*

Abstract: Alzheimer's disease (AD) is an extremely complicated neurodegenerative disease that results in memory loss and a progressive deterioration in cognitive function. While significant strides have been made in understanding its underlying mechanisms, the intricate molecular pathways of AD pose substantial challenges in developing effective treatments. This chapter explores the potential of integrative molecular approaches in targeted AD therapy, with a focus on the current pharmacological treatments available. Additionally, it highlights research into natural products related to the disease. By examining the interconnected network of molecular signalling pathways, we delve into emerging genetic innovations such as gene editing technologies, neuroinflammation modulation, and targeting amyloid-β and tau proteins. As our understanding of AD continues to deepen, integrative approaches hold the promise of not only enhancing treatment options but also fostering a more holistic approach to managing the disease. The future of AD treatment lies in combining molecular insights with innovative therapies, paving the way for more effective and personalized care for patients.

Keywords: Alzheimer's disease, Amyloid-β, Acetylcholine, Natural products, NMDA receptor antagonists.

[*] **Corresponding author Swarupananda Mukherjee:** Department of Pharmaceutical Technology, NSHM Knowledge Campus, Kolkata-Group of Institutions, Kolkata, West Bengal, India; E-mail: swarupananda.mukherjee@nshm.com

Swarupananda Mukherjee, Souvik Roy & Dipanjan Karati (Eds.)

INTRODUCTION

Alzheimer's disease (AD) is the leading cause of dementia and the most prevalent neurodegenerative disorder. It is characterized by a deterioration in short-term memory and cognitive function, which affects daily activities. The number of Americans affected by AD is rapidly increasing. In 2024, approximately 6.9 million people aged 65 and older are living with Alzheimer's, with nearly 73% of them being 75 or older [1]. This means that roughly 1 in 9 people in this age group, or 10.9%, have the disease. Women make up almost two-thirds of those diagnosed, and older Black and Hispanic Americans are disproportionately affected, with Black Americans being about twice as likely, and Hispanics one and a half times as likely, to develop Alzheimer's or other dementias compared to older Whites. As the U.S. population continues to age, the number of people living with Alzheimer's is expected to grow significantly, potentially reaching 12.7 million by 2050, unless significant medical breakthroughs are made to prevent or cure the disease [1].

The complexity of AD is reflected in the intertwining of these various factors, where genetic predispositions may set the stage for the disease, but environmental and lifestyle factors may influence its progression and severity. Understanding these interconnections is crucial for developing more effective prevention and treatment strategies.

There are several hypotheses that attempt to explain the underlying mechanisms and causes of AD. These hypotheses are based on the observed pathological features of the disease and the factors that might contribute to its development [2]. The major ones have been illustrated in Fig. (**1**).

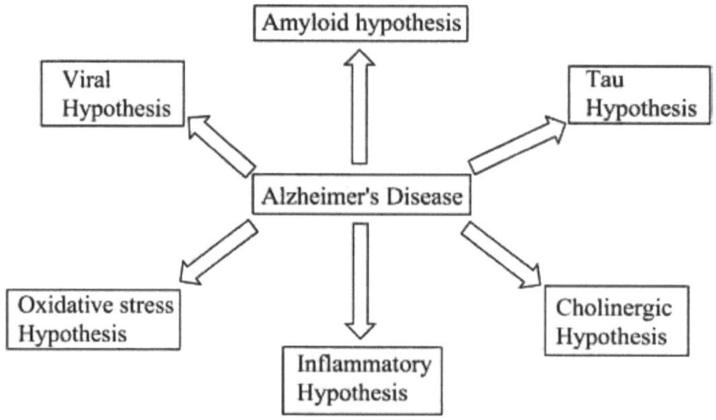

Fig. (1). Predominant hypotheses of Alzheimer's disease.

PHARMACOLOGICAL TREATMENT LANDSCAPE

Traditional AD medications are generally classified into two main groups: acetylcholinesterase inhibitors (AChEIs) and NMDA receptor antagonists [3]. The AChEIs—such as tacrine, donepezil, rivastigmine, and galantamine—work by elevating the concentration and prolonging the duration of acetylcholine (ACh) activity at the synapse, which helps improve cognitive and behavioral symptoms in patients [4]. Tacrine, the first AChEI approved for the treatment of AD in 1993, was taken off the global market in 2013 mainly because its usage was linked to liver toxicity. Despite this, tacrine remains of interest in research, particularly in the development of multitarget-directed therapies [5 - 7].

Second-generation acetylcholinesterase inhibitors (AChEIs), such as donepezil, rivastigmine, and galantamine, are more selective than their predecessors [8, 9]. These drugs tend to have fewer side effects and enhanced pharmacokinetic properties, making them the preferred choice for treating AD. Despite their widespread use, current research is dedicated to refining aspects such as optimal dosing, formulation, administration methods, and development of combination therapies in order to reduce side effects and lead to the improvement of patient adherence to treatment [10 - 12]. In 2022, the FDA approved the donepezil transdermal patch, Adlarity, for the treatment of mild, moderate, and severe AD-related dementia [13]. This patch, which is applied weekly, proved to be bioequivalent to the oral version taken daily at the same dosage, while also resulting in significantly less gastrointestinal side effects compared to oral administration. Moreover, using a combination of suitable cholinesterase inhibitors like donepezil and galantamine, or pairing AChEIs with some other neurological medications, metal chelators, or potent antioxidants, can result in unexpected benefits in managing cholinergic drugs for AD therapy, including improved efficacy, safety, and tolerability [11, 14].

Memantine, an NMDA receptor antagonist approved by the FDA, is used to treat moderate to severe AD. By regulating glutamate transmission and dopamine receptors, it has shown effectiveness in enhancing cognitive function, daily living skills, and behavior in patients [15, 16]. Namzaric, a fixed dose combination of extended-release memantine and donepezil, offers an additional therapeutic option for individuals with moderate to severe AD [17]. Medications like these mainly work by adjusting the neurotransmitter levels, though they do not alter the progression of the disease [15, 18]. This limitation has helped guide the development of new treatments. In 2017, a review [19] introduced the concept of "disease-modifying therapy for AD, which seeks to target the core physiological mechanisms of the disease to stop its progression and provide lasting benefits for patients.

Aducanumab, lecanemab, and donanemab are some monoclonal antibodies aimed at selectively targeting amyloid beta, each showing different results: Aducanumab received controversial FDA accelerated approval in 2021 [20, 21]; lecanemab earned full approval in 2023 [22]; and donanemab received FDA approval in July 2024 for the treatment of early symptomatic AD [23]. Aducanumab targets 3-7 amino acids of Aβ, focusing on soluble oligomers and insoluble fibrils [24, 25]. Lecanemab, in conjunction with the E22G Aβ variant, demonstrated a stronger affinity for soluble Aβ aggregates (including oligomers and protofibrils) compared to aducanumab [26]. Donanemab specifically targets pyroglutamate-modified Aβ, binding directly to plaques [25]. All three antibodies have demonstrated effectiveness in reducing Aβ plaques and slowing cognitive decline. However, the risks associated with amyloid-related imaging abnormalities and the high costs of treatment are important considerations [27 - 29].

The oligosaccharide sodium oligomannate (GV-971), which is obtained from marine algae, received conditional approval in China in 2019, despite constant debates about its action mechanism as well as therapeutic effectiveness [30, 31]. It was initially suggested that GV-971 could combat AD through the reduction of neuroinflammation caused by gut dysbiosis and interfering with the development of Aβ fibrils [32, 33]. Subsequent studies revealed that GV-971 modified the gut microbiome's composition and abundance in the animal models of 5xFAD and APPPS1-21 in a sex-dependent manner. This adjustment affected microbial metabolism as well as peripheral inflammation, influenced the microglial activation and its functioning, and consequently helped reduce neuroinflammation and amyloid buildup [34]. Two phase IV clinical trials are now in progress (NCT05181475 and NCT05058040) to further explore both the efficacy and safety of the treatment, with plans to continue through 2025.

Brexpiprazole, typically used to treat depression and schizophrenia, works by targeting serotonin, dopamine, and norepinephrine receptors [35 - 37]. It has also been found to aid in the reduction of agitation in AD patients.

These groundbreaking treatments explore new aspects of AD mechanisms and offer a range of potential targets, with the promise of potentially halting or reversing the disease's progression. However, additional research is necessary to better understand the drug's mechanisms, evaluate its long-term effectiveness, and establish its safety. Additionally, the challenging risk-to-benefit profile in AD has made the repurposing of drugs a popular strategy. The lengthy, expensive, and resource-intensive procedure of the development of new AD treatments, along with their greater failure rates, has sparked increased interest in the repurposing of drugs originally developed for other diseases, such as cardiovascular diseases, diabetes, cancer, psychiatric disorders, and different neurological conditions.

There are several approved pharmacological treatment options available for patients with AD, which are illustrated in Fig. (**2**).

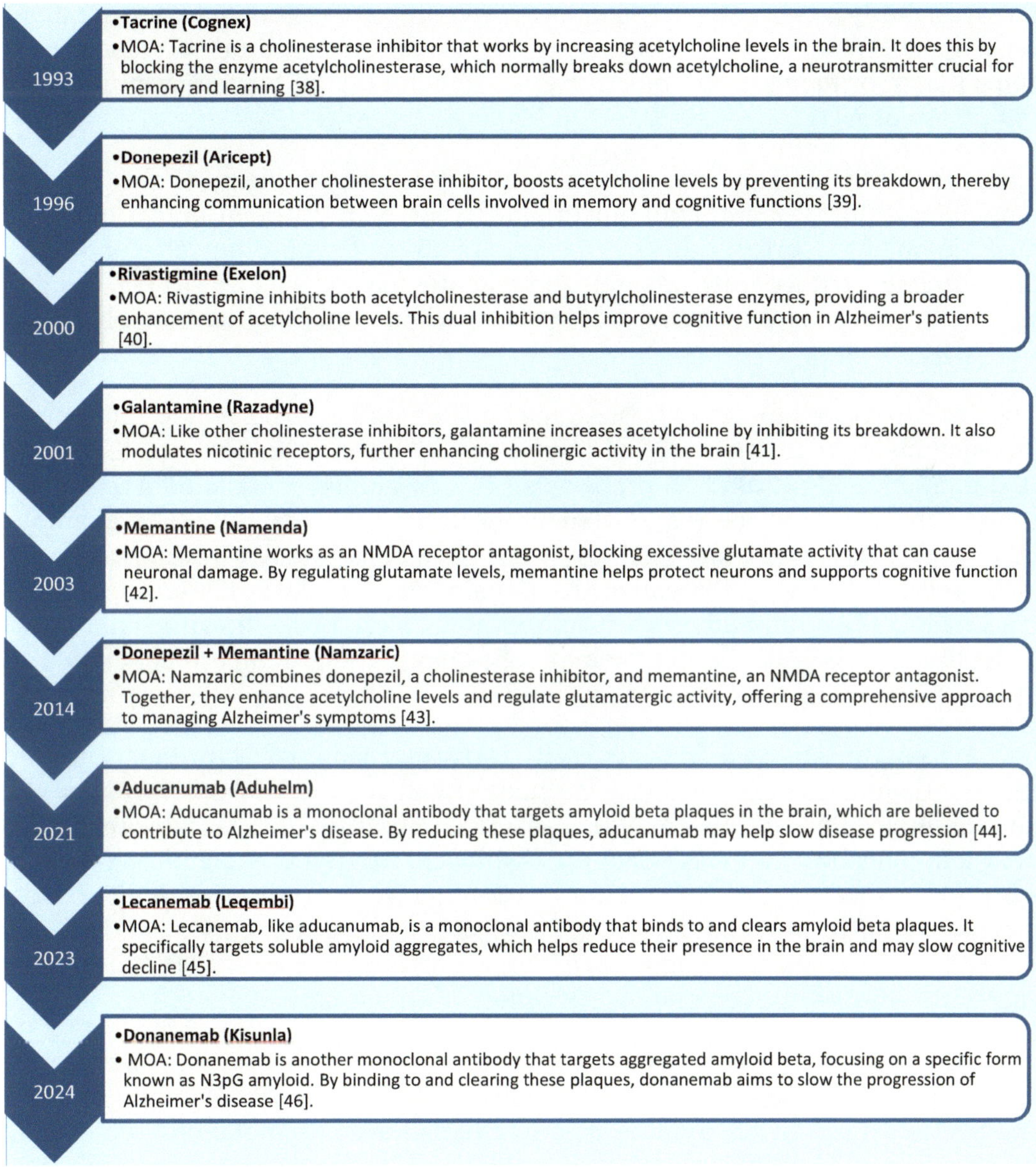
1993
•Tacrine (Cognex)
•MOA: Tacrine is a cholinesterase inhibitor that works by increasing acetylcholine levels in the brain. It does this by blocking the enzyme acetylcholinesterase, which normally breaks down acetylcholine, a neurotransmitter crucial for memory and learning [38].
1996
•Donepezil (Aricept)
•MOA: Donepezil, another cholinesterase inhibitor, boosts acetylcholine levels by preventing its breakdown, thereby enhancing communication between brain cells involved in memory and cognitive functions [39].
2000
•Rivastigmine (Exelon)
•MOA: Rivastigmine inhibits both acetylcholinesterase and butyrylcholinesterase enzymes, providing a broader enhancement of acetylcholine levels. This dual inhibition helps improve cognitive function in Alzheimer's patients [40].
2001
•Galantamine (Razadyne)
•MOA: Like other cholinesterase inhibitors, galantamine increases acetylcholine by inhibiting its breakdown. It also modulates nicotinic receptors, further enhancing cholinergic activity in the brain [41].
2003
•Memantine (Namenda)
•MOA: Memantine works as an NMDA receptor antagonist, blocking excessive glutamate activity that can cause neuronal damage. By regulating glutamate levels, memantine helps protect neurons and supports cognitive function [42].
2014
•Donepezil + Memantine (Namzaric)
•MOA: Namzaric combines donepezil, a cholinesterase inhibitor, and memantine, an NMDA receptor antagonist. Together, they enhance acetylcholine levels and regulate glutamatergic activity, offering a comprehensive approach to managing Alzheimer's symptoms [43].
2021
•Aducanumab (Aduhelm)
•MOA: Aducanumab is a monoclonal antibody that targets amyloid beta plaques in the brain, which are believed to contribute to Alzheimer's disease. By reducing these plaques, aducanumab may help slow disease progression [44].
2023
•Lecanemab (Leqembi)
•MOA: Lecanemab, like aducanumab, is a monoclonal antibody that binds to and clears amyloid beta plaques. It specifically targets soluble amyloid aggregates, which helps reduce their presence in the brain and may slow cognitive decline [45].
2024
•Donanemab (Kisunla)
• MOA: Donanemab is another monoclonal antibody that targets aggregated amyloid beta, focusing on a specific form known as N3pG amyloid. By binding to and clearing these plaques, donanemab aims to slow the progression of Alzheimer's disease [46].

Fig. (2). Chronological order of approved drugs (till 2024) and their mechanism of action (MOA) for the treatment of Alzheimer's disease.

NATURAL PRODUCTS IN AD

Natural products have long been explored as potential treatments for AD due to their availability, diverse bioactivity, and fewer side effects compared to synthetic drugs. Several plant-derived compounds, herbs, and other natural substances have been studied for their neuroprotective effects and potential to slow or prevent the progression of AD.

Curcumin, derived from the rhizomes of the Curcuma plant, is the primary compound within the curcuminoid group. It has demonstrated antioxidant and anti-inflammatory effects [47]. In the context of neurological conditions, curcumin helps reduce inflammation and reactive oxygen species (ROS). It might improve cognitive and memory performance when combined with aerobic yoga (NCT01811381).

Meganatural-Az grape seed extract, grape powder, and elderberry juice all include anthocyanins as their main active ingredients, which are known for their anti-inflammatory and antioxidant properties [48]. In animal models of Alzheimer's disease, anthocyanins have shown neuroprotective effects [49]. For example, anthocyanins extracted from black soybeans have been found to reverse oxidative stress induced by lipopolysaccharide, D-galactose, or Aβ1–42, and to reduce levels of ROS. Additionally, other anthocyanins have been shown to inhibit the hyperactivation of GSK-3_ and the hyperphosphorylation of tau protein caused by amyloid plaques and oxidative stress [50, 51].

Omega-3 polyunsaturated fatty acids (PUFAs) are recognized for their ability to reduce inflammation and mitigate vascular risk factors. PUFAs help lower cell adhesion molecules, and this may be causing cerebral small vessel disorder. This condition contributes to the buildup of white matter hyperintensities, which in turn can lead to cognitive decline. Additionally, certain metabolites have demonstrated neuroprotective effects. For instance, icosapent ethyl, an ethyl ester derived from eicosapentaenoic acid (EPA), which is an omega-3 PUFA, enhances synaptic function while causing the reduction of inflammation [52, 53].

Huperzine A, derived from Huperzia serrata, a Chinese club moss, is a selective and reversible acetylcholinesterase inhibitor [54]. It has higher binding affinity and specificity for AChE than other drugs like tacrine, galantamine, donepezil, and physostigmine, with a very low dissociation rate from the enzyme [55 - 59]. Both the (+)- and (-)-huperzine A enantiomers exhibit similar neuroprotective features, though in a model of amyloid-peptide toxicity, the (+)-enantiomer inhibits AChE 50 times less effectively [60]. In a separate study, both enantiomers provided similar protection against amyloid toxicity [61]. The neuroprotective effects of huperzine A are attributed to its ability to safeguard cells from hydrogen peroxide, amyloid toxicity, glutamate, ischemia, and staurosporine-induced cytotoxicity and apoptosis [55 - 57].

Toxicological studies in various animal species and clinical trials in China have shown that huperzine A causes fewer cholinergic side effects than other AChE inhibitors, with nausea being the most common side effect [62 - 65]. Additionally, huperzine A has been shown to improve memory in both elderly individuals and Alzheimer's patients. It is available as a dietary supplement.

The standardized extract derived from the dry leaves of Ginkgo biloba, known as Ginkgo biloba extract (GBE), has neuroprotective properties and is commonly used to treat memory impairment and dementia [66, 67]. GBE is composed of 5–10% organic acids, 24% flavonoid glycosides, and 6% terpenoids [68]. The terpenoids further contain ginkgolides A, B, C, and J. Both flavonoids and terpenoids are the key physiologically active components of GBE [69, 70]. Research has shown that GBE can cause a reduction in the expression of transgenic human APP (amyloid precursor protein) in murine brains and help normalize the brain's glucose metabolism changes caused by the treatment of streptozotocin in rats [71].

In summary, natural products hold significant promise as adjunctive therapies for AD, with many compounds exhibiting neuroprotective, anti-inflammatory, and antioxidant effects. Ingredients like curcumin, Ginkgo biloba, omega-3 fatty acids, and huperzine A have been investigated for their potential to enhance brain health, alleviate oxidative stress, and reduce cognitive decline. Although some of these natural substances have shown encouraging results in early studies, more research is necessary to fully understand their mechanisms, efficacy, and safety. While these natural options could supplement standard treatments, they should be used with caution and under the guidance of healthcare professionals, given the complexity of Alzheimer's and the variation in individual responses. Ultimately, a combined approach that integrates both conventional and natural treatments, supported by continued scientific investigation, could offer a more effective strategy for managing or slowing AD progression.

MULTI-TARGETED DIRECTED LIGANDS

The complex nature of AD has spurred the development of innovative therapeutic strategies focused on multitargeted treatments aimed at specific areas of the brain affected by the disease. While traditional "one-target, one-molecule" approaches have shown some effectiveness in influencing pathogenic processes, they often result in only limited clinical benefits. As a result, a more promising approach may involve a single compound designed to target multiple critical molecular sites. One common strategy is the creation of hybrid therapeutic complexes, which combine several active compounds into one treatment. Compared to separate co-treatment or "single pill" combinations, these multitarget strategies have shown significant advantages, including fewer side effects and enhanced pharmacokinetic and pharmacodynamic profiles, along with optimized absorption, distribution, metabolism, and excretion (ADME). However, the development of "multi-target-directed ligands" remains a challenging area that requires ongoing research and innovation [72].

GENETIC APPROACHES IN THE TREATMENT OF AD

Genetic strategies for treating AD focus on altering or correcting the genetic elements that play a role in the development and progression of the disease. These approaches specifically target genetic mutations, pathways, and risk factors related to AD, including the formation of Aβ plaques, tau protein dysfunction, and neuroinflammatory processes [73]. Below are some key genetic approaches to AD treatment:

Gene Therapy and Editing

- **CRISPR-Cas9 Technology:** CRISPR gene editing holds the promise of directly altering the genetic code to address specific mutations linked to familial AD, including those in the amyloid precursor protein (APP), PSEN1, or PSEN2 genes. Scientists are investigating how CRISPR can beused to correct thesegenetic defects at the DNA level, with the potential to slow or even reverse the disease's progression in individuals with inherited forms of AD [74, 75].
- **Gene Silencing:** Emerging techniques like RNA interference are being developed to downregulate or silence genes that contribute to AD, such as those responsible for amyloid precursor protein or tau production [76]. By lowering the levels of amyloid-β or tau, these methods may help slow or prevent the buildup of toxic proteins in the brain.

Modulating Risk Genes

- **APOE Gene:** The APOE ε4 allele is one of the most significant genetic risk factors for AD [77]. Targeted genetic therapies designed to alter or counteract the effects of APOE ε4 hold considerable promise. Current research is investigating the use of gene therapies or small molecules to modify the function of the APOE protein, which may help reduce its detrimental impact on neuroinflammation and the buildup of amyloid-β plaques [78].
- **SIRT1 and Other Longevity Genes:** Genes such as SIRT1, which are linked to aging and neuroprotection, have been shown to play a role in the progression of AD [79]. Approaches aimed at boosting the activity of these genes could present

a promising therapeutic strategy to slow neurodegeneration and enhance cognitive function [80].

Gene-based Delivery Systems

- **Viral Vectors:** A major challenge in gene therapy is effectively delivering genetic material to the brain. Researchers are exploring the use of viral vectors, like adenoviruses and lentiviruses, to directly transport therapeutic genes into the central nervous system. These vectors could potentially introduce genes that help protect neurons, reduce neuroinflammation, or stimulate repair processes [81].
- **Non-viral Delivery Methods:** Researchers are also investigating nanoparticle- and lipid-based delivery systems that can effectively transport genetic material across the blood-brain barrier and into neurons, enabling more targeted treatment of genes associated with AD [82].

Gene Expression Modulation

- **Epigenetic Modifications:** In addition to genetic mutations, epigenetic factors like DNA methylation and histone modifications can affect gene expression in AD. Strategies that target these epigenetic changes aim to reactivatebeneficialgenes or suppress harmfulones, providing a more refined approach to treating AD [83].
- **Transcriptional Regulation:** Boosting the expression of neuroprotectivegenes, particularly those involved in synapticplasticity, mitochondrial function, and neurotrophic signalling, may help slow or even reverse the neuronal damage associated with AD [84].

Targeting Neuroinflammation through Genetic Pathways

- Neuroinflammation plays a central role in AD, and specific genetic approaches aim to regulate the brain's immune response. For instance, modifying microglial genes—cells responsible for the brain's immune function—could help reduce neuroinflammation and enhance neuronal health. Genetic strategies may also target signaling pathways, such as TREM2, a gene linked to microglial activity, to better control their response to amyloid-β plaques [85].

Personalized Genetic Approaches

- **Precision Medicine:** Genetic profiling of individuals with AD enables the identification of specific mutations and risk factors, allowing for more personalized treatment strategies based on each person's genetic makeup [86, 87]. For instance, individuals with mutations in genes like APP or PSEN1 may require different therapies than those with more common risk factors such as

APOE ε4. This personalized approach ensures that genetic treatments are tailored to the individual, enhancing their effectiveness.

CHALLENGES AND FUTURE DIRECTIONS OF GENETIC THERAPIES

While genetic therapies offer a propitious future for AD treatment, several challenges still exist that must be overcome:

- **Delivery Challenges:** One of the major hurdles in gene therapy is successfully delivering genetic material across the blood-brain barrier [72, 81].
- **Long-Term Safety and Effectiveness:** The long-term impact of genetic modifications requires careful evaluation to avoid unintended consequences, such as immune reactions or off-target effects [72, 81].
- **Ethical Considerations:** As with any form of genetic modification, there are ethical concerns, particularly regarding the potential use of gene editing in humans, especially in germline cells, which could affect future generations [72, 81].

Genetic strategies for treating AD hold great promise for enhancing our understanding and treatment of the condition. Whether through gene therapy, gene editing, or the modulation of risk-related genes, these approaches have the potential to offer more precise, personalized, and effective treatments. However, substantial efforts are still required to overcome technical, ethical, and safety challenges associated with these therapies. With ongoing research and technological progress, genetic approaches could ultimately lead to groundbreaking treatments for AD, providing hope for both patients and their families [88].

CONCLUSION

In conclusion, the treatment landscape for AD is at a critical juncture, with significant advancements in our understanding of the disease's complex molecular mechanisms. Although challenges remain in developing effective therapies, integrative molecular approaches show considerable promise in overcoming these obstacles. By combining insights from pharmacological treatments, genetic innovations, natural products, and the modulation of molecular pathways such as neuroinflammation and amyloid-β and tau targeting, we are moving closer to more personalized and effective interventions. The future of AD treatment lies in the convergence of these diverse approaches, which will likely offer more tailored and comprehensive solutions to manage and, potentially, slow the progression of the disease. As research continues to expand, these innovations could transform the way we treat Alzheimer's, improving outcomes and quality of life for those affected.

REFERENCES

[1] Alzheimer's Association. Alzheimer's disease facts and figures [Internet]. Alzheimer's & Dementia. 2024. Available from: https://www.alz.org/alzheimers-dementia/facts-figures

[2] Naughton SX, Raval U, Pasinetti GM. The viral hypothesis in alzheimer's disease: novel insights and pathogen-based biomarkers. J Pers Med 2020; 10(3): 74. [http://dx.doi.org/10.3390/jpm10030074] [PMID: 32751069]

[3] Galimberti D, Scarpini E. Old and new acetylcholinesterase inhibitors for Alzheimer's disease. Expert Opin Investig Drugs 2016; 25(10): 1181-7. [http://dx.doi.org/10.1080/13543784.2016.1216972] [PMID: 27459153]

[4] Masters CL, Bateman R, Blennow K, Rowe CC, Sperling RA, Cummings JL. Alzheimer's disease. Nat Rev Dis Primers. 2015; 1: 15056. [http://dx.doi.org/10.1038/nrdp.2015.56]

[5] Thakral S, Yadav A, Singh V, *et al.* Alzheimer's disease: Molecular aspects and treatment opportunities using herbal drugs. Ageing Res Rev. 2023; 88: 101960. [http://dx.doi.org/10.1016/j.arr.2023.101960]

[6] Akıncıoğlu H, Gülçin İ. Potent acetylcholinesterase inhibitors: Potential drugs for Alzheimer's disease. Mini Rev Med Chem. 2020; 20(8): 703–715. [http://dx.doi.org/10.2174/1389557520666200103100521]

[7] Simunkova M, Alwasel SH, Alhazza IM, *et al.* Management of oxidative stress and other pathologies in Alzheimer's disease. Arch Toxicol 2019; 93(9): 2491-513. [http://dx.doi.org/10.1007/s00204-019-02538-y] [PMID: 31440798]

[8] Chen ZR, Huang JB, Yang SL, Hong FF. Role of cholinergic signaling in Alzheimer's disease. Molecules. 2022; 27(6): 1816. [http://dx.doi.org/10.3390/molecules27061816]

[9] Thompson S, Lanctôt KL, Herrmann N. The benefits and risks associated with cholinesterase inhibitor therapy in Alzheimer's disease. Expert Opin Drug Saf. 2004; 3(5): 425–440. [http://dx.doi.org/10.1517/14740338.3.5.425]

[10] Nunes D, Loureiro JA, Pereira MC. Drug delivery systems as a strategy to improve the efficacy of FDA-approved Alzheimer's drugs. Pharmaceutics. 2022; 14(11): 2296. [http://dx.doi.org/10.3390/pharmaceutics14112296]

[11] Kabir MdT, UddinMdS, Mamun AA, *et al.* Combination drug therapy for the management of alzheimer's disease. International Journal of Molecular Sciences [Internet]. 2020 May 5; 21(9). Available from: https://www.ncbi.nlm.nih.gov/pmc/articles/PMC7246721/

[12] E J, Jm R. Cognitive symptoms of alzheimer's disease: Clinical management and prevention [Internet]. BMJ (Clinicalresearched.). 2019. Available from: https://pubmed.ncbi.nlm.nih.gov/31810978/

[13] Larkin HD. First donepeziltransdermal patch approved for alzheimer disease. JAMA 2022; 327(17): 1642.

[14] Amat-ur-Rasool H. Ahmed M, Hasnain S, Carter WG. Anti-cholinesterase combination drug therapy as a potentialtreatment for alzheimer's disease. Brain Sci 2021; 11(2): 184. [http://dx.doi.org/10.3390/brainsci11020184] [PMID: 33540879]

[15] Miculas DC, Negru PA, Bungau SG, Behl T, Hassan SS ul, Tit DM. Pharmacotherapy evolution in alzheimer's disease: Current framework and relevant directions. Cells [Internet]. 2022 Dec 28; 12(1): 131. Available from: https://www.mdpi.com/2073-4409/12/1/131/pdf

[16] Pardo-Moreno T, González-Acedo A, Rivas-Domínguez A, García-Morales V, García-Cozar FJ, Ramos-Rodríguez JJ, *et al.* Therapeutic approach to alzheimer's disease: current treatments and new perspectives. Pharmaceutics [Internet]. 2022 May 24; 14(6): 1117. Available from:

https://www.ncbi.nlm.nih.gov/pmc/articles/PMC9228613/

[17] Greig SL. Memantine er/donepezil: A review in alzheimer's disease. CNS Drugs 2015; 29(11): 963-70.
[http://dx.doi.org/10.1007/s40263-015-0287-2] [PMID: 26519339]

[18] Huang LK, Chao SP, Hu CJ. Clinical trials of new drugs for Alzheimer disease. Journal of Biomedical Science [Internet]. 2020 Jan 6; 27(1). Available from: https://jbiomedsci.biomedcentral.com/articles/10.1186/s12929-019-0609-7
[http://dx.doi.org/10.1186/s12929-019-0609-7]

[19] Cummings J, Fox N. Definingdiseasemodifyingtherapy for alzheimer's disease. The Journal of Prevention of Alzheimer's Disease [Internet]. 2017; 4(2): 109–15. Available from: https://www.ncbi.nlm.nih.gov/pubmed/29071250

[20] Liu KY, Howard R. Can we learn lessons from the FDA's approval of aducanumab? Nat Rev Neurol 2021; 17(11): 715-22.
[http://dx.doi.org/10.1038/s41582-021-00557-x] [PMID: 34535787]

[21] Lythgoe MP, Jenei K, Prasad V. Regulatory decisions diverge over aducanumab for Alzheimer's disease. BMJ 2022; 376: e069780.
[http://dx.doi.org/10.1136/bmj-2021-069780] [PMID: 35091420]

[22] Harris E. Alzheimer drug lecanemab gains traditional FDA approval. JAMA 2023; 330(6): 495.
[http://dx.doi.org/10.1001/jama.2023.12548] [PMID: 37466999]

[23] Sims JR, Zimmer JA, Evans CD, *et al.* Donanemab in Early Symptomatic Alzheimer Disease. JAMA 2023; 330(6): 512-27.
[http://dx.doi.org/10.1001/jama.2023.13239] [PMID: 37459141]

[24] Sevigny J, Chiao P, Bussière T, *et al.* The antibodyaducanumabreduces Aβ plaques in Alzheimer's disease. Nature [Internet]. 2016 Aug 31; 537(7618): 50–6. Available from: https://www.nature.com/articles/nature19323

[25] Karran E, De Strooper B. The amyloid hypothesis in Alzheimer disease: new insights from new therapeutics. Nat Rev Drug Discov 2022; 21(4): 306-18.
[http://dx.doi.org/10.1038/s41573-022-00391-w] [PMID: 35177833]

[26] Vitek GE, Decourt B, Sabbagh MN. Lecanemab (BAN2401): an anti–beta-amyloid monoclonal antibody for the treatment of Alzheimer disease. Expert Opin Investig Drugs 2023; 32(2): 89-94.
[http://dx.doi.org/10.1080/13543784.2023.2178414] [PMID: 36749830]

[27] Golde TE, Levey AI. Immunotherapies for Alzheimer's disease. Science 2023; 382(6676): 1242-4.
[http://dx.doi.org/10.1126/science.adj9255] [PMID: 38096276]

[28] Boxer AL, Sperling R. Accelerating Alzheimer's the rapeutic development: The past and future of clinical trials. Cell [Internet]. 2023 186(22): 4757–72. Available from: https://www.sciencedirect.com/science/article/pii/S0092867423010772

[29] Couzin-Frankel J. Side effects loom over Alzheimer's drugs. Science 2023; 381(6657): 466-7.
[http://dx.doi.org/10.1126/science.adk0830] [PMID: 37535727]

[30] Syed YY. Sodium Oligomannate: First Approval. Drugs 2020; 80(4): 441-4.
[http://dx.doi.org/10.1007/s40265-020-01268-1] [PMID: 32020555]

[31] Yeo-Teh NSL, Tang BL. A review of scientific ethics issues associated with the recently approved drugs for alzheimer's disease. Sci Eng Ethics 2023; 29(1): 2.
[http://dx.doi.org/10.1007/s11948-022-00422-0] [PMID: 36625928]

[32] Xiao S, Chan P, Wang T, *et al.* A 36-week multicenter, randomized, double-blind, placebo-controlled, parallel-group, phase 3 clinical trial of sodium oligomannate for mild-to-moderate Alzheimer's dementia. Alzheimers Res Ther 2021; 13(1): 62.
[http://dx.doi.org/10.1186/s13195-021-00795-7]

[33] Wang X, Sun G, Feng T, *et al.* Sodium oligomannate therapeutically remodels gut microbiota and suppresses gut bacterial amino acids-shaped neuroinflammation to inhibit Alzheimer's disease progression. Cell Res 2019; 29(10): 787-803. [http://dx.doi.org/10.1038/s41422-019-0216-x] [PMID: 31488882]

[34] Bosch ME, Dodiya HB, Michalkiewicz J, *et al.* Sodium oligomannate alters gut microbiota, reduces cerebral amyloidosis and reactive microglia in a sex-specific manner. Mol Neurodegener 2024; 19(1): 18-8. [http://dx.doi.org/10.1186/s13024-023-00700-w] [PMID: 38365827]

[35] Cao Y, Yu F, Lyu Y, Lu X. Promising candidates from drug clinical trials: implications for clinical treatment of Alzheimer's disease in China. Front Neurol. 2022; 13: 1034243. [http://dx.doi.org/10.3389/fneur.2022.1034243]

[36] Ballard C. Brexpiprazole for the treatment of agitation and aggression in alzheimer disease. JAMA Neurol 2023; 80(12): 1272-3. [http://dx.doi.org/10.1001/jamaneurol.2023.3967] [PMID: 37930677]

[37] Almeida OP, Ford AH. Are we getting better at managing agitation in dementia? Am J Geriatr Psychiatry 2020; 28(4): 401-3. [http://dx.doi.org/10.1016/j.jagp.2019.11.004] [PMID: 31812357]

[38] Tacrine [Internet]. DrugBank Online. Available from: https://go.drugbank.com/drugs/DB00382

[39] Kumar A, Gupta V, Sharma S. Donepezil. StatPearls [Internet]. Treasure Island (FL): StatPearls Publishing; 2023 Aug 17 [cited 2026 Apr 20]. Available from: https://www.ncbi.nlm.nih.gov/books/NBK513257/

[40] Müller T. Rivastigmine in the treatment of patients with Alzheimer's disease. Neuropsychiatr Dis Treat 2007; 3(2): 211-8. [http://dx.doi.org/10.2147/nedt.2007.3.2.211] [PMID: 19300554]

[41] Galantamine [Internet]. DrugBank Online. Available from: https://go.drugbank.com/drugs/DB00674

[42] Johnson JW, Kotermanski SE. Mechanism of action of memantine. Curr Opin Pharmacol. 2006; 6(1): 61–67. [http://dx.doi.org/10.1016/j.coph.2005.09.007]

[43] Memantine/donepezil (oral) [Internet]. WebMD. Available from: https://www.webmd.com/drugs/2/drug-168253/memantine-donepezil-oral/details

[44] Padda IS, Parmar M. Aducanumab. StatPearls [Internet]. Treasure Island (FL): StatPearls Publishing; 2021. Available from: https://www.ncbi.nlm.nih.gov/books/NBK573062/

[45] Johannesson M, Söderberg L, Zachrisson O, *et al.* Lecanemab demonstrates highly selective binding to Aβ protofibrils isolated from Alzheimer's disease brains. Mol Cell Neurosci 2024; 130: 103949. [http://dx.doi.org/10.1016/j.mcn.2024.103949] [PMID: 38906341]

[46] Donanemab [Internet]. DrugBank Online. Available from: https://go.drugbank.com/drugs/DB16647

[47] Bhat A, Mahalakshmi AM, Ray B, *et al.* Benefits of curcumin in brain disorders. Biofactors 2019; 45(5): 666-89. [http://dx.doi.org/10.1002/biof.1533] [PMID: 31185140]

[48] Khan MS, Ali T, Kim MW, *et al.* Anthocyanins protect against LPS-induced oxidative stress-mediated neuroinflammation and neurodegeneration in the adult mouse cortex. Neurochem Int 2016; 100: 1-10. [http://dx.doi.org/10.1016/j.neuint.2016.08.005] [PMID: 27522965]

[49] Khan MS, Ali T, Kim MW, Jo MH, Chung JI, Kim MO. Anthocyanins Improve Hippo campus-Dependent Memory Function and Prevent Neurodegeneration *via* JNK/Akt/GSK3β Signaling in LPS-Treated Adult Mice. Molecular Neurobiology [Internet]. 2018; 56(1): 671–87. Available from: https://link.springer.com/article/10.1007/s12035-018-1101-1

[50] Rehman SU, Shah SA, Ali T. Jong Il Chung, myeong ok kim. Anthocyanins reversed d-galactos--induced oxidative stress and neuro inflammation mediated cognitive impairment in adult rats. Mol Neurobiol 2016; 54(1): 255-71.
[http://dx.doi.org/10.1007/s12035-015-9604-5] [PMID: 26738855]

[51] Ali T, Kim T, Rehman SU, *et al.* Natural dietary supplementation of anthocyanins *via* PI3K/Akt/Nrf2/HO-1 pathways mitigate oxidative stress, neurodegeneration, and memory impairment in a mouse model of alzheimer's disease. Mol Neurobiol 2018; 55(7): 6076-93.
[http://dx.doi.org/10.1007/s12035-017-0798-6] [PMID: 29170981]

[52] Wang Q, Liang X, Wang L, *et al.* Effect of omega-3 fattyacidssupplementation on endothelialfunction: ameta-analysis of randomizedcontrolled trials. Atherosclerosis [Internet]. 2012 Apr 1; 221(2): 536–43. Available from: https://pubmed.ncbi.nlm.nih.gov/22317966/

[53] Bowman GL, Silbert LC, Dodge HH, *et al.* Randomized trial of marine n-3 polyunsaturated fatty acids for the prevention of cerebral small vessel disease and inflammation in aging (PUFA Trial): Rationale, design and baseline results. Nutrients 2019; 11(4): 735.
[http://dx.doi.org/10.3390/nu11040735] [PMID: 30934894]

[54] Tang XC, Han YF. Pharmacological profile of huperzine a, a novel acetylcholinesterase inhibitor from chinese herb. CNS Drug Rev 1999; 5(3): 281-300.
[http://dx.doi.org/10.1111/j.1527-3458.1999.tb00105.x]

[55] Rathmann KL, Conner CS. Alzheimer's disease: clinical features, pathogenesis, and treatment. Drug intelligence & clinical pharmacy. 1984; 18(9): 684-91.

[56] Wang YE, Yue DX, Tang XC. Anti-cholinesterase activity of huperzine A. Zhongguo Yao Li Xue Bao (Acta Pharmacol Sin). 1986; 7(2): 110–113.
[PMID: 2946143]

[57] Wang R, Tang XC. Neuroprotective effects of huperzine A. Neurosignals 2005; 14(1-2): 71-82.
[http://dx.doi.org/10.1159/000085387] [PMID: 15956816]

[58] McKinney M, Miller JH, Yamada F, Tuckmantel W, Kozikowski AP. Potencies and stereoselectivities of enantiomers of huperzine A for inhibition of rat cortical acetylcholinesterase. Eur J Pharmacol 1991; 203(2): 303-5.
[http://dx.doi.org/10.1016/0014-2999(91)90730-E] [PMID: 1800123]

[59] Dvir H, Jiang HL, Wong DM, *et al.* X-ray structures of *Torpedo californica* acetylcholinesterase complexed with (+)-huperzine A and (-)-huperzine B: structural evidence for an active site rearrangement. Biochemistry 2002; 41(35): 10810-8.
[http://dx.doi.org/10.1021/bi020151+] [PMID: 12196020]

[60] Zhang HY, Liang YQ, Tang XC, He XC, Bai DL. Stereoselectivities of enantiomers of huperzine A in protection against β-amyloid25–35-induced injury in PC12 and NG108-15 cells and cholinesterase inhibition in mice. Neurosci Lett 2002; 317(3): 143-6.
[http://dx.doi.org/10.1016/S0304-3940(01)02437-5] [PMID: 11755260]

[61] Zhang HY, Brimijoin S, Tang XC. Apoptosis induced by beta-amyloid25–35 in acetylcholinesterase-overexpressing neuroblastoma cells. Acta Pharmacol Sin. 2003; 24(9): 853–858.

[62] Yan XF, Lu WH, Lou WJ, Tang XC. Effects of huperzine A and B on skeletal muscle and the electroen cephalogram. Zhong guoyao li xue bao = Acta pharmacologica Sinica [Internet]. 1987 Mar; 8(2): 117–23. Available from: https://pubmed.ncbi.nlm.nih.gov/2958995/

[63] Zhang RW, Tang XC, Han YY, Sang GW, Zhang YD, Ma YX, Zhang CL, Yang RM. Drug evaluation of huperzine A in the treatment of senile memory disorders. Zhongguo Yao Li Xue Bao (Acta Pharmacol Sin). 1991; 12(3): 250–252.
[PMID: 1781288]

[64] Xu SS, Gao ZX, Weng Z, et al. Efficacy of tablet huperzine-A on memory, cognition, and behavior in Alzheimer's disease. Zhongguo Yao Li Xue Bao (Acta Pharmacol Sin). 1995; 16(5): 391–395.

[PMID: 8701750]

[65] Xu SS, Cai ZY, Qu ZW, et al.. Huperzine-A in capsules and tablets for treating patients with Alzheimer disease. Zhongguo Yao Li Xue Bao (Acta Pharmacol Sin). 1999; 20(6): 486–490. [PMID: 10678137]

[66] Oken BS, Storzbach DM, Kaye JA. The Efficacy of Ginkgo biloba on Cognitive Function in Alzheimer Disease. Archives of Neurology [Internet]. 1998 Nov 1; 55(11): 1409. Available from: https://jamanetwork.com/journals/jamaneurology/article-abstract/774397 [http://dx.doi.org/10.1001/archneur.55.11.1409]

[67] Vellas B, Coley N, Ousset PJ, *et al.* Long-term use of standardised Ginkgo biloba extract for the prevention of Alzheimer's disease (GuidAge): arandomised placebo-controlled trial. The Lancet Neurology [Internet]. 2012; 11(10): 851–9. Available from: https://www.ncbi.nlm.nih.gov/pubmed/22959217 [http://dx.doi.org/10.1016/S1474-4422(12)70206-5]

[68] Singh SK, Srivastav S, Castellani RJ, Plascencia-Villa G, Perry G. Neuroprotective and antioxidant effect of Ginkgo biloba extract against Alzheimer's disease and other neurological disorders. Neurotherapeutics. 2019; 16(3): 666–674. [http://dx.doi.org/10.1007/s13311-019-00767-8] [PMID: 31376068]

[69] Smith PF, Maclennan K, Darlington CL. The neuroprotective properties of the Ginkgo biloba leaf: A review of the possible relationship to platelet-activating factor (PAF). J Ethnopharmacol 1996; 50(3): 131-9. [http://dx.doi.org/10.1016/0378-8741(96)01379-7] [PMID: 8691847]

[70] Shi C, Liu J, Wu F, Yew D. Ginkgo biloba extract in Alzheimer's disease: From action mechanisms to medical practice. Int J Mol Sci 2010; 11(1): 107-23. [http://dx.doi.org/10.3390/ijms11010107] [PMID: 20162004]

[71] Augustin S, Rimbach G, Augustin K, Schliebs R, Wolffram S, Cermak R. Effect of a short- and long-term treatment with Ginkgo biloba extract on Amyloid Precursor Protein Levels in a transgenic mouse model relevant to Alzheimer's disease. Arch Biochem Biophys 2009; 481(2): 177-82. [http://dx.doi.org/10.1016/j.abb.2008.10.032] [PMID: 18996078]

[72] Bajda M, Guzior N, Ignasik M, Malawska B. Multi-target-directed ligands in Alzheimer's disease treatment. Curr Med Chem 2011; 18(32): 4949-75. [http://dx.doi.org/10.2174/092986711797535245] [PMID: 22050745]

[73] Nilsson P, Iwata N, Muramatsu S, Tjernberg LO, Winblad B, Saido TC. Gene therapy in Alzheimer's disease: potential for disease modification. J Cell Mol Med. 2010; 14(4): 741–757. Available from: https://www.ncbi.nlm.nih.gov/pmc/articles/PMC3823109/

[74] Bhardwaj S, Kesari KK, Rachamalla M, *et al.* CRISPR/Cas9 gene editing: new hope for Alzheimer's disease therapeutics. J Adv Res. 2021; 40: 207–221. [http://dx.doi.org/10.1016/j.jare.2021.07.001]

[75] Addgene. CRISPR used to edit disease out of the genome [Internet]. Available from: https://blog.addgene.org/crispr-used-to-edit-disease-out-of-the-genome

[76] Emm A. Clinical trials show promise for first "gene silencing" treatment for Alzheimer's disease [Internet]. Genomics Education Programme; 2024. Available from: https://www.genomicseducation.hee.nhs.uk/blog/clinical-trial-show-promise-for-first-gene-silencing-treatment-for-alzheimers-disease

[77] Serrano-Pozo A, Das S, Hyman BT. APOE and Alzheimer's disease: advances in genetics, pathophysiology, and therapeutic approaches. Lancet Neurol. 2021;20(1):68–80. Available from: https://www.ncbi.nlm.nih.gov/pmc/articles/PMC8096522/

[78] Troutwine BR, Hamid L, Lysaker CR, Strope TA, Wilkins HM. Apolipoprotein E and Alzheimer's disease. Acta Pharmaceutica Sinica B [Internet]. 2022 Feb 1 [cited 2022 Mar 12]; 12(2): 496–510. Available from: https://www.ncbi.nlm.nih.gov/pmc/articles/PMC8897057/

[79] Mehramiz M, Porter T, Laws SM, Rainey-Smith SR. Sleep, Sirtuin 1 and Alzheimer's disease: A review. Aging Brain 2022; 2: 100050. [http://dx.doi.org/10.1016/j.nbas.2022.100050] [PMID: 36908890]

[80] Donmez G. The effects of SIRT1 on alzheimer's disease models. Int J Alzheimers Dis 2012; 2012: 1-3. [http://dx.doi.org/10.1155/2012/509529] [PMID: 23251824]

[81] Doshi V, Joshi G, Sharma S, Choudhary D. Gene therapy: an alternative to treat Alzheimer's disease. Naunyn Schmiedebergs Arch Pharmacol 2024; 397(6): 3675-93. [http://dx.doi.org/10.1007/s00210-023-02873-z] [PMID: 38078920]

[82] Williams L, Larsen J. Nanoparticle-mediated delivery of non-viral gene editing technology to the brain. Prog Neurobiol 2024; 232: 102547-7. [http://dx.doi.org/10.1016/j.pneurobio.2023.102547] [PMID: 38042249]

[83] Pandey D, Pal T, Sharma A, Flora SJS. Potential epigenetic targets for combating Alzheimer's disease. Mini Rev Med Chem. 2021; 21(12): 1527–1540. [http://dx.doi.org/10.2174/1389557521999201228191427] [PMID: 33371834]

[84] Chen XF, Zhang Y, Xu H, Bu G. Transcriptional regulation and its misregulation in Alzheimer's disease. Mol Brain 2013; 6(1): 44. [http://dx.doi.org/10.1186/1756-6606-6-44] [PMID: 24144318]

[85] Ardura-Fabregat A, Boddeke EWG, Boza-Serrano A, *et al.* Targeting neuroinflammation to treat Alzheimer's disease. CNS Drugs. 2017; 31(12): 1057-1082. [http://dx.doi.org/10.1007/s40263-017-0483-3] [PMID: 29260466]

[86] Arafah A, Khatoon S, Rasool I, *et al.* The future of precision medicine in the cure of Alzheimer's disease. Biomedicines. 2023; 11(2): 335. [http://dx.doi.org/10.3390/biomedicines11020335]

[87] Behl T, Kaur I, Sehgal A, *et al.* The road to precision medicine: eliminating the "one size fits all" approach in Alzheimer's disease. Biomed Pharmacother. 2022; 153: 113337. [http://dx.doi.org/10.1016/j.biopha.2022.113337]

[88] Pardo-Moreno T, González-Acedo A, Rivas-Domínguez A, *et al.* Therapeutic approach to Alzheimer's disease: current treatments and new perspectives. Pharmaceutics 2022; 14(6): 1117. [http://dx.doi.org/10.3390/pharmaceutics14061117] [PMID: 35745693]

SUBJECT INDEX

A

B

C

D

E

F

Swarupananda Mukherjee, Souvik Roy & Dipanjan Karati (Eds.)

G

H

I

K

L

M

N

O

P

Q

R

S

T

V

X

www.ingramcontent.com/pod-product-compliance
Lightning Source LLC
LaVergne TN
LVHW070944210926
848482LV00002B/89